Workbook *to accompany*

Mosby's

PARAMEDIC TEXTBOOK

Revised Second Edition

About the Authors

Kim D. McKenna, RN, BSN, CEN, EMT-P is the Chief Medical Officer for the Florissant Valley Fire Protection District in Florissant, Missouri, and an Adjunct Instructor for St. Louis Community College in St. Louis, Missouri. Her past experiences include intensive care and emergency nursing. She has been involved in prehospital education since 1985, including 4 years as the primary instructor of a paramedic training program.

Mick J. Sanders, MSA, EMT-P received his paramedic training in 1978 from St. Louis University Hospitals. He earned a Bachelor of Science degree in 1982 and a Master of Science degree in 1983 from Lindenwood College in St. Charles, Missouri. He has worked in various health care systems as a field paramedic, emergency department paramedic, and EMS instructor. For 12 years, Mr. Sanders served as Training Specialist with the Bureau of Emergency Medical Services, Missouri Department of Health, where he oversaw EMT and paramedic training and licensure in St. Louis City and the surrounding metropolitan area.

Workbook *to accompany*

Mosby's

PARAMEDIC TEXTBOOK

Revised Second Edition

Kim D. McKenna, *RN, BSN, CEN, EMT-P*
Chief Medical Officer
Florissant Valley Fire Protection District
Florissant, Missouri;
Adjunct Instructor
St. Louis Community College
St. Louis, Missouri

Mick J. Sanders, *MSA, EMT-P*
EMS Training Specialist
St. Charles, Missouri

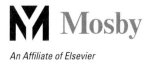 Mosby

An Affiliate of Elsevier

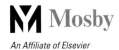 Mosby

An Affiliate of Elsevier

Executive Editor: Claire Merrick
Project Manager: Linda McKinley
Production Editor: Rich Barber, Jennifer Furey
Designer: Stephanie Foley

Credits for illustrations appear on p. 487

REVISED SECOND EDITION

Mosby, Inc.
An Affiliate of Elsevier
11830 Westline Industrial Drive
St. Louis, Missouri 63146
Printed in the United States of America

International Standard Book Number 0-323-01421-6

03   04   05   TG/RDC   9   8   7   6   5   4   3

To my children—Ginny, Becky, Maggie, Grant—and to my husband, Don.
Thanks for helping me remember to enjoy life.

KDM

Preface

The *Workbook to accompany Mosby's Paramedic Textbook,* revised second edition, has been written to enhance the paramedic student's understanding and retention of the material presented in the textbook. This has been accomplished using a variety of questions designed to encourage the various levels of learning necessary in this field, from recall and memorization to application of concepts. Some of the features of this workbook include the following:

- A special section on studying and test-taking skills (see p. vii) so that good habits can begin early in the program
- Format that follows *Mosby's Paramedic Textbook,* revised second edition, chapter by chapter, with answers referenced to the appropriate objective
- Matching questions that reinforce key terms or content within the chapters
- Extensive use of case study–based questions to help visualize the "real-life" application of information
- Self-assessment sections that offer the opportunity to review material using multiple-choice questions, a testing format often used by instructors for examinations
- Complete rationale for all answers that ensures understanding of material
- A programmed review of basic math skills that precedes the drug dose calculation section
- Illustrations for student identification of anatomy, patient management techniques, and special equipment
- Paramedic career options section (see p. 371) that introduces some of the choices in the paramedic profession

ECG and drug flashcards at the end of the book can be removed for easy reference and study purposes. Flashcards are completed by the students and are keyed to questions in the workbook. The ECG flashcards show actual patient rhythms, and the drug flashcards are based on patient-care scenarios. Three blank drug flashcards will allow students to create cards for regional drugs.

Before completing each chapter of the workbook, you should read the accompanying chapter in *Mosby's Paramedic Textbook,* revised second edition, and review the learning objectives. When areas of difficulty are encountered while completing the questions, reread the text and attempt the questions again. We hope that this workbook, when used effectively, will facilitate mastery of the complex knowledge necessary to become a paramedic. Enjoy!

● ACKNOWLEDGMENTS

This workbook would, of course, never have been possible without the terrific manuscript of *Mosby's Paramedic Textbook,* revised second edition, written by Mick J. Sanders. His commitment to excellence is reflected throughout the text, and his encouragement and suggestions made the completion of the workbook possible.

Many thanks to Catherine Parvensky, who wrote the studying and test-taking tips and the paramedic career options sections of the workbook.

Thanks to Mark Wieber for his illustrations and Don McKenna for the photographs included in this text. For the original patient ECG strips, I am indebted to the staff of the intensive care unit and especially to my former colleagues in the emergency department at St. John's Mercy Medical Center. A debt of gratitude goes to Gary Denton of Acute Coronary Syndrome Consultants, Inc., and to Wolff for the 12-lead ECG tracings included in this edition of the text.

To all of my paramedic students, past and present, I sincerely appreciate all that you have taught me and your suggestions for the content of this workbook.

And to the fellow paramedics and EMTs I have worked with in the field, thanks for showing me where the textbook ends and reality begins.

I am also grateful to the reviewers, Bob Nixon, BA, EMT-P; Monroe Yancie, NREMT-P; Jeff DeGraffenreid, Johnson County Medical Action Emergency Medical Services, Olathe, Kansas; and Janet Fitts, RN, EMT-P for their suggestions and fresh ideas.

Thanks to the staff at Mosby, especially Elaine Steinborn who worked so diligently to make this project happen; to Claire Merrick for surviving a second edition with us; to Rich Barber whose attention to detail is evident throughout the text; and to Derril Trakalo in marketing who cheered us all on. We are forever grateful.

Kim D. McKenna
Mick J. Sanders

STUDY TIPS

For all the emphasis placed on furthering education, little guidance is given for how to be a good student. Learning the following studying and test-taking tips can help you get the most out of your paramedic course and other classes in the future.

● STUDY SESSIONS

The way that an individual studies may determine the likelihood of successful completion of a training program. You need to develop a routine pattern for studying and stick to it. The following are methods to increase the effectiveness of study sessions:

- Set a regular time for studying each day.
- Pace yourself by scheduling a specific amount of time for each subject or chapter.
- Take periodic breaks to prevent burnout.
- Read lesson information before each session and review notes immediately after the class.
- Do not wait until the last minute and expect to cram information and do well. Instead, pace yourself throughout the course.
- Be aware of distractions, both internal and external:
  - Internal distractions include hunger, tension, fatigue, illness, glucose levels, and day-dreaming and getting side-tracked.
  - External distractions include room temperature (hot or cold), noise levels, and lighting.
- Make a game of it; drill the information by using the following:
  - Flash cards for memorizing facts
  - Jeopardy cards
  - Trivial Pursuit cards
- When frustration sets in, do the following:
  - Take a break.
  - Have a snack. (Sugar helps.)
  - Take a walk. (Increased cardiovascular activity increases blood flow to the brain.)
  - Take a few deep breaths and relax.

● WHERE AND WHEN DO YOU STUDY BEST?

Everyone has a particular time and place in which they are most productive. For some it is late at night, and for others it is early in the morning. Determine when you are at your peak and study daily at that time.

- Where do you do the best work?
  - At a desk or table?
  - In front of the television? (Some people need background noise to focus.)

- Decide if you work better studying alone or in work groups. Sometimes, work sessions are a great motivation for studying.
- Decide what form of studying works best for you:
  - Writing notes from the book
  - Highlighting information in the book
  - Taking copious notes
  - Listening to the instructor and asking questions

● INCREASING RETENTION

There are many ways to increase retention of material, including association, mnemonics, imagery, and recitation. Try them all and see what works best for you:

Association—Relate information to something you understand. Build new information on what is already known.

Mnemonics—Use letters or words to remember facts. For example, use "AVPU" to determine a patient's level of consciousness: *Alert, Verbal, Painful stimuli,* or *Unconscious.*

Imagery—Visualize a picture of the information. Memorize a chart or picture of the body and associated organs, and then remember that picture for questions on anatomy.

Recitation—Read notes out loud or discuss the information with peers. Hearing information repeatedly helps retention.

● TEST-TAKING TIPS

Test taking is a skill that can be learned. Most state examinations are multiple-choice questions and graded solely on the number of correct answers. There is no penalty for guessing, so do not leave any questions unanswered because they will be marked incorrect.

Multiple-choice questions are made up of two parts, the stem (question) and possible answers. These types of questions can be factual or situational:

Factual: During one-person CPR, the ratio of compressions to ventilations is:

a. 15 to 2
b. 5 to 1
c. 10/min
d. 20/ min

Situational: A 55-year-old man was shoveling his driveway when he developed shortness of breath and pain in the middle of his chest. He is most likely suffering from which of the following?

    a. Myocardial infarction
    b. Congestive heart failure
    c. Emphysema
    d. Angina pectoris

When answering a question, thoroughly analyze it. To accomplish this, do the following:

- Read the stem without looking at the answers. Evaluate the question looking for key words such as *not, except, first,* or *final.*
- Identify key content words such as *one rescuer, adult victim, radiating pain, slurred speech,* or *conscious victim.*
- Think of a correct answer and then look at all the choices to see whether your answer is there. If not, find the next *best answer.*
- Do not read into the question.
- Eliminate obviously wrong answers and select from those remaining.
- Do not change answers. Your first hunch is usually correct.

● PREPARING FOR TESTS

You can take some simple steps to prepare yourself for a test:

- Get a good night's sleep before the examination.
- Avoid milk products because they tend to induce sleep.
- Eat a good meal but not too much before the examination. (Blood flow is forced to the digestive tract the first hour after eating a large meal, which tends to induce sleep.)
- Exercise moderately to increase blood supply to the brain.
- Layer clothes so that you can add or remove layers as necessary to be comfortable during the examination.
- Use a wristwatch to pace yourself.
- Sit away from friends or other distractions.
- Be prepared and be positive. If you have studied properly, you know the material and will do well on the examination.

● STRATEGIES FOR INCREASING TESTING PERFORMANCE

If you use the following strategies, you are sure to improve your performance during tests:

- Pace yourself to make certain that you have enough time to answer all questions.
- Use scrap paper to work through questions.
- At the end, make certain you have answered *all* questions. Do not change answers unless you initially misread the question.
- Make sure that you complete the answer sheet correctly. Fill in circles completely, and do not leave stray marks. Make certain that you check the number on the answer sheet against the number on the test every 10 questions to avoid the unnecessary stress of finding yourself on the wrong line.

Contents

Division Five Medical

Division Six Special considerations

Division Seven Assessment-based management

Division Eight Operations

QUESTIONS

DIVISION ONE
PREPARATORY

EMS SYSTEMS: ROLES AND RESPONSIBILITIES

● READING ASSIGNMENT
Chapter 1, pages 2-27, in *Mosby's Paramedic Textbook*, ed 2

● OBJECTIVES
As a paramedic, you should be able to:
1. Outline key historical events that influenced the development of emergency medical services systems.
2. Identify the key elements necessary for effective emergency medical services systems operations.
3. Differentiate training and roles and responsibilities of the four nationally recognized levels of EMS licensure and certification: first responder, EMT-B, EMT-I, and EMT-P.
4. List the benefits of membership in a professional EMS association.
5. Describe the benefits of continuing education.
6. Differentiate between professionalism and professional licensure, certification, and registration.
7. Apply to a patient care situation the components of the paramedic's role as defined by the Department of Transportation.
8. Describe the benefits of each aspect of offline and online medical direction.
9. Outline the role and components of an effective continuous quality improvement program.
10. Identify the key components of prehospital research and its benefit.
11. Describe how to address ethical considerations related to research.

● REVIEW QUESTIONS
1. While working late, a 56-year-old man develops chest pain. The man is alone in his office when the chest pain increases and he falls to the floor, suffering a cardiac arrest.

   Identify the missing components of the EMS system in Fig. 1-1 that are necessary to effectively resuscitate this victim and return him to a productive role in society.

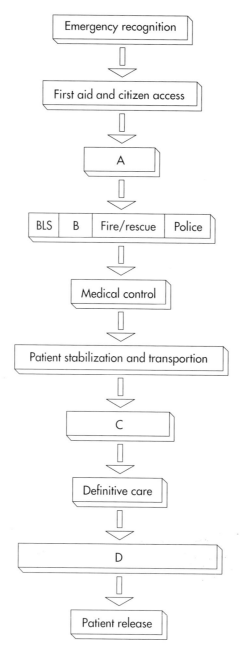

Figure 1-1

Questions 2 and 3 pertain to the following case study:

After attending a continuing education lecture on Advances in Trauma Care, you report to work for your 12-hour shift. You carefully check out your vehicle for equipment and mechanical readiness for a call and then head to the company fitness room to exercise. Just as you finish your workout, the tones sound and you are dispatched to a nursing home for a person with "difficulty breathing." The street alarm is activated, and as you pull out, you carefully glance to ensure that traffic has come to a stop before proceeding onto the busy roadway in front of your station. As you obtain a rapid history from the nursing home staff, you begin your patient assessment of the 87-year-old patient. She is in obvious respiratory distress, and you recognize the need for rapid interventions to prevent further deterioration of her condition. Your partner applies oxygen and prepares to initiate an intravenous (IV) line as you contact online medical direction. You briefly describe your patient's condition and request orders for nitroglycerin and furosemide. The physician advisor agrees with your treatment plan, and as soon as your partner secures the IV line, you administer the drugs, carefully checking for allergies and appropriate dosing before giving them. A repeat assessment of the patient in 5 minutes shows some improvement. You continue plans to transfer her into the ambulance. The nursing home staff indicates that she should be transported to the city hospital. This is consistent with your medical protocols, so you agree and as you depart, another evaluation demonstrates even more improvement. On arrival at the hospital, you give a report and transfer care of the patient to the nursing staff and then complete your patient report. You ask the physician about another drug that you had considered requesting, but she agrees that in this patient's circumstance, the treatment plan you had chosen was appropriate. Back at base, you restock the vehicle with the drugs and equipment used on the call and then head down to the classroom to help teach the 8 PM community CPR class being held in the department.

2. List 10 primary responsibilities of the paramedic that were demonstrated in this simulated call.
   a.
   b.
   c.
   d.
   e.
   f.
   g.
   h.
   i.
   j.
3. List 2 additional responsibilities of the paramedic that were demonstrated in this scenario.
   a.
   b.

Match the historical role in EMS described in Column I with the appropriate person or event listed in Column II. Use each answer only once.

	Column I		Column II
4. _____	First use of helicopter for medical evacuation during an armed conflict	a.	American Red Cross
5. _____	Demonstrated the value of mouth-to-mouth ventilation	b.	Belfast—1966
6. _____	Twentieth century battlefield ambulance corps developed	c.	Korean conflict
7. _____	Dr. Eugene Nagel trains firefighters as paramedics	d.	Miami, Fla—1967
8. _____	Earliest documented mobile coronary unit performs prehospital defibrillation	e.	Napoleonic Wars
9. _____	Clara Barton performs battlefield emergency medical care and brings this organization to the United States	f.	Peter Safar, MD—1958
		g.	World War I
10. _____	Jean Larry transports wounded in covered cart	h.	World War II
11. _____	Fixed-wing medical transports were developed in this conflict	i.	Vietnam conflict

Match the description in Column I with the appropriate licensure and certification level in Column II. Use each answer only once.

	Column I		Column II
12. _____	Trained in basic life support, including defibrillation	a.	EMT-B
13. _____	Trained in all aspects of basic and advanced life support	b.	EMT-I
14. _____	Trained in all aspects of basic life support and IV therapy	c.	EMT-P
		d.	First Responder

Match the activities listed in Column I with the appropriate term in Column II. You may use each term *more* than once.

	Column I		Column II
15. _____	Education and training of EMS personnel	a.	Continuing education
16. _____	Personnel selection for employment	b.	Continuous quality improvement
17. _____	Appropriate equipment choice selection	c.	Medical direction
18. _____	Clinical protocol guidance and direction	d.	Professional associations
19. _____	Clinical problem resolution		
20. _____	Interface among EMS systems		
21. _____	Advocacy within medical community		
22. _____	Online communication with physicians and EMS		
23. _____	Patient care report reviews		

24. _____ Establish standards of care
25. _____ Serve as resource experts
26. _____ Introduction of new information

Questions 27-35 pertain to the following research abstract, which was published in *Prehospital Emergency Care*, July/Sept 1998, Vol 2/No 3. Read the abstract carefully and then respond to each question.

Efficacy of Midazolam for Facilitated Intubation by Paramedics

Authors: Edward T. Dickinson, MD, NREMT-P
Jason E. Cohen, BA, EMT-P
C. Crawford Mechem, MD

Affiliation: Department of Emergency Medicine, University of Pennsylvania School of Medicine, Philadelphia, Pennsylvania

Objective: The use of pharmacologic agents by paramedics to facilitate endotracheal intubation (ETI) is becoming increasingly common. This study was done to determine the efficacy of intravenous midazolam, a short-acting benzodiazepine, as a drug to facilitate ETI in patients resistant to conventional ETI.

Methods: The study was conducted in a suburban municipal EMS system over a 22-month period. All paramedics were trained in the use of midazolam for facilitated intubation prior to allowing the use of midazolam in the system. All calls where midazolam was used were reviewed on a monthly basis by investigators via retrospective review of the prehospital care reports.

Results: During the study period, 13,212 emergency responses occurred, resulting in 154 ETIs by paramedics. Midazolam was used to facilitate 20 (13%) of these ETIs. "Clenched teeth" and failed intubation attempt were the most commonly cited indications for facilitated intubation. Eleven patients had medical complaints and nine were trauma patients. Successful ETI with midazolam was achieved in 17 of 20 (85%) cases. In 88% (15 of 17) of these cases, a single dose of midazolam was sufficient for ETI; mean dose 3.6 mg (SD 1.1 mg). The three patients with failed ETI received multiple doses of midazolam; mean dose 5.0 mg (SD 2.0 mg).

Conclusion: The prehospital use of single-dose IV midazolam is generally effective in accomplishing facilitated ETI in patients resistant to conventional (nonpharmacologic) endotracheal intubation.

27. What was the purpose of this study (i.e. what problem or question are they trying to solve)?

_____

_____

28. Is the hypothesis stated in this abstract? _____ If you answered yes, what is it? If you answered no, what do you think it is?

_____

29. What is the study population?

_____

30. What is the sample and sample size for this research?

_____

31. Was a random sampling procedure used? Yes No
Explain your answer

_____

32. Did this study use a qualitative or quantitative approach?

_____

33. The study indicates a standard deviation for the mean dose of 1.1 mg. What does that mean?

_____

34. What are some weaknesses or unanswered questions related to this research?

_____

35. Are the findings of this study important to the EMS community?

_____

● STUDENT SELF-ASSESSMENT

36. Which federal law enabled creation of the U.S. Department of Transportation and the National Highway Traffic Safety Administration and provided funding for EMS?
 a. Accidental Death and Disability Act
 b. Consolidated Omnibus Reconciliation Act
 c. Emergency Medical Services Systems Act
 d. Highway Safety Act

37. Which of the following is _not_ a component of the EMS system?
 a. Disaster planning   c. Intensive care units
 b. Insurance providers   d. Paramedic training

38. How has health care reform affected emergency medical services?
 a. It results in larger reimbursement amounts for each call
 b. It may increase the distance for transport based on insurance restrictions for hospitals
 c. It has caused a decrease in emergency ambulance transports
 d. It will restrict the scope of practice for the EMS provider

39. Which of the following describes the manner in which a paramedic follows the practice, guidelines, and ethical considerations within the practice of prehospital emergency care?
 a. Certification   **c.** Professionalism
 b. Licensure   **d.** Registration

40. Which of the following is _not_ a role of the paramedic as defined by the Department of Transportation?
 a. Assessing and providing emergency patient care
 b. Coordinating collection of outstanding patient bills
 c. Documenting and communicating patient care
 d. Ensuring the ambulance is adequately stocked

41. The EMS physician medical director is responsible for which of the following:
 a. Ensuring maintenance of ambulances and equipment
 b. Monitoring the quality of EMS care
 c. Negotiating staff salary and benefit disputes
 d. Providing patient care in the field on advanced life-support units

42. A man who claims to be an emergency department physician is attempting to direct care in an inappropriate manner on a cardiac arrest call. You should do which of the following:
 a. Contact online medical direction for instructions
 b. Follow his orders because he has appropriate credentials
 c. Ignore him and carry on as you see appropriate
 d. Immediately ask the police to arrest him

43. Which of the following demonstrates a prospective method of a continuous quality improvement model?
   a. Continuing education programs
   b. Listening to audio tapes of EMS reports
   c. Observation of prehospital care by the medical director
   d. Reviewing prehospital patient care records
44. You are conducting research for a drug to treat cardiac arrest. Only you and your partner have been trained to gather the data, so the drug will only be used on days that you work. This type of subject selection is called which of the following:
   a. Alternative time sampling
   c. Statistical table sampling
   b. Convenience sampling
   d. Systemic sampling
45. You are performing a study on variability of scene response times according to time of day. Here is the data you collected (in minutes) for one group: 1, 2, 3, 4, 4, 4, 4, 5, 5, 5, 5, 6, 6, 6, 7, 7, 8, 9. What is the mode for this set of data?
   a. 4
   b. 5
   c. 6
   d. 7
46. Before your research is approved by an Institution Review Board, what must you prove?
   a. Consent will be obtained
   b. The hypothesis is true
   c. There will be no risks
   d. Your sample is large enough

CHAPTER 2
THE WELL-BEING OF THE PARAMEDIC

● READING ASSIGNMENT
Chapter 2, pages 28-53, in *Mosby's Paramedic Textbook,* ed 2

● OBJECTIVES
As a paramedic, you should be able to:
1. Describe the components of wellness and their benefits.
2. Discuss the paramedic's role in promoting wellness.
3. Outline the benefits of specific lifestyle choices that promote wellness, including proper nutrition, weight control, exercise, sleep, and smoking cessation.
4. Identify risk factors and warning signs of cancer and cardiovascular disease.
5. Identify preventive measures to minimize the risk of work-related illness or injury associated with exposure, the lifting and moving of patients, hostile environments, vehicle operations, and rescue situations.
6. List signs and symptoms of addiction and addictive behavior.
7. Distinguish between normal and abnormal anxiety and stress reactions.
8. Give examples of stress reduction techniques.
9. Outline the 10 components of critical incident stress management.
10. Given a scenario involving death or dying, identify therapeutic actions you may take based on your knowledge of the dynamics of this process.
11. List measures that may be taken to reduce the risk of infectious disease exposure.
12. Outline actions that should be taken after a significant exposure to a patient's blood or other body fluids.

● REVIEW QUESTIONS
Complete the following table to describe your wellness behaviors, analyze risks or benefits associated with those behaviors, and identify opportunities to improve them.

Behavior	Present practice	Risk/benefit of this behavior	Improvement plan
Diet: Fats, vitamins, carbohydrates			
Weight			
Cardiovascular endurance			
Strength/flexibility			
Sleep (hr/day)			
Cardiovascular disease risk factors			
Cancer risk factors			
Injury prevention			
Substance abuse			
Smoking			

Match the defense mechanism in Column II with its appropriate example in Column I. Use each defense mechanism only once.

Column I

1. _____ A rape victim who cannot recall anything from the time she was abducted until the police find her
2. _____ A paramedic who, when passed over for a promotion, states that the boss always plays favorites
3. _____ A paramedic who is upset by a violent death and washes all the vehicles in the garage
4. _____ An automobile accident victim refuses to acknowledge that he cannot move his legs
5. _____ An EMT who gave poor care complains about the patient's hospital treatment
6. _____ A 10-year-old who begins to suck his thumb en route to the hospital after sustaining a fracture from a fall

Column II

a. Compensation
b. Denial
c. Isolation
d. Projection
e. Rationalization
f. Reaction formation
g. Regression
h. Repression
i. Substitution

Questions 7-11 pertain to the following case study:

You respond to a call for an assault. Police on the scene tell you an 18-year-old man has been stabbed. You find him at a party on the 4th floor of an apartment complex that has no working elevators. The patient, your nephew, is alert and crying and has a briskly bleeding puncture wound in the midaxillary line. He is complaining of severe difficulty breathing and abdominal pain and has a rapid radial pulse. Oxygen is applied, and as you prepare for rapid transport and treatment, some party-goers begin to get belligerent.

7. Describe three measures that you should take to reduce the risk of work-related illness and injury on this type of call in each of the following areas:
   a. Infectious disease

   _____

   b. Lifting and moving

   _____

   c. Hostile environments

   _____

   d. Vehicle operation

   _____

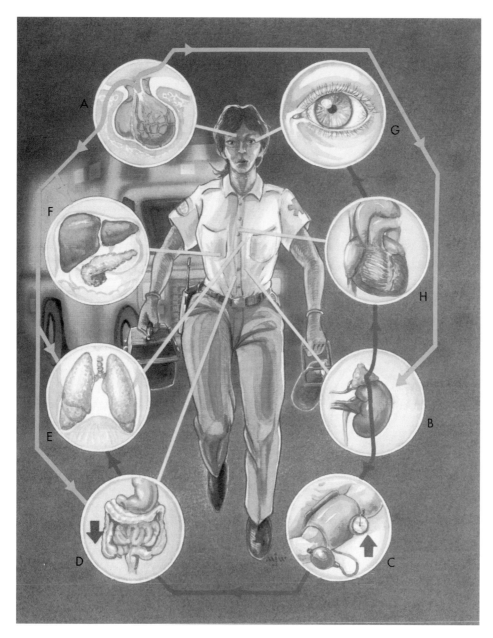

Figure 2-1

8. Briefly explain how each area of the body labeled in Fig. 2-1 responds to stress during the alarm reaction in this type of situation.

a.

b.

c.

d.

e.

_____

f.

_____

g.

_____

h.

_____

9. Describe two daily wellness practices that may benefit you as a paramedic when you respond to this type of situation.
   a.
   b.

10. List two reasons you, your crew, or both might use the services of the critical incident stress debriefing team after this call.

_____

11. Which of the services that can be provided by a critical incident stress debriefing team may be of benefit after this call?

_____

12. List five causes of stress that are job related and five that are non–job related.
   a. Job-related stressors:

_____

_____

   b. Non–job-related stressors:

_____

_____

13. List three potential symptoms of decompensation from the effects of long-term stress.
   a.
   b.
   c.

14. Name five effective stress-management techniques that can minimize the effects of EMS job-related stress. (After you complete this, survey paramedics you know to see what strategies they use.)
   a.
   b.
   c.
   d.
   e.

Questions 15-17 pertain to the following case study:

   You arrive at a family gathering where you find a 46-year-old man in full cardiopulmonary arrest. His mother is crying and begging, "Please, Lord, don't take him, take me." His wife is distraught, pacing and saying, "It's going to be OK; it's not as bad as it seems." The brother yells at you as you enter, "What took you so long? Hurry up! What are you waiting for?"

15. Identify which of the stages of grief described by Dr. Kubler-Ross each family member is exhibiting in this situation.
  a. Mother:
  b. Wife:
  c. Brother:

16. How should you care for these family members to promote normal grieving?

_____

_____

_____

17. How can you deal with the pent-up emotions you must suppress while caring for dying patients and their families on calls like this?

_____

_____

18. Identify which of the following situations represents an exposure to blood or body fluids. If there is an exposure, describe a measure that could have prevented it.
  a. After you use a lancet to obtain a blood sample for dextrose from your patient, you puncture your hand with the lancet. Exposure?

_____

  Prevention: _____
  b. Blood sprays from a patient's endotracheal tube, hitting you in the face. You aren't sure if any got in your eyes or mouth. Exposure?

_____

  Prevention: _____
  c. Your bare forearm brushes against a bloody sheet. You have no open wounds on your arm. Exposure?

_____

  Prevention: _____
  d. You put the IV bag in your mouth to hold it up as you move the patient, and then your partner points out that there is blood splattered over the bag. Exposure?

_____

  Prevention: _____
19. At the scene of a motor vehicle collision, glass punctures your glove and your finger. The patient's blood penetrates the glove and is on your cut. List at least four actions that you should take after this exposure.
  a.
  b.
  c.
  d.

20. Which of the following is true regarding a healthy diet?
    a. Amino acids are produced by the body in the liver.
    b. Fats should be completely eliminated from the diet.
    c. Vitamin supplements are necessary for normal health.
    d. Water is one of the most important nutrients.

21. Which of the following is true regarding a routine physical fitness program?
    a. A decrease in muscle mass and metabolism will occur.
    b. A decrease in resting blood pressure may occur.
    c. A decrease in resistance to injury will occur.
    d. It should not be done if you have any preexisting illness.

22. Which of the following is a lifestyle modification that is associated with a decreased risk of heart disease?
    a. Decreasing cigarette smoking
    b. Estrogen therapy for postmenopausal women
    c. Decreasing the VLDL triglyceride level to 400 mg/dl
    d. Maintaining LDL cholesterol levels at 190 mg/dl

23. Which of the following signs or symptoms is commonly listed as a warning sign of cancer?
    a. Indigestion or change in bowel habits
    b. Irregular heart beats or palpitations
    c. Lifelong presence of warts or moles
    d. Persistent nasal congestion

24. Actions that may prevent you from becoming infected with a communicable disease while practicing as a paramedic include which of the following?
    a. Annual skin testing for tuberculosis
    b. Frequent handwashing during all patient care activities
    c. Recapping of needles after patient use
    d. Use of body substance isolation for high-risk patients

25. How can you minimize your risk of injury while lifting or moving patients?
    a. Bend at the hips and knees.
    b. Hold the load 18 inches from your body.
    c. Lift with your back, not your legs.
    d. Move backward rather than forward.

26. Which of the following may indicate the potential for addiction or addictive behavior?
    a. Your partner asks you to drive him home from a bar because he feels he has had too much to drink.
    b. Your partner tells her husband that she only had 6 beers instead of the 12 she actually drank.
    c. Your partner mentions that he is going out to have a few beers with some friends after work.
    d. Your partner says she can't handle booze the way she used to and now prefers beer to hard liquor.

27. You are called to a scene to assume care from a rescue unit. You immediately recognize the paramedic who is caring for the patient as an individual whom you consistently disagree with over patient care issues. What type of stress is this call likely to produce?
    a. Environmental   c. Personality
    b. Managerial   d. Psychosocial

28. Generalized feelings of apprehension are known as:
    a. Anxiety   c. Reaction formation
    b. Phobias   d. Stress

29. A paramedic student has just failed his practical examination station because of improper airway-management technique and states, "Well, I would have done it, but we never practiced it in class this way." This is an example of which defense mechanism?
   a. Projection
   c. Regression
   b. Rationalization
   d. Sublimation
30. Critical incident stress debriefing is most helpful for which of the following?
   a. New employees after every critical patient situation
   b. Selected high-risk employees with psychological problems
   c. Mass casualty incidents involving more than 10 patients
   d. Situations in which a high degree of stress is perceived
31. When dealing with the family of a patient who is dying, you can best interact with them by doing which of the following?
   a. Reassuring them that no one you ever care for dies
   b. Changing the subject every time someone brings up death
   c. Allowing the family to remain with the patient if possible
   d. Avoiding direct communication with the immediate family
32. Which response to the death of a close family member would not be expected in a preschool child?
   a. The child acts as though nothing has happened.
   b. The child asks when the family member will come back.
   c. The child fears that other family members will die too.
   d. The child thinks that he/she was responsible for the death.
33. School-age children (7 to 12 years) feel that death:
   a. Is temporary and reversible
   b. Happens to others, not themselves
   c. Is punishment for their bad thoughts
   d. Is the same as severe illness
34. Which is an appropriate action to take after a needlestick injury of the finger?
   a. Complete the exposure report and turn it in at the end of your shift.
   b. Determine whether the patient is high risk to see whether you need to report the incident.
   c. Report the exposure to your supervisor and the receiving facility immediately.
   d. Squeeze as much blood out as possible and suck on your finger.

INJURY PREVENTION

● READING ASSIGNMENT

Chapter 3, pages 54-65, in *Mosby's Paramedic Textbook*, ed 2

● OBJECTIVES

As a paramedic, you should be able to:

1. Identify roles of the EMS community in injury prevention.
2. Describe the epidemiology of trauma in the United States.
3. Outline the aspects of the EMS system that make it a desirable resource for involvement in community health activities.
4. Describe community leadership activities that are essential to enable the active participation of EMS in community wellness activities.
5. List areas with which paramedics should be familiar to participate in injury prevention.
6. Evaluate a situation to determine opportunities for injury prevention.
7. Identify resources necessary to conduct a community health assessment.
8. Relate how alterations in the epidemiological triangle can influence injury or disease patterns.
9. Differentiate among primary, secondary, and tertiary health prevention activities.
10. Describe strategies to implement a successful injury prevention program.

● REVIEW QUESTIONS

Questions 1-9 pertain to the following case study:

> At 1400 the tones sound and you are dispatched to the home of an elderly resident who has slipped and fallen. On the patient's arrival to the emergency department, the physician confirms your suspicion, the patient's hip is broken. As you ride back to the base, you remark to your partner how this is the fourth patient you've transported this month with a broken hip. These calls really bother you because your own grandmother was institutionalized and then died of pneumonia shortly after a similar injury just 6 months ago. By the time you arrive back at your station, you have resolved to do something about the problem. You approach the chief and he listens to your idea and then tells you to return when you have some solid information about the target population, magnitude of the problem, your goals, and the cost involved.

1. What percentage of emergency department visits in the United States are related to injury? _____
2. The initial visit to the emergency department for this type of injury has a high price. List two other "costs" that are associated with this type of injury.

   _____, _____

3. Why is EMS ideally suited to perform community prevention activities with the elderly (list at least three reasons)?
   a.
   b.
   c.

4. What additional information would you need to be able to provide prevention for this type of injury to this group?

_____

5. What will you need from your boss before moving ahead with this project?

_____

6. List three community resources that you may need to contact to identify the number of elderly persons living in your district, the incidence of hip fractures, morbidity and mortality rates associated with this injury, and costs associated with this injury.

a.

b.

c.

7. You decide that the causes of fall injury in the elderly are most likely the result of the host and environmental factors of the epidemiological triangle. List two host and two environmental factors that may contribute to falls in the elderly.

Host: **a.** _____

      b. _____

Environmental: **a.** _____

      b. _____

After a careful evaluation of the problem, you decide that the best plan would be to have EMS crews visit elderly residents' homes with a checklist that would identify risk factors for falls present in the home. A brief education pamphlet with specific recommendations would then be given to the resident.

8. Is your plan an example of a primary, secondary, or tertiary intervention?

_____

9. List at least four factors that you should consider when you prepare your written education materials to distribute to the community.

_____

Each of the examples in questions 10-18 represents a factor that could cause or increase susceptibility to illness and injury. Indicate whether the example indicates an _agent_ (causative), _host_ (influence on exposure, susceptibility, or response to agents), or _environmental_ (influence on existence of the agent, exposure, or susceptibility) factor.

Example	Agent, Host, or Environmental
10. Fatigue	
11. Firefighter	
12. Carbon monoxide	
13. Gender	
14. Hepatitis	
15. Malnutrition	
16. Poor personal hygiene	
17. Flood	
18. Cholesterol	

19. A total of 10 people in your EMS district were killed in a motor vehicle collisions this year. Where do deaths from unintentional causes such as this rank in the United States?
    a. 1st   c. 5th
    b. 3rd   d. 7th
20. Your community has experienced an increase in drownings during the past year. The health department asks your EMS agency to assist with an education plan to reduce the incidence of these injuries. Why are EMS providers ideal for this type of program?
    a. They have more time than other health care providers to teach these programs.
    b. Paramedics and EMTs will be welcomed into homes and public places for education.
    c. EMS agencies have abundant financial resources to fund these programs.
    d. EMS providers are the best authorities on preventing injuries such as these.
21. How can EMS safety be enhanced during emergency care and transportation?
    a. Educate the public to pull to the right when they see emergency traffic.
    b. Ticket people who fail to yield to emergency traffic.
    c. Establish a policy to park upwind from all hazmat spills.
    d. Ensure that police assume all responsibility for scene safety.
22. How can EMS agencies promote positive involvement of staff in community wellness programs?
    a. Penalize those who decline to participate.
    b. Ask everyone on duty to participate.
    c. Offer it as an alternative to a less desirable chore.
    d. Provide salary for off-duty injury prevention work.
23. You respond to a call for domestic violence. You find a woman with bruising around her face, and she and her husband are both yelling at each other. She screams at you to leave her alone when you try to examine her and he is staggering and cursing at you. What is your primary goal in this situation?
    a. To restrain the patient and ask medical direction for permission for involuntary transport
    b. To ask the police to arrest both of them so that they can be contained in a controlled space
    c. To maintain the safety of your crew and to calmly diffuse the situation without violence
    d. To forcibly remove the man from the situation so that the woman will not be afraid of treatment
24. Which of the following would likely represent a situation where a teachable moment exists?
    a. During transport with a hysterical mother whose child has just fallen down a flight of stairs
    b. An elderly patient who refuses care after she fell in a dimly lit stairway and injured her wrist
    c. A child who has minor injuries after being struck by a car that crossed the median onto the sidewalk
    d. An unhelmeted cyclist who has fallen off his bike during a race and is confused during transport
25. You believe that you are running many more calls related to heart-related problems in the elderly. What community resources can you use to obtain information to see whether the makeup of your community is changing?
    a. Census data   c. Fire service
    b. Chamber of commerce d. Local newspaper

26. It is a cold, wintry day and the trees are glistening after the ice storm last night. Your crew alone has run four calls to the local sledding hill to care for patients with injuries ranging from broken extremities to lumbar fractures. Which element in the epidemiological triangle is most likely having the greatest influence in the injuries you are seeing in this situation?
    a. Physical environment
    c. Strength of the agent
    b. Social setting
    d. Susceptibility of the host

27. Which of the following is an example of a primary health prevention activity that a paramedic may be involved with?
    a. You check the blood pressure of residents diagnosed with hypertension each week.
    b. You coordinate a stop-smoking program for a group of your fellow employees.
    c. You coordinate a drunk-u-drama at the high school before prom week.
    d. You arrange a support group for EMS personnel who are recovering from alcohol abuse.

28. You are preparing a presentation for the youth in your area about drug use. How can you be sure that your audience will understand your message?
    a. You should test it on a teen patient during an EMS call.
    b. You should ask your crew to see whether it appeals to them.
    c. You should include slides to increase learning potential retention.
    d. You should ensure that the language and reading level suits the audience.

MEDICAL/LEGAL ISSUES

● READING ASSIGNMENT
Chapter 4, pages 66-89, in *Mosby's Paramedic Textbook*, ed 2

● OBJECTIVES
As a paramedic, you should be able to:
1. Describe the basic structure of the legal system in the United States.
2. Relate how laws affect the paramedic's practice.
3. List situations that the paramedic is legally required to report in most states.
4. Describe laws that provide protection for the paramedic.
5. Describe the four elements involved in a claim of negligence.
6. Describe measures paramedics may take to protect themselves from claims of negligence.
7. Describe the paramedic's responsibilities with regard to patient confidentiality.
8. Outline the process for obtaining expressed, informed, and implied consent.
9. Describe actions to be taken in a refusal-of-care situation.
10. Describe legal considerations related to patient transportation.
11. Outline legal issues related to specific resuscitation situations.
12. List measures the paramedic should take to preserve evidence when at a crime or an accident scene.
13. Detail the components of the narrative report necessary for effective legal documentation.
14. Define common medical-legal terms that apply to prehospital situations involving patient care.

● REVIEW QUESTIONS
Match the legal term in Column II with its definition in Column I. Use each answer only once.

Column I	Column II
1. _____ Forcefully restraining the arm of an alert, competent patient while an intravenous line is being placed	a. Abandonment
	b. Assault
	c. Battery
2. _____ As a joke, advising the emergency department staff that the patient is a prostitute	d. False Imprisonment
	e. Libel
3. _____ Telling a friend that you treated a nurse you both know for a drug overdose	f. Invasion of privacy (libel)
4. _____ Restraining an alert, conscious adult with an obvious fracture and transporting him by ambulance against his will	g. Malpractice
	h. Slander
5. _____ Documenting that the patient is homosexual and remarking, "now let's see them get insurance"	

6. _____ Leaving a patient in the emergency
department to go on another call before
you have an opportunity to give a
report to the nurse or physician on duty

7. Violations of state motor vehicle codes by a paramedic can result in civil lawsuits only. True/false. If this answer is false, why is it false?

_____

_____

8. Good Samaritan legislation may protect off-duty EMS providers from litigation if there was no negligence or reckless disregard. True/false. If this answer is false, why is it false?

_____

_____

9. Group insurance policies will protect EMS providers from having lawsuits brought against them arising from negligent acts. True/false. If this answer if false, why is it false?

_____

_____

10. List four situations that most states require a paramedic to report to the authorities.
   a.
   b.
   c.
   d.

11. List the four elements necessary to prove negligence.
   a.
   b.
   c.
   d.

12. A 40-year-old patient involved in a motor vehicle collision is complaining of mild neck pain and tingling in her fingers. She is quickly assessed and signs a refusal-of-care form at the urging of the paramedic crew. Later that day, she loses sensation and movement in all extremities, ceases breathing, and dies. Which, if any, of the four elements in Question 11 could be used to prove negligence in this situation and why?

_____

_____

_____

13. Name three effective means by which the paramedic may avoid claims of liability when providing patient care.
   a.
   b.
   c.

14. Fill in the blanks with the types of consent that best apply to the situation. You are called to treat an alert, 72-year-old patient who is experiencing chest pain. The patient exhibits classic signs and symptoms of myocardial infarction. You explain to him that he needs to go to the hospital because you feel that his symptoms could be those of a heart attack and proper medicine could be given to aid his condition. He states that he wants his wife to drive him instead of going by ambulance. You advise him that if his condition worsens in the car, his wife would be unable to help him and he might die. You again urge him to come with you. The patient can now make a(n)

a. _____ consent. He tells you that he has decided to go in the ambulance. This constitutes a(n)

b. _____ consent. If he had lost consciousness before agreeing to ambulance transport, his consent is said to be a(n)

c. _____ consent, and treatment could be rendered.

15. You respond to the scene of an automobile collision, where you find an awake, alert, 24-year-old man complaining of neck pain and tingling in his right arm. Vital signs are stable. The patient's vehicle was struck from behind and sustained considerable damage. The patient is refusing transport to the hospital. What five things should be done or explained to this patient and documented on the patient care report regarding his refusal of care?

a.

b.

c.

d.

e.

Questions 16-21 refer to the following case study:

> You are dispatched to an expensive rural home for an "accidental injury." When you arrive, you find two patients. The first is a man, approximately 30 years of age, who has apparently been shot at close range in the head and was found pulseless and breathless by the family member who found the patients 20 minutes before your arrival. There is a large exit wound with brain matter extruding. After your initial assessment, you decide not to resuscitate him. The second patient is a woman who you recognize as a local celebrity. She has a gunshot wound to the abdomen, is unconscious, and has no radial pulse. You note a plastic bag of white powder and a hypodermic needle next to the woman. A handgun is lying on the floor next to the man. The family wants you to take the patient to the closest local hospital so that they can "keep things quiet." The nearest trauma center is an equal distance.

16. What type of consent applies in this situation?

_____

17. List four facts you must document about the male patient to ensure legal compliance.

a.

b.

c.

d.

18. Describe actions you should take to preserve evidence at this scene relative to the following:

a. Clothing:

_____

b. Weapon:

_____

c. Blood on the floor:

_____

d. Documentation of the scene:

_____

e. Positioning your ambulance:

_____

19. Should you transport the patient to the hospital the family wishes or to the trauma center? (Explain your answer.)

_____

20. Why shouldn't you document "Drugs found lying next to patient?"

_____

_____

21. To which of the following personnel is it appropriate to tell the facts of this case?
   a. Police officers assigned to the case   Yes/No
   b. A paramedic from another service   Yes/No
   c. Press   Yes/No
   d. Medical personnel caring for patient   Yes/No
   e. Hospital staff in the smokers' area   Yes/No

● STUDENT SELF-ASSESSMENT

22. Which branch of law is also referred to as *tort law?*
   a. Administrative law   c. Criminal law
   b. Civil law   d. Legislative law
23. In which of the following situations may abandonment be alleged when a paramedic relinquishes care to an EMT?
   a. A patient being transferred with an infusion of blood
   b. A patient going from a nursing home to a hospital for a wrist injury
   c. A hysterical, uninjured patient from a mass casualty situation
   d. A dialysis patient being transported for routine care
24. Which of the following is necessary for successful prosecution of a criminal law case?
   a. Criminal intent must be proved.
   b. Injury must be demonstrated.
   c. A patient must sue for financial gain.
   d. A statute must be violated.
25. You are called to a private residence where you find an elderly man who is suffering from heat-related illness. The family evidently left this chronically confused individual at home with no air conditioning and all the windows closed. What legal issue must you remember on this call?
   a. Do not remove the patient's clothes so that you can preserve the chain of evidence.
   b. This patient can't give consent, so you must contact the next-of-kin before transport.
   c. Writing the neighbors' statements in the patient care report may constitute libel.
   d. You are required to report this situation to the appropriate legal or social agency.

26. The Ryan White Act provides protection for the paramedic related to which of the following?
    a. Good Samaritan acts
    c. Infectious disease
    b. Governmental immunity
    d. Violent acts
27. A paramedic finds an unconscious patient who has a strong odor resembling alcohol on the breath. No care is initiated, and during transport, the patient aspirates. On arrival to the hospital, the patient is found to have a dangerously low blood sugar and a lengthy hospitalization ensues. Why could this patient claim negligence?
    a. The paramedic violated a law while providing care.
    b. The paramedic committed malfeasance while providing care.
    c. The patient suffered damage from the negligent act.
    d. There was evidence of conflicting views of causation.
28. Patient confidentiality would be breached in most states if a paramedic discussed the patient's comments and care with which of the following?
    a. Lawyers in court
    b. Emergency department personnel
    c. Personal friends
    d. A quality-assurance committee
29. When a patient agrees verbally or in writing to treatment, it is known as which of the following?
    a. Expressed consent
    c. Informed consent
    b. Implied consent
    d. Referred consent
30. You are caring for an elderly patient who experienced a syncopal episode. He is now refusing care. What actions must you take to ensure legal compliance during this refusal process?
    a. You must force the patient to sign the refusal form before release.
    b. Tell the patient that if he changes his mind, he can call you again for transport.
    c. Do not give the patient any additional advice or you may be liable.
    d. Transport the patient against his will because his condition involved a loss of consciousness.
31. What do EMS traffic right-of-way privileges usually include?
    a. The right to travel as fast as necessary to get to the hospital quickly
    b. The ability to proceed without slowing through intersections
    c. The right to override the directions of a traffic officer
    d. Definitions of appropriate use of lights and sirens
32. According to the American Heart Association, what criteria must be met to stop resuscitation in the prehospital setting after you have initiated advanced life support procedures?
    a. Persistent asystole or agonal rhythm is present and no reversible causes are identified.
    b. The family assures you that there is a "do not resuscitate" order but it can't be found.
    c. Endotracheal intubation and IV access can't be established, so you are unable to give drugs.
    d. Trauma is present and your transport time will be 20 minutes or longer.
33. You respond to a stabbing at a local bar. What actions should you take during your care of the patient to preserve evidence?
    a. Cut the clothing through the knife hole to minimize other damage.
    b. Give the clothes to a bystander so that evidence will remain at the scene.
    c. Move the knife if present so that EMS personnel will not step on it.
    d. Follow the same path to and from the ambulance and patient.
34. Which of the following should be included in the narrative portion of the patient care report?
    a. Care rendered
    c. Physical findings
    b. History
    d. All of the above

ETHICS

● READING ASSIGNMENT

Chapter 5, pages 90-101, in *Mosby's Paramedic Textbook,* ed 2

● OBJECTIVES

As a paramedic, you should be able to:

1. Define *ethics* and *bioethics.*
2. Distinguish among professional, legal, and moral accountability.
3. Outline strategies that may be used to resolve ethical conflicts.
4. Describe the role of ethical tests in resolving ethical dilemmas in health care.
5. Discuss specific prehospital ethical issues, including allocation of resources, decisions surrounding resuscitation, confidentiality, and consent.
6. Identify ethical dilemmas that may occur related to care in futile situations, obligation to provide care, patient advocacy, and the paramedic's role as physician extender.

● REVIEW QUESTIONS

Match the term in Column II with its description in Column I. Use each term only once.

Column I	Column II
1. _____ Working to benefit others	**a.** Autonomy
2. _____ Study of right, wrong, and morality	**b.** Beneficence
3. _____ To do no harm	**c.** Bioethics
4. _____ A person's ability to make rational decisions independently	**d.** Confidentiality
	e. Ethics
5. _____ Moral duty or obligation related to medicine	**f.** Nonmaleficence
6. _____ Maintaining the privacy of personal patient information	**g.** Rationality

Questions 7-9 pertain to the following case study:

> A fellow paramedic who is a close friend calls you and is very upset. Her daughter was involved in a vehicle collision. She is fine, but a person in the other car was injured and has been taken to the hospital. You transported the injured patient, and your friend wants to know the extent of injuries, what the patient said, and details related to the crash.

7. **a.** What should you tell your friend about the patient's injuries? _____
   b. Is your decision ethically correct with regard to the patient and your friend?_____

> Your friend's daughter has been charged with reckless driving. You believe that the patient you transported was intoxicated; in fact, he admitted to using alcohol and cocaine before the incident. Despite his serious injuries, he was laughing and making inappropriate comments.

8. Will this affect your decision about disclosing patient information? Why?
9. Did you make your decision about this problem based on professional, legal, or moral accountability?

10. Think about how you would respond to each of the following situations, and state whether *professional, legal,* or *moral* accountability issues would prompt your actions.
   a. You are leaving the hospital after transporting a patient. You notice that your partner has picked up some towels when you didn't use any on the patient. He says, "Oh these are for me, I want to wash my car this afternoon."

   _____

   b. As you depart from a scene, you hear your partner make an inappropriate racial comment about the patient.

   _____

   c. You notice that an on-duty co-worker has an alcoholic drink while attending your annual department awards banquet.

   _____

   d. Your partner administers a slightly different dose of pain medicine than ordered by medical direction because he felt that the doctor was being "too conservative."

   _____

   e. Your teenage niece is experiencing severe vomiting in her first trimester of pregnancy. It is clear that she needs IV fluids to relieve her dehydration, but she has no insurance and you know it will cost your brother hundreds of dollars if she is seen in the emergency department. He asks whether you can get some supplies from work and come to the house to give her the fluids.

   _____

   Question 11 pertains to the following case study:

   You and your partner are caring for a 55-year-old patient who is in respiratory arrest. You have called for assistance and are told it will be 10 minutes. After intubation, the patient is stable as long as you ventilate regularly. You are preparing for transport when, suddenly, your partner collapses and is pulseless.

11. a. The circumstances will only allow you to care for one patient or the other. Who will you choose to resuscitate, and why?

   _____

   b. How did you reach that decision? Try to use the ethical tests in the rapid approach to emergency medical problems to see whether they would assist you in this situation.
      I. Have you experienced a similar problem in the past?
      II. Can you buy time for deliberation or to consult with others?
      III. Would you accept the action if you were in the patient's place?
      IV. Would you feel comfortable having the action performed in all similar circumstances?
      V. Can you provide good reasons to justify and defend your actions to others?

12. State which of the following is the cause of the ethical dilemma in each of the following situations and an action you could take.
      I. Allocation of resources
      II. Decisions surrounding resuscitation
      III. Confidentiality
      IV. Consent
      V. Care in futile situations
      VI. Obligation to provide care
      VII. Role as physician extender

   a. You request pain medicine to care for a very painful single-extremity injury that your patient has. On-line medical direction refuses.

      Cause: _____ Action: _____

   b. Your patient has a severe headache, is vomiting, and has a numb right hand. Blood pressure is 220/140 mm Hg. Despite your detailed explanations, the patient is refusing treatment or transport.

      Cause: _____ Action: _____

   c. You are triaging at a mass casualty situation. You evaluate a child, the same age as yours, whose skin is warm. Bystanders say she just stopped breathing a few moments ago.

      Cause: _____ Action: _____

   d. You respond to a private residence. The patient has a legally executed living will. Hysterical family members are begging you to resuscitate the patient.

      Cause: _____ Action: _____

● STUDENT SELF-ASSESSMENT

13. What are the standards of honorable behavior that paramedics are expected to conform to within the EMS profession?
   a. Certifications   **c.** Laws
   b. Ethics   **d.** Morals

14. Which of the following determines moral accountability in the practice of EMS?
   a. Laws and regulations
   b. Personal beliefs and values
   c. Professional licensure
   d. Standards related to education and skills

15. During a call, you find yourself in a situation that involves an ethical dilemma. What strategy can you use to resolve the problem?
   a. Let the patient's family tell you what to do.
   b. Ask yourself which action you would prefer if you were in their place.
   c. Abide by your partner's opinion in the situation.
   d. Rely on your policies and procedures for guidance.

16. Which of the ethical tests can help correct for your personal bias about a situation?
   a. Would you accept the action if you were in the patient's place?
   b. Would you feel comfortable having this action performed under similar circumstances?
   c. Can you justify and defend your actions to others?
   d. Have you experienced a similar problem in the past?

17. You are faced with an unusual situation on a call that falls just on the fringe of your legal and professional boundaries. You decide to take action because you are able to provide clear reasons to explain and defend your actions to others. What type of ethical test have you used?
    a. Autonomy
    c. Interpersonal justifiability
    b. Impartiality
    d. Universalizability
18. Which of the following situations involves an ethical decision? The patient has a living will and is pulseless.
    a. The family asks you to abide by the living will.
    b. The patient is cold and has rigor mortis.
    c. The living will has a signature misplaced on the document.
    d. The nursing home staff think there is a living will but cannot locate it.
19. You are transporting a patient and her doctor from an outpatient surgery center to the hospital after a complication has occurred. The patient's respirations are very slow, and her chest is barely moving. You indicate the need to ventilate, but the physician strongly disagrees. If you elect to proceed, you are acting on the ethical principle of which of the following?
    a. Allocation of resources
    c. Care in futile situations
    b. Autonomy
    d. Patient advocacy

OVERVIEW OF HUMAN SYSTEMS

● READING ASSIGNMENT

Chapter 6, pages 102-179, in *Mosby's Paramedic Textbook,* ed 2

● OBJECTIVES

As a paramedic, you should be able to:
 1. Discuss the importance of human anatomy as it relates to the paramedic profession.
 2. Describe anatomical position.
 3. Properly interpret anatomical directional terms and body planes.
 4. List the structures that compose the axial and appendicular regions of the body.
 5. Define the divisions of the abdominal region.
 6. List the three major body cavities.
 7. Describe the contents of the three major body cavities.
 8. Discuss the functions of the following cellular structures: the cytoplasmic membrane, the cytoplasm (and its organelles), and the nucleus.
 9. Describe the process by which human cells reproduce.
10. Differentiate and describe the following tissue types: epithelial tissue, connective tissue, muscle tissue, and nervous tissue.
11. For each of the 11 major organ systems in the human body, label a diagram of anatomical structures, list the functions of the major anatomical structures, and explain how the organs of the system interrelate to perform the specified functions of the system.
12. For the special senses, label a diagram of the anatomical structures of the special sense, list the functions of the anatomical structures of each sense, and explain how the structures of the sense interrelate to perform its specialized functions.

● REVIEW QUESTIONS

Match the cellular structure from Column II with its definition in Column I. Use each answer only once.

Column I	Column II
1. _____ Cytoplasmic "canals" that transport proteins and other substances	a. Centrioles
	b. Cytoplasm
2. _____ Phospholipid layer that forms the outer boundary of the cell	c. Cytoplasmic membrane
3. _____ Organelles that contain enzymes capable of digesting proteins and lipids	d. Endoplasmic reticulum
4. _____ Mass of cell that lies between the cytoplasmic membrane and nucleus	e. Golgi apparatus
	f. Lysosomes
5. _____ Sacs that package materials for secretion from the cell	g. Mitochondria
	h. Nucleus
6. _____ Control center of the cell that contains genetic material	i. Ribosomes

7. _____ Structures that are composed of
ribonucleic acid and protein and that
manufacture enzymes

8. _____ Powerhouse of the cell, responsible for
production of adenosine triphosphate

9. Label Fig. 6-1 with the appropriate cellular structures listed in Column II of
question 8.
   a.
   b.
   c.
   d.
   e.
   f.
   g.

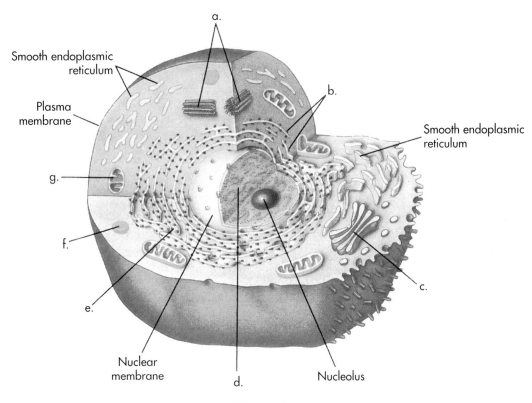

Figure 6-1

10. All human cells divide by the process of mitosis throughout the life of a human organism. True/False. If this is false, explain why.

_____

11. Describe the anatomical position.

_____

12. Circle the appropriate directional terms in boldface in the following sentences.
  a. The wrist lies **distal/proximal** to the elbow.
  b. The right nipple is located **medial/lateral** to the sternum.
  c. The cervical spine is **superior/inferior** to the lumbar spine.
  d. The umbilicus is located on the **dorsal/ventral** surface of the body.
13. List the structures that compose the following:
  a. The appendicular region of the body:

_____

  b. The axial region of the body:

_____

14. Name the anatomical landmarks that divide the abdomen into four quadrants.

_____

Questions 15-19 pertain to the following case study.

You respond to a call for a burn. You determine the scene is safe and then approach the patient. She is lying on her right side moaning, with burned sites over several areas. You begin your assessment and care and roll her supine. As you carefully remove her clothing, you can better observe the burns shown in Fig. 6-2.

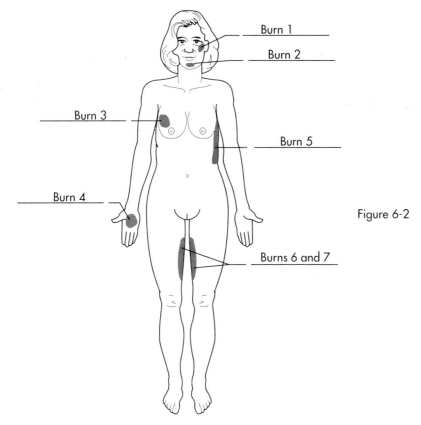

Figure 6-2

15. What directional term describes the patient's position when you arrived?

_____

16. Using appropriate directional terms, describe where:
   a. Burn (1) is located relative to the left eye

_____

   b. Burn (2) is located relative to the mouth

_____

   c. Burn (3) is located relative to the nipple

_____

   d. Burn (4) lies relative to the right hand

_____

   e. Burn (5) lies relative to the axilla

_____

   f. Burns (6 and 7) are located

_____

17. In what abdominal quadrant does burn (5) encroach?

_____

18. List the major body cavities under each wound.
   a. Burn (3)

_____

   b. Burn (5)

_____

19. Have these wounds affected the axial or appendicular region of the body?

_____

20. For each of the following subgroups of tissues, list the tissue type to which it belongs (epithelial, connective, muscle, or nervous), one area of the body where it is found, and at least one specialized function it performs.

Subgroup	Type	Body Area	Function
a. Striated voluntary			
b. Bone			
c. Epithelium			
d. Adipose			
e. Hemopoietic			
f. Striated involuntary			
g. Neurons			
h. Cartilage			
i. Areolar			
j. Nonstriated involuntary			
k. Neuroglia			

21. List the 11 major body systems:

a.

b.

c.

d.

e.

f.

g.

h.

i.

j.

k.

22. Label structures of the skin in Fig. 6-3 and list two functions of each.

Structure   **Function**

a.

b.

c.

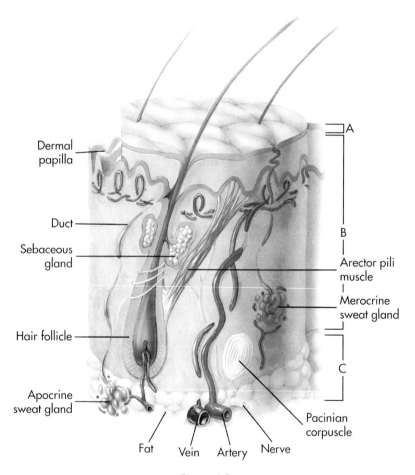

Figure 6-3

23. List three functions of the glands located in the skin.

a.

b.

c.

24. Describe what effect a large third-degree (full-thickness) burn that destroys all of the layers of the dermis will have on the skin's function.

_____

_____

25. Label the bones of the human skull in Fig. 6-4.

a.

b.

c.

d.

e.

f.

g.

h.

i.

j.

k.

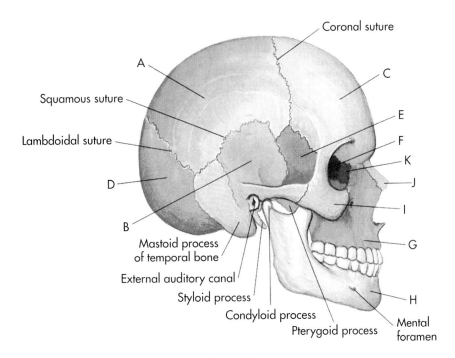

Figure 6-4

35

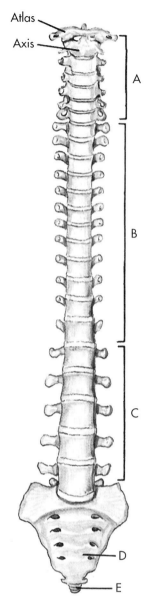

Atlas

Axis

A

B

C

D

E

Figure 6-5

26. Label the bony regions of the vertebral column shown in Fig. 6-5 and indicate the number of vertebrae in each region.

            Region   **Number of vertebrae**

a.

b.

c.

d.

e.

27. List two functions of the thoracic cage.

a.

b.

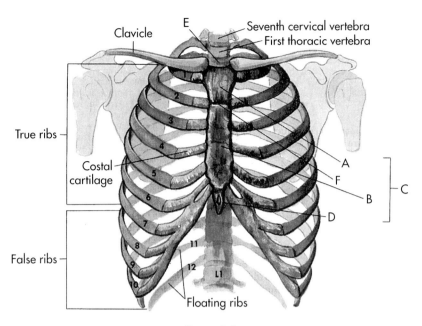

Figure 6-6

28. Label the structures of the thoracic cage shown in Fig. 6-6.
   a.
   b.
   c.
   d.
   e.
   f.

29. What problems can occur when a patient sustains a traumatic injury that results in a fractured sternum and multiple fractured ribs?

_____

30. Complete the following sentences that relate to the skeletal system:

The pectoral girdle is composed of the (a) _____

and (b) _____. Its function is to (c) _____

_____.

The point of attachment of the appendicular and axial skeleton occurs at

the (d) _____ joint.

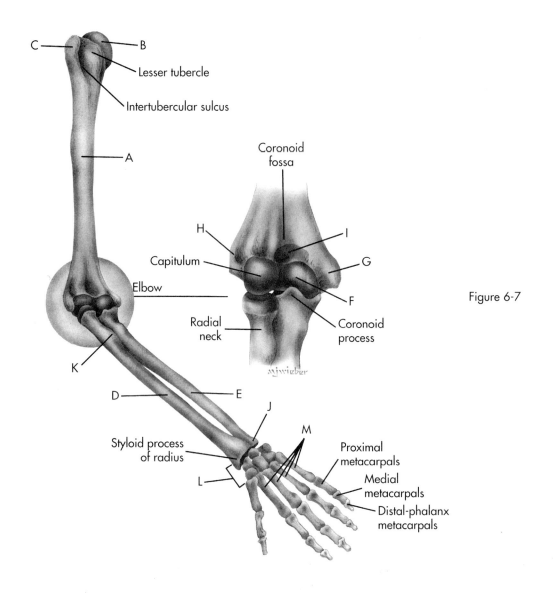

C

B

Lesser tubercle

Intertubercular sulcus

A

Coronoid
fossa

H

Capitulum

Elbow

Radial
neck

I

G

F

Coronoid
process

Figure 6-7

K

D

E

J

M

Styloid process
of radius

L

Proximal
metacarpals

Medial
metacarpals

Distal-phalanx
metacarpals

mjwieber

31. Label the diagram of the upper extremity shown in Fig. 6-7.

    a.

    b.

    c.

    d.

    e.

    f.

    g.

    h.

    i.

    j.

    k.

    l.

    m.

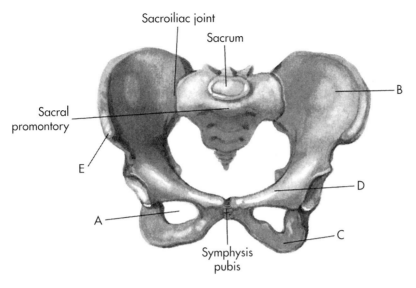

Sacroiliac joint

Sacrum

Sacral promontory

Symphysis pubis

Figure 6-8

32. Label the pelvic girdle shown in Fig. 6-8.
   a.

   b.

   c.

   d.

   e.

33. What are the functions of the pelvic girdle?

34. Label the bones of the lower extremity shown in Fig. 6-9.

a.
b.
c.
d.
e.
f.
g.
h.
i.
j.
k.
l.
m.
n.
o.
p.
q.

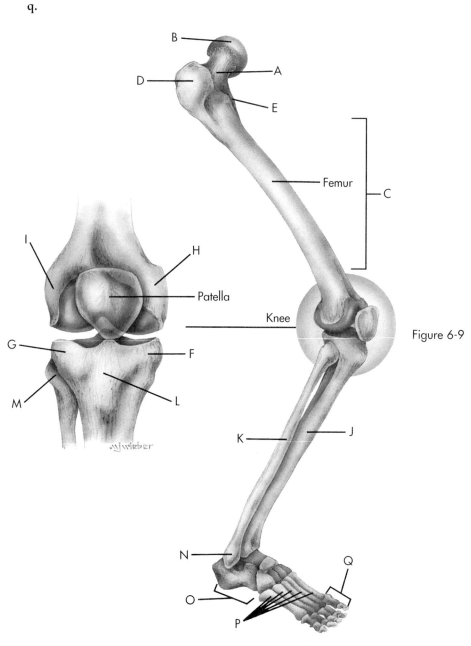

Figure 6-9

35. Complete the blanks in the following statements regarding joints:

The three major classifications of joints are (a) _____,

_____, and _____. Fibrous

joints have (b) _____ movement. Fibrous joints can

be further divided into sutures found in the (c) _____,

syndesmoses found between the (d) _____ and

_____, and a gomphosis joint, which consists of a

peg in a socket such as the joints between (e) _____

and _____. A synchondrosis is a cartilaginous joint
that allows only slight movement and can be found in the chest between

the ribs and the (f) _____. Symphysis joints are an-
other example of cartilaginous joints and can be found in the chest at the (g)

_____ _____, in the pelvis at

the (h) _____ _____, and in

the spine at the (i) _____ _____.
Synovial joints are classified into six divisions, all of which contain (j)

_____ _____. Joints consisting
of two opposed, flat surfaces, such as the articular processes between

vertebrae, are (k) _____ joints. Joints that consist of
two saddle-shaped, articulating surfaces that allow movement in two
planes and include the carpometacarpal joint in the thumb are (l)

_____ _____. Joints that con-
sist of a convex cylinder of bone that fits into a corresponding concavity in
another bone and permit movement in one plane, such as the elbow and

knee, are known as (m) _____ joints. A cylindrical
bony process that rotates within a ring composed of bone and ligament,
such as the head of the radius where it articulates with the ulna, is a(n) (n)

_____ joint. A wide range of motion is permitted by
shoulder and hip joints, where the head of one bone fits into the socket of

an adjacent bone. These are known as (o) _____

_____ _____ joints. The
atlantooccipital joint is an example of a modified ball-and-socket joint

known as a(n) (p) _____ joint.

36. Replace the boldface words in the following sentences with the correct terms from the following list. Use each term only once.

Abduction	Excursion	Opposition
Adduction	Extension	Pronation
Depression	Flexion	Rotation
Eversion	Inversion	Supination

  a. The patient has sustained an injury to his elbow and is unable **to rotate his forearm so that the anterior surface is up** or **rotate his forearm so that the anterior surface is down.**
  _____ or _____
  b. To determine whether the patient had an intact neurological function, the paramedic had **her move her thumb and little finger toward each other.**
  _____

  c. After he injured his knee, the soccer player had pain when he **bent** and **stretched out** his lower leg.
  _____ and _____
  d. An older woman with a hip fracture has a leg that looks shortened and shows **external movement about its axis.** _____
  e. A person with a shoulder separation has a limited ability to **move the arm from the midline.** _____
  f. A patient with a posterior hip dislocation has the following physical findings: the leg is shortened, internally rotated, and slightly **moved toward the midline.** _____
  g. Ankle sprains are frequently produced by **turning the ankle inward** or **turning the ankle outward.**
  _____ or _____
  h. Newer splints for the foot can sometimes make casting unnecessary when the desired effect is to prevent **movement from side to side.**
  i. The blow to the head with a baseball bat **produced movement of the temporal bone in an inferior direction.** _____

37. List the three primary functions of the muscular system.
  a.
  b.
  c.

38. Complete the following sentences pertaining to the muscular system:

The specialized contractile cells of the muscles are called (a) _____

_____. Each muscle fiber is filled with thick and

thin threadlike structures known as (b) _____.

These are composed of the proteins (c) _____ and

_____. The contractile unit of skeletal muscle fibers

is the (d) _____. During muscle contraction, the two myofilaments slide toward each other and shorten the sarcomere fueled

with energy from (e) _____.

39. Define the following terms:

a. Isometric muscle contraction:

_____

b. Isotonic muscle contraction:

_____

c. Muscle tone:

_____

40. Describe the role that the muscular system plays in maintaining body temperature.

_____

_____

41. Briefly describe the function of the nervous system.

_____

42. List the primary components of the following:

a. The central nervous system:

_____

b. The peripheral nervous system:

_____

43. List the two subdivisions of the efferent division of the nervous system and briefly describe the function of each.

_____

a.

_____

b.

_____

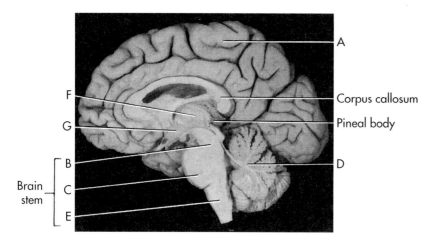

Figure 6-10

44. Label the brain shown in Fig. 6-10.
    a.
    b.
    c.
    d.
    e.
    f.
    g.
45. Briefly describe the functions of each of the following areas of the brain stem:
    a. Medulla:

_____

    b. Pons:

_____

    c. Midbrain:

_____

    d. Reticular formation:

_____

    e. Hypothalamus:

_____

    f. Thalamus:

_____

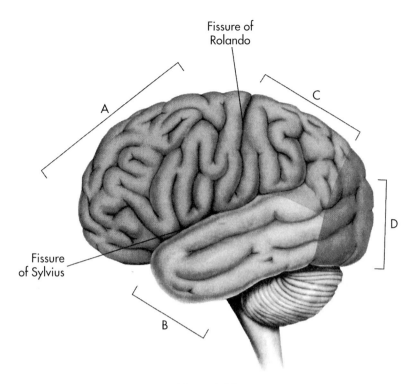

Fissure of
Rolando

A

C

D

Fissure
of Sylvius

B

Figure 6-11

46. Label the cerebrum shown in Fig. 6-11 and list one important function of each area.

	Area	Function
a.		
b.		
c.		
d.		

47. Briefly describe the major functions of the cerebellum.

48. List two functions of the spinal cord.
    a.
    b.

49. Complete the following sentences about the meninges:

Cerebrospinal fluid bathes and cushions the (a) _____

and _____. It is formed in a network of brain capillar-

ies known as the (b) _____.

50. List the three functional categories of the 12 cranial nerves.

   a.

   b.

   c.

51. For each of the following organs or body systems, describe the effects of stimulation by each division of the autonomic nervous system.

Affected Organ	Sympathetic	Parasympathetic
Heart		
Lungs		
Pupils		
Intestine		
Blood vessels		

52. Describe the function of the endocrine system.

_____

_____

53. For each of the following hormones, list the primary target tissue and one action the hormone may have on that tissue.

Hormone	Target	Action
a. Epinephrine		
b. Aldosterone		
c. Antidiuretic		
d. Parathyroid		
e. Calcitonin		
f. Insulin		
g. Glucagon		
h. Testosterone		
i. Thymosin		
j. Oxytocin		
k. Thyroid		

54. Describe how hormones reach their target tissues.

_____

_____

55. List five functions of the circulatory system.

   a.

   b.

   c.

   d.

   e.

56. Complete the following sentences regarding the components of blood:

About 95% of the formed elements in blood are red blood cells, also known

as (a) _____. The primary component of red blood

cells is (b) _____. This gives blood its red color and

allows it to transport (c) _____ from the lungs to the

tissues and to transport (d) _____ _____

_____ from the tissues to the lungs. The remaining 5% of the formed elements in blood consists of white blood cells called (e)

_____ and platelets known as (f) _____.

The primary function of white blood cells is (g) _____.

Platelets help prevent blood loss by activating the formation of (h)

_____ to seal off wounds in the blood vessels. The

pale yellow fluid that surrounds these formed elements is (i) _____.

_____

57. Label the structures indicated on Fig. 6-12 of the heart and draw arrows to show the path taken by the blood from the point that it enters the heart from the body until it returns to the body from the heart.

a.   g.
b.   h.
c.   i.
d.   j.
e.   k.
f.   l.

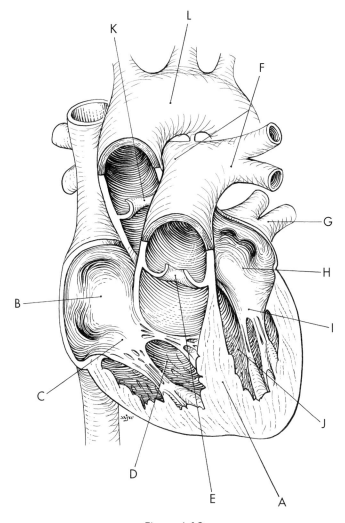

Figure 6-12

58. Name the branches of the circulatory system from the aorta to the cellular level and back to the vena cava.

_____

_____

59. Briefly describe the characteristics of blood vessels that permit vasodilation and vasoconstriction.

_____

_____

60. What structural feature of some veins inhibits the backflow of blood?

_____

61. What is the purpose of an arteriovenous anastomosis (arteriovenous shunt)?

_____

_____

62. List the three basic functions of the lymphatic system.
   a.
   b.
   c.

63. Describe the flow of lymph from its beginning in the tissues until it empties in the circulatory system.

_____

_____

_____

64. Label the upper airway in Fig. 6-13 of and list one function of each structure named.

Structure	Function
a.	
b.	
c.	
d.	
e.	
f.	

65. Label the larynx shown in Fig. 6-14.
   a.
   b.
   c.
   d.
   e.

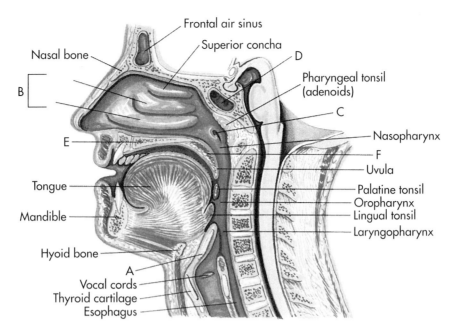

Figure 6-13

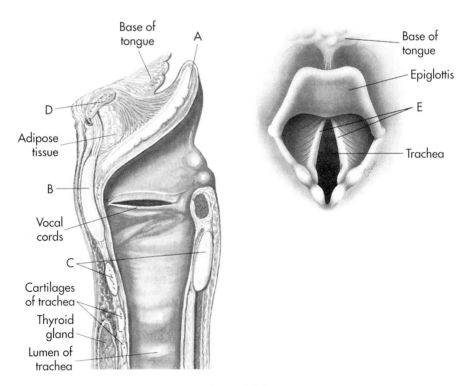

Figure 6-14

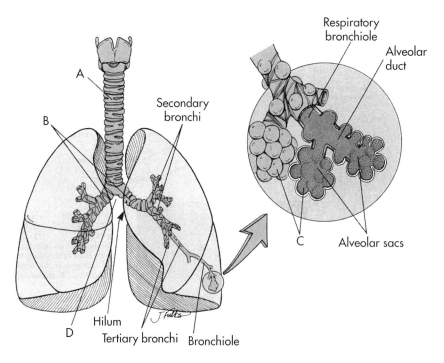

Figure 6-15

66. Label the lower airway shown in Fig. 6-15.
    a.
    b.
    c.
    d.
67. Describe how the structure of the trachea protects the airway.

_____

_____

68. Describe what happens to the bronchioles that causes wheezing during an asthma attack.

_____

_____

69. Describe the anatomical feature of the alveoli that does the following:
    a. Permits the movement of oxygen to the blood and CO_2 from the blood:

_____

    b. Prevents collapse of the alveoli:

_____

70. Describe the location of the lungs in the chest cavity.

_____

71. List the divisions of the following:
    a. The right lung:

    _____

    b. The left lung:

    _____

72. Describe the functions of the following:
    a. The pleural space:

    _____

    b. The pleural fluid:

    _____

73. List the functions of the digestive system.

    _____

74. As a cheeseburger passes through the digestive tract, many digestive juices act on it to convert the food into a usable form for the body. For each area of the digestive tract listed, name a digestive juice excreted and briefly describe its function.

Area	Digestive Juice	Function
a. Mouth		
b. Stomach		
c. Pancreas		
d. Liver		
e. Large intestine		

75. List the functions of the urinary system.

    _____

76. List two specific functions of the kidneys in addition to urine production.
    a.
    b.
77. The basic functional unit of the kidney is the (a) _____.

    It produces urine by a three-step process: (b) _____,

    (c) _____, and (d) _____.
78. State whether each of the following increases or decreases urine production.
    a. Aldosterone:
    b. Atrial natriuretic factor:
    c. Large increase in blood pressure:
    d. Shock:

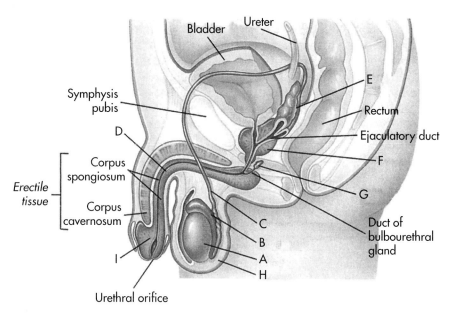

Figure 6-16

79. Label the male reproductive system shown in Fig. 6-16.
    a.
    b.
    c.
    d.
    e.
    f.
    g.
    h.
    i.

80. Label the female reproductive system shown in Fig. 6-17.
    a.
    b.
    c.
    d.
    e.
    f.

81. Label the female perineum shown in Fig. 6-18.
    a.
    b.
    c.
    d.
    e.
    f.
    g.

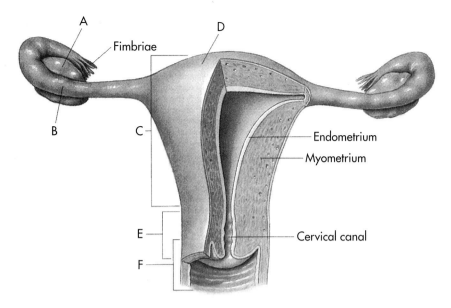

Figure 6-17

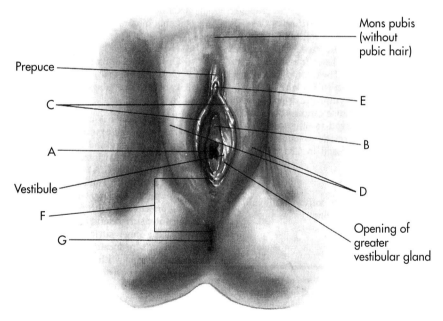

Figure 6-18

82. Complete the following sentences pertaining to the olfactory sense:
Receptors for the olfactory nerves lie in the upper part of the (a)

_____ cavity. When olfactory cells are stimulated by airborne molecules, the nerve impulses travel in the olfactory bulb and

(b) _____ _____. The brain

interprets the impulses as specific odors in the (c) _____

and (d) _____ centers.

83. Complete the following sentences pertaining to the sense of taste:
Sensory structures that detect taste stimuli in the mouth are

(a)_____ _____. Taste buds

are most commonly found in the mouth on the (b) _____.

However, they are also found on the (c) _____,

_____, and _____.

The four basic tastes that are detected are (d) _____,

_____, _____, and

_____.

84. Complete the following sentences pertaining to the sense of vision:
The sensation of vision is transmitted from the eye to the brain by way of

the (a)_____ nerve. Impulses that travel from the brain to control the movements of the eye are relayed by the

(b)_____ nerve. The avascular, transparent struc-

ture that bends and refracts light as it enters the eye is the (c) _____

_____. The size of the pupil and therefore the

amount of light that enters the eye through it is controlled by the

(d) _____. The inner sensory layer of the retina con-
tains two types of photoreceptor cells. The receptors that are responsible

for night vision are the (e) _____, and the receptors

that permit daytime and color vision are the (f) _____.

The eye has two compartments. The anterior chamber is filled with (g)

_____ humor, and the posterior chamber contains

(h) _____ humor. The humor in both chambers

helps maintain (i) _____ _____.

85. List the function of each of the following accessory structures of the eye.
   a. Eyebrows:

   _____

   b. Eyelids:

   _____

   c. Lacrimal glands:

   _____

86. Complete the following sentences pertaining to the tissues associated with hearing and balance:

   The external and middle ear are involved in (a)_____,

   and the inner ear plays a role in (b)_____ and

   _____. The senses of hearing and balance are trans-

   mitted by the (c) _____ nerve. Sound is picked up by

   the external ear prominence known as the (d) _____
   and transmitted through the external auditory meatus into the (e)

   _____ canal. At the end of this canal, vibration of the (f)

   _____ _____ is produced. These vibra-
   tions are picked up and transmitted to the oval window by the auditory

   ossicles of the middle ear. These three bones are the (g) _____

   _____, _____, and

   _____. Finally, in the inner ear inside the cochlea

   lies the hearing sense organ called the (h) _____

   _____. The two other structures within the inner

   ear involved in balance are the (i) _____ and (j)

   _____.

● **STUDENT SELF-ASSESSMENT**

87. You find your patient lying face-up on his back. This is which position?
   a. Anatomical   **c.** Prone
   b. Lateral recumbent   **d.** Supine
88. A teenage football player has collapsed after a sharp blow to the left upper quadrant of the abdomen. You suspect injury to which of the following?
   a. Appendix   **c.** Liver
   b. Gallbladder   **d.** Spleen
89. Which of the following structures is located in the mediastinum?
   a. Diaphragm   **c.** Thyroid
   b. Lungs   **d.** Trachea
90. Cardiac muscle cells are which of the following?
   a. Striated voluntary   **c.** Nonstriated voluntary
   b. Striated involuntary   **d.** Nonstriated involuntary

91. The actual conducting cells of the nervous system are which of the following?
    a. Dendrites c. Neurons
    b. Neuroglia d. Synapses
92. Which of the following is a function of the integumentary system?
    a. Collection of lymph c. Production of vitamin C
    b. Movement d. Temperature regulation
93. The scapula and clavicle comprise which of the following?
    a. Pectoral girdle c. Thorax
    b. Pelvic girdle d. Vertebral disks
94. An indoor soccer player has sustained an injury resulting in marked swelling and pain at the inner aspect of the ankle. You would describe this to an online physician as pain and swelling in which area?
    a. Lateral malleolus c. Olecranon
    b. Medial malleolus d. Patella
95. Muscle fiber contractions are initiated when stimulated by which of the following?
    a. Actin and myosin c. Myofilaments
    b. Motor neurons d. Sarcomeres
96. The primary action of the frontal lobe of the cerebral cortex is which of the following?
    a. To receive and integrate visual input
    b. To evaluate olfactory and auditory input
    c. To receive and interpret sensory information
    d. To initiate voluntary motor function
97. The spinal cord ends at which vertebrae?
    a. Twelfth thoracic c. Sacral
    b. Second lumbar d. Coccygeal
98. The innermost meningeal layer, which adheres to the brain and spinal cord, is which mater?
    a. Arachnoid c. Dura
    b. Choroid d. Pia
99. Which component of the endocrine system transmits information from the gland to its target body part?
    a. Enzyme c. Neurotransmitter
    b. Hormone d. Synapse
100. The formed element in blood that contains hemoglobin and carries oxygen is which of the following?
    a. Erythrocyte c. Leukocyte
    b. Immunoglobulin d. Platelet
101. Which blood vessel(s) carries(y) blood from the heart to the systemic circulation?
    a. Aorta c. Pulmonary veins
    b. Pulmonary arteries d. Vena cava
102. Cardiac electrical impulse conduction is normally initiated in which structure?
    a. Atrioventricular node c. Purkinje fibers
    b. Bundle of His d. Sinoatrial node
103. Lymph nodes filter foreign substances and are located in all of the following body regions except which?
    a. Axillary c. Inguinal
    b. Cervical d. Temporal
104. The airway division that is involved in the production of speech and serves as a protective sphincter to prevent liquids and solids from entering the lungs is which of the following?
    a. Larynx c. Pharynx
    b. Retropharynx d. Trachea

105. The functional unit of the respiratory system where gas exchange occurs between the lungs and the blood is which of the following?
    a. Alveolus
    c. Capillary
    b. Bronchus
    d. Trachea
106. The major site of nutrient absorption in the intestines is which of the following?
    a. Colon
    c. Ileum
    b. Duodenum
    d. Jejunum
107. Liver function includes all of the following actions except:
    a. Bile production
    c. Hormone secretion
    b. Drug detoxification
    d. Plasma protein synthesis
108. Which of the following statements is true with regard to renal function?
    a. All fluid filtered from the glomerulus becomes urine.
    b. Healthy people produce 180 L of urine per day.
    c. Water and other nutrients are reabsorbed in the tubules.
    d. Potassium and ammonia are secreted into the blood.
109. Which of the following hormones influences urine production?
    a. Aldosterone
    c. Oxytocin
    b. Glucagon
    d. Testosterone
110. Where does sperm production occur?
    a. Epididymis
    c. Seminal vesicle
    b. Prostate
    d. Testes
111. When the nasal receptors of the olfactory neurons are stimulated, messages are sent for interpretation to the olfactory and _____ centers of the brain.
    a. Frontal
    c. Pontine
    b. Medullary
    d. Thalamic
112. The hearing sense organ is which of the following?
    a. Cochlea
    c. Semicircular canal
    b. Organ of Corti
    d. Vestibule

GENERAL PRINCIPLES OF PATHOPHYSIOLOGY

● **READING ASSIGNMENT**

Chapter 7, pages 180-231, in *Mosby's Paramedic Textbook,* ed 2

● **OBJECTIVES**

As a paramedic, you should be able to:

1. Describe the normal characteristics of the cellular environment and the key homeostatic mechanisms that strive to maintain a fluid and electrolyte balance.
2. Outline pathophysiological alterations in water and electrolyte balance and their effect on body functions.
3. Describe treatment of patients who have selected fluid or electrolyte imbalances.
4. Describe the mechanisms within the body that maintain normal acid-base balance.
5. Outline pathophysiological alterations in acid-base balance.
6. Describe the management of a patient with an acid-base imbalance.
7. Describe alterations in cells and tissues related to cellular adaption, injury, neoplasia, aging, and death.
8. Outline the effects of cellular injury on local and systemic body functions.
9. Describe alterations in body functions related to genetic and familial disease factors.
10. Outline the causes, adverse systemic effects, and compensatory mechanisms associated with hypoperfusion.
11. Describe how the body's inflammatory and immune responses respond to cellular injury and antigenic stimulation.
12. Explain how alterations in immunity and inflammation can cause harmful effects on body functions.
13. Describe the impact of stress on the body's response to illness and injury.

● **REVIEW QUESTIONS**

Match the mechanism of cellular injury listed in Column I with the appropriate cause listed in Column II.

Column I	Column II
1. _____ Skin burns resulting from prolonged contact with gasoline	a. Chemical injury
2. _____ Bruising from a blow from a tire iron	b. Genetic factors
3. _____ Unconsciousness resulting from decreased blood sugar	c. Hypoxic injury
4. _____ Death occurring secondary to septic shock	d. Immunological injury
5. _____ Tissue in the leg dying after occlusion of a blood vessel	e. Infectious injury
6. _____ Severe wheezing occurring after a bee sting	f. Nutritional imbalances
	g. Physical agents

7. Complete the following sentences relating to the fluid compartments of the body:

The water found outside the cells that includes the water in plasma, bone, tendon, and fascia is the (a) _____ fluid. The water outside the vascular bed that lies between the tissue cells is known as

(b) _____ fluid. The fluid found inside the cells of the skeletal muscle, intestine, viscera, bone marrow, glands, and red blood

cells is the (c) _____ fluid.

8. For each of the following ions, state its name, indicate whether it is a cation or an anion, and state where it is most plentiful in the body (extracellular fluid [ECF] or intracellular fluid [ICF]).

Ion	Name	Cation or Anion	ECF or ICF
a. PO_4-			
b. $K+$			
c. $Na+$			
d. HCO_3-			
e. $Mg++$			
f. $Cl-$			

9. Briefly define the following terms:
   a. Cell membrane permeability:

_____

   b. Diffusion:

_____

   c. Concentration gradient:

_____

   d. Osmosis:

_____

   e. Active transport:

_____

   f. Facilitated diffusion:

_____

10. For each of the following patient situations, choose the suspected fluid or electrolyte imbalance from a given list and describe appropriate assessments and/or interventions for the patient.

a. You are transporting an older patient for chest pain. After the IV is started, 500 ml is accidently infused rapidly. The patient becomes very short of breath and evaluation reveals moist crackles in the lungs.
Imbalance: Hyponatremia, hypermagnesemia, or overhydration?

_____

Management: _____

b. Your patient is a 65-year-old adult who complains of vomiting and diarrhea. Home medications include a diuretic. The physical examination reveals a blood pressure of 100/70 mm Hg, a weak pulse, decreased reflexes, and shallow respirations.
Imbalance: Hyperkalemia, hypocalcemia, or hypokalemia?

Management: _____

c. You are called to the airport to evaluate an obviously malnourished child flown to the United States from India for adoption. The chaperone reports that the child has been displaying abnormal behavior and complaining of muscle cramps, abdominal cramps, and tingling of the extremities. As you begin to assess vital signs, the patient has a grand mal seizure.
Imbalance: Hypernatremia, hypocalcemia, or hypomagnesemia?

_____

Management: _____

d. A father calls you to evaluate an infant who has been vomiting for 36 hours. He states that the child has not had a wet diaper in 8 hours. The anterior fontanelle is depressed, and the skin and mucous membranes are dry.
Imbalance: Hypercalcemia, hypermagnesemia, or isotonic dehydration?

_____

Management: _____

e. Your patient is a 13-year-old bulimic who admits to frequent use of water enemas for weight control. You were called for a chief complaint of abdominal pain but on arrival find the patient diaphoretic with a rapid, thready pulse and cyanosis. There is no indication of bleeding.
Imbalance: Hyperkalemia, hyponatremic dehydration, or overhydration?

_____

Management: _____

f. The family of an older patient with chronic renal failure says that she is confused and very weak. The physical examination reveals shallow, slow respirations that become progressively worse.
Imbalance: Hypermagnesemia, hypocalcemia, or hypokalemia?

_____

Management: _____

11. Describe the mode of action of the three acid-base buffer systems in the body. Begin with the fastest and end with the slowest mechanism.

a.

_____

_____

b.

_____

_____

c.

_____

_____

12. For each case presented, select one of the four acid-base disturbances listed. State at least one prehospital intervention for management of the imbalance.

Respiratory acidosis   Respiratory alkalosis
Metabolic acidosis   Metabolic alkalosis

a. A 17-year-old teenager complains of dizziness and tingling in the hands and around the mouth during a college entrance examination. The medical history and physical examination are unremarkable. The respiratory rate is 28 and deep.

Imbalance: _____ Intervention: _____

b. A 72-year-old adult in an extended care facility has been treated with gastric suction.

Imbalance: _____ Intervention: _____

c. A 30-year-old diabetic has had influenza. She has taken no insulin in 2 days and appears dehydrated. Respirations are deep and rapid.

Imbalance: _____ Intervention: _____

d. A 46-year-old barbiturate overdose patient has shallow respirations at a rate of 8/min.

Imbalance: _____ Intervention: _____

13. State whether each of the following arterial blood gas values drawn on a patient who has had a stroke are normal or abnormal. Discuss any action that may be taken in the field to correct any identified abnormalities.

a. pH, 7.25
b. Po_2, 60
c. Pco_2, 53

14. For each of the following cellular adaptations, describe the cause, the effect on the cells, and an example of each.

Adaptation	Cause	Effect on Cells	Example
a. Atrophy			
b. Dysplasia			
c. Hyperplasia			
d. Hypertrophy			
e. Metaplasia			

15. For each of the following diseases, list a factor that may contribute to its development. Identify whether the factor is environmental or genetic.

Disease	Factor	Environmental or Genetic
a. Stroke		
b. Cervical cancer		
c. Oral cancer		
d. Melanoma (skin cancer)		
e. Depression		

16. For each of the following situations, describe why the cardiac output will increase or decrease in an otherwise healthy individual.

a. Patient has had a myocardial infarction with necrosis of 50% of the heart muscle.

_____

b. A dehydrated patient is given 500 ml of normal saline intravenously.

_____

c. The patient's normal heart rate is 80 and suddenly drops to 40.

_____

d. A paramedic student enters a testing station.

_____

17. Describe the physiological effects of the baroreceptor response in each of the following situations:

a. A 47-year-old adult has a sudden increase in blood pressure to 170/110 mm Hg.

_____

b. A 22-year-old adult is thrown from a horse and sustains a pelvic fracture. There is significant internal bleeding and a sudden drop in blood pressure to 60 mm Hg by palpation.

_____

18. Describe the physiological effects of chemoreceptor stimulation in the following situations:

a. A 36-year-old adult has a massive hemothorax from a gunshot wound. Blood pressure is 76/60 mm Hg.

_____

b. A 17-year-old drug overdose patient has a shallow respiratory rate of 8/min. Arterial blood gas tests reveal a P_{CO_2} of 60.

_____

19. A 47-year-old adult who sustains a large inferior myocardial infarction has progressively deteriorated. He is now unconscious with a weak carotid pulse and no obtainable blood pressure. Describe the physiological effects when the central nervous system ischemia response is initiated.

_____

20. A 65-year-old alcoholic states that he had a sudden onset of vomiting. The emesis contains bright red blood, and he continues to vomit. Vital signs are blood pressure, 94/78 mm Hg; pulse, 132; and respirations, 28. Describe the effects of the following three hormonal mechanisms that will be activated:

a. Adrenal medullary mechanism:

_____

_____

b. Renin-angiotensin-aldosterone mechanism:

_____

_____

c. Vasopressin mechanism:

_____

_____

21. Multiple organ dysfunction syndrome (MODS) begins with (a) _____

_____ _____ damage caused

by (b) _____ and _____ that

are released into the circulation. This causes the vascular (c) _____

_____ to become (d) _____,

which allows fluid and cells to leak into the (e) _____

spaces, increasing the (f) _____ and _____

_____. Then, three plasma enzyme cascades are acti-

vated. They are (g) _____, _____,

and _____/_____. Phago-
cytes cause further damage to the endothelium, causing uncontrolled (h)

_____ and formation of microvascular (i)

_____ and tissue ischemia. Bradykinin contributes to

low (j) _____ _____ _____.
The overall effect of the three complement systems is to cause (k)

_____ formation, (l) _____

_____ and (m) _____

_____. Initially, the body will compensate for these

changes, but ultimately tissue hypoxia causes (n) _____

_____ and _____ _____,

and finally multiple (o) _____ failure occurs.

22. Your partner is off sick with a diagnosis of strep throat. Describe whether the following signs and symptoms experienced during this illness are local or systemic and name at least one inflammatory mechanism that causes the sign or symptom.

Sign or Symptom	Local or Systemic Response	Cause
a. Edematous throat		
b. Purulent drainage		
c. Fever		
d. Red throat		
e. Difficulty swallowing		

23. For the following patient blood types, list all safe donor types.

Patient	Donors
a. A positive	
b. O negative	
c. AB positive	
d. B negative	

24. For each statement below, note which of the following types of altered immunologic reaction has occurred: allergy, autoimmunity, or isoimmunity.

    a. Your patient is agitated and complains of severe low back pain a few moments after you begin to transfuse a unit of blood. _____

    b. You are dispatched to a private residence to care for a 46-year-old woman who began to experience dyspnea, a swollen face, and hives after taking a penicillin tablet prescribed by her dentist. _____

    c. You are transferring a patient to a dialysis center for care after his body rejected his kidney transplant. _____

    d. You notice that your eyes water and get puffy and your hands become very red and itchy when you wear latex gloves at work. _____

    e. Your 30-year-old female patient is having chest pain. The family tells you she has systemic lupus erythematosus and has cardiac and pulmonary involvement. _____

Match the probable cause of immune suppression listed in Column II with the statement in Column I.

Column I	Column II
25. _____ An elderly woman develops pneumonia several months after the death of her husband	**a.** Acquired immune deficiency syndrome
26. _____ A cancer patient becomes septic after a course of chemotherapy	**b.** Deficiencies caused by stress
27. _____ A young girl suffering from anorexia nervosa repeatedly becomes ill with viral illness.	**c.** Deficiencies caused by trauma
28. _____ An HIV-positive patient develops Kaposi's sarcoma	**d.** Iatrogenic deficiencies
	e. Nutritional deficiencies

29. Fill in the missing information relating to the stress response:

Hormone or Receptor	Location	Action
a.	Found in plasma	Stimulates gluconeogenesis Suppresses immune cell activity
Alpha-1 receptors	Postsynaptic located on effector organs	b.
Beta-1 receptors	c.	Increased pulse rate
d.	Lungs and arteries	Bronchodilation

● STUDENT SELF-ASSESSMENT

30. Which mechanism of cellular transport moves substances against a concentration gradient and requires the use of energy?
   a. Active transport   **c.** Facilitated diffusion
   b. Diffusion   **d.** Osmosis

31. Which of the following electrolytes is found predominantly in the intracellular fluid?
   a. Bicarbonate   **c.** Potassium
   b. Chloride   **d.** Sodium

32. A solution that has a concentration of solute particles equal to that inside the cells is a(n) _____ solution.
   a. Atonic   **c.** Hypotonic
   b. Hypertonic   **d.** Isotonic

33. Which of the following causes the normal flow of fluid through the interstitial space?
   a. Capillary hydrostatic pressure filters fluid from the interstitial space through the capillary wall.
   b. Oncotic pressure exerted by blood proteins attracts fluid from the vascular space back into the interstitial space.
   c. Capillary permeability determines the ease with which fluid can pass through the capillary wall.
   d. The lymphatic channels close to prevent entry of capillary fluid pushed out by hydrostatic pressure.

34. Your patient is being transferred from a nursing home for admission for an intestinal obstruction. His skin is dry and there are furrows of his tongue. What fluid and electrolyte imbalance do you suspect?
   a. Hypernatremic dehydration   **c.** Isotonic dehydration
   b. Hyponatremic dehydration   **d.** Osmotic dehydration

35. You are called to transport a 56-year-old patient with a history of renal failure who missed his last dialysis session. He is complaining of nausea, abdominal distention, weakness, and irritability. You suspect which of the following?
   a. Hypercalcemia   **c.** Hypernatremia
   b. Hyperkalemia   **d.** Hyperuria

36. Which of the following is true regarding hypomagnesemia?
   a. It is often accompanied by hypercalcemia.
   b. It results from antacid abuse.
   c. It causes hypoactive reflexes.
   d. It causes cardiac dysrhythmias.

37. Your patient has metabolic acidosis. Which of the following compensatory mechanisms uses proteins in an attempt to rapidly restore normal acid-base balance?
   a. Carbonic-acid-bicarbonate buffering
   b. Excretion of hydrogen ions to acidify the urine
   c. Exhalation of excess carbon dioxide
   d. Recovery of bicarbonate in the renal tubules

38. Which acid-base disturbance would you anticipate in a patient with severe flail chest?
   a. Metabolic acidosis   c. Respiratory acidosis
   b. Metabolic alkalosis   d. Respiratory alkalosis

39. Lactic acidosis is harmful to the body because it:
   a. Increases the basal metabolic rate
   b. Decreases the force of cardiac contraction
   c. Increases the response to catecholamines
   d. Can cause severe hypertension

40. Increasing the rate of ventilations for a patient with metabolic acidosis and inadequate stroke volume will typically cause which of the following?
   a. Decreased pH and decreased P_{CO_2}
   b. Decreased pH and increased P_{CO_2}
   c. Increased pH and decreased P_{CO_2}
   d. Increased pH and increased P_{CO_2}

41. This cellular change that may occur with aging results in shrinkage of the brain and may cause a delay in the signs and symptoms associated with subdural hematoma (blood clot on the brain).
   a. Atrophy   c. Metaplasia
   b. Dysplasia   d. Hypertrophy

42. The process of cellular self-destruction is known as which of the following?
   a. Autolysis   c. Necrosis
   b. MODS   d. Osmosis

43. Which of the following changes would be expected early after cellular injury?
   a. Accelerated cellular reproduction
   b. Decreased intracellular hydrostatic pressure
   c. Increased intracellular oxygen accumulation
   d. Swelling of cells from increased osmosis

44. Sympathetic vasoconstriction during shock will result in which of the following?
   a. Tachycardia   c. Increased container size
   b. Pupil dilation   d. Pale, cool skin

45. The central nervous system ischemic response is initiated when:
   a. Blood pressure falls below 90 mm Hg
   b. Aortic and carotid chemoreceptors are stimulated
   c. Bradycardia and vasodilation are present
   d. Blood flow decreases in the vasomotor center

46. Which of the following hormonal mechanisms will increase urine production?
   a. Adrenal medullary mechanism
   b. Atrial natriuretic mechanism
   c. Renin-angiotension-aldosterone mechanism
   d. Vasopressin mechanism

47. An elderly patient calls 9-1-1 complaining of chest discomfort and difficulty breathing. Electrocardiographic changes on arrival to the hospital are consistent with acute myocardial infarction. The patient is showing signs of hypoperfusion. What type of shock does this likely represent?
   a. Anaphylactic   c. Hypovolemic
   b. Cardiogenic   d. Septic

48. Which of the following situations represents natural immunity in a fellow paramedic?
 a. Immunity to feline leukemia virus
 b. Immunity to measles after immunization
 c. Immunity to chicken pox after having them
 d. Immunity to hepatitis after immunoglobulin administration

49. Which of the following is true regarding hypersensitivity?
 a. It only occurs when foreign antigens are introduced to the body.
 b. Its response always occurs immediately after exposure to the antigen.
 c. It may produce either minor or life-threatening consequences.
 d. It is a normal immune response resulting from exposure to an antigen.

50. Which hormone increases the level of blood glucose and acts as an immunosuppressant by reducing the number of selected leukocytes?
 a. Cortisol   **c.** Epinephrine
 b. Dopamine   **d.** Norepinephrine

PHARMACOLOGY

● READING ASSIGNMENT
Chapter 8, pages 232-303, in *Mosby's Paramedic Textbook*, ed 2

● OBJECTIVES
As a paramedic, you should be able to:
1. Describe what a drug is.
2. Identify the four different types of drug names.
3. Outline drug standards and legislation and enforcement agencies pertinent to the paramedic.
4. Describe the paramedic's responsibilities relative to drug administration.
5. Distinguish among drug forms.
6. Differentiate among the four types of allergic reactions to drugs.
7. Outline autonomic nervous system functions that may be altered using drug therapy.
8. Discuss factors that influence drug absorption, distribution, and elimination.
9. Describe how drugs react with receptors to produce their desired effects.
10. Outline variables that can influence drug interactions.
11. Identify special considerations for administering pharmacological agents to pregnant, pediatric, and older patients.
12. Outline drug actions and considerations for care of the patient who is given drugs that affect the nervous, cardiovascular, respiratory, endocrine, and gastrointestinal systems.
13. Explain the meaning of drug terms necessary to safely interpret information in drug-reference sources.

● REVIEW QUESTIONS
Match the appropriate drug form in Column 2 with its description in Column 1. Use each drug form only once.

Column I	Column II
1. _____ Semisolid medicine in a greasy base externally applied to the skin	a. Capsule
2. _____ A sweetened alcohol and water solution	b. Elixir
3. _____ Drug ground into loose granules	c. Emulsion
4. _____ Drug compressed into small disks	d. Extract
5. _____ Drug dissolved in sugar and water suspension (magma)	e. Liniment
6. _____ Flat or round medicine held in mouth until dissolved	f. Lotion
7. _____ Gelatin-covered, dry drug preparation	g. Aqueous
8. _____ Suspension of fat or oil in water with an agent that decreases surface tension	h. Ointment
9. _____ Suspension of insoluble particles in water	i. Tablets
	j. Powder
	k. Aqueous solution
	l. Troche

10. Complete the following sentences by listing the appropriate drug name:
The precise composition and molecular structure of a drug is described in its

(a) _____ name. The name that is not protected by law and denotes pharmacologically similar drugs is known as the (b)

_____ name. The copyrighted name of the drug designated by the company that manufactures it is the (c) _____

_____ name. The initials USP or NF follow the (d)

_____ name.

11. In one sentence, describe how the following drug standards or legislation influence medication administration and distribution in the United States:
a. Pure Food and Drug Act (1906):

_____

b. Federal Drug and Cosmetic Act (1938):

_____

c. Harrison Narcotic Act (1914):

_____

12. List the agency responsible for each of the following aspects of drug control:
a. It has the power to suppress false or misleading advertising regarding drugs to the general public.

_____

b. It is responsible for enforcing the federal Food, Drug, and Cosmetic Act.

_____

c. It monitors the distribution of controlled substances.

_____

d. It regulates biological products like antitoxins.

_____

13. Refer to the *Physician's Desk Reference (PDR)* or *Mosby's GenRx*, common drug reference sources, to find the answers to the following questions.
a. What is the indication for the drug beclomethasone?

_____

b. List the contraindications and side effects of this drug.

_____

Questions 14-17 pertain to the following case study:

_____

Dispatch alerts you to respond to a call for an "accidental injury." When you arrive on the scene, you find a 35-year-old man who stumbled and fell, injuring his wrist. There is deformity, swelling, crepitus, and tenderness proximal to his right hand. After application of the appropriate splint and ice, you decide that medication for pain is indicated.

14. What eight points are critical to ensure that you meet your legal, moral, and ethical obligations for safe, effective medication administration to this patient?

a.

b.

c.

d.

e.

f.

g.

h.

> After eliciting a careful history and consultation with medical direction, you initiate an intravenous line in the uninjured extremity and administer ketorolac tromethamine (Toradol) intravenous push. Several moments after administration, the patient becomes anxious and states that he feels like "his throat is going to close in." His skin appears very flushed, and a large, flat, raised rash is erupting. The patient states he has never taken this drug before.

15. What type of hypersensitivity reaction is this patient having?

_____

16. List two chemical mediators released from mast cells during this type of reaction to cause this patient's signs and symptoms. _____

_____

> After you arrive at the emergency department, the patient admits to the physician that he has had a reaction to aspirin in the past (although during your history, he denied allergic reaction). The physician tells you that there is a reported cross-reactivity between aspirin and ketorolac tromethamine.

17. What did he mean by the term *cross-reactivity*?

_____

18. Select the appropriate drug term from the following list to complete the sentences:

Antagonism	Potentiation
Contraindications	Side effect
Cumulative action	Stimulant
Depressant	Summation
Drug allergy	Synergism
Drug dependence	Therapeutic action
Drug interaction	Tolerance
Idiosyncrasy	Untoward effect

a. An abnormal or peculiar response to a drug that is possibly caused by

a genetic deficiency is _____.

b. Caffeine and Ritalin are examples of drugs that exhibit a(n) _____

_____ effect.

c. A drug action caused by an immunological response to a previous exposure is a(n) _____ reaction.

d. Naloxone's desired effect on narcotics is attributed to _____

_____.

e. The enhancement of the effects of one drug caused by the concurrent administration of a second drug is _____.

f. An undesirable effect of a drug that is harmful to the patient is a(n)

_____.

g. The combined action of two drugs that is greater than the sum of each individual agent acting independently is _____.

h. The intense physical or emotional disturbance possibly resulting when a narcotic is withheld from a person who frequently uses it is a result of

_____.

i. A drug that diminishes a person's central nervous system function is a

_____.

j. The ability of atropine to increase the heart rate is known as the desired

effect, or _____.

k. The list of factors used to describe situations when medication administration would be harmful is the _____.

l. Concurrent administration of drugs such that one agent modifies the actions of the other is _____.

m. A decreased response to a drug after repetitive doses, which necessitates

higher doses to achieve the desired effect, is _____

_____.

n. When repeat administration of drugs results in absorption that exceeds metabolism and excretion, the increased effect that results is known as

_____.

19. List six factors that influence the rate and extent to which a drug is absorbed in the body.
 a.
 b.
 c.
 d.
 e.
 f.

20. List four groups of drugs that are associated with a high incidence of drug-drug interactions.
 a.
 b.
 c.
 d.

21. You need to administer acetaminophen to a child who has been vomiting repeatedly. What enteral route will you choose?

22. When giving epinephrine to an asthmatic patient, a slow and sustained effect is desirable to minimize side effects and prolong the drug's effects. You

will administer the drug by the _____ route.

23. Your 76-year-old patient has a heart rate of 34 and a blood pressure of 70 by palpation. You wish to give atropine to increase the heart rate. What route

will you choose? _____

24. A 3-month-old infant is in hemorrhagic shock after sustaining a gunshot wound to the abdomen. After intravenous attempts are unsuccessful, what

route will you consider for fluid volume resuscitation? _____

_____

25. Is the rate of drug absorption by the pulmonary route faster or slower than

the subcutaneous route? _____

26. List the two physiological barriers to drug distribution within the body.
    a.
    b.

27. Circle the appropriate response regarding drug effects in children.
    a. The blood brain barrier in infants is less/more effective than in adults; therefore the central nervous system effects of drugs will be less/more.
    b. The newborn has a(n) decreased/increased ability to metabolize drugs; therefore drug toxicity is less/more likely to occur.

28. List three physiological factors that may result in altered drug absorption, distribution, biotransformation, or elimination in the older adult.
    a.
    b.
    c.

29. You are called to a sparsely furnished, one-room apartment to care for a 79-year-old woman complaining of difficulty breathing. She states that she has a history of heart disease and "swelling," and she hands you a sack of empty medication bottles that contained furosemide, digoxin, and potassium. She thinks she last took them approximately 5 or 6 days ago. Discuss three possible reasons for the patient's medication noncompliance.
    a.
    b.
    c.

● DRUG CLASSIFICATIONS

30. When given the following description and drug name, identify the drug group to which it belongs and give one additional example of another drug from the same group.
    a. Your patient says he takes lorazepam (Ativan) to help him relax.

    Drug group: _____ Example: _____

    b. You arrive in the emergency department with a 65-year-old woman experiencing an acute myocardial infarction. Immediately, the emergency department staff administers tissue plasminogen activator in an attempt to dissolve the clot.

    Drug group: _____ Example: _____

c. Before your Mediterranean cruise, you take dimenhydrinate (Dramamine) to prevent seasickness.

Drug group: _____ Example: _____

d. During a cardiopulmonary arrest or in selected cases of shock, drugs such as epinephrine (Adrenalin) may be used to stimulate the heart.

Drug group: _____ Example: _____

e. Your 45-year-old patient is complaining of chest pain. His only home medications are minoxidil (Loniten) and hydrochlorothiazide (HydroDiuril) for hypertension.

Drug group: _____ Example: _____

f. An older patient is taking digoxin (Lanoxin) for his "weak heart."

Drug group: _____ Example: _____

g. A 30-year-old patient with a seizure disorder is taking phenobarbital (Luminal).

Drug group: _____ Example: _____

h. A 52-year-old hospice patient is taking hydromorphone (Dilaudid) to control his pain.

Drug group: _____ Example: _____

i. Diltiazem (Cardizem) is used by a patient who states that she takes it to control a fast heart rhythm.

Drug group: _____ Example: _____

j. A person at risk for developing clots that may cause heart attack or stroke may be prescribed dipyridamole (Persantine).

Drug group: _____ Example: _____

k. Asthmatics may have a large number of home medicines that may include isoetharine hydrochloride (Bronkosol) or theophylline (Bronkodyl).

Drug group: _____ Example: _____

l. You observe a patient in the emergency department who is drowsy and having difficulty speaking moments after she has been given etomidate (Amidate).

Drug group: _____ Example: _____

m. You will have increased vigilance for evidence of bleeding if a patient tells you he is taking warfarin sodium (Coumadin).

Drug group: _____ Example: _____

n. A 35-year-old patient is experiencing complications secondary to an outpatient surgical procedure. Her only home medication is pentazocine (Talwin).

Drug group: _____ Example: _____

o. Asthmatic patients may be on a variety of drugs besides bronchodilators in an attempt to control their disease. Examples of these include cromolyn sodium (Intal), beclomethasone dipropionate (Vanceril Inhaler), and ipratropium (Atrovent).

Drug group: _____ Example: _____

p. You are dispatched to a call for an unconscious person. The patient is awake but confused and combative when you arrive and has a medication list that includes ethosuximide (Zarontin).

Drug group: _____ Example: _____

q. You are treating a young woman with chest pain. She states that 2 years ago, she regularly took fenfluramine and phentermine ("fen-Phen").

Drug group: _____ Example: _____

r. When you arrive at the emergency department with a combative, psychotic patient in restraints, the nurse gives the patient an intramuscular injection of haloperidol (Haldol).

Drug group: _____ Example: _____

s. A patient with a chronic pain disorder is taking amitriptyline (Elavil).

Drug group: _____ Example: _____

t. Medications for management of an ulcer may include dicyclomine (Bentyl).

Drug group: _____ Example: _____

u. During your annual physical a blood test reveals that you have high cholesterol. The doctor prescribes probucol (Lorelco).

Drug group: _____ Example: _____

v. A patient with cancer is taking cyclosporine.

Drug group: _____ Example: _____

w. Your patient is vomiting blood. His home medicines include ranitidine (Zantac).

Drug group: _____ Example: _____

31. List the generic name of one drug and its general mechanism of actions for each of the following groups of antidysrhythmic drugs.

Group	Generic Name	Actions
I-A		
I-B		
I-C		
II		
III		
IV		

32. Fill in the missing information about hypertensive medications in the following table:

Classification	Generic Name	Actions
	Furosemide, hydrochlorothiazide, Aldactazide	
Beta-blocking agents		
		Block sympathetic stimulation, have multiple sites of action
	Diazoxide, hydralazine, minoxidil (arteriolar dilator), sodium nitroprusside, amyl nitrite, isosorbide dinitrate, nitroglycerin (arteriolar and venous dilator drugs)	
ACE inhibitors	Captopril, enalapril, lisinopril	
Calcium channel blockers		Decrease peripheral resistance by inhibiting blockers, decreasing the contractility of vascular smooth muscle

33. Match the drug listed in Column II with the endocrine gland that it affects in Column I. Use each drug only once.

Column I	Column II
_____ Adrenal cortex	**a.** Clomid
_____ Ovary	**b.** Decadron
_____ Pancreas	**c.** Iodine products
_____ Parathyroid	**d.** Metandren
_____ Pituitary	**e.** Tolinase
_____ Testes	**f.** Vasopressin
_____ Thyroid	**g.** Vitamin D

● STUDENT SELF-ASSESSMENT

34. Any substance taken by mouth; injected into a muscle, blood vessel, or cavity of the body; or applied topically to treat or prevent a disease or condition is a(n):

a. Antidote   **c.** Parenteral
b. Drug   **d.** Vaccine

35. Meperidine is regulated under the Controlled Substance Act of 1970 and is a Schedule _____ drug.

a. I   **c.** III
b. II   **d.** IV

36. The blood-brain barrier and placental barrier will allow passage of only:

a. Antibiotics   **c.** Undissociated drugs
b. Lipid-soluble drugs   **d.** Water-soluble drugs

37. Agonists are drugs that do which of the following?
    a. Bind to a receptor and cause a specific response
    b. Bind to a receptor and cause no response
    c. Cause duplication of specific receptors
    d. Prevent chemicals from reaching the receptor sites
38. The measurement of the relative safety of a drug is which of the following?
    a. Biological half-life
    b. Effective dose 50
    c. Lethal dose 50
    d. Therapeutic index
39. Which of the following drugs is recommended for administration by endo-tracheal tube?
    a. Bretylium
    b. Hydroxyzine
    c. Diazepam
    d. Naloxone
40. Which of the following drug administration routes will deliver the most rapid effects?
    a. Oral
    b. Intramuscular
    c. Subcutaneous
    d. Transtracheal
41. Your patient is in profound shock secondary to myocardial infarction. The route of choice for drug administration will be which of the following?
    a. Intramuscular
    b. Intravenous
    c. By mouth
    d. Subcutaneous
42. Which of the following is an opioid antagonist?
    a. Butorphanol tartrate
    b. Naloxone hydrochloride
    c. Oxycodone hydrochloride
    d. Pentazocine hydrochloride
43. All of the following drugs have anticonvulsant properties except which one?
    a. Diazepam
    b. Magnesium sulfate
    c. Nalbuphine
    d. Phenytoin
44. You are transporting a patient with a history of narcolepsy. What drugs might you find he is taking to reduce his symptoms of this disorder?
    a. Methamphetamine (Desoxyn)
    b. Methylphenidate (Ritalin)
    c. Pemoline (Cylert)
    d. Phenmetrazine (Preludin)
45. Drugs such as levodopa (Larodopa) and carbidopa-levodopa (Sinemet) enhance brain dopamine levels and are used to treat which of the following?
    a. Depression
    b. Hypotension
    c. Myasthenia gravis
    d. Parkinson's disease
46. You are experiencing severe muscle spasms after injuring your back at work. Which of the following is an antispasmodic medication that may be prescribed for you?
    a. Carbamazepine (Tegretol)
    b. Chlordiazepoxide (Librium)
    c. Chlorpromazine (Thorazine)
    d. Cyclobenzaprine (Flexeril)
47. The drugs vecuronium (Norcuron) and succinylcholine (Anectine) may be used for rapid sequence induction of intubation in a person who has sustained severe head trauma. The primary action of these drugs in this situation is which of the following?
    a. To decrease intracranial pressure
    b. To dry oral secretions
    c. To paralyze the muscles
    d. To provide pain relief
48. An indirect-acting cholinergic drug that may be used in the management of poisoning from atropine is which of the following?
    a. Glucagon
    b. Lorazepam
    c. Physostigmine
    d. Verapamil
49. What is the chief neurotransmittor for the parasympathetic nervous system?
    a. Acetylcholine
    b. Adrenalin
    c. Aramine
    d. Norepinephrine

50. Stimulation of the beta-2 adrenergic receptors will cause which of the following?
    a. Negative inotropic effect on the heart
    b. Positive inotropic effect on the heart
    c. Bronchiolar dilation
    d. Peripheral vasoconstriction
51. Epinephrine has which of the following?
    a. Alpha effects only
    b. Beta effects only
    c. Alpha and beta effects
    d. Neither alpha nor beta effects
52. Drugs that increase the contractility of the heart have a positive _____ effect.
    a. Chronotropic
    b. Cholinergic
    c. Dromotropic
    d. Inotropic
53. You are called to the home of an older man complaining of dizziness, nausea, vomiting, weakness, and yellow vision. When questioned about his home medications, he states that he takes a small tablet to help his "weak heart." His pulse is 45/min. You suspect he is suffering from which of the following?
    a. Digoxin overdose
    b. Isoproterenol overdose
    c. Tricyclic antidepressant overdose
    d. Verapamil overdose
54. Which of the following is a group IV antidysrhythmic drug?
    a. Bretylium tosylate
    b. Lidocaine
    c. Procainamide
    d. Verapamil
55. The primary mechanism by which antihypertensives reduce blood pressure is by decreasing which of the following?
    a. Cardiac output
    b. Intravascular blood volume
    c. Myocardial contractility
    d. Peripheral vascular resistance
56. Which of the following drugs acts by dissolving a clot that has already formed?
    a. Aspirin
    b. Coumadin
    c. Heparin
    d. Streptokinase
57. An example of a beta-2–specific bronchodilator is which of the following?
    a. Albuterol
    b. Aminophylline
    c. Ephedrine
    d. Isoproterenol
58. All of the following are indications for antihistamines except which one?
    a. Allergic reactions
    b. Asthma
    c. Motion sickness
    d. Nausea and vomiting
59. An elderly patient has a disorder necessitating the use of pilocarpine drops. What is he suffering from?
    a. Conjunctivitis
    b. Glaucoma
    c. Keratitis
    d. Pain
60. Which of the following is true about insulin?
    a. It is secreted by the adrenal glands.
    b. It is secreted only during stress.
    c. It will increase the use of fat for fuel.
    d. It will move glucose into the cells.
61. Your patient states she is allergic to penicillin. Which of the following drugs can she take safely?
    a. Amoxicillin (Amoxil)
    b. Cefazolin (Ancef)
    c. Dicloxacillin (Dynapen)
    d. Tetracycline (Achromycin)
62. Which of the following is an antiviral drug used in treatment of patients infected with HIV?
    a. Acyclovir (Zovirax)
    b. Pyrimethamine (Daraprim)
    c. Quinine (Quinamm)
    d. Zidovudine (Retrovir)
63. Isoniazid (Izonid) and rifampin (Rifadin) are drugs used to treat which of the following?
    a. HIV infection
    b. Leprosy
    c. Malaria
    d. Tuberculosis

VENOUS ACCESS AND MEDICATION ADMINISTRATION

● READING ASSIGNMENT
Chapter 9, pages 304-313, in *Mosby's Paramedic Textbook*, ed 2

● OBJECTIVES
As a paramedic, you should be able to:
1. Convert selected units of measurement among the household, apothecary, and metric systems.
2. Identify steps to use to perform drug dosage calculations.
3. Calculate the correct volume of drug to be administered in a given situation.
4. Compute the correct rate for an infusion of drugs or intravenous fluids.
5. List measures that should be employed to ensure safe administration of medications.
6. Describe actions the paramedic should take if a medication error occurs.
7. Relate measures that should be taken to preserve asepsis during parenteral drug administration.
8. Explain techniques of drug administration by enteral and parenteral routes.
9. Describe the steps to safely initiate intravenous infusion.
10. Identify complications and adverse effects associated with intravenous access.
11. Describe the steps to safely initiate intraosseous infusion.
12. Explain techniques of drug administration by percutaneous routes.
13. Identify special considerations for administering pharmacological agents to pediatric patients.
14. Explain the technique for obtaining a venous blood sample.
15. Describe how to safely dispose of contaminated items and sharps.

● MATH SKILLS
The following questions are a brief review of basic math skills necessary for drug dose calculation. It is intended as a refresher. If these concepts are not understood, references should be consulted or tutoring sought before proceeding to the next section.

Fractions
A fraction is part of a whole number or one number divided by another number. A fraction consists of two parts, the numerator and the denominator:

$$\frac{a}{b} \quad \begin{array}{l} \text{a is the numerator} \\ \text{b is the denominator} \end{array}$$

The denominator indicates the number of equal parts into which the whole is separated. The numerator tells how many parts are being considered (Fig. 9-1).

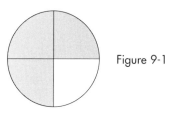

Figure 9-1

Example: $\dfrac{3}{4}$ $\dfrac{\text{Numerator is 3, so 3 parts are being used}}{\text{Denominator is 4, so there are four equal parts}}$

A fraction that has the same numerator and denominator equals the whole number 1 (Fig. 9-2).

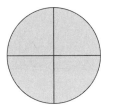

Figure 9-2

Example: $\dfrac{4}{4} = 1$

1. Identify the numerator and denominator of the following fractions.

   a. $\dfrac{7}{8}$ = _____   **b.** $\dfrac{6}{13}$ = _____

When the numerator and denominator of the fraction are multiplied by the same number, the value of the fraction remains unchanged.

Example: $\dfrac{1 \times 2}{2 \times 2} = \dfrac{2}{4} = \dfrac{1}{2}$

A fraction may be reduced to lower terms by dividing the numerator and denominator by the largest whole number that will go evenly into both of them.

Example: $\dfrac{100}{1000} \times \dfrac{100 \div 100}{1000 \div 100} = \dfrac{1}{10}$

2. Reduce the following fractions to lowest terms.

   a. $\frac{7}{28}$ **d.** $\frac{9}{36}$ **g.** $\frac{24}{120}$ **j.** $\frac{10}{25}$
   b. $\frac{9}{12}$ **e.** $\frac{25}{125}$ **h.** $\frac{9}{25}$ **k.** $\frac{17}{23}$
   c. $\frac{4}{8}$ **f.** $\frac{18}{72}$ **i.** $\frac{1000}{10,000}$ **l.** $\frac{16}{24}$

   An improper fraction has a larger numerator than denominator.

Example: $\dfrac{8}{4}$

To change an improper fraction to a whole number, divide the numerator by the denominator:

   Example: $\frac{8}{4} = 8 \div 4 = 2$ (Whole number)

   $\frac{7}{4} = 7 \div 4 = 1\frac{3}{4}$ (This is a mixed number because it has a whole number plus a fraction.)

3. Convert the following to whole numbers or mixed fractions.

   a. $\frac{75}{5}$ **b.** $\frac{24}{12}$ **c.** $\frac{12}{4}$ **d.** $\frac{15}{6}$

To change a mixed number into an improper fraction, multiply the whole number by the denominator of the fraction and add the numerator of the fraction to the result.

Example: $4\frac{1}{2} = \dfrac{(4 \times 2) + 1}{2} = \dfrac{9}{2}$

79

4. Change each of the following mixed numbers to improper fractions:

    a. $5\frac{3}{8}$ **b.** $1\frac{1}{4}$ **c.** $3\frac{1}{12}$ **d.** $15\frac{2}{3}$

To change a fraction to equivalent fractions in which both terms are larger, multiply the numerator and denominator by the same number.

    Example: Enlarge $\frac{2}{5}$ to the equivalent fraction in tenths.

$$\frac{2}{5} \times \frac{2}{2} = \frac{4}{10}$$

5. Change the following fractions to the equivalent fraction indicated.

    a. $\dfrac{6}{8} = \dfrac{x}{24}$ **b.** $\dfrac{12}{15} = \dfrac{x}{60}$ **c.** $\dfrac{79}{100} = \dfrac{x}{100{,}000}$

To compare fractions with different denominators, find the lowest common denominator. The lowest common denominator is the smallest number that is divisible by the denominators.

    Example 1:   What is the lowest common denominator of $\frac{1}{2}$, $\frac{3}{5}$, and $\frac{7}{10}$? The denominators are 2, 5, and 10. Because 10 is divisible by 2 and 5, it is the lowest common denominator.

    Example 2:   What is the lowest common denominator of $\frac{1}{5}$ and $\frac{2}{3}$? Because 5 is not divisible by 3, multiply the larger denominator by 2, 3, 4, and so on. Each time, determine whether the product is divisible by 3:

    $5 \times 2 = 10$ 10 is not divisible by 3.
    $5 \times 3 = 15$ 15 is divisible by 3, so 15 is the lowest common denominator.

6. Find the lowest common denominator.

    a. $\frac{1}{6}$ and $\frac{1}{5}$ **b.** $\frac{2}{3}$ and $\frac{1}{12}$ **c.** $\frac{1}{3}$, $\frac{3}{5}$, and $\frac{3}{4}$

7. Circle the correct response:

    a. $\frac{3}{8}$ is greater than, less than, or equal to $\frac{9}{24}$.
    b. $\frac{5}{6}$ is greater than, less than, or equal to $\frac{5}{8}$.
    c. $\frac{2}{3}$ is greater than, less than, or equal to $\frac{7}{10}$.

To add or subtract fractions, do the following:

    1. Convert all fractions to equivalent fractions using the lowest common denominator.
    2. Add or subtract the numerator and place over the common denominator.
    3. Simplify to the lowest terms.

    Example: $\dfrac{5}{9} + \dfrac{2}{6} = \dfrac{5(2)}{9(2)} + \dfrac{2(3)}{6(3)} = \dfrac{10}{18} + \dfrac{6}{18} = \dfrac{16}{18} \div \dfrac{2}{2} = \dfrac{8}{9}$

8. Add the following fractions and mixed numbers:

    a. $\frac{7}{8} + \frac{2}{3} + \frac{1}{10}$ **b.** $1\frac{1}{4} + 2\frac{2}{3}$

9. Subtract the following fractions and mixed numbers:

    a. $1\frac{3}{5} - \frac{9}{10}$ **b.** $2\frac{1}{4} - \frac{5}{6}$

To multiply fractions, do the following:

    1. Change mixed numbers to improper fractions.
    2. Multiply numerators.
    3. Multiply denominators.
    4. Simplify to the lowest terms.

    Example: $\dfrac{3}{4} \times \dfrac{4}{5} = \dfrac{12}{20} \div \dfrac{4}{4} = \dfrac{3}{5}$

10. Multiply the following fractions and mixed numbers:

    a. $\frac{5}{16} \times \frac{11}{13}$ **c.** $6\frac{1}{8} \times 2$
    b. $8\frac{1}{2} \times 3$ **d.** $\frac{1}{3} \times \frac{7}{8}$

To divide fractions, do the following:
1. **Change mixed numbers to improper fractions.**
2. **Turn the number after the division sign (÷) upside down.**
3. **Follow the steps for multiplication of fractions.**
4. **Simplify to the lowest terms.**

Example: $\dfrac{4}{5} \div \dfrac{2}{3} = \dfrac{4}{5} \times \dfrac{3}{2} = \dfrac{12}{10} \div \dfrac{2}{2} = \dfrac{6}{5} = 1\frac{1}{5}$

11. Divide the following fractions:
 a. ⅜ ÷ ³⁄₁₀   **b.** 2½ ÷ ⁷⁄₁₁

Decimals
All whole numbers are to the left of the decimal; all decimal fractions are to the right of the decimal (Fig. 9-3).

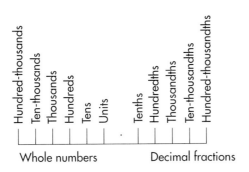

Figure 9-3

12. Write the decimal notation for the following examples:
 a. 3 and 4 tenths   **b.** 5 and 35 hundredths   **c.** 62 thousandths

To convert a fraction into a decimal, do the following:
1. **Divide the numerator by the denominator.**
2. **Place the decimal point in the proper position.**

Example: $\dfrac{3}{5} = 3 \div 5 = 5\overline{)3.0}^{\,0.6}$

13. Change the following fractions to decimals:
 a. ¼   **b.** ⁷⁄₂₅   **c.** ³⁄₁₅₀

To convert a decimal to a fraction, do the following:
1. **Write the numerator of the fraction as the numbers expressed in the decimal.**
2. **Write the denominator of the fraction as the number 1 followed by the number of zeros as there are places to the right of the decimal point.**
3. **Simplify the fraction to the lowest terms.**

Example: 0.234 = x
Numerator = 234
Denominator = 1 + 3 zeros = 1000
Simplify: $\dfrac{234}{1000} = \dfrac{234}{1000} \div \dfrac{2}{2} = \dfrac{117}{500}$

14. Change the following decimals to fractions.
 a. 0.5   **b.** 3.24   **c.** 6.007

81

To add or subtract decimals, do the following:
1. **Line up the decimal points.**
2. **Add zeros to make all decimal numbers equal length.**
3. **Add or subtract as with whole numbers.**
4. **Place the decimal point in the sum.**

$$
\begin{array}{rl}
\text{Example:} & 0.6 + 4.23 + 1.123 = x \\
\text{Line up the decimal points:} & 0.6 \\
& 4.23 \\
& \underline{1.123} \\
\text{Add zeros:} & 0.600 \\
& 4.230 \\
& \underline{1.123} \\
\text{Add as whole numbers:} & 5.953 \\
\end{array}
$$

Place the decimal point in the sum

15. Add the following decimals.
   a. $0.03 + 0.12 + 0.32$ **b.** $0.26 + 0.01 + 0.75$

16. Subtract the following decimals.
   a. $91.5 - 62.5$ **b.** $17 - 3.42$

To multiply decimals, do the following:
1. **Multiply as with whole numbers.**
2. **Count the total number of decimal places in the decimals multiplied.**
3. **Place the decimal point in the answer to the left of the total decimal places calculated in step 2.**
4. **When multiplying a decimal by a power of 10, move the decimal point the same number of places to the right as there are zeros in the multiplier.**

$$
\begin{array}{rl}
\text{Example:} & 1.25 \times 3.3 = x \\
& 1.25 \quad \text{(two decimal places)} \\
& \underline{\times\ 3.3} \quad \text{(one decimal place)} \\
& 4.125 \text{ (The decimal point is placed to the left} \\
& \qquad \text{of three decimal places.)}
\end{array}
$$

Example: $3.46 \times 10 = 3\underset{\vee}{.4}6 = 34.6$

17. Multiply the following decimals.
   a. 3.62×0.02 **c.** 7.25×0.03 **e.** 2.9×10
   b. 27×0.04 **d.** 4.256×100 **f.** 7.052×1000

To divide decimals, do the following:
1. **If the divisor (number you are dividing by) is a whole number, divide as you would with whole numbers. Place the decimal place in the answer in the same place it was in the number to be divided.**
2. **If the divisor (number you are dividing by) is a decimal, make it a whole number by moving the decimal place to the end of the divisor. Move the decimal in the number being divided by the same number of places.**
3. **If the divisor is a power of 10, move the decimal point to the left as many places as there are zeros in the divisor.**

Example: $25.5 \div 5 = 5\overline{)25.5} = 5.1$ with quotient 5.1

Example: $25.5 \div 0.5 = 0.5\overline{)25.5} = 5\overline{)255} = 51$ with quotient 51

Example: $25.5 \div 10 = 2.55\ (2\underset{\vee}{.5}5)$

18. Divide the following.
   a. $0.25 \div 5$ **d.** $0.16 \div 0.04$
   b. $5.16 \div 2$ **e.** $14.237 \div 100$
   c. $4 \div 0.5$ **f.** $0.17 \div 10$

Rounding decimal fractions: Most drug calculations require rounding to the hundredth or greater. This depends on the individual example. To round off, consider the number in the next position to the right. If the number is greater than or equal to 5, increase the number being considered by 1. If it is less than 5, do not increase the number being considered.

Example: Round off 0.74 to the nearest tenths. Because the number in the hundredths column is less than 5, the answer will be 0.7.

Example: Round off 0.24555 to the nearest hundredths. Because the number in the thousandths column is 5, the answer will be 0.25.

19. Round off the following examples to the nearest tenth:
    a. 7.6245   b. 0.081   c. 0.851
20. Round off the following examples to the nearest hundredth:
    a. 0.10423   b. 5.6258   c. 892.02975

Ratios

Ratios indicate the relationship of one quantity to another. They indicate division and may be expressed as the following:

$$\frac{a}{b}, \text{a to b, or a:b}$$

Example: 5 gallons of gas for 6 dollars means the ratio of gas to dollars is:

$$\frac{5}{6}, \text{5 to 6, or 5:6}$$

21. Write the ratio for the following examples.
    a. The heart ejects approximately 5000 ml of blood every 60 seconds.
    b. Approximately 6000 cc of air is moved in and out of the lungs every 60 seconds.
    c. The intravenous line delivers 100 ml every 30 minutes.
    d. There are 100 mg of the drug in 10 ml of solution.

To simplify a ratio that compares two measures, divide the denominator into the numerator to calculate the unit rate.

Example: On a routine transfer, we traveled 120 miles in 2 hours.

$$\text{The unit rate} = \frac{120 \text{ miles}}{2 \text{ hours}} = 60 \text{ miles per hour}$$

22. Calculate the unit rate for each of the following (based on the examples in Question 21).
    a. How many milliliters of blood are ejected from the heart each second?
    b. How much air is moved in and out of the lungs each second?
    c. How much fluid is being delivered each minute?
    d. How many milligrams are in each milliliter?

A proportion shows the relationship between two different ratios. To determine whether a proportion is true (equivalent), do the following:

1. If the proportion is expressed as a fraction, ($\frac{1}{2}$ = $\frac{2}{4}$), multiply the cross products and then determine whether the proportion is equivalent.

Example: $\frac{1}{2} = \frac{2}{4}$ $\frac{1}{2}$ $\frac{2}{4}$ $1 \times 4 = 4$ and $2 \times 2 = 4$;

4 = 4; therefore the proportion is true.

2. If the proportion is expressed as a ratio (2:5::4:10), multiply the two inside numbers ($5 \times 4 = 20$) and the two outside numbers ($2 \times 10 = 20$). 20 = 20; therefore the proportion is equivalent.

23. Determine whether each of the following proportions is true:
    a. $\frac{5}{10} = \frac{1}{2}$ b. $\frac{4}{6} = \frac{8}{10}$ c. $\frac{25}{75} = \frac{1}{3}$

To solve a proportion problem when one of the numbers is unknown (x), do the following:

1. Use either proportion methods demonstrated previously.
2. Make x stand alone by dividing both sides of the equation by the number on the side of x.
3. Solve for x.

Example: $\dfrac{17}{20} = \dfrac{x}{100}$ $20x = 17 \times 100 = \dfrac{20x}{20} = \dfrac{17 \times 100}{20}$

$$x = \dfrac{17 \times 100}{20}$$

$$x = 85$$

Example: 17:20::x:100 $20x = 17 \times 100$

$$\dfrac{20x}{20} = \dfrac{17 \times 100}{20}$$

24. Solve for x in the following problems:

    a. ¾ = ⅚   **c.** ⅔ = ⁷⁄   **e.** 3:5::x:45   **g.** x:35::80:100

    b. ¼ = ⁄₁₆   **d.** ¾ = ⁄₁₂   **f.** 4:9::16:x   **h.** 1.5:3::x:18

Simplifying a problem by cancelling common elements will make problem solving easier.

Example: $x = \dfrac{12 \times 10}{20} = 6$ Zeros cancel. Then 2 divides into 12 six times.

Example: $x = \dfrac{1\ mg \times 1\ ml}{1\ mg} = 1\ ml$ *mg* cancels *mg*. 1 ml is left.

25. Simplify the following problems as much as possible and then solve.

    a. $x = \dfrac{10 \times 150}{50}$

    b. $x = \dfrac{25 \times 2}{50}$

    c. $x = \dfrac{2500 \times 500}{20,000}$

    d. $x = \dfrac{1\ g \times 1\ L}{1\ g}$

    e. $x = \dfrac{2\ mg \times 1\ cc}{10\ mg}$

    f. $x = \dfrac{10\ mg \times 10\ ml}{100\ mg}$

Percentages

Percent (%) is a portion of a whole divided by 100.

1. To change a percent to a decimal, drop the percent sign and move the decimal two places to the left.

    Example: 15.0% = 0.15

2. To change a decimal to a percent, move the decimal two places to the right and add the percent sign.

    Example: 0.76 = 76%

3. To change a fraction to a percent, convert it to a decimal and follow rule 2 above.

    Example: 2/5 = 0.2   0.2 = 20%

26. Change the following percentages to decimals.
   a. 25%   **b.** 110%   **c.** 0.5%
27. Convert the following decimals to percentages.
   a. 0.34   **b.** 2.29   **c.** 0.07
28. Express the following as percentages:
   a. $\frac{34}{50}$ **b.** $\frac{100}{500}$ **c.** $\frac{3}{7}$
29. Rewrite the following fractions as ratios, decimals, and percentages:

Fraction	Ratio	Decimal	Percentage
a. $\frac{5}{6}$			
b. $\frac{1}{20}$			
c. $\frac{7}{33}$			

30. Solve the following:
   a. 15% of 75   **b.** 0.5% of 250
   This concludes the refresher.

● **MATHEMATICAL EQUIVALENTS AND DRUG DOSE CALCULATIONS**

31. In the metric system the primary unit of volume is the (a) _____

   _____, the primary unit of mass (weight) is the

   (b) _____, and the primary unit of length is the

   (c) _____.
32. List the four metric weight units commonly used in the prehospital environment, beginning with the largest and ending with the smallest.
   a.
   b.
   c.
   d.
33. Each of the units listed in Question 32 differs in value from the next unit

   by _____.
34. To convert from one unit to the next smallest unit in Question 32, you must

   move the decimal point three places to the right or left? _____
35. To convert from one unit to the previous unit (example unit 32d to unit 32c), one must move the decimal point three places to the right or left?

   _____

36. Convert the following units of weight to the units indicated.
   a. 2 kg = _____ g   **e.** 400 mcg = _____ mg
   b. 4 mg = _____ mcg   **f.** 350 mg = _____ g
   c. 2 g = _____ mg   **g.** 0.25 mg = _____ mcg
   d. 600 mg = _____ kg   **h.** 12.5 g = _____ mg
37. Convert the following units of volume to the units indicated.
   a. 1 cc = _____ ml   **c.** 250 ml = _____ L
   b. 10 ml = _____ cc   **d.** 0.33 L = _____ ml
38. The primary unit of mass in the apothecary system is the _____

   _____.

39. The primary unit of volume in the apothecary system is the _____

_____.

40. If the physician orders acetaminophen gr X, how many milligrams will

you give? _____

41. Your patient has chest pain, and medical direction orders nitroglycerin gr ¹⁄₁₅₀. How many milligrams will you administer?

(a) _____ When it is time for a second nitroglycerin, the patient's blood pressure is slightly low, so this time the physician orders nitroglycerin gr ¹⁄₂₀₀. How many milligrams will you give?

(b) _____

42. Convert the following measures in the household system to the units indicated:

a. 1 T = _____ t	**c.** 1 pt = _____ oz	**e.** 1 f oz = _____ T
b. 1 lb = _____ oz	**d.** 1 gl = _____ qt	**f.** 1 c = _____ f oz

43. Convert the following measures in the household system to the appropriate metric units.

a. 1 tsp = _____ ml	**c.** 1 f oz = _____ ml	**e.** 22 lb = _____ kg
b. 1 T = _____ ml	**d.** 1 qt = _____ ml	**f.** 110 lb = _____ kg

44. Convert the following measures to the appropriate units indicated.

a. A patient's family tells you that he lost about a cup of blood from a head wound. You will relay to medical direction that the estimated blood loss is approximately _____ ml.

b. A patient vomits about a quart of coffee-grounds emesis. This is equal to _____ ml.

c. The patient took 1 ounce or _____ ml of antacid. Then she drank 16 oz of milk. This is equal to _____ ml of milk.

d. A parent reads a drug label and, instead of administering 2 ml of a drug, accidentally gives 2 oz of a drug. How many milliliters in excess of the prescribed dose did they give? _____ ml

e. The human body normally contains about 5 L of blood, or _____ qt.

f. A pregnant woman states that her membranes have ruptured and about a pint of amniotic fluid leaked out. This is equal to _____ ml.

g. A premature newborn you have just delivered weighs 2 pounds, or _____ kg (_____ g).

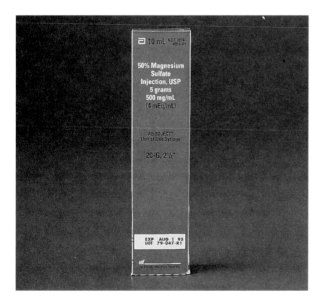

Figure 9-4

45. Identify the following information from the drug label or package in Fig. 9-4.

    a. Drug name: **d.** Total drug:

    b. Expiration date: **e.** Concentration of drug:

    c. Total volume:

46. Convert the following drug concentrations into the total number of grams.

    a. Calcium chloride 10% solution = _____ g in 100 ml.

    b. Epinephrine 1:1000 solution = _____ g in 1000 ml.

    c. Magnesium sulfate 10% solution = _____ g in 100 ml.

    d. Epinephrine 1:10,000 solution = _____ g in 10,000 ml.

    e. Lidocaine 0.4% solution = _____ g in 100 ml.

    f. Mannitol 25% solution = _____ g in 100 ml.

    g. Dextrose 50% solution = _____ g in 100 ml.

47. Calculate the concentration per milliliter of the following drugs using the following formula: Concentration = Total dose of drug (mg) ÷ Total volume (ml). For example, a 10-ml vial of lidocaine contains 100 mg of the drug. Concentration = 100 mg ÷ 10 ml = 10 mg/ml.

    a. A 40-mg vial of furosemide is in a 4-ml vial. Concentration = _____.

    b. A 10-ml vial of epinephrine contains 1 mg of the drug. Concentration = _____.

    c. You have 25 g of D50W in 50 ml. Concentration = _____.

    d. A 2-ml vial of diphenhydramine contains 50 mg of the drug. Concentration = _____.

    e. There is 1 g of lidocaine in a 250-ml bag. Concentration = _____.

48. Calculate the total dose of a drug to be administered.

    a. Lidocaine 1 mg/kg is ordered for a 100-kg patient who is having many premature ventricular contractions each minute. Dose = _____ mg.

    b. The maximum dose of procainamide is 17 mg/kg and the patient weighs 60 kg. Total dose = _____ mg.

    c. Push sodium bicarbonate 1 mEq/kg during a lengthy cardiac arrest. The patient weighs 80 kg. Dose = _____ mEq.

    d. Hang a dopamine drip at 5 mcg/kg/min on a hypotensive patient who weighs 50 kg. Dose = _____ mcg/min.

    e. Give epinephrine 0.01 mg/kg to an 11-lb child who is in cardiopulmonary arrest. Dose = _____ mg.

    f. Administer mannitol 1 g/kg to a 176-lb patient with rising intracranial pressure. Dose = _____ g.

49. Solve the following problems using the following formula:

$$\text{Volume (x)} = \frac{\text{Desired dose (D)} \times \text{Volume on hand (Q)}}{\text{Dose on hand (H)}}$$

    a. You wish to give furosemide 20 mg. It is supplied in a 4-ml vial containing 40 mg of the drug. Volume = _____ ml.

    b. You wish to administer morphine 3 mg. You have a 1-ml Tubex containing 10 mg of the drug. Volume = _____ ml.

    c. You wish to give amiodarone 300 mg. You have a 3-ml vial containing 150 mg of the drug. Volume = _____ ml.

    d. You must give 2.5 mg of diazepam. It is supplied in a 2-ml vial containing 10 mg. Volume = _____ ml.

    e. You have 50 mg of meperidine in a 1-ml Tubex. You need to give 12.5 mg of the drug. Volume = _____ ml.

    f. Your patient needs 0.3 mg of epinephrine (1:1000). You have a 1-ml vial containing 1 mg. Volume = _____ ml.

    g. Your patient needs 0.5 mg of dopamine. You have a 500-ml bag containing 400 mg of the drug. Volume = _____ ml.

50. Solve the following drug dose problems using the following equation:
Desired dose: Desired volume::Dosage on hand:Volume on hand.

Example: Give 50 mg of procainamide. It is supplied in a 10-ml vial
containing 1000 mg.

50 mg:x = 1000 mg:10 ml   Set up the ratio.

$$\frac{1000 \text{ mg} \times x}{1000 \text{ mg}} = \frac{50 \text{ mg} \times 10 \text{ ml}}{1000 \text{ mg}}$$ Multiply inside (means) and then
outside (extremes) numbers.

$$x = \frac{50 \text{ mg} \times 10 \text{ ml}}{1000 \text{ mg}}$$ Solve for x

x = 0.5 ml

    a. Administer adenosine 6 mg. It is supplied in a 2-ml vial containing 6 mg
of the drug. Desired volume = _____ ml.
    b. Administer diphenhydramine 25 mg. You have a 2-ml vial containing 50
mg of the drug. Desired volume = _____ ml.
    c. Give 2.5 mg of verapamil. It is supplied in a 2-ml vial containing 5 mg of
the drug. Desired volume = _____ ml.
    d. Give 1000 mg of mannitol. You have a 20% solution. Desired volume
= _____ ml.

51. Calculate the drops/min needed to deliver the following volumes of fluid
over the required time.
    a. The physician orders an intravenous fluid to run at 30 cc/hr (drop factor,
60 drops/ml). Drops/min = _____.
    b. You want to give a fluid challenge of 200 ml over 20 min (drop factor, 10
drops/ml). Drops/minute = _____.
    c. You need to infuse a drug mixed in 50 ml of fluid over 15 min (drop fac-
tor, 15 drops/ml). Drops/min − _____.
    d. Online medical direction orders 150 ml of lactated Ringer's solution to in-
fuse in 2 hours (drop factor, 15 drops/ml). Drops/min = _____.
    e. You are told to give 275 ml over 2 hours (drop factor, 10 drops/ml).
Drops/min = _____.
    f. The intravenous drug must run in at 0.5 ml/min (drop factor, 60
drops/ml). Drops/min = _____.
    g. You have delivered a baby, and medical direction advises you to add 10
units (1 ml) of oxytocin to 1000 ml of normal saline and infuse it at 200
ml/hr (drop factor, 10 drops/ml). Drops/min = _____.
    h. You have added magnesium sulfate to D5W for a total volume of 100 ml.
You must infuse it over 2 min to treat your patient's ventricular arryth-
mia (drop factor, 10 drops/ml). Drops/min = _____.
    i. A severely acidotic patient needs bicarb. You have added 50 mEq of
sodium bicarbonate (50 ml) to 1000 ml of normal saline and are to infuse
it over 2 hours (drop factor, 15 drops/ml). Drops/min = _____.
    j. You have added 2 mg (2 ml) of epinephrine to a 250-ml bag of normal
saline and wish to infuse it at 1 ml/min to your severely bradycardic patient (drop factor, 60 drops/ml). Drops/min = _____.
    k. Your patient has just converted from ventricular fibrillation. You are
hanging a lidocaine drip at 3 mg/min. You have mixed 1 g of lidocaine
in 250 ml normal saline. How many drops/min will you set your IV to
deliver the 0.75 ml/min necessary for this dose of drug (drop factor, 60
drops/ml)? Drops/min = _____.

52. Calculate the following problems using any of the methods demonstrated.
Ensure that all units are compatible. If the dosage is given in mg/kg, make
the appropriate calculation.

a. You wish to give lidocaine 1 mg/kg to a 75-kg man. It is supplied in a 10-ml syringe containing 100 mg of the drug. How many milliliters will you administer?

b. You must give bretylium 10 mg/kg to a 60-kg woman. You have a 10-ml Tubex containing 500 mg of the drug. How much will you give?

c. You must give 0.5 mg of glucagon to a 90-kg patient. When you mix it up, you have 1 mg in 1 ml of solution. How much will you give?

d. You have diluted your phenobarbital so that you have 130 mg in 10 ml. You need to give 100 mg. The patient weighs 100 kg. How much will you give?

e. You must give 1 g/kg of mannitol. The patient weighs 70 kg. You have a 20% solution. How many milliliters will you give?

f. You need to administer 150 mg of aminophylline. You have 500 mg in a 20-ml ampule. How many milliliters will you give?

g. Your patient needs a dopamine drip at 5 mcg/kg/min. He weighs 100 kg. You have 400 mg of dopamine in 500 ml of D5W. How many ml/min will you administer and at how many drops/min will you set the microdrip intravenous line?

h. You wish to administer a lidocaine drip at 2 mg/min. You have an intravenous bag containing a 0.4% solution of lidocaine. How many milliliters will you give each minute and how fast will you set your microdrip tubing to deliver this rate?

53. For each of the following situations, calculate the correct volume of solution to be administered using the drug package information illustrated.

a. Give 0.5 mg of atropine (Fig. 9-5). Desired volume = _____ ml.

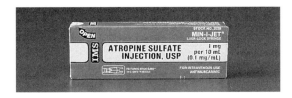

Figure 9-5

b. Give 0.3 mg of epinephrine (Fig. 9-6). Desired volume = _____ ml.

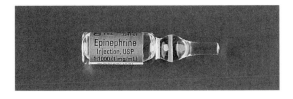

Figure 9-6

c. Give lidocaine 0.5 mg/kg to an 80-kg patient (Fig. 9-7). Desired volume = _____ ml.

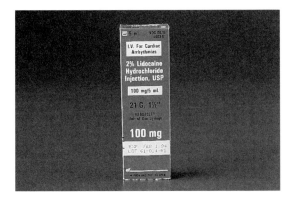

Figure 9-7

89

54. After determining the correct volume of drug to be administered in the following examples, shade the corresponding syringe in Fig. 9-8 to illustrate the proper amount to be given.

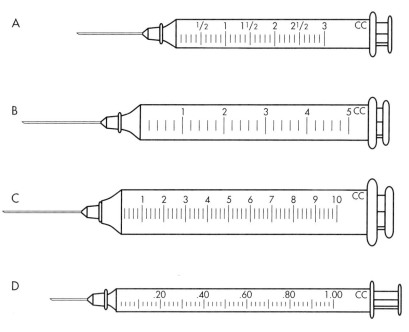

Figure 9-8

a. Adenosine 6 mg must be given to a patient with paroxysmal supraventricular tachycardia. You have a 2-ml vial containing 3 mg/ml of the drug. How many milliliters will you give?

b. Your patient has had a seizure and needs phenytoin 200 mg. You have a 5-ml vial containing 250 mg of the drug. How much will you give?

c. You have a 10-ml vial of furosemide containing 10 mg/ml of the drug. A total of 70 mg is indicated for your patient, who is in congestive heart failure. What volume will you administer?

d. You wish to administer epinephrine 0.3 mg to a patient experiencing an allergic reaction. It is supplied in a 1-ml ampule containing 1 mg of a 1:1000 solution of the drug. How much will you give?

● DRUG ADMINISTRATION

55. List at least 10 general steps to be taken when administering any drug to avoid errors.

a.

b.

c.

d.

e.

f.

g.

h.

i.

j.

56. You intended to deliver the lidocaine drip at 1 ml/min during your 15-min transport, but when you look at the 250-ml bag, the roller clamp has been opened and almost 150 ml has been infused. List five actions that you should take after this error.

    a.

    b.

    c.

    d.

    e.

57. List two methods to ensure medical asepsis when you administer an intramuscular injection.

    a.

    b.

58. Complete the following sentences regarding drug administration routes:

Oral medications should be given with the patient in the (a) _____

position. The drug should be swallowed with (b) _____

ounces of fluid to ensure it reaches the (c) _____.

Sublingual medications should be placed under the (d) _____

and allowed to (e) _____. They should not be (f) _____

because this will delay action of the drug. Parenteral drug administration

may cause (g) _____, (h) _____,

or (i) _____. The correct needle length and size is important. For subcutaneous injections a (j) _____

-inch, (k) _____ -gauge needle should be used. When

administering an intramuscular shot, you should select a (l) _____

_____ -inch, (m) _____

-gauge needle. To minimize the risk of needle stick injury, you should understand that the use of two-handed needle recapping is (n)

_____. Also, all sharp items, including needles, should

be placed in (o) _____. When withdrawing medication from a multidose vial, you should cleanse the stopper with alcohol and

then inject the same amount of (p) _____ as drug to be withdrawn before aspirating the appropriate amount of medicine into the syringe. To minimize the risk of glass particles entering the injection

when aspirating from a glass ampule, use a (q) _____

needle. Subcutaneous injections should be administered at a (r) _____

_____ -degree angle. Sites of administration for this

route include (s) _____, _____,

and _____. Intramuscular injections should be administered at a (t) _____ -degree angle. Administration sites for this route include the (u) _____ and

_____ . To prevent drug effects on the rescuer, you should always wear (v) _____ when administering transdermal medicines. Dilution with at least (w) _____

ml of fluid is recommended to ensure maximum absorption of drugs administered by the endotracheal route. Two advantages of drugs administered by inhalation are (x) _____ and fewer _____

_____.

59. List three complications of intravenous line placement for each of the following approaches:
   a. Peripheral site:

   b. Internal jugular and subclavian sites:

   c. Femoral site:

60. You respond to care for a 3-year-old child who is in cardiac arrest. Attempts to intubate and secure IV access are unsuccessful, so you elect to attempt intraosseous infusion. After applying gloves and preparing your equipment,

   you select the preferred site, located (a) _____

   _____.

   The needle is then inserted using a (b) _____ motion

   and advanced until (c) _____. The next step involves

   aspirating marrow into a syringe. Then, a syringe filled with (d) _____

   _____ should be used to ensure that free flow occurs without

   resistance. If correct placement is detected, the (e) _____

   should be connected and infused at the appropriate rate. To prevent the

   needle from being dislodged, you should (f) _____

   the needle.

● **STUDENT SELF-ASSESSMENT**

61. Your patient's mother states her child's temperature is 38.5° Celcius. What is her temperature in degrees Fahrenheit?
   a. 69.9   c. 101.3
   b. 99.6   d. 103.6

62. You must administer a drug that is calculated based on mg/kg. The patient tells you that he weighs 144 pounds. How many kg does that convert to (rounded to the nearest pound)?
    a. 65   **c.** 80
    b. 72   **d.** 86

63. You wish to administer mannitol 500 mg/kg to a 100-kg woman. You have a 10% solution of the drug. How many milliliters will you give?
    a. 2   **c.** 20
    b. 5   **d.** 500

64. You are going to give epinephrine 0.01 mg/kg to a 6-kg child. It is supplied as 1 mg in a 10-ml syringe. How many ml will you administer?
    a. 0.006   **c.** 0.6
    b. 0.06   **d.** 6.0

65. Which syringe will you use to withdraw the drug volume that you calculated in Question 64?
    a. 1 ml   **c.** 5 ml
    b. 3 ml   **d.** 10 ml

66. Which measure should be taken to ensure safe administration of drugs?
    a. Learn a rapid dose calculation method that you can always perform in your head.
    b. Set unlabeled syringes in a consistent place so that you will know what is in them.
    c. Verify the label of the drug selected once before administration.
    d. Monitor the patient for drug effects closely for the first 5 minutes after you give them.

67. Your patient suddenly vomits and has chest pain after you administer epinephrine intravenously instead of subcutaneously as ordered for his anaphylaxis. How should this be recorded in the patient care report?
    a. Document the correct route only.
    b. Document the route ordered and the incorrect route.
    c. Document the incorrect route only.
    d. Omit the route in the report.

68. What parenteral route would you use to test for allergies?
    a. Intradermal   **c.** Intravenous
    b. Intramuscular   **d.** Subcutaneous

69. Which muscle is appropriate for an intramuscular injection in a 2-year-old child?
    a. Deltoid   **c.** Ventrogluteal site
    b. Dorsogluteal site   **d.** Vastus lateralis

70. You suspect that your patient has a ruptured ectopic pregnancy. She is in profound shock. Which intravenous catheter will you select?
    a. 14 gauge, 1½ inch   **c.** 18 gauge, 1½ inch
    b. 14 gauge, 3 inch   **d.** 18 gauge, 3 inch

71. You are transferring a patient with a jugular central line. Suddenly, the patient becomes unconscious, cyanotic, and tachycardic. You note that the IV tubing has been disconnected from the central line catheter. The patient should immediately be positioned on his:
    a. Left side with his head down   **c.** Right side with his head down
    b. Left side with his head up   **d.** Right side with his head up

72. You wish to administer normal saline intravenous at 30 ml/hr. The infusion set delivers 60 drops/ml. How fast will you run it?
    a. 1 drop/min   **c.** 100 drops/min
    b. 30 drops/min   **d.** 400 drops/min

73. A 200-ml fluid challenge is to be infused over 15 minutes. The drop factor is 10 drops/ml. How fast will you run it?
    a. 35 drops/min   **c.** 133 drops/min
    b. 75 drops/min   **d.** 150 drops/min

74. Which of the following statements is true regarding intraosseous infusion?
    a. It is generally recommended for children between 1 and 18 years of age.
    b. It is associated with a risk of air embolism if the tubing is disconnected.
    c. Absorption of drugs is irregular and slow through this route.
    d. The procedure should only be considered in critically ill children.
75. Which of the following is true regarding sublingual drug administration?
    a. The patient may have a sip of water after administration.
    b. Nifedipine may be administered by this route.
    c. The drug should be permitted to dissolve under the tongue.
    d. Swallowing the drug will increase its effects.
76. When administering medication into a 2-year-old child's ear, you should pull the ear:
    a. Down and back   c. Up and back
    b. Down and forward   d. Up and forward
77. Which is true regarding administration of medication to young children?
    a. Tell the child not to cry or make noise.
    b. Avoid any physical restraint.
    c. Give injections slowly and firmly.
    d. Be honest about painful techniques.
78. Which of the following describes an appropriate procedure for obtaining a blood sample for glucose on an adult patient?
    a. Disconnect the IV infusion, insert the vacutainer into the hub of the IV catheter, and withdraw.
    b. Insert the intraosseoous needle, flush with normal saline, attach a syringe, and pull back.
    c. Enter the vein with a 24-gauge needle attached to a syringe and withdraw.
    d. Push blood collection tubes into the barrel of the vacutainer and allow to fill.

THERAPEUTIC COMMUNICATIONS

● READING ASSIGNMENT
Chapter 10, pages 344-357, in *Mosby's Paramedic Textbook,* ed 2

● OBJECTIVES
As a paramedic, you should be able to:
1. Define therapeutic communication.
2. Outline the elements in effective therapeutic communication.
3. Identify internal factors for effective communication.
4. Describe external factors for effective communication.
5. Outline the elements of an effective patient interview.
6. Summarize strategies to get appropriate patient information.
7. Discuss methods to assess mental status during the interview.
8. Describe techniques to enhance communications when interviewing a patient unmotivated to talk, a hostile patient, a child, an older adult, a hearing-impaired patient, a blind patient, a patient under the influence of drugs or alcohol, a sexually aggressive patient, or a patient with different cultural traditions.

● REVIEW QUESTIONS
Match the communication response in Column II with the description in Column I. Use each response only once.

Column I		Column II
1. _____ Making associations or implying a cause		a. Clarification
2. _____ Paraphrasing a patient's words		b. Confrontation
3. _____ Pausing for several moments		c. Empathy
4. _____ Reviewing with open-ended questions		d. Explanation
5. _____ Having the patient rephrase a word		e. Interpretation
6. _____ Providing information		f. Reflection
7. _____ Refocusing on one aspect of the interview		g. Silence
		h. Summary

8. Identify selected elements of the communication process in the following example:
   You tell your patient that you plan to take his temperature. He says, "where are you going to take it to?" You clarify that you are going to put a thermometer under his tongue to see whether he has a fever.
   a. Who is the source?
   b. Who did the encoding in the initial message?
   c. Was the decoding effective?
   d. Who was the receiver?
   e. Why was feedback needed?

9. You are caring for a patient who is very emotionally upset. List six actions that you can use to convey that you are actively listening to the patient.
   a.
   b.
   c.
   d.
   e.
   f.

10. A patient was assaulted and is found in the midst of a large crowd. How can you control external factors to enable effective communication with this patient?

_____

_____

11. Rewrite the following questions into an open-ended format:
  a. Do you feel bad?

_____

  b. Does your chest hurt here?

_____

  c. Did this problem start today?

_____

  d. Are you taking any medicine on a daily basis?

_____

12. Can you identify the problem in each of the following statements if they were made by a paramedic?
  a. I know you can't move your legs right now, but don't worry; everything will be just fine.

_____

  b. You know you won't have this trouble breathing if you quit smoking.

_____

  c. We believe your substernal chest pain may be causing an ischemic area in your myocardium that is going to result in myocardial infarction.

_____

  d. Why didn't you take your blood-pressure medicine?

_____

13. You are called to a residence for a woman who fell down the stairs. You begin your assessment and patient management, and by the time you get in the back of the ambulance, you realize that her injuries are not consistent with the mechanism of injury she describes. The patient is reluctant to give you much information, and you strongly suspect domestic violence was the cause of her injuries.
  a. What reasons may this patient have for resistance regarding information?

_____

  b. What statements might you make to begin to talk about this issue?

_____

  c. If she tells you she was beaten up by her husband but doesn't want to leave him or have him arrested, how should you respond?

_____

14. You are called to a college dorm for an "overdose." As you arrive on the scene, the patient is walking toward you.
    a. What is the first step in your mental status examination of this patient?

    _____

    b. As you begin your conversation with the patient, what observations will you make regarding mental status?

    _____

15. For each of the following difficult situations, identify three strategies that you may use to attempt to communicate with the patient:
    a. A 72-year-old man has paralysis on the right side. He appears to be awake and alert, but he is not responding to your questions appropriately.

    _____

    b. You have been called to a jail to care for a patient who has expressed a wish to kill a number of people. He is sitting with his arms folded, and his voice is getting progressively louder.

    _____

16. Describe your approach when interviewing a 3-year-old and his father.

    _____

17. You are caring for a patient in the ambulance who makes inappropriate and sexually suggestive remarks. What should you do?

    _____

● STUDENT SELF-ASSESSMENT

18. Which of the following best describes therapeutic communication?
    a. Verbal and nonverbal behavior that conveys a message
    b. Planned act to communicate and obtain information
    c. Spoken or written words to express ideas or feelings
    d. Decoding and encoding from a messenger to a receiver
19. When a message is put into an understandable format, it is considered which of the following?
    a. Decoded   c. Received
    b. Encoded   d. Sourced
20. When you try to see the situation from another person's point of view, you are demonstrating which of the following?
    a. Cultural imposition   c. Ethnocentrism
    b. Empathy   d. Sympathy
21. Which of the following would convey a confident, open attitude during the patient interview in the prehospital setting?
    a. Speaking loudly and quickly
    b. Standing with your arms folded on your chest
    c. Looking at the patient's eyes as the patient speaks
    d. Not invading the patient's personal space
22. Which of the following would demonstrate an effective patient communication strategy?
    a. Beginning questions with "how"
    b. Demonstrating personal bias
    c. Interrupting to get to the point
    d. Using medical terminology

23. Which of the following is a normal finding during the mental status examination?
    a. The patient demonstrates long pauses and rapid shifts in conversation.
    b. The patient has an upright posture and is well groomed.
    c. You repeat questions several times before the patient understands you.
    d. The patient is trembling and clenching and unclenching the fists.
24. Which of the following is the most effective method to communicate with a hearing-impaired patient in the prehospital setting?
    a. Lip reading
    b. Sign language
    c. Whatever method the patient prefers
    d. Note writing

DIVISION TWO
AIRWAY MANAGEMENT AND VENTILATION

CHAPTER 11
AIRWAY MANAGEMENT AND VENTILATION

● READING ASSIGNMENT
Chapter 11, pages 360-429, in *Mosby's Paramedic Textbook,* ed 2

● OBJECTIVES
As a paramedic, you should be able to:
1. Distinguish among respiration, pulmonary ventilation, and external and internal respiration.
2. Explain the mechanics of respiration.
3. Relate the partial pressures of gases in the blood and lungs to atmospheric gas pressures.
4. Describe pulmonary circulation.
5. Explain the process of exchange and transport of gases in the body.
6. Describe voluntary, chemical, and nervous regulation of respiration.
7. Discuss the assessment and management of medical or traumatic obstruction of the airway.
8. Outline the causes, preventive measures, and effects of pulmonary aspiration.
9. Outline essential parameters to evaluate the effectiveness of airway and breathing.
10. Describe the indications, contraindications, and techniques for supplemental oxygen delivery.
11. Discuss methods for patient ventilation based on knowledge of their indications, contraindications, potential complications, and use.
12. Describe the use of manual airway maneuvers and mechanical airway adjuncts based on knowledge of their indications, contraindications, potential complications, and techniques.
13. Describe assessment techniques and devices used to ensure adequate oxygenation and ventilation and correct placement of the endotracheal tube.
14. Explain variations in assessment and management of airway and ventilation problems in pediatric patients.
15. Given a patient scenario, identify potential alterations in oxygenation and ventilation based on a knowledge of gas exchange and mechanics of breathing.

● REVIEW QUESTIONS

1-5 Match the lung volume in Column II with its description in Column I. Use each answer only once.

Column I	Column II
1. _____ The air inhaled and exhaled during a normal respiratory cycle (500 to 600 ml)	a. Expiratory reserve volume
2. _____ Quantity of air moved on deepest inspiration and expiration	b. Inspiratory reserve volume
3. _____ Tidal volume multiplied by respiratory rate	c. Minute volume
4. _____ Air remaining in respiratory passages after a forceful exhalation	d. Residual volume
5. _____ Amount of air that can be forcefully exhaled after a normal breath is exhaled	e. Tidal volume
	f. Vital capacity

6. Pulmonary ventilation is the movement of oxygen and carbon dioxide into and out of the lungs. True/false. If this is false, why is it false?

_____

7. pH is a measurement that reflects hydrogen ion concentration. True/false. If this is false, why is it false?

_____

8. The pressure regulator attached to an oxygen cylinder permits administration of a specific amount of oxygen. True/false. If this is false, why is it false?

_____

9. Describe the *mechanical* process by which air is moved into and out of the lungs.

_____

_____

10. Complete the sentences in the following paragraph: At sea level, atmospheric pressure is **(a)** _____. The pressure in the alveoli is known as the **(b)** _____ pressure. Changes in this pressure are caused by changes in the **(c)** _____ size. During inspiration the pressure in the alveoli will **(d)** _____ _____ approximately 1 mm Hg relative to atmospheric pressure, whereas during exhalation the pressure will **(e)** _____ _____ by 1 mm Hg. The ability of the lungs to expand during changes in pressure is known as **(f)** _____. This ability can be impaired by diseases such as **(g)** _____, _____, and _____.

11. The major blood vessels that carry deoxygenated blood to the lungs are the

(a) _____. Oxygenated blood is carried away from

the lungs by the (b) _____ _____.

12. Your patient is a 70-year-old man with chronic bronchitis and emphysema who experienced an acute onset of shortness of breath while at the grocery store. Describe your ongoing assessment of this patient's head, neck, chest, and abdomen. Be specific when describing the muscle groups that you will inspect to help determine his degree of distress.

_____

_____

13. The partial pressure of nitrogen (P_{N_2}) = (a) _____ % × atmospheric pressure (b) _____ mm Hg = (c) _____ mm Hg. The partial pressure of oxygen (P_{O_2}) = (d) _____ % × atmospheric pressure (e) _____ mm Hg = (f) _____ mm Hg.

14. List 3 physiological factors that can increase the work of breathing.
    a.
    b.
    c.

15. Describe the *structural* aspects of the lung that explain the following:
    a. Normal lung expansion:

_____

_____

    b. Alveolar collapse that occurs secondary to decreased surfactant in a premature infant:

_____

_____

    c. Poor ventilation during an asthma attack:

_____

_____

16. Each of the diagrams in Fig. 11-1 represents solutions separated by a semi-permeable membrane. In each illustration, indicate whether the process of diffusion will cause a net movement of solute particles to the *left, right,* or *not at all.*

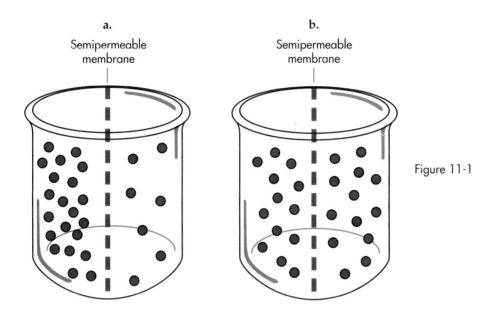

Figure 11-1

17. Complete the missing values for PCO_2 and PO_2 in the following. Then draw an arrow indicating the direction of movement of each of the gases across the respiratory membrane.

Alveolar Gas	Direction of Movement of Gas	Venous Blood (Pulmonary Capillaries)
PCO_2 _____ torr		PCO_2 _____ torr
PO_2 _____ torr		PO_2 _____ torr

18. Complete the following sentences:
    a. The primary way that oxygen is transported in the blood is by a chemical bond to _____.
    b. PO_2 describes the oxygen level dissolved in blood _____

    _____.

    c. The amount of carbon dioxide present in the venous blood is influenced

    by the rate and type of _____.
    d. Carbon dioxide is transported in the blood in three forms: _____

    _____, _____ _____,

    and _____.

19. In one sentence describe the physiological basis for poor blood oxygenation in the following patients:

    a. A 23-year-old woman who is completely paralyzed from Guillain-Barré syndrome:

_____

    b. A 52-year-old patient with pneumonia:

_____

    c. An 8-year-old who is having an acute asthma attack:

_____

    d. A 42-year-old with massive head trauma caused by a motor vehicle crash:

_____

20. Briefly explain the origin or site of stimulation, location of effect, and action of each of the following mechanisms that control respiration:

Mechanism	Origin or Stimulus	Location of Effect	Action
Inspiratory centers			
Expiratory centers			
Hering-Bruer reflex			
Pneumotaxic center			
Apneustic center			

21. For each of the following scenarios, briefly explain why the patient's respirations will increase or decrease or be unchanged.

    a. A 3-year-old who loses consciousness from breath-holding secondary to a temper tantrum:

_____

    b. A 34-year-old with a morphine overdose:

_____

    c. A 17-year-old football player with a dislocated shoulder:

_____

    d. A hostage with no apparent injuries who has just been freed:

_____

    e. A student who is sleeping in class:

_____

    f. An individual who suffers from chronic obstructive pulmonary disease who has fallen and for whom an oxygen level of 10 L/min is being administered by nonrebreather mask:

_____

    g. A lost snow skier who has a core temperature of 84° F (28.9° C):

_____

22. Briefly describe the benefit of the following modified forms of respiration:

a. Cough:

_____

b. Sneeze:

_____

c. Hiccough:

_____

d. Sigh:

_____

23. For each of the following scenarios identify the pathological condition or injury you would suspect and list the signs and symptoms the patient may develop:

a. A 50-year-old man unable to speak after choking on a piece of steak:

_____

b. A nursing home patient with shortness of breath after "inhaling" some food:

_____

c. A 17-year-old hockey player who has difficulty speaking after being struck across the neck by a stick:

_____

d. A 2-year-old with croup:

_____

e. A 23-year-old who reportedly overdosed, is unconscious, and has vomitus draining from the side of her mouth.

_____

24. You are transporting a patient with severe asthma to a medical center 40 minutes away. What are the advantages of using a pulse oximeter in this scenario?

_____

25. For each of the following scenarios, circle the best oxygen-delivery device and explain why you made that selection:

a. A 76-year-old patient with chronic obstructive pulmonary disease complains of right-sided chest pain and a nosebleed after a fall. Vital signs are normal. Nasal cannula at 2 L/min oxygen or Venturi mask at 24% oxygen?

_____

b. A 25-year-old patient involved in a motor vehicle crash has ineffective respirations, cyanosis, and signs of a flail chest segment. Simple face mask at 8 L/min oxygen or bag-valve-mask with reservoir device at 15 L/min oxygen?

_____

c. A 45-year-old patient with slight chest pain (SaO$_2$ on room air is 98%). Simple face mask at 4 L/min oxygen or nasal cannula at 4 L/min oxygen?

---

d. A 17-year-old patient who sustained a crush injury to the abdomen in a farming accident is pale, with cyanosis around the lips and decreased blood pressure. Simple mask at 6 L/min oxygen or complete nonrebreather mask at 10 L/min oxygen?

---

26. For each of the following scenarios, choose the airway adjunct from the list that is most appropriate after initial manual airway maneuvers have been used. Explain why you selected your answer.

Oral airway   Nasal airway
Oral endotracheal intubation   Nasal endotracheal intubation
Percutaneous tracheal ventilation   Esophageal obturator airway

a. Your patient is a 17-year-old victim of a snowmobiling accident who struck a concealed barbed wire fence, injuring his neck. The airway is not patent. All attempts to secure the airway, including oral and nasal intubation, are unsuccessful.

---

b. You are called to evaluate a 34-year-old patient who is postictal after a single grand mal seizure. He has snoring respirations and no gag reflex.

---

c. Your patient was pulled from a swimming pool after an unsuccessful dive into the shallow end. He has ineffective shallow respirations and flaccid paralysis of all limbs.

---

d. A 32-year-old woman with a history of diabetes has taken her insulin but has not eaten. She has snoring respirations and can be aroused with painful stimulus.

---

e. A 19-year-old ejected from his all-terrain vehicle has an obviously severe head injury and shallow agonal respirations.

---

f. A 79-year-old is in cardiac arrest of medical origin.

---

27. Describe your actions if you discover the following physical findings after endotracheal intubation of a patient:

a. The carbon dioxide detector fades from purple to yellow as the patient exhales.

_____

b. Breath sounds are present bilaterally.

_____

c. Gurgling is auscultated over the epigastric region during ventilation.

_____

d. Breath sounds are markedly diminished over the left lung.

_____

e. The patient's color deteriorates and the abdomen becomes distended.

_____

f. The bulb of the esophageal detector device fills in 8 seconds after placement on the end of the endotracheal tube.

_____

28. Fill in the blanks with the appropriate airway adjunct(s) from the following list:

Esophageal obturator   Esophageal gastric tube
  airway (EOA)   airway (EGTA)
Pharyngeal tracheal lumen (PtL) airway   None

a. _____ Permits direct gastric suction
b. _____ May be used if placed in trachea or esophagus
c. _____ May cause regurgitation on removal
d. _____ Permits ventilation that is as effective as with an endotracheal tube
e. _____ Requires 5 to 8 ml of air to inflate a balloon
f. _____ Requires a tight mask seal for effective use

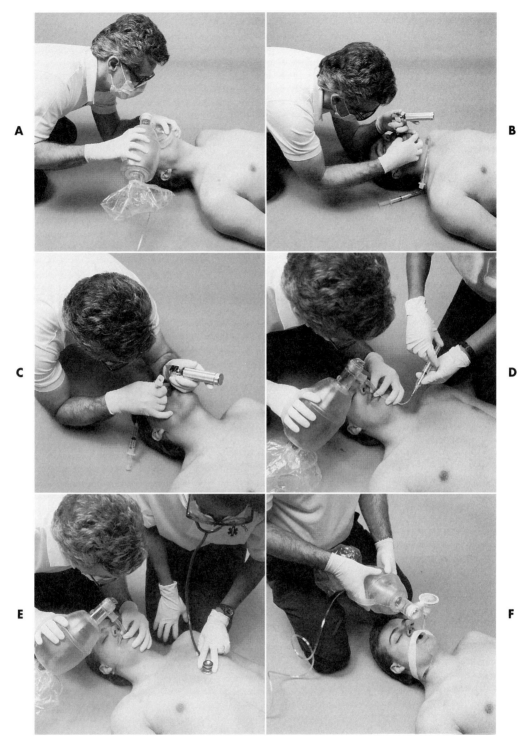

Figure 11-2

29. Briefly describe each step of the orotracheal intubation procedure illustrated
in Fig. 11-2.
    a.
    b.
    c.
    d.
    e.
    f.

30. List one advantage and one disadvantage for each of the following ventilation adjuncts:

Adjunct	Advantage	Disadvantage
a. Mouth to mouth		
b. Mouth to mask		
c. Bag-valve-mask		

31. List three patient situations in which use of tonsil-tip suction is indicated:
    a.
    b.
    c.

32. What precautions should be taken to prevent complications when using a whistle-tip suction device for tracheal suctioning?

_____

_____

33. Explain the anatomical basis for the following variations in pediatric airway management:
    a. The oral airway should be inserted only with direct visualization with a tongue blade, never upside down and then rotated:

_____

    b. Uncuffed endotracheal tubes should be used for children under 8 years of age:

_____

    c. The endotracheal tube may "hang up" in the newborn, necessitating use of the Sellick maneuver to attain successful placement:

_____

34. You are called to the home of an 86-year-old patient who fell down 12 steps. Her chief complaint is rib pain and shortness of breath. On physical examination, you note crepitus and bruising on the lower rib cage. Why is it important to provide rapid, aggressive intervention for this older patient?

_____

_____

● **STUDENT SELF-ASSESSMENT**

35. What is the term for the transfer of oxygen and carbon dioxide between the peripheral blood capillaries and tissue cells?
    a. External respiration   c. Pulmonary ventilation
    b. Internal respiration   d. Respiration

36. In what structure must continuous negative pressure be maintained to maintain lung expansion?
    a. Alveoli   c. Pleural space
    b. Mediastinum   d. Thoracic cage

37. When you arrive at the hospital, blood gasses on your 18-year-old patient indicate that the P_{O_2} is 70 mm Hg. What does this mean?
    a. 70% of the hemoglobin is filled with oxygen.
    b. The patient is adequately oxygenated.
    c. Less than 3 ml of oxygen is dissolved in 1 L of blood.
    d. The blood sample must have been venous.
38. Which of the following factors will result in an *increased* energy requirement for breathing?
    a. Loss of pulmonary surfactant
    c. An increase in lung compliance
    b. A decrease in airway resistance
    d. Bronchodilation
39. Which of the following patients is most likely to have a decreased minute volume?
    a. A 17-year-old with deep respirations and signs of hyperventilation
    b. A 20-year-old patient with a head injury with shallow, slow respirations
    c. An alert 45-year-old with a possible myocardial infarction
    d. A 30-year-old in early shock with an increased respiratory rate
40. Your patient is on a pulse oximeter, and the reading is 100% saturation. What does this mean?
    a. The patient is on 100% oxygen by mask.
    b. The partial pressure of oxygen is 100.
    c. All hemoglobin has converted to oxyhemoglobin.
    d. The blood will not carry any more oxygen.
41. Which of the following conditions causes decreased oxygenation secondary to increased resistance in the airways?
    a. Asbestosis
    c. Poliomyelitis
    b. Asthma
    d. Tuberculosis
42. Why might the tissues of a patient with anemia not be well oxygenated?
    a. The blood does not reach all tissue to off-load oxygen.
    b. The respiratory drive in the brain is depressed.
    c. There are insufficient red blood cells to carry oxygen.
    d. The pulmonary vessels are not well perfused with blood.
43. Respiratory chemoreceptors in the medulla, aortic bodies, and carotid bodies are stimulated by changes in all of the following except which one?
    a. Blood pressure
    c. Oxygen
    b. Carbon dioxide
    d. pH
44. If a person appears to be choking but can still speak and cough, what should the rescuer do?
    a. Deliver five back blows.
    b. Perform the Heimlich maneuver.
    c. Administer five chest thrusts.
    d. Not intervene but just observe.
45. What is the most frequent cause of airway obstruction in the unconscious adult?
    a. Hot dogs
    c. Tongue
    b. Steak
    d. Vomitus
46. You arrive at a private residence, where you find an unconscious 52-year-old man. You open his airway and determine that he is not breathing. You attempt to ventilate his lungs, but the airflow is blocked. What is your next step?
    a. Assess the pulse.
    b. Reposition the head.
    c. Administer five abdominal thrusts.
    d. Perform a cricothyrotomy.

47. Which of the following represents the *most* effective measure to prevent aspiration of stomach contents?
   a. Applying cricoid pressure during bag-valve-mask ventilation
   b. Frequent suctioning of the mouth using a tonsil-tip suction
   c. Inserting an oropharyngeal airway and nasogastric tube
   d. Positioning the patient in the modified Trendelenberg position
48. Your patient attempted suicide by hanging. She is hoarse and has hemoptysis and stridor. What do you suspect?
   a. Laryngeal fracture   c. Foreign body obstruction
   b. Laryngeal spasm   d. Tracheal injury
49. All of the following are potential complications of nasopharyngeal airway insertion except which one?
   a. It is poorly tolerated by sedated patients with gag reflexes.
   b. It may enter the esophagus if it is of excessive length.
   c. It may cause injury and bleeding to the nasal mucosa.
   d. It may become obstructed with blood or mucus.
50. To ensure adequate ventilation when an esophageal obturator airway is used, you must be certain that:
   a. The tube passes into the trachea.
   b. There is a tight mask seal.
   c. The patient is less than 5 feet tall.
   d. Breath sounds are audible over the gastric area.
51. The pharyngeal tracheal lumen airway may be used successfully if the tube is placed in which structure?
   a. The esophagus   c. The right mainstem bronchus
   b. The trachea   d. The esophagus or trachea
52. If 30 seconds have elapsed from the last ventilation and tracheal intubation has not been accomplished, what should you do?
   a. Remove the tube, hyperventilate, and try again.
   b. Continue if intubation can be done in a few more seconds.
   c. Insert an esophageal obturator airway.
   d. Have another paramedic attempt the skill.
53. Which of the following statements is true regarding percutaneous transtracheal ventilation?
   a. Demand valves may be used to provide adequate ventilations.
   b. It is a good long-term airway-management device.
   c. It minimizes the risk of aspiration.
   d. The high pressures generated may cause pneumothorax.
54. Which of the following is *not* an advantage of the bag-valve-mask device?
   a. It allows delivery of high oxygen concentrations.
   b. It can give the rescuer a sense of the patient's lung compliance.
   c. It is easily used by one rescuer to deliver ventilations.
   d. It can provide a wide range of inspiratory pressures.
55. Which of the following indicates a properly placed endotracheal tube?
   a. End tidal CO_2 shows purple during ventilation.
   b. Gurgling is heard during auscultation over the stomach.
   c. Esophageal detection bulb refills in 10 seconds.
   d. Oxygen saturation changes from 79% to 94%.
56. Which of the following statements is true regarding patient suctioning?
   a. Hyperventilation for 2 minutes should precede suctioning.
   b. Suction should be applied for a maximum of 30 seconds.
   c. Coughing may cause decreased intracranial pressure.
   d. Suction should be set between 200 and 300 mm Hg.

57. The patient who is on a nasal cannula at 5 L/min is receiving approximately how much oxygen?
    a. 36%   c. 44%
    b. 40%   d. 50%

58. Your patient has been removed from a smoky building and is confused and tachycardic. What is the appropriate oxygen-delivery device for this person?
    a. Nasal cannula   c. Simple face mask
    b. Nonrebreather mask   d. Venturi mask

59. Why might lidocaine be administered during rapid sequence induction for intubation?
    a. To minimize the potential for ventricular dysrhythmias
    b. To reduce the incidence of vomiting during the procedure
    c. To minimize the increase in ICP and prevent laryngospasm
    d. To anesthetize the airway structures and minimize the cough reflex

60. Which of the following complications related to cricothyrotomy will result in the absence of breath sounds when ventilation begins?
    a. Aspiration   c. Injury to the vocal cords
    b. False passage   d. Perforation of a great vessel

DIVISION THREE
PATIENT ASSESSMENT

HISTORY TAKING

● READING ASSIGNMENT
Chapter 12, pages 432-441, in *Mosby's Paramedic Textbook*, ed 2

● OBJECTIVES
As a paramedic, you should be able to:
1. Describe the purpose of effective history taking in prehospital patient care.
2. List components of the patient history as defined by the Department of Transportation.
3. Outline effective patient interviewing techniques to facilitate history taking.
4. Identify strategies to manage special challenges in obtaining a patient history.

● REVIEW QUESTIONS
Questions 1 and 2 pertain to the following case study:

> You are dispatched to a home to care for a 75-year-old woman who is having chest pain.

1. What additional questions will you need to ask related to her history?
   a. Present illness:

   _____

   _____

   b. Significant past medical history:

   _____

   _____

   c. Personal habits and environmental conditions:

   _____

   _____

   d. Family history:

   _____

   _____

2. What is her chief complaint?

---

3. Your elderly patient fell and has a painful wrist. Discuss any finding in each of the following elements of the SAMPLE history that may explain a reason for her fall.

S—

A—

M—

P—

L—

E—

4. For each of the following patient complaints, list any personal habits and environmental conditions that are important to know during the patient history:

  a. A 4-year-old child awakens suddenly with a sore throat, fever, muffled voice, dysphagia, and pain on swallowing:

---

  b. A 25-year-old soldier complains of fever, night sweats, weight loss, and hemoptysis:

---

  c. A 40-year-old is injured in a motor vehicle collision:

---

  d. An 18-year-old female is complaining of abdominal pain:

---

  e. A 72-year-old has slurred speech:

---

  f. A 45-year-old is complaining of depression:

---

  g. A 27-year-old has a heart rate of 50:

---

  h. A 77-year-old is dirty and has bruises in various stages of healing on the back and arms:

---

  i. A 16-year-old is extremely thin and frail looking:

---

5. Describe one technique to use when dealing with each of the following situations during the patient interview:
   a. Your elderly patient is clearly distraught and has a lengthy pause in his conversation as he relates a painful story to you:

   _____

   b. The patient begins a very long and complex history in much more detail than necessary:

   _____

   c. Within the first 60 seconds of your interview, your patient has related at least five different problems of varying severity:

   _____

   d. The patient is trembling and tearful despite a relatively minor injury:

   _____

   e. The patient asks you to tell her everything will be all right, when you know her condition is critical, and perhaps even lethal:

   _____

   f. A patient is verbally venting his anger and frustration about his illness:

   _____

   g. The patient strokes your leg in a sexually suggestive manner:

   _____

   h. The patient does not speak or understand your language:

   _____

● STUDENT SELF-ASSESSMENT

6. What is the purpose of obtaining a patient history?
   a. To obtain billing information
   b. To detect signs of injury
   c. To establish priorities of patient care
   d. To make the patient comfortable

7. Which of the following is a routine component of the patient history?
   a. Age   c. Religion
   b. Insurance information   d. Vital signs

8. Which of the following is true regarding the chief complaint in the patient history?
   a. It is always stated by the patient.
   b. It is usually the reason that EMS was called.
   c. It includes significant past medical history.
   d. It will remain the same throughout the call.

9. What might be a good question to ask during the history of present illness for a patient who is experiencing difficulty breathing?
   a. Did it start today?
   b. Is your difficulty breathing pretty bad?
   c. Where is your difficulty breathing?
   d. What makes your breathing better or worse?

10. Your patient is complaining of headache and chest tightness after an exposure to an unknown gas at work. What personal habits should you ask about for this patient?

    a. Exercise
    c. Sleep patterns
    b. Immunizations
    d. Smoking history

11. You plan to administer ketorolac tromethamine (Toradol) to a patient. You will not give it if your patient reports anaphylactic reaction to which drug?

    a. Acetaminophen (Tylenol)
    c. Meperidine (Demerol)
    b. Aspirin
    d. Penicillin

12. In which of the following situations is determination of last oral intake important?

    a. An adult with a corneal abrasion
    b. An adult with a small laceration on the forearm
    c. An adult with dizziness
    d. An adult with shoulder pain

13. Which of the following illnesses is not hereditary?

    a. Diabetes
    c. Sickle cell anemia
    b. Kidney disease
    d. Tuberculosis

14. You are called to care for a patient who is very depressed. Which statement may be most helpful?

    a. "Don't worry, we'll take good care of you."
    b. "Everything will be okay when we get you to the hospital."
    c. "My friend was depressed and he's just fine now."
    d. "It seems as though you are really sad, I'm here to listen."

15. What is a good approach when you are managing the angry or intoxicated patient who does not pose an immediate danger to self or the EMS crew?

    a. Physical restraint
    c. Threaten
    b. Set limits
    d. Yell

16. When interviewing the patient who has developmental delays, you should do which of the following?

    a. Clarify answers
    c. Omit most questions
    b. Not ask the patient
    d. Speak loudly

TECHNIQUES OF PHYSICAL EXAMINATION

● READING ASSIGNMENT

Chapter 13, pages 442-481, in *Mosby's Paramedic Textbook,* ed 2

● OBJECTIVES

As a paramedic, you should be able to:
1. Describe physical examination techniques commonly used in the prehospital setting.
2. Describe the examination equipment commonly used in the prehospital setting.
3. Describe the general approach to physical examination.
4. Outline the steps of a comprehensive physical examination.
5. Detail the components of the mental status examination.
6. Distinguish between normal and abnormal findings in the mental status examination.
7. Outline the steps in the general patient survey.
8. Distinguish between normal and abnormal findings in the general patient survey.
9. Describe physical examination techniques used for assessment of specific body regions.
10. Distinguish between normal and abnormal findings when assessing specific body regions.
11. State modifications to the physical examination that are necessary when assessing children.
12. State modifications to the physical examination that are necessary when assessing the older adult.

● REVIEW QUESTIONS

1-8 Match the sign in Column II with its definition in Column I. Use each answer only once.

Column I	Column II
1. _____ Persistent respiratory rate less than 12 breaths/min	a. Biot's
2. _____ Normal breath sounds heard over most lung fields	b. Bradypnea
3. _____ Low-pitched, rumbling expiratory sounds	c. Cheyne-Stokes
4. _____ Crowing sound associated with upper airway narrowing	d. Crackles
5. _____ Crescendo-decrescendo sequence of respirations followed by apnea	e. Rhonchi
6. _____ Irregular respirations interrupted by apneic periods	f. Stridor
7. _____ End inspiratory sounds associated with fluid in the small airways	g. Vesicular
8. _____ High-pitched airway noise resulting from lower airway narrowing	h. Wheezes

9-18 Match the term in Column II with the appropriate statement in Column I. Use each answer only once.

Column I

9. _____ The child with Down syndrome had a slanted opening between the upper and lower eyelids.
10. _____ The patient said the aliens were controlling him.
11. _____ The third degree burns affect the skin's resiliency.
12. _____ Malnutrition had caused the man to be very thin.
13. _____ The older patient staggered when he tried to walk.
14. _____ The paralyzed patient had a persistent erection.
15. _____ You see a semicircle of blood over the iris.
16. _____ The patient's cirrhosis made him look pregnant.
17. _____ After her stroke she had trouble making the muscles of her mouth form words.
18. _____ The alcoholic's wife told you the history he gave you was untrue.

Column II

a. Affect
b. Ascites
c. Ataxia
d. Confabulation
e. Delusions
f. Dysarthria
g. Emaciated
h. Hyphema
i. Hypopyon
j. Macula
k. Palpebral fissures
l. Priapism
m. Turgor

19. Describe the correct method to perform each of the following patient assessment techniques:

   a. Inspection:

   _____

   b. Palpation:

   _____

   c. Auscultation:

   _____

20. For each of the following deviations from normal pupil response, list a cause:

Abnormality	Cause
a. Dilated/unresponsive	
b. Constricted/unresponsive	
c. Unequal/one dilated and unresponsive	
d. Dull/lackluster	

21. Your patient is a teenage assault victim who was struck repeatedly on the head with a baseball bat.

   a. List the 10 steps in the comprehensive physical examination.

   1.
   2.
   3.
   4.
   5.
   6.
   7.
   8.
   9.
   10.

b. List the components of the mental status examination for this patient.

_____

_____

c. Describe your physical examination of this patient's head and neck, detailing specific examination techniques and the types of normal or abnormal findings you would look for (include ophthalmoscopic and otoscopic examination techniques).

_____

_____

_____

_____

22. You are called to evaluate a patient whose chief complaint is difficulty breathing. Explain your assessment of the thorax.

_____

_____

23. Your 56-year-old patient has a history of right upper quadrant abdominal pain, malaise, nausea, and vomiting. He is jaundiced and complains of itching. Past history reveals heavy alcohol use. You suspect hepatitis. Describe your physical examination of this patient's abdomen.

_____

_____

24. You are examining a patient involved in a motor vehicle collision whose automobile was struck on his side. The patient complains of considerable pain in the pelvic area. The primary survey has been completed. The patient's pulse is elevated but blood pressure is within normal limits. Describe your examination of this patient's pelvic area.

_____

_____

25. Your crew arrives at the home of an older patient whose family states that she complained of weakness on one side, stumbled, and fell down five steps. No life-threatening conditions are found in the primary survey, and vital sign assessment reveals a moderately elevated blood pressure and pulse. The patient is slightly confused but cooperative. You suspect a stroke. Describe your assessment of this patient's extremities.

_____

_____

26. A painter has fallen approximately 20 feet, striking a scaffold rail with his lower back. Primary survey and vital signs are normal. Outline your physical examination of this patient's back.

_____

_____

27. Complete the information that is missing in the following, which outlines examination techniques for cranial nerves.

Cranial Nerve Number(s)	Cranial Nerve Name(s)	Assessment Technique
I		Test smell with ammonia inhalants
II		
	Optic	
III	Oculomotor	Test EOMs by asking the patient to look up and down, to the left and right, and diagonally up and down to the left and right
IV	Trochlear	
VI		
V		
	Facial	Note facial symmetry, tics, or abnormal movement; have patient raise eyebrows, frown, show upper and lower teeth, smile, and puff out cheeks; have patient close eyes tightly and resist while you try to open lids
VIII		
IX		
X		
	Spinal accessory	
XII		

28. List four general guidelines that are helpful when approaching a pediatric patient.
    a.
    b.
    c.
    d.

29. Describe two specific developmental differences of the children in each of the following age groups that influence patient assessment:
    a. Birth to 6 months:

    _____

    b. 7 months to 3 years:

    _____

    c. 4 to 10 years:

    _____

    d. Adolescence:

    _____

30. Describe two special considerations and techniques that may be useful when caring for an older patient.

_____

_____

● **STUDENT SELF-ASSESSMENT**

31. Auscultation is the examination technique that involves which of the following?
   a. Listening with a stethoscope
   b. Feeling for masses and assessing for crepitus
   c. Looking for signs of illness
   d. Tapping the body with your finger

32. Which instrument is used to evaluate the retina, macula, and optic nerve disc?
   a. Ophthalmoscope   **c.** Penlight
   b. Otoscope   **d.** Sphygmomanometer

33. Using an adult blood pressure cuff to evaluate a child's blood pressure can result in which of the following?
   a. False low reading   **c.** Normal reading
   b. False high reading   **d.** Inability to inflate cuff

34. What is the most important information to guide your physical examination of the patient?
   a. Medications and specific doses
   b. Past medical history
   c. Present illness and chief complaint
   d. Vital signs, including blood pressure

35. Which of the following is a component of the comprehensive physical examination?
   a. Chief complaint   **c.** Vascular access
   b. History of present illness **d.** Vital signs

36. Which of the following is a component of the mental status examination?
   a. Distal pulses   **c.** Speech and language
   b. Pupil reaction   **d.** Visual acuity

37. Which of the following is the clearest way to report an altered level of consciousness?
   a. The patient is obtunded.
   b. The patient is semiconscious.
   c. The patient is stuporous.
   d. The patient is unresponsive to pain.

38. Patient memory and attention can be assessed with which of the following?
   a. AVPU method   **c.** General survey
   b. Digit span   **d.** Glasgow coma scale

39. Your patient walks with a limp. What is this known as?
   a. An abnormal gait   **c.** Bizarre posture
   b. Ataxia   **d.** Cranial nerve palsy

40. An odor of acetone on the breath is associated with which condition?
   a. Alcohol use   **c.** Diabetic conditions
   b. Bowel obstruction   **d.** Poor dental hygiene

41. A patient who tells you that he is very depressed and suicidal but has an expressionless face may be said to have which condition?
   a. Altered affect   **c.** Altered attention
   b. Altered appearance   **d.** Altered emotion

42. Which sign of distress may be found in a patient who has cardiorespiratory insufficiency, pain, or anxiety?
    a. Bradycardia   c. Sweating
    b. Cough   d. Wincing
43. Skin color is best assessed by observing the skin on what part of the body?
    a. Arms   c. Legs
    b. Face   d. Nailbeds
44. When you are assessing an axillary temperature using a standard mercury thermometer, what is the minimum time the thermometer should be in place to obtain an accurate temperature?
    a. 4 minutes   c. 8 minutes
    b. 5 minutes   d. 10 minutes
45. What is the proper sequence for examination of the abdomen?
    a. Auscultation, inspection, palpation
    b. Inspection, palpation, auscultation
    c. Inspection, auscultation, palpation
    d. Auscultation, palpation, inspection
46. Which of the following findings during examination of the nails is consistent with chronic respiratory or cardiac disease?
    a. Beau's lines   c. Paronychia
    b. Clubbing   d. Terry's nails
47. What should you do to verify that vision is present?
    a. Assess bilateral pupil response to light.
    b. Ask the patient to count fingers at a distance.
    c. Lightly touch the cornea with a cotton swab.
    d. Palpate the globe for firmness.
48. To perform an effective otoscopic examination of the ear, you should pull the ear in what direction?
    a. Down and back in adults   c. Down and back in infants
    b. Down and forward in adults   d. Down and forward in infants
49. What physical finding may be encountered in patients who are pregnant, have leukemia, or are taking phenytoin?
    a. Enlarged gums   c. Swollen eyelids
    b. Nasal bleeding   d. Tonsillar exudate
50. Chest wall diameter may be increased in patients with what condition?
    a. Heart disease
    b. Implanted cardiac pacemaker
    c. Obstructive pulmonary disease
    d. Rib fractures
51. Which sound may be heard during percussion if there is hyperinflation due to pulmonary disease, pneumothorax, or asthma?
    a. Dullness   c. Resonance
    b. Flatness   d. Hyperresonance
52. Which of the following is true regarding assessment of breath sounds?
    a. Normal breath sounds are louder on exhalation.
    b. The stethoscope bell is used to auscultate the lungs.
    c. The patient's mouth should be open.
    d. The patient should be in the supine position.
53. For maximal effectiveness, where should heart sounds be auscultated?
    a. Over the left anterior axillary line
    b. Over the left fifth intercostal space
    c. Over the sternal angle
    d. Over the xiphoid process
54. Simultaneous palpation of the apical and carotid pulses whereby each apical beat is not transmitted is known as which of the following?
    a. Mean arterial pressure   c. Pulsus paradoxus
    b. Pulse deficit   d. Pulse pressure

55. All of the following may cause muffled heart sounds except which one?
    a. Cardiac tamponade
    c. Obstructive lung disease
    b. Obesity
    d. Myocardial infarction

56. What is a palpable tremor over a blood vessel called?
    a. Bruit
    c. Thrill
    b. Murmur
    d. Vibration

57. During the vascular examination, the anterior surface of the foot should be palpated to detect which pulse?
    a. Brachial pulse
    c. Popliteal pulse
    b. Dorsalis pedis pulse
    d. Posterior tibial pulse

58. If a deformity and point tenderness are noted on examination of the pelvis, what condition should you consider?
    a. Appendicitis
    c. Ruptured ectopic pregnancy
    b. Internal hemorrhage
    d. Spinal cord injury

59. To evaluate motor function in the lower extremities, you should instruct the patient to do what?
    a. Flex and extend the feet and lower and upper legs.
    b. Lift and hold both legs in the air while lying supine.
    c. Move the legs laterally as far as possible bilaterally.
    d. Push the soles of the feet against the paramedic's palms.

60. Which of the following is an example of a test to evaluate gait?
    a. Have the patient hop in place.
    b. Have the patient do the Romberg test.
    c. Have the patient touch each heel to the opposite shin.
    d. Have the patient touch the finger to the nose, alternating hands.

61. Your patient is a 2-year-old in respiratory distress. Level of consciousness, spontaneous movement, respiratory effort, and skin color can be most effectively evaluated when the child is in which position?
    a. Held by the paramedic
    c. On the stretcher
    b. Held by the parent
    d. Sitting in a chair

62. A young child has an obviously fractured lower leg. Which of the following statements is *false* regarding care of this patient?
    a. Remain calm and confident.
    b. Separate the parents from the child.
    c. Establish rapport with the parents.
    d. Be honest with the child and parents.

63. Which of the following statements is *true* regarding the physical examination of a 2-year-old child?
    a. Abdominal breathing is normal in this age group.
    b. Patient modesty should be a primary concern.
    c. Explanations should be given for each activity.
    d. Separation anxiety will not be a problem.

64. When examining the older patient, what should you do?
    a. Always speak loudly because most of these patients are deaf.
    b. Assume that memory impairment is present.
    c. Anticipate numerous health problems and medications.
    d. Not expect any variation in the examination.

CHAPTER 14
PATIENT ASSESSMENT

● READING ASSIGNMENT

Chapter 14, pages 482-491, in *Mosby's Paramedic Textbook*, ed 2

● OBJECTIVES

As a paramedic, you should be able to:
1. Identify the components of the scene size-up.
2. Identify the priorities in each component of patient assessment.
3. Outline the critical steps in initial patient assessment.
4. Describe findings in the initial assessment that may indicate a life-threatening condition.
5. Discuss interventions for life-threatening conditions that are identified in the initial assessment.
6. Identify the components of the focused history and physical examination for medical patients.
7. Identify the components of the focused history and physical examination for trauma patients.
8. List the components of the detailed physical examination.
9. Describe the ongoing assessment.
10. Distinguish priorities in the care of the medical versus trauma patient.

● REVIEW QUESTIONS

Questions 1-15 pertain to the following case study:

> You are dispatched from your base on a cold, snowy winter night, to a motor vehicle crash with injuries on the highway.

1. After ensuring safety, list five priorities during your scene size-up/assessment on this call.
   a.
   b.
   c.
   d.
   e.

> You find one patient, the driver of a car involved in a single-car collision. He was not restrained and has been ejected approximately 15 feet from the car. You find him lying motionless in a safe location.

2. What are three goals of your initial assessment of this patient?
   a.
   b.
   c.
3. What information have you already gathered to form your general impression of this patient?

4. What mnemonic can be used to quickly assess his level of consciousness?

As you approach the patient you see some slight movement and note a gurgling sound in his mouth. He responds to pain only.

5. What could be causing gurgling in his airway?

_____

_____

6. What personal protective equipment should you be wearing?

_____

_____

7. What measures will you use to secure this patient's airway?

_____

_____

8. How should the breathing be evaluated?

_____

_____

_____

The patient has a dusky color and slow, agonal respirations.

9. What care should be initiated based on this finding?

_____

_____

10. What assessment techniques will you use in the initial assessment to evaluate circulatory status?

_____

_____

You palpate a very rapid carotid pulse but *cannot* detect a radial pulse. His skin is pale and cool, and capillary refill is very slow.

11. What criteria for priority patients does this patient meet?

_____

_____

12. List the components of the focused history and physical examination that you will perform on this patient.

_____

_____

You note numerous facial lacerations and crepitus of the facial bones. He has an abrasion on the lateral chest and abdominal area. His left lower arm is deformed, and his left ankle is swollen.

13. What care should be provided before transport for this patient?

_____

14. What should be your goal for scene time on this type of call?

_____

15. Outline the components of the reassessment and the time interval at which they should be performed.

_____

Questions 16-20 pertain to the following case study:

You are dispatched to a home for a call of a patient with "difficulty breathing." Your initial scene assessment reveals no hazards and you enter the patient's bedroom to begin your assessment and care.

16. What information will you gather as you enter the room that will help form your general impression of the patient?

_____

_____

The patient, an elderly black female, is awake and appears to be in respiratory distress.

17. How will you further assess the following to determine her condition?
    a. Airway

_____

    b. Breathing

_____

    c. Circulation

_____

You note that the patient is speaking in broken sentences because she must stop often to catch her breath. She has wheezes throughout her lungs and intercostal muscle retractions and her mucous membranes and nailbeds are blue. Her pulse is 124 (regular and strong in the radial artery), and her skin is damp.

18. List two criteria that she meets indicating she is a priority patient who needs stabilization and rapid transport.
    a.
    b.

19. List four types of information that should be gathered in the focused history portion of this patient's examination.
    a.
    b.
    c.
    d.

20. How might the care of this patient differ from that given to a critically ill trauma patient?

---

21. You arrive on the scene of a rollover motor vehicle crash involving a small sports car. Which of the following is a component in scene size-up/assessment on this call?
    a. Begin definitive patient care activities.
    b. Contact medical direction with an initial report.
    c. Initiate a mass casualty plan if indicated.
    d. Notify dispatch to send more resources if needed.

22. During which phase of the patient assessment will the first vital signs be assessed?
    a. Detailed physical examination
    b. Focused physical examination
    c. Initial assessment
    d. Ongoing assessment

23. During the initial assessment of a trauma patient, what is the most appropriate method to assess the neurological status?
    a. AVPU
    b. Determination of EOM function
    c. Pupil assessment
    d. Reflex examination

24. Which of the following patient situations represents a life threat identified in the initial assessment of an adult?
    a. Blood pressure in the right arm is much greater than in the left arm.
    b. Heart rate increases by 30 beats/min when the patient stands up.
    c. Stridor is audible.
    d. Temperature is 105.8°F (41°C).

25. You detect that the patient has agonal respirations and a radial pulse during your initial assessment. How should your care and assessment proceed?
    a. Auscultate the chest to determine the proper intervention.
    b. Continue assessment and then manage respiratory failure.
    c. Initiate airway management and ventilation and then proceed.
    d. Treat the respiratory difficulty and transport with no further examination.

26. What should be the primary determinant of the extent of the focused history and physical examination of the patient?
    a. Patient's overall condition and level of consciousness
    b. Age and preexisting illness
    c. Response time to the closest appropriate hospital
    d. Results of the initial vital sign assessment

27. You respond to a call to aid a person who has fallen 25 feet and is complaining of severe pain in the finger. Which of the following is a component of the focused history and physical examination for this patient?
    a. Continued spinal immobilization
    b. Detailed examination of the finger
    c. Initiation of intravenous fluid therapy
    d. Otoscopic examination of the eyes

28. In which of the following cases is the paramedic most likely to perform a detailed physical examination?
    a. A 2-year-old is acutely dyspneic and cyanotic.
    b. A pale 40-year-old was shot in the chest.
    c. A 59-year-old is weak and diaphoretic.
    d. A 67-year-old patient is in cardiac arrest.

29. What should be included in the ongoing assessment of the patient?
   a. Detailed physical examination
   b. Head-to-toe examination
   c. Repetition of the initial assessment
   d. Vital sign assessment only

30. What should *not* be included in the scene management of the critical trauma patient?
   a. Airway control
   b. Intravenous fluid therapy
   c. Major fracture stabilization
   d. Spinal immobilization

CHAPTER 15
CLINICAL DECISION MAKING

● **READING ASSIGNMENT**

Chapter 15, pages 492-499, in *Mosby's Paramedic Textbook,* ed 2

● **OBJECTIVES**

1. List the key elements of paramedic practice.
2. Discuss the limitations of protocols, standing orders, and patient care algorithms.
3. Outline the key components of the critical thinking process for paramedics.
4. Identify elements necessary for an effective critical thinking process.
5. Describe situations that may necessitate the use of the critical thinking process while delivering prehospital patient care.
6. Describe the six elements required for effective clinical decision making in the prehospital setting.

● **REVIEW QUESTIONS**

1. List the four key elements of paramedic practice described in this chapter.
   a.
   b.
   c.
   d.
2. Why is it difficult to follow standard protocols, standing orders, and patient care algorithms in the following situations?
   a. A patient does not speak your language. He appears very ill, is pale and diaphoretic, and has a very slow, irregular heartbeat. He gets very anxious and pulls away when you attempt to establish an intravenous line to give medications.

   b. A patient with chronic obstructive pulmonary disease has signs and symptoms of heart failure and is wheezing.

   c. An elderly patient with severe kyphosis (hunchback posture) has fallen but screams in pain when you attempt to immobilize him on the spine board.

   d. A child choked on a toy and is stridorous. Each time you approach to assess her, she begins to cry and has increased distress.

Question 3 pertains to the following case study:

An elderly patient is complaining of chest pain that began 30 minutes ago. She tells you that it began suddenly when she was reading the paper. It is crushing and substernal, rating an "8" on a 1 to 10 scale. It does not radiate, but she feels nauseated and is diaphoretic. Your assessment reveals normal vital signs, clear breath sounds, and no other obvious clinical findings. A 12-lead ECG demonstrates ST segment elevation in leads V_1 and V_2. You and your partner recognize that her presentation is consistent with septal myocardial infarction. You immediately begin oxygen, initiate an intravenous line, and administer nitroglycerin and aspirin. You notify medical direction and transmit the ECG, anticipating the need for cardiac catheterization. You reevaluate her vital signs, breath sounds, and level of pain every 5 minutes during the 15-minute transport to the hospital. During the following shift your supervisor gives you feedback on the patient's outcome. During the run critique everyone agrees that the care was good, but the scene time was somewhat long. During the ensuing discussion, you identify ways to decrease scene times on future calls.

3. Identify which parts of this scenario demonstrate each of the following phases of the critical thinking process:
   a. Concept formation:

   b. Data interpretation:

   c. Application of principle:

   d. Evaluation:

   e. Reflection on action:

4. List five steps that may be taken to help the paramedic think clearly in highly stressful situations.
   a.
   b.
   c.
   d.
   e.
5. List the six "Rs" for effective clinical decision making.
   a.
   b.
   c.
   d.
   e.
   f.

● **STUDENT SELF-ASSESSMENT**

6. To practice effectively as a paramedic, you should be able to do which of the following?
   a. Gather, evaluate, and synthesize information
   b. Know all current medical techniques
   c. Make diagnoses and provide definitive care
   d. Teach your personal values to patients
7. Which of the following is an advantage of protocols, standing orders, and patient care protocols?
   a. They don't relate well when numerous disease etiologies coexist.
   b. They may not apply to nonspecific patient complaints that do not fit the model.
   c. They promote a standardized approach to patient care for classic presentations.
   d. They promote linear thinking and cookbook medicine in all situations.

129

8. You recognize that a patient is hypoglycemic based on the history, physical examination, and blood analysis. What phase of the critical thinking process have you entered when you initiate an intravenous line and administer glucose?
   a. Application of principle   c. Data interpretation
   b. Concept formation   d. Reflection on action
9. In which of the following situations is a paramedic most likely to use critical thinking skills?
   a. The monitor shows ventricular fibrillation.
   b. The blood glucose strip reads 40 mg/dl.
   c. The patient stops breathing and becomes cyanotic.
   d. The trauma patient has severe neck pain but is dyspneic when supine.
10. Which of the following is *not* one of the six elements described in the text as being needed for effective clinical decision making?
   a. React
   b. Read the scene
   c. Request consultation with medical direction
   d. Review performance at run critique

COMMUNICATIONS

● READING ASSIGNMENT

Chapter 16, pages 500-513, in *Mosby's Paramedic Textbook,* ed 2

● OBJECTIVES

As a paramedic, you should be able to:
1. Outline the phases of EMS communications.
2. Describe the role of communications in EMS.
3. Define common EMS communication terms.
4. Describe the primary modes of EMS communication.
5. Describe the role of dispatching as it applies to prehospital emergency medical care.
6. Describe how EMS communication is regulated.
7. Outline techniques for relaying EMS communications clearly and effectively.

● REVIEW QUESTIONS

Match the communication term in Column II with the appropriate definition in Column I. Use each answer only once.

Column I	Column II
1. _____ A unit of frequency equal to one cycle per second	a. Base station
2. _____ The ability to transmit or receive in one direction at a time	b. Duplex
3. _____ A grouping of radio equipment that includes a transmitter and receiver	c. Hertz
4. _____ Radio frequencies between 300 and 3000 MHz	d. Kilohertz
5. _____ The ability to transmit and receive simultaneously through two different frequencies	e. Megahertz
6. _____ A unit of frequency equal to 1,000,000 cycles per second	f. Mobile station
7. _____ Radio frequencies between 30 and 300 MHz	g. Remote console
8. _____ A unit that receives transmissions from a mobile radio and retransmits them at higher power on another frequency	h. Repeater
	i. Simplex
	j. UHF
	k. VHF

9. A person is stabbed with a knife. List the five phases of communications that occur on most EMS calls such as this.
   a.
   b.
   c.
   d.
   e.

10. A man is seriously injured at a rural site. Describe the communication process from the time of his injury until the EMS crew returns to service.

_____

_____

_____

_____

_____

11. List three common causes of interference with radio transmissions.
    a.
    b.
    c.
12. Briefly describe four responsibilities of an EMS dispatcher.
    a.
    b.
    c.
    d.
13. List three essential pieces of information that the dispatcher must obtain from a bystander who calls in to report a motor vehicle crash.
    a.
    b.
    c.
14. Identify three ways in which the Federal Communications Commission directly influences EMS.
    a.
    b.
    c.
15. Describe six actions the paramedic may take to ensure clear and understandable radio transmissions.
    a.
    b.
    c.
    d.
    e.
    f.

Johnny Smith, a paramedic who works on City Unit 7, is called to an industrial site. He finds a 30-year-old patient lying on his back on the grass, where he landed after falling 20 feet from a painting platform. On the paramedic's arrival at 1:00 PM, the patient's vital signs are as follows: blood pressure 120/80, pulse 116, and respiration 20. He states he became dizzy and fell. When Smith palpates, the patient complains of pain in the lumbar region of the back and on both heels, which are swollen. Distal pulses, sensation, and movement are present in all extremities. Lung sounds are clear and equal bilaterally. The patient gives Smith his name and knows the date and time and where he is. His skin is warm and dry. The patient weighs approximately 100 kg and takes ibuprofen prescribed by Dr. Jones for back pain. Smith places him on 100% oxygen via nonrebreather mask, positions him on a backboard with cervical collar, and notifies Dr. Kane, the online medical physician, of the patient's condition and the 15-minute estimated arrival time to City Hospital. Vital signs at 1:25 PM are unchanged. The patient's condition remains the same en route.

16. Write a concise, complete radio report to communicate the appropriate information regarding this patient to the base hospital.

_____

_____

_____

_____

_____

_____

_____

_____

_____

_____

_____

_____

_____

● STUDENT SELF-ASSESSMENT

17. What is manipulation of the intended idea for communication known as?
    a. Decoding   **c.** Feedback
    b. Encoding   **d.** Receiving

18. After being called to an airplane crash with two seriously injured patients, the first arriving EMS crew tells online medical direction, "There are people (meaning bystanders) everywhere." The physician interprets this to indicate a mass casualty situation and activates the MCI plan. What type of communication error occurred here?
    a. Attributes of the receiver   **c.** Semantic problems
    b. Selective perception   **d.** Time pressures

19. Which of the following is a component of a simple communication system?
    a. Remote console   **c.** Mobile unit
    b. Microwave links   **d.** Satellite receivers

20. What is a radio receiver circuit used for suppressing the audio portion of unwanted radio noises or signals called?
    a. Decibel   **c.** Squelch
    b. Frequency modulation   **d.** Tone

21. What is the term for the number of repetitive cycles per second completed by a radio wave?
    a. Amplitude modulation   c. Range
    b. Frequency   d. Wattage
22. What is transmission and reception of electrocardiograms over the radio or telephone called?
    a. Coverage   c. Patch
    b. Hotline   d. Telemetry
23. What are the HEAR and EACOM radios used to tie hospitals together and receive and transmit tone pulses known as?
    a. Cellular telephones   c. Microwave transmitters
    b. Decoders and encoders   d. Satellite dishes
24. Which component of a communication system receives transmissions from a low-power portable radio on one frequency and simultaneously retransmits it at a higher power on another frequency?
    a. Mobile transceivers   c. Remote console
    b. Portable radios   d. Repeaters
25. How is the strongest signal selected when numerous satellite receivers are used?
    a. Base stations   c. Decoders
    b. Cellular lines   d. Voting systems
26. What are dispatch services located away from base stations that facilitate communications with field personnel known as?
    a. Complex systems   c. Portable transceivers
    b. Mobile transceivers   d. Remote consoles
27. What is an advantage of communication with cellular telephones?
    a. They allow unlimited channel access.
    b. They permit uninterrupted communication.
    c. They provide a secure link between EMS and the hospital.
    d. They transmit simultaneous calls in disaster situations.
28. Which of the following is not a responsibility of the dispatcher?
    a. Dispatching EMS resources
    b. Coordinating with public safety services
    c. Receiving calls for assistance
    d. Providing offline medical control
29. What is a function of prearrival instructions?
    a. To allow EMS personnel to be disregarded
    b. To determine whether the call is unfounded
    c. To provide life-saving instructions
    d. To allow the EMS crew more time to respond
30. What is the role of the FCC?
    a. To consult with EMS agencies regarding radio equipment
    b. To develop new radio technologies
    c. To monitor frequencies for appropriate usage
    d. To train dispatchers in prearrival instructions
31. Which of the following is a technique for effective radio communication?
    a. Speak at a range of 6 to 8 inches from the microphone
    b. Speak slowly and clearly and enunciate words distinctly
    c. Show emotion to demonstrate the urgency of critical situations
    d. Take your time and include all patient information available
32. Which is *not* a component of the SOAP format for patient reports?
    a. Assessment data   c. Patient information
    b. Objective data   d. Subjective information

DOCUMENTATION

● **READING ASSIGNMENT**

Chapter 17, pages 514-523, in *Mosby's Paramedic Textbook*, ed 2

● **OBJECTIVES**

1. Identify the purpose of the prehospital care report.
2. Describe the uses of the prehospital care report.
3. Outline the components of an accurate, thorough prehospital care report.
4. Describe the elements of a properly written EMS document.
5. Describe an effective system for documentation of prehospital patient care.
6. Identify differences necessary when documenting special situations.
7. Describe the appropriate method to make revisions or corrections to the prehospital care report.
8. Recognize consequences that may result from inappropriate documentation.

● **REVIEW QUESTIONS**

Questions 1 and 2 pertain to the following case study:

> You are a paramedic working on Unit 4017 and are dispatched to a private residence on a call for a "person down." On arrival at the scene at 14:00, you find a 20-year-old woman lying on the lawn in front of the house. She is awake but is saying inappropriate words. The patient's husband tells you that his wife is diabetic and takes insulin, but she missed lunch. He says he found her confused in the yard. Her skin is pale, cool, and diaphoretic, respiratory rate is 20 and unlabored with clear breath sounds in all fields, radial pulse is 120, and her blood pressure is 110/70 mm Hg. While your partner initates an IV in the right antecubital space at 14:06, you measure the patient's blood blood glucose level, which is 50 mg/dl. Following your standing orders, you begin an IV of normal saline and then at 14:08 25 g (50 ml) of D50W is administered through the IV. Within 2 minutes the patient looks at you and asks, "Why are you here?" She is now alert and answering appropriately, and by the time her husband reminds her what has happened, she is completely oriented to person, place, and time. She agrees to be transported to General Hospital, and the ambulance departs the scene at 14:13. While en route, you call a report to Dr. Smith, and at 14:16 another set of vital signs reveals the following: BP 118/74, P 96/min, R 20/min with warm, dry pink skin. She denies allergies to medicine and states she took 10 units of regular and 20 units of lente insulin at 07:00. On arrival to the hospital at 14:20, there is no change in the patient's condition and you note that 100 ml of the IV fluid has been infused. Your partner restocks your bag with the supplies used, which include a 250 ml bag of normal saline, macrodrip IV tubing, an 18G IV catheter, and D50W.

1. Write a narrative documenting your findings on this patient as you would on your state patient care report (assuming there is no check-box format on your report).

_____

_____

_____

_____

_____

_____

_____

_____

_____

_____

_____

_____

2. List at least four activities your patient care report from this call may be used for.

_____

_____

3. Describe the appropriate method to complete documentation for each of the following situations:
   a. Your patient lacerated his hand. The wound is deep and gaping and he cannot move two of his fingers. He is refusing care and says he will go to his doctor tomorrow.

_____

_____

   b. You are responding to a call for a "full arrest." Before you arrive on scene, the dispatcher notifies you to disregard the call. You go back in service and return to your station.

_____

_____

   c. More than 100 patients are complaining of burning eyes and throats and difficulty breathing after an industrial gas release. You are providing care in the treatment sector.

_____

_____

_____

   d. You have just returned to your engine house from the hospital when you realize that you did not document some essential information about the patient's history on the patient care report.

_____

_____

_____

4. What is a possible consequence of failure to document the following information in a patient care report?
   a. The trauma patient reports an allergy to tetanus vaccine. He is unconscious when you arrive in the emergency department.

_____

_____

_____

   b. You administered the maximum dosage of lidocaine to a patient who was in ventricular tachycardia but neglected to document it on your patient care report.

_____

_____

_____

   c. The patient fell earlier in the day and is unconscious on arrival to the emergency department. You do not document that the patient takes warfarin (Coumadin) daily.

_____

_____

_____

   d. You fail to note that a patient had numbness in his arm before spinal immobilization.

_____

_____

_____

5. What is the purpose of the patient care report?
   a. To document patient assessment
   b. To document patient care
   c. To document patient transport
   d. To document all of the above

6. Which of the following is not an appropriate use of the patient care report?
   a. Administrative and billing information
   b. Legal record of sequence of care provided
   c. Research document for the local press
   d. Supply inventory tracking

7. Which of the following should *not* be documented on the patient care report?
   a. Chronological description of events that occurred during the call
   b. Circumstances documenting that the paramedic fell during care of this patient
   c. Difficulties encountered during patient care, treatment, and transport
   d. Time of call, dispatch, arrival at scene, arrival at hospital, and back in service

8. If the respiratory rate section is not completed on the ambulance reporting form, what should the physician assume about patient respirations?
   a. They were not an important vital sign assessment
   b. They were not pertinent in this patient section
   c. They were not specifically assessed by the paramedic
   d. They were within normal limits for the patient age group

9. When a patient refuses care, what must the paramedic document?
   a. Advice given to the patient regarding the condition
   b. Nothing is needed as long as the patient was alert and oriented.
   c. The detailed physical examination
   d. The patient's insurance information

10. What should you document when your response is canceled en route to the scene?
    a. Canceling authority and time of cancellation
    b. No documentation is needed in this situation.
    c. Scene size-up information
    d. You must still respond and obtain an AMA.

11. You are leaving work and suddenly realize you forgot to document a crucial piece of information about patient care on a patient record. What should you do?
    a. Ask your supervisor to fill in the essential information.
    b. Note the date and time the correction was made on the appropriate form.
    c. Wait until you return to work after your 4-day break to finish it.
    d. You may not add anything after the report is complete.

DIVISION FOUR
TRAUMA

CHAPTER 18
TRAUMA SYSTEMS AND MECHANISM OF INJURY

● READING ASSIGNMENT
Chapter 18, pages 526-549, in *Mosby's Paramedic Textbook*, ed 2

● OBJECTIVES
As a paramedic, you should be able to:
1. Describe the incidence and scope of traumatic injuries and deaths.
2. Identify the role of each component of the trauma system.
3. Predict injury patterns based upon a knowledge of the laws of physics related to forces involved in trauma.
4. Describe injury patterns that should be suspected when injury occurs related to a specific type of blunt trauma.
5. Describe the role of restraints in injury prevention and injury patterns.
6. Discuss how organ motion may contribute to injury in each body region depending on the forces applied.
7. Identify selected injury patterns associated with motorcycle and ATV collisions.
8. Describe injury patterns associated with pedestrian collisions.
9. Identify injury patterns associated with sports injuries, blast injuries, and vertical falls.
10. Describe factors that influence tissue damage related to penetrating injury.

● REVIEW QUESTIONS
Match the appropriate energy law listed in Column II with its description in Column I.

	Column I		Column II
1. _____	Force is equal to mass times acceleration or deceleration.	a.	Newton's first law of motion
2. _____	Equal to ½ mass × velocity².	b.	Newton's second law of motion
3. _____	An object at rest or in motion remains in that state unless force is applied.	c.	Conservation of energy law
4. _____	Energy can neither be created nor destroyed; it can only change form.	d.	Joule's law
		e.	Kinetic energy law

5. Identify three causes of death for each of the periods of the trimodal distribution of traumatic death; for each period, identify prehospital interventions that may increase patient survival.

    a. Immediate:

    b. Early:

    c. Late:

6. A 17-year-old female falls asleep at the wheel, rides the median for 50 feet, and then strikes a concrete bridge abutment head-on.

    a. Identify the three collisions that occur in this situation.

    b. Assuming that this driver took the down-and-under pathway during the collision, what injuries should you anticipate?

7. Aside from speed and size, what factor affects the injury pattern found in a lateral impact collision?

8. In which of the following rear-end collisions will damage be greater, assuming that mass and other factors are equal? Why?

    a. A vehicle traveling 50 mph is struck by a vehicle traveling 70 mph.

    b. A vehicle traveling 5 mph is struck by a vehicle traveling 40 mph.

9. For each of the body regions, list the injury or injuries that may occur during sudden rapid deceleration.

    a. Head and neck injuries:

    b. Thoracic injuries:

    c. Abdominal injuries:

10. You are called to the scene of a high-speed frontal crash caused by a cross-over accident. The driver of one of the vehicles complains of severe dyspnea and has a large circular bruise on her chest. You note markedly decreased lung sounds on the right side of the chest and suspect a pneumothorax.
   a. What traumatic mechanism can cause a pneumothorax in this example?

   b. The driver of the other vehicle has severe abdominal pain and is exhibiting signs of hypovolemic shock. Which abdominal organs or structures can be injured from sudden compression of the abdomen?

11. Identify the type of motorcycle collision most frequently associated with the pattern of injuries listed:
   a. A seasoned biker has a severely angulated fracture of the right forearm and extensive abrasions to the right side of the body.

   b. A 47-year-old executive has bilateral fractured femurs and facial injuries.

   c. A traffic officer has a severe crush injury to the left lower leg.

12. Identify the injuries to be anticipated in the following situations:
   a. A motorist swerves across the highway and is struck by an oncoming vehicle.

   b. As a young child hurries to avoid being late to school, he is struck by a full-size automobile.

13. When evaluating a sports injury, what principles of kinematics must be considered to determine probable areas of injury?

14. A suitcase filled with plastic explosives detonates in a locker at a busy urban airport. Describe the type of injuries the paramedic should anticipate in each of the following categories:
   a. Primary blast injuries:

   b. Secondary blast injuries:

   c. Tertiary blast injuries:

15. You are called to a home to care for a person who has fallen.

    a. List three things you must determine to predict injuries associated with this fall.

_____

    b. What age of patient is most likely to fall?

_____

    c. If the person who fell is an adult, how is she likely to land?

_____

16. Briefly describe the way each of the following ballistic properties influences injury patterns in penetrating trauma:

    a. Character of the penetrating object:

_____

_____

    b. Speed of penetration:

_____

_____

    c. Distance from patient that a bullet is fired:

_____

_____

● STUDENT SELF-ASSESSMENT

17. Trauma is the leading cause of death in persons of which of the following ages?

    a. Less than 1 year   **c.** 35 to 65 years
    b. 1 to 34 years   **d.** More than 65 years

18. What actions can a paramedic take to intervene at the incident phase of trauma?

    a. Educate the community   **c.** Promote safety legislation
    b. Decrease scene time   **d.** Wear personal restraint systems

19. Which of the following is a component of a trauma system as defined in the National Standard Paramedic Curriculum?

    a. EMS education   **c.** Pain management
    b. Fire suppression   **d.** Rehabilitation

20. What factor influences trauma triage guidelines?

    a. Mechanism of injury   **c.** Paramedic preference
    b. Patient's ability to pay   **d.** Patient preference

21. What is the process of predicting injury patterns that may result from the forces and motions of energy known as?

    a. Force of energy applied   **c.** Kinematics
    b. Index of suspicion   **d.** Mechanism of injury

22. Injury resulting from blunt trauma is most often caused by which of the following forces?

    a. Compression   **c.** Distraction
    b. Deceleration   **d.** Torsion

23. Your patient was restrained when her car was struck on the right side on her door at a high rate of speed. What injuries do you predict?
    a. Aortic injury   c. Pancreatic injury
    b. Liver injury   d. Splenic injury
24. Which injuries are more likely if the lap belt is improperly applied?
    a. Duodenal injuries   c. Pelvic fractures
    b. Maxillofacial injuries   d. Sternal fractures
25. Which of the following is true regarding ejection from a vehicle?
    a. It will not happen if the person is restrained.
    b. It usually happens before impact.
    c. Spinal injuries are very common.
    d. There is little risk of death.
26. Steering wheel/dash air bags are designed to reduce injuries in which of the following collisions?
    a. Frontal collisions   c. Rollover collisions
    b. Lateral collisions   d. All of the above
27. Which of the following are predictable injuries from ATV crashes?
    a. Abdominal injuries   c. Thoracic injuries
    b. Kidney injuries   d. Upper extremity injuries
28. Which of the following is more likely to occur when a child is struck by a car, compared with an adult?
    a. The child may strike the hood of the vehicle.
    b. The child may be dragged under the vehicle.
    c. The child may land on the ground.
    d. The child may strike the bumper of the vehicle.
29. A roofer falls from the top of a two-story residence. What type of injuries do you anticipate?
    a. Minor injuries to the feet and spine
    b. Severe injuries to the feet and spine
    c. Minor injuries to the head and neck
    d. Major injuries to the head and neck
30. A 2-year-old child falls from a second-story window. What area of the body is most likely to be injured?
    a. Head and neck   c. Leg
    b. Arm   d. Pelvis
31. Which of the following is a high-energy weapon with the potential to cause the greatest injury to tissues?
    a. M-16   c. 12-gauge shotgun
    b. .357 magnum   d. Knife
32. Which organ is likely to experience the most severe injury from tissue crushing caused by cavitation after a gunshot wound?
    a. Bowel   c. Lung
    b. Liver   d. Muscle

CHAPTER 19

HEMORRHAGE AND SHOCK

● READING ASSIGNMENT

Chapter 19, pages 550-571, in *Mosby's Paramedic Textbook*, ed 2

● OBJECTIVES

As a paramedic, you should be able to:

1. Describe how to recognize signs and symptoms of internal or external hemorrhage.
2. Define shock.
3. Outline the factors necessary to achieve adequate tissue oxygenation.
4. Describe how the diameter of resistance vessels influences preload.
5. Describe the function of the components of blood.
6. Outline the changes in the microcirculation during the progression of shock.
7. List the causes of hypovolemic, cardiogenic, neurogenic, anaphylactic, and septic shock.
8. Describe pathophysiology as a basis for signs and symptoms associated with the progression through the stages of shock.
9. Describe key assessment findings to distinguish the etiology of the shock state.
10. Outline the prehospital management of the patient in shock based upon knowledge of the pathophysiology associated with each type of shock.
11. Discuss how to integrate the assessment and management of the patient in shock.

● REVIEW QUESTIONS

Match the blood component in Column II with its definition in Column I. Use each answer only once.

Column I	Column II
1. _____ Provides oxygen to and removes carbon dioxide from cells	a. Albumin
2. _____ Forms sticky plugs and initiates clotting	b. Erythrocytes
3. _____ Destroys red blood cells and bacteria	c. Fibrinogen
4. _____ Large protein that moves water from tissues into the blood	d. Gamma globulin
5. _____ Important in human immune response	e. Leukocyte
6. _____ Blood's solvent through which salts, minerals, and fats travel	f. Plasma
	g. Platelet

7. You are called to evaluate a 20-year-old butcher who sustained a stab wound to the femoral artery. Evaluation of the patient reveals a large amount of blood loss from an inguinal wound that is spurting bright red blood. The patient is very anxious and confused. Vital signs are as follows: blood pressure 86/70 mm Hg, pulse 136, respirations 28, and lungs clear. The patient's lips and nailbeds are pale and cyanotic, and capillary refill is greater than 2 seconds. List the three physiological components necessary for normal cellular oxygenation as measured by the Fick principle and determine whether each has been met.

a.

b.

c.

8. Describe the structural elements of the vascular system that enable it to adjust its size and adapt to pressure changes.

_____

_____

9. Complete the following sentences: The pressure that blood exerts against the vessel walls is known as (a) _____ pressure. Pressure that results from contraction of the ventricles is (b) _____

_____ pressure, whereas the residual pressure between contractions is (c) _____ pressure. The pulse felt in an artery resulting from the difference in (b) and (c) pressure is known as (d) _____ pressure. Pressure in the vessels is greatest at the (e) _____ and least at the (f) _____

_____.

10. State the effect that each of the following patient situations has on the size of the patient's vascular container and on preload:
a. A patient with a cervical spine injury from a motor vehicle collision has the following vital signs: blood pressure 80/60 mm Hg, pulse 60, and respirations 28. His skin is cool and pale above the level of the injury and warm and dry below it.

_____

b. A 55-year-old woman with heavy vaginal bleeding has been very dizzy. Vital signs are as follows: blood pressure 106/92 mm Hg, pulse 116, and respirations 20.

_____

11. For each of the following intravenous fluids, indicate whether the solution is isotonic, hypotonic, or hypertonic. Indicate whether there will be immediate net movement of fluid into or out of the intravascular space if this fluid is given, or whether no movement is observed.

Intravenous Fluid	Isotonic, Hypotonic, or Hypertonic	Fluid Movement
$D_{50}W$		
Lactated Ringer's		
Normal saline		
0.45% normal saline		
D_5W		

12. A 65-year-old complains of severe abdominal pain that radiates to the back. A large pulsatile mass is evident in the abdomen. Vital signs are as follows: blood pressure 80/70 mm Hg, pulse 128, and respirations 28. Predict the pathophysiological changes and associated signs and symptoms that will occur during the stages of shock for this patient.

   a. Stage 1: Vasoconstriction

   b. Stage 2: Capillary and venule opening

   c. Stage 3: Disseminated intravascular coagulation

   d. Stage 4: Multiple organ failure

13. For each of the following situations, list the type of shock and briefly describe interventions necessary for patient management:

   a. You are called to evaluate a 72-year-old man whose wife states that he had chest pain all day yesterday and earlier today. He has no pain when you arrive, but he is confused, pale, and diaphoretic. No bleeding is evident. Lung sounds reveal crackles in the bases. Vital signs are as follows: blood pressure 86/76 mm Hg, pulse 128 and irregular, and respirations 28.

    Classification:

    Interventions:

   b. Your 17-year-old patient was unrestrained in a motor vehicle collision. He has no sensation below the nipple line and is confused. He has a large laceration on the parietal area and complains of neck pain. No other injuries are evident. His skin is pale and cool above the nipple line and warm and dry below. Vital signs are as follows: blood pressure 84 mm Hg by palpation, pulse 56, and respirations 28 and very shallow.

    Classification:

    Interventions:

c. A 26-year-old woman who states that her last menstrual period was 8 weeks ago is complaining of severe right lower quadrant abdominal pain. She is pale, cool, and diaphoretic. Vital signs are as follows: blood pressure 106/78 mm Hg, pulse 120, and respirations 20 while supine; blood pressure 88/76 mm Hg, pulse 136, and respirations 28 while standing also are noted.

   Classification:

   Interventions:

d. A 42-year-old woman experiences acute shortness of breath, urticaria, nausea, and dizziness after ingesting a penicillin tablet prescribed by her dentist. Vital signs are as follows: blood pressure 80 mm Hg by palpation, pulse 140, and respirations 40 and labored.

   Classification:

   Interventions:

e. A 72-year-old resident of a nursing home has a fever and is restless and agitated. The urine in the indwelling catheter collection bag is milky and green in color. Vital signs are as follows: blood pressure 94/60 mm Hg, pulse 132, and respirations 30.

   Classification:

   Interventions:

f. A 55-year-old office worker has complained of a pounding sensation in his chest and has fallen from his chair, striking his head on the desk. You note a 5-cm laceration on the frontal area that is freely oozing dark red blood (approximately 20 ml on the floor). The patient is unconscious and vital signs are as follows: blood pressure 60 mm Hg by palpation, pulse 180, and respirations 28.

   Classification:

   Interventions:

14. For each of the following situations, identify whether the patient is in compensated or uncompensated shock and explain why:

 a. A 48-year-old has sustained second- and third-degree burns to 70% of his body. He is pale, cool, and diaphoretic. His nailbeds are cyanotic, and his vital signs are as follows: blood pressure 84/76 mm Hg, pulse 136, and respirations 32.

_____

_____

 b. A 22-year-old passenger in a high-speed motor vehicle crash was restrained with a lap belt. She complains of severe abdominal pain. Her skin is cool and pale. Vital signs are as follows: blood pressure 110/86 mm Hg, pulse 128, and respirations 28.

_____

_____

15. Describe the characteristics of irreversible shock.

_____

16. List three conditions, situations, or characteristics that decrease a patient's ability to compensate in shock.

_____

17. For each of the following scenarios, select the appropriate intervention(s) from the following list. Briefly justify your answer.

Pneumatic antishock garment   Drug therapy
Rapid fluid replacement   Blood transfusions
Intraosseous infusion

 a. A 72-year-old after experiencing a myocardial infarction with pulmonary edema and vital signs as follows: blood pressure 86/60 mm Hg, pulse 124, and respirations 28.

_____

_____

 b. A 2-year-old was struck by an automobile and you suspect that he has numerous pelvic and abdominal injuries and vital signs as follows: blood pressure unobtainable, pulse 170 carotid and very weak, and respirations 40 and shallow.

_____

_____

 c. A 44-year-old with a sudden onset of dizziness followed by syncope and vital signs as follows: blood pressure 86/68 mm Hg, pulse 44, and respirations 20.

_____

_____

148

d. An 18-year-old stung by a bee at a park has generalized redness and hives and is acutely short of breath. Vital signs are as follows: blood pressure 70 mm Hg by palpation, pulse 132, and respirations 36.

   e. A 53-year-old woman with heavy abdominal bleeding for 1 week became lethargic and confused. Vital signs are as follows: blood pressure 66 mm Hg by palpation, pulse 136, and respirations 32.

   f. A 19-year-old sustained a gunshot wound to the chest. Vital signs are as follows: blood pressure 106/88 mm Hg, pulse 128, and respirations 24.

● **STUDENT SELF-ASSESSMENT**

18. Your patient is passing bright red blood through the rectum. What is this called?
   a. Coffee-ground emesis
   b. Epistaxis
   c. Hematochezia
   d. Melena

19. Which of the following is the best definition of shock?
   a. Systolic blood pressure less than 90 mm Hg
   b. Greater than 25% loss of circulating blood
   c. Inadequate perfusion of the capillaries
   d. Blood flow deficit to the myocardium

20. Which of the following is true according to the Fick principle?
   a. Glucose must be available for cellular oxygenation.
   b. Precapillary and postcapillary sphincters must be open for adequate flow.
   c. Red blood cells must be able to load and unload oxygen.
   d. The pH should be at least 6.5 for adequate perfusion to occur.

21. Which of the following blood characteristics is the greatest determinant of afterload (peripheral vascular resistance)?
   a. Vessel diameter
   b. Vessel length
   c. Viscosity
   d. Volume

22. A decrease in peripheral vascular resistance will cause the container size of the body to _____ and the blood pressure to _____.
   a. decrease, decrease
   b. decrease, increase
   c. increase, increase
   d. increase, decrease

23. Which blood vessels act as collecting channels and storage (capacitance) vessels?
   a. Arterioles
   b. Arteries
   c. Capillaries
   d. Venules/veins

24. Which of the following blood cells are responsible for transporting approximately 99% of the oxygen carried to body tissues?
   a. Erythrocytes
   b. Leukocytes
   c. Plasma proteins
   d. Platelets

25. At what phase of shock does the microcirculation develop the leaky capillary syndrome?
    a. Capillary and venule opening
    b. Disseminated intravascular coagulation
    c. Multiple organ failure
    d. Vasoconstriction
26. What happens to fluid in stage two of the progression of shock?
    a. It is pulled into the intravascular space because of vasoconstriction.
    b. It leaks out of the intravascular space because of vasoconstriction.
    c. It is pulled into the intravascular space because of increased hydrostatic pressure.
    d. It leaks out of the intravascular space because of decreased hydrostatic pressure.
27. What occurs when there is dilation of the precapillary sphincter while the postcapillary sphincter remains constricted during lactic acidosis?
    a. No net movement of fluid between the fluid compartments
    b. Loss of vascular fluid into the interstitial spaces
    c. Movement of fluid from the interstitial spaces to the intravascular spaces
    d. Fluid shunting around the capillaries through the arterioles
28. What is shock caused by heart (pump) failure known as?
    a. Anaphylactic shock   c. Hypovolemic shock
    b. Cardiogenic shock   d. Neurogenic shock
29. Which of the following shock states does *not* produce vasodilation?
    a. Anaphylactic   c. Neurogenic
    b. Cardiogenic   d. Septic
30. Your patient was stabbed in the abdomen 20 minutes ago. Vital signs are as follows: blood pressure 80/50 mm Hg, pulse 136, and respirations 26. He is anxious and very pale. He is probably in which stage of shock?
    a. Compensated   c. Transitional
    b. Irreversible   d. Uncompensated
31. Increases in peripheral vascular resistance can be indirectly measured by noting which of the following?
    a. Diastolic blood pressure   c. Pulse rate
    b. Jugular distention   d. Systolic blood pressure
32. For which of the following conditions is the pneumatic antishock garment considered helpful?
    a. Cardiogenic shock   c. Penetrating chest injuries
    b. Pelvic fractures   d. Pulmonary edema
33. Which of the following fluids is a colloid solution?
    a. Dextran   c. Lactated Ringer's solution
    b. 0.45% sodium chloride   d. Normal saline
34. Which of the following blood products has the greatest oxygen-carrying capacity per volume?
    a. Fibrinogen   c. Plasma
    b. Packed red blood cells   d. Whole blood
35. You arrive at the emergency department with a patient who has been vomiting bright red blood and is exhibiting signs and symptoms of shock. Which fluid is most beneficial to him at this time?
    a. Blood plasma   c. Packed red blood cells
    b. Dextran   d. Plasmanate
36. Your patient has fallen 30 feet from scaffolding and is anxious, confused, and in obvious shock. Which of the following is your priority of care, in the proper order?
    a. Rapid transport, oxygen, intravenous therapy
    b. Oxygen, intravenous therapy, rapid transport
    c. Intravenous therapy, rapid transport, oxygen
    d. Oxygen, rapid transport, intravenous therapy

37. In the absence of spinal or head injury, in what position should the hypovolemic patient in shock be placed?
    a. Lateral recumbent
    c. Supine hypotension
    b. Modified Trendelenberg
    d. Trendelenberg
38. Which of the following is *not* an appropriate initial prehospital management technique for the patient in hypovolemic shock?
    a. Crystalloid fluid replacement
    c. Pneumatic antishock garment
    b. External hemorrhage control
    d. Vasoactive drug therapy
39. Fluid therapy in cardiogenic shock should be slowed to the to-keep-open rate in which of the following cases?
    a. If lung crackles (rales) increase.
    b. If jugular vein distention decreases.
    c. If heart rate decreases.
    d. If peripheral edema increases.
40. Which of the following is the treatment of choice for the patient in severe anaphylactic shock?
    a. Antihistamines
    c. Fluid challenge
    b. Epinephrine
    d. Pneumatic antishock garments
41. You suspect that your patient has a ruptured ectopic pregnancy. She is in profound shock. Which intravenous catheter will you select?
    a. 14 gauge, 1½ inch
    c. 18 gauge, 1½ inch
    b. 14 gauge, 3 inch
    d. 18 gauge, 3 inch
42. A 200-ml fluid challenge is to be infused over 20 minutes. The drop factor is 10 drops/ml. How fast will you run it?
    a. 1 drop/min
    c. 100 drops/min
    b. 33 drops/min
    d. 400 drops/min
43. Which of the following is *not* a goal of prehospital care for the patient with severe hemorrhage and shock?
    a. Definitive care for internal hemorrhage
    b. Initiation of treatment
    c. Rapid recognition of the event
    d. Rapid transport to the appropriate hospital

SOFT TISSUE TRAUMA

● **READING ASSIGNMENT**

Chapter 20, pages 572-595, in *Mosby's Paramedic Textbook*, ed 2

● **OBJECTIVES**

As a paramedic, you should be able to:

1. Describe the normal structure and function of the skin.
2. Describe the pathophysiologic responses to soft tissue injury.
3. Discuss pathophysiology as a basis for key signs and symptoms and describe the mechanism of injury and signs and symptoms of specific soft tissue injuries.
4. Outline management principles for prehospital care of soft tissue injuries.
5. Describe, in the correct sequence, patient management techniques for control of hemorrhage.
6. Identify the characteristics of six general categories of dressings.
7. Describe prehospital management of specific soft tissue injuries not requiring closure.
8. Discuss factors that increase the potential for wound infection.
9. Describe the prehospital management of selected soft tissue injuries.

● **REVIEW QUESTIONS**

Match the type of dressing listed in Column II with its description in Column I. Use each answer only once.

Column I	Column II
1. _____ Air does not pass through this dressing.	**a.** Adherent dressing
2. _____ Bacteria has been eliminated from this dressing.	**b.** Nonadherent dressing
3. _____ This dressing can be used when infection is not a concern.	**c.** Nonocclusive dressing
4. _____ This dressing sticks to the wound surface.	**d.** Nonsterile dressing
5. _____ This dressing allows air to pass through to the wound.	**e.** Occlusive dressing
6. _____ This dressing does not stick to the wound.	**f.** Sterile dressing

7. List at least six structures or tissues located in the dermis.
   a.
   b.
   c.
   d.
   e.
   f.
8. Identify at least three functions of the integumentary system.
   a.
   b.
   c.
9. Identify the three crucial steps in the clotting mechanism.
   a.
   b.
   c.

10. Why are redness, swelling, warmth, and pain found at the site of an inflammatory response?

_____

_____

11. List six types of drugs that can impair normal wound healing.
    a.
    b.
    c.
    d.
    e.
    f.

12. List six types of wounds that are likely to require closure.
    a.
    b.
    c.
    d.
    e.
    f.

13. For each of the following scenarios, list the soft tissue injury described and key prehospital interventions to manage the trauma.
    a. A 45-year-old woman is being transported for care after her husband repeatedly struck her head and face with his fist. You note numerous swollen, ecchymotic areas on the face and head.
       Injury:
       Interventions:

_____

_____

    b. Rescuers have just removed a victim who had been trapped in a concrete structure for 2 days. The patient's lower torso had been pinned under a concrete piling. During the rescue phase the patient was alert but somewhat confused. Vital signs were within normal limits. Shortly after extrication the patient's physiological status begins to deteriorate.
       Injury:
       Interventions:

_____

_____

    c. A wallpaper hanger has sustained a deep linear wound after cutting himself with an Exacto knife. The wound is oozing dark red blood and fatty tissue is visible at the edges of the injury.
       Injury:
       Interventions:

_____

_____

d. A motorcyclist wearing only her swimsuit had to lay the bike down to avoid a collision. The patient states that the bike slid approximately 100 feet along the asphalt road. She has huge scrape-type injuries on her entire left side. She denies pain or tenderness anywhere else.
Injury:
Interventions:

---

e. Neighbors direct you to a yard where a young child has been attacked by a large dog. No one is sure of the dog's present location. The child is screaming and his left arm has many puncture wounds and lacerations.
Injury:
Interventions:

---

f. A hunter has been impaled with an arrow. The arrow has penetrated the right upper quadrant of the abdomen. She is pale and cool.
Injury:
Interventions:

---

g. A mechanic reports an injury to her right hand while working with a high-pressure grease gun. You note a small puncture wound with a drop of grease on it at the distal end of the left thumb.
Injury:
Interventions:

---

h. A butcher slices off the distal tip of his index finger.
Injury:
Interventions:

---

i. A factory employee catches his hair in some large machinery and avulses a large portion of the posterior aspect of his scalp.
Injury:
Interventions:

---

j. A weekend handyman severs his right index finger with a skill saw. He drives himself to a nearby firehouse but does not have the digit with him.

Injury:

Interventions:

___

Questions 14 and 15 pertain to the following case study:

Your patient was treated and released from the emergency department with a diagnosis of tibial fracture after a fall. He has a plaster splint that was applied there and is complaining of pain so severe "I just can't take it anymore."

14. What further assessments should you perform on this patient's leg to look for compartment syndrome?

___

15. If he has compartment syndrome, what could a delay in treatment cause?

___

Questions 16 and 17 pertain to the following case study:

You are called to the scene of a construction site, where a 57-year-old workman has lacerated his left hand.

16. What questions should you ask to obtain the wound history on this patient?

___

17. Outline the physical examination of the wound and hand.

___

18. You are called to a rural farm, where a 17-year-old has sustained a partial amputation of his left lower arm after tangling it in a corn picker. There is extensive soft tissue damage and deformity of the extremity, which is squirting bright red blood. Your estimated time of arrival to the nearest hospital is 30 minutes. Describe in the proper sequence six measures you can use to control the bleeding in this patient and briefly describe the proper technique for using each skill.

a.

___

b.

___

c.

___

d.

_____

_____

e.

_____

_____

f.

_____

_____

_____

For questions 19-23, circle **(a)** or **(b)** to indicate the wound that is at *greater risk* for infection. Explain why you chose your answer in **(c)**.

19. **a.** A farmer lacerates his hand on a combine.
    b. A chef cuts his hand on a butcher knife.
    c.
20. **a.** A 25-year-old athlete is stabbed.
    b. A 79-year-old nursing home resident is stabbed.
    c.
21. **a.** The patient cut his abdomen.
    b. The patient's laceration is on his hand.
    c.
22. **a.** Your patient reports to the emergency department for sutures 18 hours after the injury.
    b. The patient drives to the emergency department 2 hours after injury.
    c.
23. **a.** His finger was split open after he jammed it in a door.
    b. He sliced his finger on a piece of metal on the door.
    c.

● **STUDENT SELF-ASSESSMENT**

24. What is the avascular layer of the skin called?
    a. Dermis   **c.** Sebaceous
    b. Epidermis   **d.** Subcutaneous tissue
25. Which of the following does *not* play a role in normal hemostasis?
    a. Activation of platelets   **c.** Thrombin formation
    b. Aldosterone synthesis   **d.** Vasoconstriction
26. Which medications can interfere with hemostasis?
    a. Acetaminophen   **c.** Decongestants
    b. Aspirin   **d.** Insulin
27. Which of the following medical conditions is associated with delayed healing?
    a. Alcoholism   **c.** Cardiac dysrhythmias
    b. Asthma   **d.** Stroke
28. Which of the following wound forces is least likely to be associated with a high risk for infection?
    a. Foreign bodies   **c.** Injection injuries
    b. Human and animal bites   **d.** Paring knife wounds

29. Which of the following is considered a closed injury?
    a. Avulsion
    c. Hematoma
    b. Bite
    d. Puncture
30. High-pressure injection injuries can be limb-threatening. Why is the severity of this wound difficult to assess in the prehospital environment?
    a. The light is too poor to evaluate the wound adequately.
    b. The location of the wound is difficult to visualize.
    c. The equipment needed for assessment is not available.
    d. The wound is very small with minimal external signs.
31. What is the appropriate prehospital care for avulsed body tissue?
    a. Placing it directly on ice
    b. Sealing it in a plastic bag
    c. Soaking it in a cup of lactated Ringer's solution
    d. Debridement of all dirt
32. Which type of soft tissue injury may result in abscesses, lymphangitis, cellulitis, osteomyelitis, tenosynovitis, tuberculosis, hepatitis B, and tetanus?
    a. Amputation
    c. Bites
    b. Avulsion
    d. Crush injury
33. Which of the following is an early finding in crush injury?
    a. Paralysis
    c. Paresthesia
    b. Paresis
    d. Pulselessness
34. Where is compartment syndrome most likely to be found?
    a. Abdomen
    c. Head
    b. Upper arm
    d. Thorax
35. What causes life-threatening symptoms in patients with crush syndrome after being released from entrapment?
    a. Circulatory overload when blood rushes back to the central circulation
    b. Hypokalemia, hypouricemia, hypercalcemia, and hypophosphatemia
    c. Myoglobin is released and filtered through the liver, causing liver failure.
    d. Toxic substances from anaerobic metabolism are released into the blood.
36. Blast injuries can cause rupture in air-filled organs such as which of the following?
    a. Bladder
    c. Lungs
    b. Heart
    d. Pancreas
37. Which wound is least likely to require physician evaluation if tetanus immunization is up to date?
    a. A needle fragment imbedded in the wound.
    b. Weakness in the finger distal to the laceration.
    c. Laceration extending of over the border of the lip.
    d. A painful abrasion on the leg oozing slightly.
38. Who would *not* be a candidate for tetanus toxoid if they report they have not had one in more than 10 years?
    a. A patient who takes insulin for diabetes.
    b. A patient whose baby is due in 3 weeks.
    c. A patient whose arm was sore the last time he had one.
    d. A patient whose home medicines include lanoxin.

BURNS

● READING ASSIGNMENT

Chapter 21, pages 596-623, in *Mosby's Paramedic Textbook,* ed 2

● OBJECTIVES

1. Describe the incidence, patterns, and sources of burn injury.
2. Describe the pathophysiology of local and systemic responses to burn injury.
3. Classify burn injury according to depth, extent, and severity based on established standards.
4. Discuss the pathophysiology of burn shock as a basis for key signs and symptoms.
5. Outline the physical examination of the burned patient.
6. Describe the prehospital management of the patient who has sustained a burn injury.
7. Discuss pathophysiology as a basis for signs, symptoms, and management of the patient with an inhalation injury.
8. Outline the general assessment and management of the patient with a chemical injury.
9. Describe specific complications and management techniques for selected chemical injuries.
10. Describe the physiological effects of electrical injuries as they relate to each body system based on an understanding of principles of electricity.
11. Outline assessment and management of the patient with electrical injury.
12. Describe the distinguishing features of radiation injury and considerations in the prehospital management of these patients.

● REVIEW QUESTIONS

Match the chemicals listed in Column II with the appropriate description in Column I.

	Column I	Column II
1. _____	Chemical used to clean fabric and metal, can cause hypocalcemia and severe burns	**a.** Alkali
2. _____	Noxious gas that, when in solution, can cause blindness if it contaminates the eye	**b.** Ammonia
3. _____	Chemical that causes burns after prolonged exposure and also may result in lead poisoning	**c.** Hydrofluoric acid
4. _____	Chemical that produces heat if exposed to water and should be removed or covered with oil	**d.** Petroleum
5. _____	Exposure to this chemical that may be painless and result in dysrhythmias and central nervous system depression	**e.** Phenol

6. Identify the four major sources of burn injury.
   a.
   b.
   c.
   d.

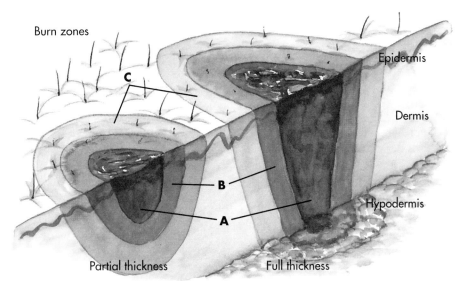

Burn zones

Epidermis

Dermis

Hypodermis

C

B

A

Partial thickness

Full thickness

Figure 21-1

7. Label the three zones of burn injury on Fig. 21-1 and briefly describe the characteristics of the tissue in each.

A.

_____

_____

B.

_____

_____

C.

_____

_____

8. Explain two mechanisms that cause swelling in the burned tissue.
   a.
   b.

9. Describe the response in each of the following body systems to a major burn injury:
   a. Cardiovascular:

_____

   b. Pulmonary:

_____

   c. Gastrointestinal:

_____

   d. Musculoskeletal:

_____

e. Neuroendocrine:

f. Metabolic:

g. Immune:

h. Emotional:

10. For each of the following situations, classify the burn according to depth (first-, second-, or third-degree), extent (body surface area), and severity (according to the American Burn Association). Identify those patients who meet the American Burn Association criteria for referral to a burn center.

    a. A chef at a local restaurant has spilled hot grease down the anterior surface of his body. The wound is extremely painful, moist, and red, with many blisters. The burns cover the anterior surface of his chest, abdomen, arms, and left leg.
      Depth:
      Extent:
      Severity:
      Referral:

    b. On a hot summer day a young motorist opens his radiator cap and sprays hot steam and fluid over the upper half of his torso. The wounds are painful, moist, and red, with some blistering, and they blanch to the touch. The burns cover his face, anterior chest, and abdomen.
      Depth:
      Extent:
      Severity:
      Referral:

    c. An 80-year-old woman steps into a tub of extremely hot water. Because of her severe arthritis, she takes a long time to get out. She has circumferential burns around the right lower extremity up to the knee. The burn wound appears white and leathery and has no capillary refill.
      Depth:
      Extent:
      Severity:
      Referral:

11. As you arrive at the scene of a residential fire, rescue workers carry out an approximately 40-year-old, 80-kg man who is unconscious and has white, leathery burns. The burns cover the entire body surface except the posterior surface of both legs. He has shallow respirations at a rate of 24/min, and his blood pressure is 106/70 mm Hg. Patchy pieces of his smoldering clothing remain.

    a. Describe your initial assessment of this patient, including depth, extent, and severity of burns.

b. Describe the prehospital care, including airway and fluid resuscitation, with type of fluid and rate.

_____

_____

12. Describe the specific interventions to be used when the following third-degree burns are present:
    a. Burns to the face:

_____

    b. Extremity burns:

_____

    c. Circumferential burns:

_____

Questions 13-16 pertain to the following case study:

> A 13-year-old boy uses gasoline to start a bonfire and ignites his clothing. As he attempts to pull his flaming jacket over his head, it gets stuck while continuing to burn. On your arrival, he is alert after an initial brief loss of consciousness. He has extensive burns on his face, neck, and chest. The burns are white and dry, with charred patches. They do not blanch when touched. His nasal hair is singed, and he is coughing up black, sooty sputum.

13. What aspects of the mechanism of injury and history of the event lead you to believe that this patient may have an inhalation injury?

_____

14. What physical findings suggest inhalation injury?

_____

15. At what point would you consider intubation?

_____

16. Do you suspect an inhalation injury above or below the glottis, and why?

_____

17. You are responding to a call for a person who has a chemical burn. En route to the industrial complex, you review the questions you will ask to determine the potential seriousness of the burn.
    a. Provide two examples of these questions.

_____

_____

    b. You find your patient covered with a powder known to cause chemical burns to the skin. Describe patient decontamination techniques.

_____

_____

18. Identify two examples of chemicals that can cause burn injury in each of the following categories:

a. Acids:

_____

b. Alkalis:

_____

c. Organic compounds:

_____

19. The amount of tissue damage caused by an electrical current depends on six

factors: (a) _____, _____,

_____, _____,

_____, and _____.

Amperage is the measure of current (b) _____ per

unit time. Voltage is a continuous (c) _____ applied
to any electrical circuit causing a flow of electricity. High-voltage electrical
injuries result from contact with an electrical source of (d)

_____ or greater. Resistance to electricity depends on

four factors: (e) _____

_____, _____,

_____, and _____.

Resistance to electrical flow in the body is greatest in the (f) _____

_____ tissue. The two types of current commonly

used are (g) _____ and _____.

Direct current flows in (h) _____ direction. It is used

in (i) _____. Alternating current periodically reverses

(j) _____ of flow. This reversal may cause muscle

contractions that may (k) _____ the patient to the
source. In general, the current pathway in low-voltage current follows the

path of (l) _____ _____, and

high-voltage current follows the (m) _____ path. As
the duration of contact with the patient increases, tissue damage (n)

_____.

20. Name the three burn patterns that can result from electrical current.

    a.

    b.

    c.

21. Briefly describe the potential effects of electrical injury on each of the following body regions.

    a. Cutaneous:

---

    b. Cardiovascular:

---

    c. Neurological:

---

    d. Vascular:

---

    e. Muscular:

---

    f. Renal:

---

    g. Pulmonary:

---

    h. Orthopedic:

---

    i. Ocular and otic:

---

22. A homeowner was trimming his trees when he came into contact with overhead electrical wires. On your arrival, he is still in contact with the electrical source.

    a. What must be done before treatment commences?

    The patient falls 10 feet from the tree to the ground. The scene is now safe. He is conscious and alert. You note multiple small, round, white burns on his right hand. When his clothing is removed, you discover significant burns and tissue injury to both feet.

    b. Describe your history and physical examination of this patient.

---

    c. Describe treatment, including fluid resuscitation (rate and type).

---

23. Describe the appearance of wounds characteristically associated with lightning burns.

_____

24. For each of the following classes of lightning injury, list two physical signs:
 a. Minor:

_____

 b. Moderate:

_____

 c. Severe:

_____

25. Describe the characteristics of the following three types of radiation particles:
 a. Alpha:

_____

 b. Beta:

_____

 c. Gamma:

_____

26. Describe the physical effects that can be expected at the following levels of radiation exposure:
 a. Less than 100 rem:

_____

 b. 100 to 200 rem:

_____

 c. Greater than 450 rem:

_____

Questions 27-29 pertain to the following case study:

You arrive at a clinical laboratory, where a significant amount of radioactive material reportedly was released when a worker fell 1 foot from a platform.

27. Describe your approach to the emergency scene.

_____

_____

28. The victim must be accessed. Describe how the crew members designated to perform the rescue can minimize their radiation exposure.

_____

_____

_____

29. Describe any special measures that you should use to care for this patient after you reach him or her.

_____

_____

● STUDENT SELF-ASSESSMENT

30. Which is an example of a thermal mechanism of injury?
    a. Arcing   **c.** Ionizing agents
    b. Alkali agents   **d.** Scalding

31. Which of the following risk factors is associated with a high incidence of burn fatality?
    a. Female gender   **c.** Industrial setting
    b. Child   **d.** High-income family

32. The most common source of burn injury is:
    a. Chemical   **c.** Radiation
    b. Electrical   **d.** Thermal

33. Which of the following is a systemic response to burn injury?
    a. Hypoventilation
    b. Hyperactive gastrointestinal tract
    c. Decreased metabolic rate
    d. Depressed inflammatory response

34. A burn characterized by a moist, red appearance with blisters is probably what degree?
    a. First   **c.** Third
    b. Second   **d.** Fourth

35. A 5-year-old patient with third-degree burns of the anterior and posterior surfaces of both legs would be estimated to have a (n) _____ burn.
    a. 18%   **c.** 28%
    b. 24%   **d.** 36%

36. Hypovolemia in burn injury occurs secondary to which of the following?
    a. Blood loss
    b. Condensation of tissue fluid
    c. Increased capillary permeability
    d. Decrease in fluid intake

37. When calculating the extent of burn injury to ensure accurate fluid resuscitation, the paramedic should do which of the following?
    a. Calculate the burn size after arriving at the hospital.
    b. Estimate size before cooling the burn.
    c. Not include first-degree burns.
    d. Use the Lund and Browder chart.

38. To cool the burn of a patient burned on 50% of the body surface area, the paramedic should do which of the following?
    a. Apply ice intermittently in 15-minute cycles.
    b. Leave the patient exposed to air and apply a fan.
    c. Apply cool water and then cover the patient with sheets and blankets.
    d. Continuously apply cool water while en route to the hospital.

39. Using the consensus burn formula, calculate the minimum fluid requirement during the first hour for a 100-kg patient who has 60% third-degree burns covering his body.
    a. 250 ml   **c.** 750 ml
    b. 500 ml   **d.** 6000 ml

40. Which of the following is *not* a reason to suspect inhalation injury?
  a. Burns involving petroleum products
  b. Documented loss of consciousness
  c. Hoarseness or stridor
  d. Burns in an enclosed space

41. Which of the following statements is true regarding carbon monoxide poisoning?
  a. Oxygen saturation on the pulse oximeter is 80 or less.
  b. Skin color is cyanotic and often mottled.
  c. Respiratory rate is depressed in the early stages.
  d. Oxygen administration reduces the half-life of carbon monoxide.

42. What is the treatment of choice for almost all chemical injuries?
  a. Vigorous drying of the chemical
  b. Application of a chemical antidote
  c. Copious irrigation with water
  d. Delayed treatment until arrival at the hospital

43. Severity of chemical injury is related to all of the following except which one?
  a. Chemical concentration
  c. Environmental temperature
  b. Duration of contact
  d. Type of chemical agent

44. Calcium gluconate gel and solution are used to treat which of the following chemical injuries?
  a. Ammonia
  c. Petroleum
  b. Hydrofluoric acid
  d. Phenol

45. Electrical burns that result when the heat of the electric current ignites the patient's clothing are what type of burns?
  a. Alternating
  c. Direct
  b. Arc
  d. Flame

46. Which tissue does electrical current flow through most easily?
  a. Bone
  c. Muscle
  b. Blood
  d. Nerve

47. Death in lightning injury most frequently results from which of the following?
  a. Cardiac or respiratory arrest
  c. Coagulation of the blood
  b. Central nervous system injury
  d. Severe burn shock

48. Which type of radiation requires a lead shield to stop penetration?
  a. Alpha
  c. Gamma
  b. Beta
  d. Nonionizing

HEAD AND FACIAL TRAUMA

● READING ASSIGNMENT
Chapter 22, pages 624-655, in *Mosby's Paramedic Textbook,* ed 2

● OBJECTIVES
As a paramedic, you should be able to:
1. Describe mechanisms of injury, assessment, and management of maxillofacial injuries.
2. Describe mechanisms of injury, assessment, and management of ear, eye, and dental injuries.
3. Describe mechanisms of injury, assessment, and management of anterior neck trauma.
4. Describe mechanisms of injury, assessment, and management of injuries to the scalp, cranial vault, and cranial nerves.
5. Distinguish among types of traumatic brain injury based on an understanding of pathophysiology and assessment findings.
6. Outline the prehospital management of the patient with cerebral injury.
7. Calculate a Glasgow coma scale, trauma score, revised trauma score, and pediatric trauma score when the appropriate patient information is provided.

● REVIEW QUESTIONS
Match the type of skull fracture listed in Column II with the appropriate description in Column I. Use each answer only once.

Column I	Column II
1. _____ Associated with Battle's sign and raccoon's eyes	**a.** Basilar
2. _____ Most common skull fracture; has low complication rate	**b.** Depressed
3. _____ Direct communication between scalp laceration and brain tissue	**c.** Linear
4. _____ Fracture when bone is pushed downward; often associated with scalp laceration	**d.** Open vault

Match the cranial nerve in Column II with the abnormal sign or symptom associated with it in Column I. Use each cranial nerve only once.

Column I	Column II
5. _____ Hearing loss	**a.** Olfactory
6. _____ Loss of vision in one eye	**b.** Optic
7. _____ Weakness of one side of the face	**c.** Oculomotor
8. _____ Double vision	**d.** Facial
9. _____ Loss of sense of smell	**e.** Acoustic
	f. Glossopharyngeal

10. A 6-year-old unrestrained child strikes his face on the stick shift of a truck in a head-on collision. On arrival, you find him seated in the cab of the truck, alert, crying, and complaining of pain in his face. Blood is oozing from his mouth.

   a. Describe your focused assessment of his head and face.

   _____

   _____

   b. On physical examination, you note the child's difficulty closing his mouth and an apparent space between the two lower front teeth, as well as a laceration that extends down through the gums. The bleeding continues, and you note excessive oral secretions. Vital signs are stable. Describe how you would transport and manage this child.

   _____

   _____

11. Briefly describe the evaluation of a suspected eye injury on a patient with no life threats.

   _____

   _____

12. For each of the following patients, identify the injury you suspect and list prehospital management techniques:

   a. A 10-year-old complains of severe pain in the right eye after he was struck in the face with a handful of sand. The right eye is reddened and tearing.

   _____

   b. A 35-year-old has sustained a partially avulsed right upper lid.

   _____

   _____

   c. A fish hook is embedded in the eye of a 42-year-old woman.

   _____

   _____

   d. A handball player is struck directly in the eye by the ball. He is having difficulty seeing from the injured eye. You note blood in the anterior chamber of the eye.

   _____

   _____

   e. During hockey playoffs a high stick strikes a player in the eye. You note an irregular pupil on the affected side. A jellylike substance extrudes from an apparent laceration to the globe.

   _____

   _____

Questions 13 and 14 pertain to the following case study:

> You are en route to a domestic disturbance in which a 45-year-old man has reportedly been stabbed in the neck with an ice pick.

13. Identify possible signs and symptoms of penetrating neck trauma that you should anticipate.

_____

> On arrival, you note an ashen-colored unconscious patient who is breathing and has a weak pulse. A large pool of blood surrounds him, and a large amount of blood is coming from his neck.

14. List the steps in management of this patient with respect to the neck wound.

_____

_____

15. Briefly list the signs and symptoms associated with the following brain injuries and state whether the injury is a diffuse axonal injury or focal brain injury:
    a. Concussion:

_____

    b. Contusion:

_____

    c. Subdural hematoma:

_____

    d. Epidural hematoma:

_____

    e. Severe diffuse axonal injury:

_____

16. A man has been struck on the head with a baseball bat during a barroom brawl. He is alert and oriented, with an obvious depression and laceration at the right temporal area. Describe the signs and symptoms you will see if his intracranial pressure progressively rises en route to the hospital.

_____

_____

17. You are transporting by air a patient who has sustained an isolated head injury in a motorcycle accident. Initially, he was awake and talking, but over the past 10 minutes, his condition has deteriorated rapidly. He now has a fixed, dilated right pupil; irregular respirations; a blood pressure of 170/100 mm Hg; and a pulse of 64. Identify treatment modalities you would provide for this patient.

_____

_____

18. Calculate the score indicated (Glasgow Coma scale [GCS], revised trauma score [RTS], pediatric trauma score [PTS]) for each of the following patient examples:

   a. Your patient opens her eyes to voice, is confused, and pulls her hand away when you start intravenous therapy. Her vital signs are blood pressure, 90/70; pulse, 120; and respirations, 24 and unlabored. Capillary refill is 1 second. GCS _____ RTS _____

   b. Your patient opens his eyes to deep pain, moans some unrecognizable sounds, and withdraws slightly from pain. His vital signs are blood pressure, 70 mm Hg by palpation; pulse, 136; and respirations, 30 and very shallow. His capillary refill is 4 seconds.
   GCS _____ RTS _____

   c. Your 10-day-old, 4-kg patient fell to the floor. She is crying vigorously. You note a small abrasion on her head, with a slight amount of swelling but no palpable crepitus. No other injuries are noted. Her blood pressure is 80 mm Hg. PTS _____

● **STUDENT SELF-ASSESSMENT**

19. Which of the following is a sign of midface fracture?
   a. Diplopia
   c. Mastoid ecchymosis
   b. Lengthening of the face
   d. Numbness of the forehead

20. Your patient has signs and symptoms of midface fractures with a Glasgow Coma score of 6. Which of the following is an appropriate prehospital intervention?
   a. Elevation of the head of the cot
   c. Orotracheal intubation
   b. Nasogastric intubation
   d. Pressure dressing over the nares

21. What is the name of the bone that, when fractured, often is associated with signs and symptoms similar to orbital fractures?
   a. Frontal
   c. Maxilla
   b. Mandible
   d. Zygoma

22. Your patient has been struck in the eye with a ball. She has diplopia, subconjunctival ecchymosis, enophthalmos, and numbness in the cheek. Which of the following bone fractures is consistent with these findings?
   a. Mandible
   c. Orbit
   b. Maxilla
   d. Zygoma

23. Displaced nasal fractures are most significant when they:
   a. Are displaced to one side
   b. Are associated with bleeding
   c. Depress the dorsum of the nose
   d. Occur in children

24. The upper segment of the patient's pinna was avulsed in an MVC. Which of the following treatments is appropriate for this patient?
   a. Approximate the edges of the avulsed tissue to the ear and apply a pressure dressing.
   b. Care for the remaining ear only. No chance exists to reimplant avulsed ear tissue.
   c. Scrub the avulsed tissue before wrapping it for transport to prevent infection.
   d. Wrap the avulsed tissue in moist gauze, seal it in a plastic bag, and place the bag on ice.

25. Prehospital management of ear pain secondary to barotrauma may include which of the following?
    a. Administration of nitrous oxide by inhalation
    b. A request that the patient perform the Valsalva maneuver
    c. Oxygen delivery to increase the absorption of trapped air
    d. Placement of the patient in the lateral recumbent position
26. Which of the following is an acceptable way to transport an avulsed tooth?
    a. In a mild soap solution
    c. In a dry gauze dressing
    b. In sterile water
    d. In fresh whole milk
27. Why are zone I neck injuries associated with the highest mortality? They contain which of the following?
    a. Brainstem, carotid artery, and nasopharynx
    b. Carotid artery, jugular vein, trachea, larynx, esophagus, and cervical spine
    c. Distal carotid arteries, salivary glands, and pharynx
    d. Subclavian and jugular vessels, lung, esophagus, trachea, C spine, cervical nerve roots
28. Which sign or symptom may indicate compromise of the upper airway associated with a hematoma in the neck?
    a. Cough
    c. Stridor
    b. Dysphagia
    d. Wheezing
29. Intubation of the patient with laryngeal or tracheal trauma may be difficult due to which of the following?
    a. Absence of spontaneous respirations
    b. Collapse of the trachea and bronchial tubes
    c. The presence of acute hypoxia
    d. Distorted and invisible vocal cords
30. Which of the following is an injury associated with focal brain injury?
    a. Concussion
    b. Contusion
    c. Minute petechial bruising of brain tissue in several areas
    d. Mechanical disruption of axons in both cerebral hemispheres
31. Which of the following is the most reliable indicator of increasing intracranial pressure?
    a. Deteriorating level of consciousness
    b. Nausea and vomiting
    c. Increased blood pressure and decreased pulse
    d. Unilateral dilated pupil
32. Which of the following breathing patterns is *not* likely to be exhibited by the patient with a brain injury?
    a. Ataxic breathing
    c. Hypoventilation
    b. Cheyne-Stokes respirations
    d. Kussmaul respirations
33. Characteristic signs and symptoms of subarachnoid hemorrhage include which of the following?
    a. Clinical signs of unexplained hypovolemia
    b. Gradual onset of unilateral weakness of the arms
    c. Intermittent pain and double vision in both eyes
    d. Sudden onset of "the worst headache I've ever had"
34. Which is the most rapid and effective intervention to decrease intracranial pressure in a patient with a severe head injury and a Glasgow Coma score of 6?
    a. Elevation of the head of the bed
    b. Intravenous administration of mannitol
    c. Intubation and adequate ventilation
    d. Massive doses of steroids

35. You wish to give 40 g of mannitol to a patient who has a head injury. You have a 20% solution of the drug. How many milliliters do you give?
    a. 8
    c. 80
    b. 50
    d. 200
36. Which drug may be administered before intubation to prevent a sudden increase in intracranial pressure?
    a. Atropine
    c. Mannitol
    b. Lidocaine
    d. Midazolam

CHAPTER 23

SPINAL TRAUMA

● **READING ASSIGNMENT**

Chapter 23, pages 656-685, in *Mosby's Paramedic Textbook*, ed 2

● **OBJECTIVES**

As a paramedic, you should be able to:
1. Describe the incidence, morbidity, and mortality related to spinal injury.
2. Predict mechanisms of injury that are likely to cause spinal injury.
3. Describe the anatomy and physiology of the spine and spinal cord.
4. Outline the general assessment of a patient with suspected spinal injury.
5. Distinguish among types of spinal injury.
6. Describe prehospital evaluation and assessment of spinal cord injury.
7. Identify prehospital management of the patient with spinal injuries.
8. Distinguish among spinal shock, neurogenic shock, and autonomic hyper-reflexia syndrome.
9. Describe selected nontraumatic spinal conditions and the prehospital assessment and treatment of them.

● **REVIEW QUESTIONS**

Match the spinal illness/injury in Column II with the description in Column I. Use each term only once.

Column I	Column II
1. _____ A tear in the capsule that encloses the center of the disk	a. Anterior cord syndrome
2. _____ Nontraumatic structural defect that involves the lamina or vertebral arch	b. Autonomic hyperreflexia syndrome
3. _____ Paralysis and decreased pain and temperature sensation below a flexion injury	c. Brown-Sequard syndrome
4. _____ Sprain causing partial dislocation of intervertebral joints	d. Central cord syndrome
5. _____ Hemitransection of cord with weakness on the injured side	e. Herniated nucleus pulposus
6. _____ Whiplash from a low-speed, rear-end collision	f. Hyperextension strain
7. _____ Sudden rapid increase in blood pressure, relieved by emptying of the bladder	g. Neurogenic hypotension
8. _____ Bradycardia, warm skin, and low blood pressure	h. Spinal cord tumors
9. _____ Abnormal tissue growth in the spine that may cause spasticity	i. Spinal shock
10. _____ Injury characterized by paralysis of the arms with sacral sparing	j. Spondylosis
	k. Subluxation

11. In each of the following situations, state whether the mechanism of injury is negative, positive, or uncertain related to your assessment of the spine:

   a. A soccer player falls and twists her knee. _____

   b. A patient is ejected during a rollover crash. _____

   c. A patient has a gunshot wound lateral to the spine. _____

   d. A young man falls 3 feet off a porch. _____
   e. A patient is the restrained driver in a motor vehicle crash, and the rear

   hood is buckled. _____

   f. A child dives off the high board and strikes the bottom of the pool with

   his head. _____

   g. A woman who was running slips and falls, striking her head on a ceramic

   tile floor. _____

12. List five preexisting conditions that can increase the risk of spine injury or complicate the injury.
   a.
   b.
   c.
   d.
   e.

13. Spinal sprains and strains usually result from (a) _____

   and (b) _____ forces. A hyperflexion sprain occurs

   when a tear is present in the posterior (c) _____

   _____ and _____

   _____, which allows partial (d) _____

   of the intervertebral joints. Hyperextension strains are common with low-velocity, rear-end automobile collisions and are commonly known as

   (e) _____. The most frequently injured spinal re-

   gions, in descending order, are (f) _____ to

   _____, (g) _____

   to _____, and (h) _____ to

   _____. The most common are wedge-shaped

   (i) _____ fractures. (j) _____

   and (k) _____ are extremely unstable injuries
   caused by a combination of severe hyperflexion and compression forces.

14. A cyclist was thrown from his bike and has severe pain in the back between his scapulae. List signs and symptoms that can indicate a complete cord lesion as a result of this injury.

_____

_____

Questions 15-17 pertain to the following case study:.

A 35-year-old was involved in a motor vehicle crash with moderate damage, which you classify as an uncertain mechanism for spine injury. She says she is fine, and just wants to be "checked out" at the hospital.

15. Which conditions or situations would make her unreliable to perform spinal examination for clinical criteria?

_____

_____

16. Describe your examination for motor findings suggestive of spine injury.

_____

_____

17. Describe how to perform the sensory exam to evaluate for spine injury on this patient.

_____

18. Identify five situations involving suspected cervical spine injury when the head should *not* be moved to a neutral inline position with manual immobilization.
   a.
   b.
   c.
   d.
   e.
19. Identify the steps involved in rolling of a supine patient (Fig. 23-1), including positioning of rescuers.

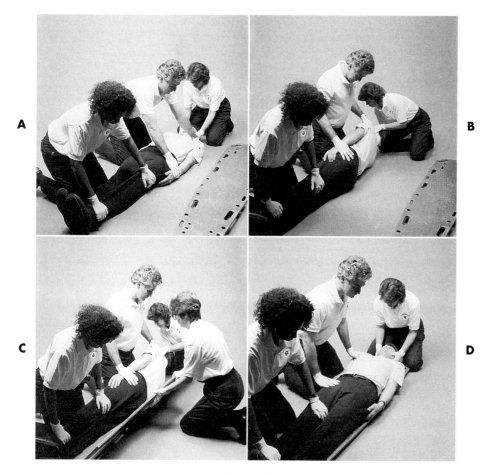

Figure 23-1

A.

B.

C.

D.

20. Identify drugs that may be used for each of the following spinal cord emergencies:

 a. Spinal cord injury with paralysis:

_____

 b. Spinal cord injury with hypotension and bradycardia:

_____

● STUDENT SELF-ASSESSMENT

21. Most spinal injuries occur as a result of which of the following?
 a. Falls
 b. Motor vehicle crashes
 c. Sports-related injuries
 d. Penetrating injuries from acts of violence

22. Which of the following classifications of mechanism of injury would be given to a fall from the roof of a single-story residence?

a. Alternative mechanism of injury
b. Negative mechanism of injury
c. Positive mechanism of injury
d. Uncertain mechanism of injury

23. Which of the following patients would be considered reliable to assess for spinal cord injury?
    a. A patient who witnessed the death of his or her child in crash.
    b. A patient with a severely angulated, partially amputated foot.
    c. A patient who can't communicate in a language you understand.
    d. A patient who is complaining of knee and hip pain with no deformity.

24. Which is the most flexible area of the spine?
    a. Cervical spine   c. Sacral spine
    b. Lumbar spine   d. Thoracic spine

25. A side-impact motor vehicle collision is most likely to produce spinal injury from extremes in which motion?
    a. Axial loading   c. Flexion
    b. Distraction   d. Lateral bending

26. Which finding on a patient with uncertain mechanism of injury should cause you to suspect spine trauma and immobilize the spine?
    a. High blood pressure
    b. History of Parkinson's disease
    c. Laceration on the scalp
    d. Pain or tenderness of the neck

27. Hyperflexion sprains can cause partial dislocation of the intervertebral joints. This condition is known as which of the following?
    a. Axial loading   c. Subluxation
    b. Herniated disks   d. Whiplash

28. Fractures at the level of S1 and S2 may lead to which of the following?
    a. Loss of bowel and bladder function
    b. Neurogenic shock
    c. Paralysis of the legs
    d. Transection of the spinal cord

29. Paralysis and loss of sensation below the umbilicus indicates an injury at the level of which of the following?
    a. C4   c. T10
    b. T4   d. S1

30. Which of the following is a sign of autonomic dysfunction resulting from spinal cord injury?
    a. Bradycardia   c. Profuse sweating
    b. Hypertension   d. Polyuria

31. Which of the following signs or symptoms is associated with central cord syndrome?
    a. Intact light touch and position sensation
    b. Greater motor weakness or paralysis in the arms than legs
    c. Loss of pain and temperature sensation on the side of injury
    d. Weakness in the upper and lower extremities on the side opposite the injury

32. Respiratory distress should be anticipated in the patient with which of the following?
    a. Brown-Sequard syndrome
    b. Herniated thoracic disk
    c. Hyperextension strain
    d. Spinal cord transection above C5 to C6

33. The purpose of immobilizing the patient suspected to have spinal injury in the prehospital setting is which of the following?
    a. To apply traction to pull apart injured bones

    b. To minimize neurogenic shock

    c. To prevent primary injury

    d. To prevent additional cord hypoxia or edema

34. When a patient on a long spine board is immobilized, which of the following body regions should be secured first?

    a. Arms   **c.** Legs

    b. Head   **d.** Torso

35. Which of the following cord injury presentations involves flaccid paralysis that usually resolves in 24 hours?

    a. Autonomic hyperreflexia syndrome

    b. Neurogenic hypotension

    c. Spinal shock

    d. Spondylosis

36. Which of the following medical conditions of the spine can increase the risk of spinal fractures?

    a. Degenerative disk disease

    b. Herniated intervertebral disk

    c. Spinal cord tumors

    d. Spondylolysis

THORACIC TRAUMA

● READING ASSIGNMENT

Chapter 24, pages 686-701, in *Mosby's Paramedic Textbook,* ed 2

● OBJECTIVES

As a paramedic, you should be able to:
1. Discuss epidemiology and mechanism of injury associated with thoracic trauma.
2. Describe mechanism of injury, signs and symptoms, and treatment of skeletal injuries to the chest.
3. Describe mechanism of injury, signs and symptoms, and prehospital treatment of pulmonary trauma.
4. Describe mechanism of injury, signs and symptoms, and prehospital treatment of injuries to the heart and great vessels.
5. Outline the mechanism of injury, signs and symptoms, and prehospital care of the patient with diaphragmatic rupture.

● REVIEW QUESTIONS

Questions 1-3 pertain to the following case study:

> You are transferring a 26-year-old woman who was a passenger in a car struck laterally on her door. She has a fractured right humerus and multiple fractures of ribs 3 to 8. En route to the trauma center, you note paradoxical movement of her chest.

1. What chest injury do you suspect?

2. Why is the patient likely to become hypoxic secondary to this injury?

3. What patient care measures should you use to improve ventilation?

4. Identify three symptoms common to all types of pneumothorax.
   a.
   b.
   c.

5. A deer hunter is accidentally shot with a 30:30 shell from a rifle. There is an open wound inferior to the right nipple, and you cannot find an exit wound.
   a. Why is this patient likely to become hypoxic?

   _____

   _____

   b. What interventions must be taken immediately to correct the hypoxia?

   _____

   _____

6. A patient from a motor vehicle crash has sustained severe blunt chest trauma. There are diminished breath sounds on the right side of the chest. He is anxious and dyspneic.
   a. What additional signs and symptoms would indicate that he has developed a tension pneumothorax?

   _____

   b. Describe the prehospital intervention for tension pneumothorax.

   _____

   _____

7. What two life-threatening conditions may be caused by hemothorax?
   a.
   b.
8. You are called to care for a worker who was momentarily crushed between a truck and a loading dock. His face and head are a bright, reddish-purple color, and his jugular veins are markedly distended.
   a. What injury do you suspect?

   _____

   b. What treatment would you provide?

   _____

9. A 28-year-old woman was involved in a frontal collision, during which her chest struck the steering wheel. She complains of crushing substernal chest pain and palpitations. Her blood pressure is normal, her pulse is 110 and irregular, and her lungs are clear.
   a. What injury do you suspect?

   _____

   b. What treatment measures should be instituted for this patient?

   _____

10. A 27-year-old was splitting wood when a metal splinter flew off the ax and penetrated his chest. On your arrival, he is confused, with a systolic blood pressure of 80 mm Hg, a narrow pulse pressure, muffled heart sounds, and distended neck veins.
    a. What chest injury do you suspect?

    _____

    b. What prehospital care should be rendered?

    _____

11. What signs should be anticipated in a patient with an aortic rupture secondary to a rapid deceleration injury?

_____

_____

● **STUDENT SELF-ASSESSMENT**

12. Which of the following is true regarding chest trauma?
   a. It is associated with a small number of deaths each year.
   b. It only occurs with motor vehicle crashes and penetrating injury.
   c. It only includes soft tissue injuries to the chest.
   d. The use of seatbelts decreases the mortality associated with it.

13. Which of the following is true regarding clavicle fractures?
   a. Clavicle fractures are unusual injuries.
   b. They are never serious injuries.
   c. They usually occur when the arm is twisted.
   d. They can be treated with a sling and swath.

14. Which of the following is true regarding rib fractures?
   a. They are more common in children.
   b. The first rib is frequently fractured.
   c. They are associated with pancreatic injury.
   d. Ribs 3 to 8 are most commonly fractured.

15. Respiratory distress in a patient with flail chest is most often associated with which of the following?
   a. Impaired mechanics of respiration
   b. Open chest wounds
   c. Severe pain that increases with respiration
   d. Underlying pulmonary contusion

16. Sternal injuries are frequently associated with which of the following?
   a. Airway compromise   **c.** Myocardial injury
   b. Flail chest   **d.** Spleen injury

17. Which is the most common cause of pneumothorax?
   a. Excessive pressure on the chest wall
   b. Penetration from a gun or knife
   c. Penetration from a rib fracture
   d. Spontaneous pneumothorax

18. When is a pneumothorax least likely to cause a life threat?
   a. It is closed.
   b. It is a tension pneumothorax.
   c. It occupies more than 40% of the hemithorax.
   d. It occurs in a patient with shock.

19. Your patient has a pneumothorax and may be developing a hemothorax. What signs or symptoms will you anticipate?
   a. Bradypnea
   b. Hypotension
   c. Tracheal deviation away from the affected side
   d. Widened pulse pressure

20. Injury to the lung tissue may occur when overexpansion of air in the lungs occurs after the primary energy wave has passed. This is known as which of the following?
   a. Implosion effect   **c.** Paper-bag effect
   b. Inertial effect   **d.** Spalding effect

21. What often occurs as a result of pulmonary contusion?
   a. Hypovolemia   **c.** Pericardial tamponade
   b. Hypoxia   **d.** Pneumothorax

181

22. Which of the following is *not* a sign associated with Beck's triad (found in pericardial tamponade)?
    a. Jugular vein distention
    b. Muffled heart sounds
    c. Narrowing pulse pressure
    d. Tracheal deviation
23. Which of the following is a complication of pericardiocentesis?
    a. Cardiac dysrhythmias
    b. Increased tamponade
    c. Laceration of a coronary artery
    d. Laceration of the ventricle
    e. All of the above
24. Your patient was involved in a high-speed motor vehicle crash. Which of the following signs may signal aortic rupture?
    a. Congestive heart failure
    b. Decreased breath sounds
    c. Hypertension
    d. Jugular venous distention
25. Your patient was in a motorcycle crash and has dyspnea and bowel sounds at the nipple line on the left side of the chest. You suspect which of the following?
    a. Pericardial tamponade
    b. Liver rupture
    c. Diaphragmatic rupture
    d. Kidney injury

ABDOMINAL TRAUMA

● READING ASSIGNMENT

Chapter 25, pages 702-709, in *Mosby's Paramedic Textbook,* ed 2

● OBJECTIVES

As a paramedic, you should be able to:
1. Identify mechanisms of injury associated with abdominal trauma.
2. Describe mechanisms of injury, signs and symptoms, and complications associated with abdominal solid organ, hollow organ, retroperitoneal organ, and pelvic organ injuries.
3. Outline the significance of injury to intraabdominal vascular structures.
4. Describe the prehospital assessment priorities for the patient suspected to have abdominal injury.
5. Outline the prehospital care of the patient with abdominal trauma.

● REVIEW QUESTIONS

1. A 12-year-old boy recovering from mononucleosis has been hit on the left side by another child. He complains of severe left upper quadrant abdominal pain and left shoulder pain. He has signs of shock.
   a. What solid organ is most likely injured in this situation?

   _____

   b. Why would he complain of shoulder pain?

   _____

   c. What care should you provide for him?

   _____

2. Describe complications that may result when hollow organs of the abdomen are injured.

   _____

3. List nine signs or symptoms associated with abdominal trauma.
   a.
   b.
   c.
   d.
   e.
   f.
   g.
   h.
   i.

4. Which of the following is true of abdominal trauma?
   a. Blunt injuries do not occur when personal restraints are used.
   b. Complications of penetrating abdominal trauma appear immediately.
   c. Penetrating injury is associated with higher mortality than blunt trauma.
   d. Shearing forces may produce a tear or rupture of solid organs or blood vessels.

5. Which is one of the most commonly injured solid organs?
   a. Adrenal gland
   c. Liver
   b. Kidney
   d. Pancreas

6. After injury to the liver, patients often experience which of the following?
   a. Bowel obstruction
   c. Peritoneal irritation
   b. Gastrointestinal bleeding
   d. Renal failure

7. Which of the following is true regarding renal trauma?
   a. Bleeding is usually minimal.
   b. Fractures often need surgical repair.
   c. It only occurs when posterior trauma occurs.
   d. Urine output will stop.

8. Which of the following mechanisms of blunt trauma is most often associated with pancreatic injury?
   a. Bicycle handlebar impalement
   b. Falls from higher than 20 feet
   c. Punch injuries from abuse
   d. Restrained passenger in head-on crash

9. What sign or symptom is a contraindication to insertion of an indwelling Foley catheter?
   a. Blood at the urinary meatus
   c. Burning during urination
   b. Bruising over the flank
   d. Microscopic hematuria

10. Intraabdominal arterial and venous injuries:
    a. Always present with a palpable mass
    b. Have the potential for massive hemorrhage
    c. Only involve the aorta or vena cava
    d. Only occur in penetrating trauma

11. The patient was involved in a high-speed motor vehicle crash. He refuses care. When he stands to leave, he becomes pale and states that he feels nauseated and dizzy. Which condition should you first assess for as a possible cause of his signs and symptoms?
    a. Hyperventilation
    c. Severe abdominal injury
    b. Preexisting medical problem
    d. Vagal reaction from pain

12. Scene care of the patient who has signs of shock from abdominal injury should include which of the following?
    a. Comprehensive physical examination
    b. Initiation of IV fluid therapy
    c. Ongoing assessment
    d. Oxygen administration

   Questions 13-15 pertain to the following case study:

   Your patient is a 30-year-old who was stabbed in the right upper quadrant of the abdomen. She is pale and restless with cool, clammy skin. Vital signs are blood pressure, 76/58; pulse, 128; and respirations, 28.

13. You would suspect injury to the (i) chest, (ii) liver, (iii) spleen, (iv) urinary bladder?
    a. i and ii
    c. ii and iv
    b. i and iii
    d. iii and iv

14. Interventions for this patient include which of the following?
   a. Oxygen 4 L/min via nasal cannula and intravenous lactated Ringer's solution to keep the vein open
   b. Oxygen 10 L/min via mask and intravenous lactated Ringer's solution to keep the vein open
   c. Oxygen 4 L/min via nasal cannula and intravenous lactated Ringer's solution via rapid infusion
   d. Oxygen 10 L/min via mask and intravenous lactated Ringer's solution via rapid infusion

15. Your *first* priority on arrival to this call would be:
   a. Airway maintenance
   b. The application of oxygen
   c. Scene safety
   d. To stop the bleeding

MUSCULOSKELETAL TRAUMA

● READING ASSIGNMENT

Chapter 26, pages 710-727, in *Mosby's Paramedic Textbook,* ed 2

● OBJECTIVES

As a paramedic, you should be able to:
1. Describe the features of each classification of musculoskeletal injury.
2. Describe the features of bursitis, tendonitis, and arthritis.
3. Given a specific patient scenario, outline the prehospital assessment of the musculoskeletal system.
4. Outline general principles of splinting.
5. Describe the significance and prehospital treatment principles for selected upper-extremity injuries.
6. Describe the significance and prehospital treatment principles for selected lower-extremity injuries.
7. Identify prehospital treatment priorities for open fractures.
8. Describe principles for realignment of angular fractures and dislocations.
9. Outline the process for referral of patients with minor musculoskeletal injury.

● REVIEW QUESTIONS

Match the type of fracture in Column II with the description in Column I. Use each answer only once.

Column I	Column II
1. _____ A cancer patient sustains a fracture from no apparent trauma.	a. Closed
2. _____ A fracture is incomplete and the bone is bent.	b. Comminuted
3. _____ There is bone sticking out of a laceration.	c. Epiphyseal
4. _____ A runner feels increased pain in the foot and is found to have a fracture.	d. Greenstick
5. _____ A patient's arm is broken after twisting it in an auger.	e. Oblique
6. _____ The skin over the deformed ankle is intact.	f. Open
7. _____ The fracture extends through the growth plate.	g. Pathological
8. _____ The x-ray reveals a shattered bone.	h. Spiral
9. _____ The fracture appears to be at a 45-degree angle across the bone.	i. Stress
	j. Transverse

Select *all* of the appropriate immobilization devices from Column II to treat the fractures in Column I. You may use each choice from Column II more than once.

Column I	Column II
10. _____ Shoulder	**a.** Buddy splint
11. _____ Humerus	**b.** Formable splint
12. _____ Elbow	**c.** Long spine board
13. _____ Forearm	**d.** Rigid splint
14. _____ Wrist	**e.** Pneumatic antishock
15. _____ Hand	garment
16. _____ Finger	**f.** Sling
17. _____ Pelvis	**g.** Swathe
18. _____ Hip	**h.** Traction splint
19. _____ Femur	
20. _____ Knee or patella	
21. _____ Tibia or fibula	
22. _____ Ankle or foot	
23. _____ Toes	

Questions 24-26 pertain to the following case study:

A 16-year-old injured his wrist after falling during a hockey game.

24. What is your primary objective when performing the initial assessment on

this patient? _____

25. What are the six "P's" of assessment for this injury?

P

P

P

P

P

P

26. As you examine this patient, you inspect and palpate the extremity to identify:

D

C

A

P

B

T

L

S

27. Identify at least 11 general principles of splinting.

a.

b.

c.

d.

e.

f.

g.

h.

i.

j.

k.

Questions 28 -29 pertain to the following case study:

A 55-year-old patient has a shortened and externally rotated hip with no pedal pulse distal to the injury. You anticipate a 45-minute transport to the nearest medical center.

28. Why is it appropriate to attempt to realign this dislocation?

_____

29. Explain the procedure to attempt to realign the hip in this situation.

_____

● **STUDENT SELF-ASSESSMENT**

30. Which of the following is true regarding sprains?
   a. It means injury to a tendon.
   b. No tissue disruption occurs, but bruising does.
   c. Severe hemorrhage can occur.
   d. Joint instability and dislocation may result.
31. A subluxation is another name for which of the following?
   a. Complete dislocation   c. Open fracture
   b. Incomplete dislocation   d. Strain
32. What is the cause of the pain associated with bursitis, tendonitis, and arthritis?
   a. Aging   c. Infection
   b. Degeneration   d. Inflammation
33. What group of drugs are often used to treat arthritis?
   a. Antibiotics   c. Muscle relaxants
   b. Antipyretics   d. NSAIDs

188

34. Signs or symptoms of extremity trauma that have a high urgency include which of the following?
    a. Absent distal pulses
    b. Crepitus
    c. Decreased range of motion
    d. Swelling and deformity

35. Your patient has been intubated and has signs of severe shock. His right wrist is swollen and deformed, and crepitus is present. How will you manage this extremity injury during your 7-minute transport time to the hospital?
    a. Elevation and application of ice
    b. Forearm splint
    c. Long spine board
    d. Sling and swathe

36. Boxer's fracture is the most common fracture of which bone?
    a. Carpals
    b. Metacarpal
    c. Phalanges
    d. Radius

37. When a patient has dislocation of the hip, the affected leg is usually which of the following?
    a. Lengthened and externally rotated
    b. Lengthened and internally rotated
    c. Shortened and externally rotated
    d. Shortened and internally rotated

38. A traction splint may be helpful for the patient with which of the following?
    a. Femur fracture
    b. Humerus fracture
    c. Tibial fracture
    d. Pelvic fracture

39. Your patient has severe deformity of the knee and a diminished pulse in the foot on the affected leg. This may be an indication of injury to which of the following?
    a. Femoral artery
    b. Dorsalis pedis artery
    c. Popliteal artery
    d. Posterior tibial artery

40. A bone is protruding through a wound on the lower leg. When you immobilize the fracture, the bone end slips back into the wound. What action should you take?
    a. Cover the wound with a dry sterile dressing.
    b. Irrigate the wound with sterile normal saline.
    c. Move the leg gently until the bone reappears.
    d. Soak the wound with Betadine solution.

41. Your patient fell and has a grossly deformed shoulder. Which of the following is a contraindication to realignment?
    a. Absent radial pulse
    b. Paresthesias
    c. Severe pain
    d. Thoracic spine injury

42. A woman injured her ankle during a skating activity. She has refused care and transport by EMS. What should you do before leaving the scene?
    a. Administer morphine intramuscularly for the pain.
    b. Instruct her to elevate the leg and apply ice.
    c. Have her try to bear weight and walk.
    d. Tell her to see a physician if pain persists for 2 days.

DIVISION FIVE
MEDICAL

CHAPTER 27
PULMONARY

● **READING ASSIGNMENT**

Chapter 27, pages 730-751, in *Mosby's Paramedic Textbook,* ed 2

● **OBJECTIVES**

As a paramedic, you should be able to:

1. Distinguish pathophysiology of respiratory emergencies related to ventilation, diffusion, and perfusion.
2. Outline the assessment of a patient with a pulmonary complaint.
3. Describe causes, complications, signs and symptoms, and prehospital management of patients with diagnoses of obstructive airway disease, pneumonia, noncardiogenic pulmonary edema, pulmonary thromboembolism, lung cancer, upper respiratory infection, spontaneous pneumothorax, and hyperventilation syndrome.

● **REVIEW QUESTIONS**

Match the description in Column I with the correct noninfectious pulmonary disease in Column II. Use each answer only once.

Column I	Column II
1. _____ Chronic production of excessive mucus, hypoxia, and inflammation of bronchi	**a.** Adult respiratory distress syndrome
2. _____ Pulmonary edema secondary to trauma, inhaled toxins, or metabolic disorders	**b.** Asthma
3. _____ Condition caused by a rupture of a bleb in the lung.	**c.** Chronic bronchitis
4. _____ Impaired oxygenation resulting from blockage of a pulmonary artery by a clot	**d.** Emphysema
5. _____ Bronchiolar smooth muscle spasm and excess mucus production resulting from allergy	**e.** Lung cancer
6. _____ Bacterial, viral, fungal lung infection	**f.** Hyperventilation syndrome
7. _____ Uncontrolled abnormal cell growth in the lung	**g.** Pneumonia
8. _____ Chronic disease resulting in decreased alveolar membrane surface area and polycythemia	**h.** Pulmonary thromboembolism
	i. Spontaneous pneumothorax

9. For each case, identify whether the respiratory problem is related to ventilation, diffusion, or perfusion or is a combination of two or more of these causes.
   a. Your patient is found unconscious with a plastic bag over her head.

   b. A 26-year-old is found semiconscious with a respiratory rate of 8/min. Track marks are found on the arms, legs, and under the tongue.

   c. An elderly woman with a history of congestive heart failure is acutely dyspneic and cyanotic. She has crackles throughout her lungs and coughs up frothy, bloody sputum.

   d. A woman has experienced vaginal bleeding for 2 weeks. She has profound fatigue and shortness of breath.

   e. A 56-year-old is choking in a restaurant.

   f. Your patient delivered a baby yesterday and has severe chest pain and dyspnea and an SaO_2 of 89% on room air.

   g. An 88-year-old has a large flail segment of the right chest and is hypoxic.

   Questions 10-12 pertain to the following case study:

   > You are dispatched to a call for "difficulty breathing." Dispatch tells you en route that the first responders report the patient is in moderate respiratory distress.

10. What conditions come to mind en route to this call?

   _____

11. What findings in your initial assessment would indicate life-threatening respiratory distress?

   _____

12. What information should be gathered during the focused history and physical examination of this patient?

   _____

   _____

13. Differentiate the signs and symptoms of chronic bronchitis and emphysema.
   a. Chronic bronchitis:

   _____

   b. Emphysema:

   _____

   Questions 14-16 pertain to the following case study:

   > Your 65-year-old patient has a history of chronic bronchitis and emphysema. She states that she has become acutely short of breath today and cannot complete a sentence without gasping for air. Loud wheezing is audible without a stethoscope.

14. How much oxygen should you administer to this patient? _____

15. List a drug other than oxygen that may be administered to alleviate this patient's dyspnea if not contraindicated by history or physical findings.

_____

16. Describe any additional patient care to be given en route to the hospital.

_____

_____

Questions 17-22 pertain to the following case study:

> You are called to a junior college to evaluate a 19-year-old who became acutely short of breath during a soccer game. He states that he has a history of asthma. On examination, you note inspiratory and expiratory wheezes throughout the lung fields. Vital signs are blood pressure, 130/80; pulse, 136; and respirations, 30. There is a pulsus paradoxus of 30 mm Hg.

17. Describe the pathophysiological changes in the lungs causing his signs and symptoms.

_____

18. Why would you perform a peak expiratory flow rate measurement on this patient?

_____

19. Other than oxygen, what drug can be administered to treat this patient? Include correct dose and route.

_____

20. Describe how you will reassess the patient after the medication has been administered and what you will find if the patient's condition is improving.

_____

21. If therapy is unsuccessful and the patient continues to deteriorate despite aggressive medication therapy, what condition might exist?

_____

22. What additional treatment measures will you use?

_____

23. You respond to a call for difficulty breathing. Your assessment reveals that the patient is wheezing. List one pathological cause of wheezes for each of the following:
   a. Upper airway obstruction:

_____

   b. Lower airway obstruction:

_____

   c. Trauma:

_____

   d. Alveolar pathology:

_____

   e. Interstitial space pathology:

_____

Questions 24-26 pertain to the following case study:

A physician places a 9-1-1 call to have you transport a patient from her office to the hospital with a diagnosis of pneumonia.

24. List four types of pneumonia.

    a.

    b.

    c.

    d.

25. List the signs and symptoms that may be present if this patient has bacterial pneumonia.

26. Describe the prehospital care for patients with known or suspected pneumonia.

27. You are transporting a 56-year-old man from a small rural hospital to a trauma center 70 miles away. Approximately 24 hours ago, he was involved in a head-on motor vehicle collision. He has been diagnosed with bilateral pulmonary contusions and two fractured ribs. Early in his care, he received a large volume of normal saline intravenously. He has been increasingly short of breath, was intubated before your arrival, and is very difficult to ventilate. Paralytic drugs and sedatives were administered immediately before your departure.

    a. What problem do you suspect?

    b. Describe the measures you will use during transport to assess and care for this patient.

28. List eight factors that increase the risk of pulmonary emboli.

    a.

    b.

    c.

    d.

    e.

    f.

    g.

    h.

29. List the signs and symptoms of pulmonary embolism.

30. List common characteristics of the patient who develops spontaneous pneumothorax.

31. Which of the following is an extrinsic factor associated with the development or exacerbation of respiratory disease?
    a. Cardiac or circulatory pathologies
    b. Smoking
    c. Genetic predisposition
    d. Stress

32. Which of the following is essential for normal ventilation to occur?
    a. Adequate blood volume
    b. Functional diaphragm and intercostal muscles
    c. Interstitial space that is not filled with fluid
    d. Pulmonary capillaries that are not occluded

33. Your patient has a chronic respiratory illness and calls you complaining of difficulty breathing. What is usually the most reliable indicator of the severity of the patient's present condition?
    a. One- or two- word dyspnea
    b. Pallor and diaphoresis
    c. Patient's description of severity
    d. Tachycardia

34. Which physical finding indicates chronic hypoxemia?
    a. Accessory muscle use
    b. Carpopedal spasm
    c. Clubbing
    d. Pursed lip breathing

35. Which of the following distinguishes chronic bronchitis from both emphysema and asthma?
    a. Cough
    b. Excessive mucus production
    c. Resistance to air flow
    d. Wheezing

36. Which of the following is evidence of chronic emphysema on physical examination?
    a. Decreased anterior-posterior chest diameter
    b. Decreased capillary refill in the nail beds
    c. Diminished breath sounds throughout the lungs
    d. Decreased diastolic blood pressure

37. Pulmonary hypertension can lead to which of the following?
    a. Pulmonary edema
    b. Pulmonary embolism
    c. Renal failure
    d. Right heart failure

38. Signs and symptoms of an acute asthma attack result from all of the following except which one?
    a. Bronchial muscle contraction
    b. Bronchial inflammation
    c. Mucus hypersecretion
    d. Pulmonary hypertension

39. Which physical finding is the most serious when found in an asthma patient who appears to be having acute respiratory distress?
    a. Expiratory wheezing
    b. Inspiratory wheezing
    c. Silent chest (no wheezing)
    d. Wheezing audible with a stethoscope

40. Pharmacological therapy to treat wheezing in patients with bronchitis or asthma will usually include which of the following?
    a. Albuterol
    b. Aminophylline
    c. Epinephrine
    d. Isoproterenol

41. Which pulmonary function test may be used in the prehospital setting to evaluate the effectiveness of patient ventilation?
    a. Peak expiratory flow rate
    b. Residual capacity
    c. Tidal volume
    d. Vital capacity

42. The most effective preventive measure for bacterial pneumonia is:
    a. Antibiotic therapy
    b. Patient positioning
    c. Strict isolation measures
    d. Vaccination

43. What is the most common factor associated with aspiration pneumonia?
   a. Age
   b. Airway pathology
   c. Decreased level of consciousness
   d. Drowning
44. Which of the following is true regarding adult respiratory distress syndrome regardless of the cause?
   a. Death always occurs as a result of this complication.
   b. Disseminated intravascular coagulation always occurs.
   c. Pneumonia will be a secondary complication.
   d. Pulmonary edema will result.
45. Which ventilation adjunct will work despite a leak and may prevent the need for intubation if used successfully?
   a. BiPAP   c. CPAP
   b. BVM   d. PEEP
46. The signs and symptoms of pulmonary embolus vary and are related primarily to:
   a. The age of the patient   c. The origin of the embolus
   b. The cause of the embolus   d. The size of the embolus
47. What is the most important action the paramedic can take to prevent the spread of upper respiratory infections?
   a. Obtain the appropriate immunizations
   b. Place a mask on the patient during transport
   c. Practice good handwashing techniques
   d. Wear a mask and goggles during patient care
48. Which of the following is associated with the development of spontaneous pneumothorax?
   a. Asthma   c. IV drug abuse
   b. Free-base cocaine use   d. Thromboembolus
49. Which of the following is *not* a cause of hyperventilation?
   a. Fever   c. Hyperglycemia
   b. Narcotic overdose   d. Hypoxia
50. What is the most common risk factor for lung cancer?
   a. Cigarette smoking   c. Exposure to coal products
   b. Exposure to asbestos   d. Exposure to ionizing radiation

CHAPTER 28
CARDIOLOGY

● READING ASSIGNMENT
Chapter 28, pages 752-909, in *Mosby's Paramedic Textbook*, ed 2

● OBJECTIVES
As a paramedic, you should be able to:
1. Identify risk factors and prevention strategies associated with cardiovascular disease.
2. Describe the normal physiology of the heart.
3. Discuss electrophysiology as it relates to the normal electrical and mechanical events in the cardiac cycle.
4. Outline the activity of each component of the electrical conduction system of the heart.
5. Outline the appropriate assessment of a patient who may be experiencing a cardiovascular disorder.
6. Describe basic monitoring techniques that permit electrocardiogram interpretation.
7. Explain the relationship of the electrocardiogram tracing to the heart's electrical activity.
8. Describe, in sequence, the steps in electrocardiogram interpretation.
9. Identify the characteristics of normal sinus rhythm.
10. When shown an ECG tracing, identify the rhythm, site of origin, possible causes, clinical significance, and prehospital treatment that is indicated.
11. Describe prehospital assessment and management of patients with selected cardiovascular disorders based on knowledge of the pathophysiology of the illness.
12. List indications, contraindications, and prehospital considerations when using selected cardiac interventions including basic life support, monitor-defibrillators, defibrillation, implantable cardioverter-defibrillators, synchronized cardioversion, and transcutaneous pacing.
13. List indications, contraindications, dose, and mechanism of action for pharmacological agents used in the treatment of cardiovascular disorders.
14. Identify appropriate actions that should be taken in the prehospital setting to terminate resuscitation.

● REVIEW QUESTIONS
Match each term in Column II with its definition in Column I. Use each answer only once.

Column I	Column II
1. _____ Heart rate × stroke volume	a. Afterload
2. _____ Volume available for ventricles to pump each contraction	b. Blood pressure
3. _____ Peripheral vascular resistance produces this pressure	c. Cardiac output
4. _____ Ventricular relaxation	d. Contractility
5. _____ Cardiac output × peripheral vascular resistance	e. Diastole
6. _____ Increased myocardial contractility in response to increased preload	f. Preload
7. _____ Ventricular ejection per heartbeat	g. Starling's law
	h. Stroke volume
	i. Systole

8. Identify a prevention strategy for each of the following risk factors for cardiovascular disease and a community resource where you can refer the patient to assist with modification of this risk factor.

Risk Factor	Prevention Strategy	Resource
a. Smoking		
b. Hypercholesterolemia		
c. Obesity		
d. Sedentary lifestyle		

9. Explain how the sympathetic and parasympathetic divisions of the autonomic nervous system influence cardiac function in the following areas.

	Sympathetic	Parasympathetic
a. Heart rate		
b. Myocardial contractility		
c. Lungs		
d. Blood vessels (peripheral)		

10. Name the two adrenal hormones and describe the effects of each on the cardiovascular system.

	Name	Function
a.		
b.		

11. Fill in the blanks in the following sentences about electrophysiology:
Within the body, separated charged particles with opposite charges have a **(a)**

_____ force of attraction that gives them **(b)**

_____ energy. This energy is released when the cell

membrane becomes **(c)** _____ to the charged particles and allows the charges to come together. The electrical charge between

the inside and outside of cells is the **(d)** _____ differ-

ence and is measured in **(e)** _____. Although there is
a relatively equal number of positively and negatively charged ions inside

and outside the cell, the intracellular area has a **(f)** _____

charge because of the **(g)** _____ charged proteins that
cannot move outside the cell. The electrical charge difference in the resting
state has the potential to do work and is known as the resting membrane

(h) _____ (RMP). During this phase the inside of the

cell is electrically **(i)** _____ relative to the outside of

the cell (approximately **(j)** _____ mV). The RMP is

primarily because of the difference between the intracellular and extracellu-

lar **(k)** _____ ion level. Because of the chemical gradient (more of these ions inside than outside of the cell), the **(l)**

_____ would move out of the cell in an attempt to achieve equilibrium. However, they remain in the cell because of the negative intracellular charge generated by the **(m)** _____ . In the RMP, sodium will not rush into the cell because the cell membrane

is not **(n)** _____ to sodium. The ability of nerve and muscle cells to produce action potentials is known as **(o)**

_____ . If this action potential results in a decreased charge difference across the cell membrane, the RMP becomes less negative,

and this is called **(p)** _____ . If a stimulus is strong enough to cause depolarization of a cell membrane to a level called the

(q) _____ _____ , a chain re-

action of permeability changes cause an **(r)** _____

_____ to spread over the entire cell membrane. Ac-

tion potentials have two phases: a **(s)** _____ phase

and a **(t)** _____ phase. During an action potential, the sodium ions rush into the cell, and RMP becomes **(u)**

_____ on the inside and **(v)** _____

on the outside of the cell membrane. This occurs during the **(w)**

_____ phase. The repolarization phase results from potassium leakage outside the cell and the return of the cell membrane to

its normal resting **(x)** _____ _____ state.

12. Answer the following questions regarding the five phases of the cardiac action potential:
   a. During phase 0 (rapid depolarization), what causes the inside of the cell to become positive?

_____

   b. What is the membrane potential during phase 1 (early rapid repolarization)?

_____

   c. How is the membrane potential held at 0 during phase 2 (plateau phase)?

_____

   d. What happens to the membrane potential of the cell during phase 3 (terminal phase of rapid repolarization)?

_____

   e. How is the balance of sodium and potassium restored during phase 4?

_____

f. Why can cardiac pacemaker cells depolarize without an external stimulus to initiate an action potential?

_____

_____

● INTRODUCTION TO ECG MONITORING

13. Circle the correct response in each of the following statements:
The ECG tracing represents an amplified view of the myocardial **(a)** action potentials or contractions. If the voltage displayed is positive, the ECG tracing will display a(n) **(b)** upward, downward, or isoelectric deflection. Cardiac pacemaker cells can spontaneously generate impulses, a property known as **(c)** automaticity or conductivity. This rhythmic activity occurs because these cells do not have a stable **(d)** action potential or resting membrane potential.

14. Label Fig. 28-1 illustrating the cardiac conduction system.

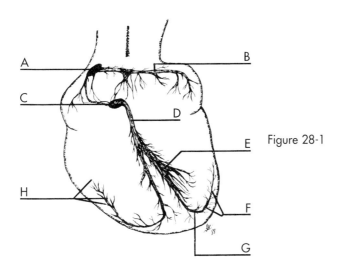

Figure 28-1

    A.
    B.
    C.
    D.
    E.
    F.
    G.
    H.

15. The sinoatrial node is the dominant pacemaker. If it fails to fire, what will happen?

_____

16. Briefly describe the mechanism for ectopic impulse formation by each of the following mechanisms:
    a. Enhanced automaticity:

_____

    b. Reentry:

_____

● ASSESSMENT OF THE CARDIAC PATIENT

17. A 62-year-old woman complains of chest pain. What questions should you ask using the OPQRST mnemonic to determine the nature and severity of her pain?

    O

    P

    Q

    R

    S

    T

18. List three chief complaints that may lead you to believe a patient has a cardiovascular problem.

    a.

    b.

    c.

19. An older man experiences a syncopal episode at a local gym. List at least two questions you should ask in an attempt to determine the nature of his syncopal episode.

    a.

    b.

20. A 34-year-old woman walks into your ambulance base complaining of a fluttering sensation in her chest. What will your history and physical examination include to determine the cause of this sensation?

Questions 21-23 pertain to the following case study:

An 87-year-old woman calls you to her home complaining of weakness and nausea. On arrival, you find her seated on the commode. She is pale, cool, and diaphoretic. Her blood pressure is 70 mm Hg by palpation, and her ECG is shown in Fig. 28-2.

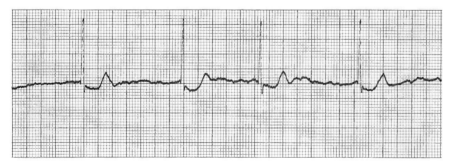

Figure 28-2

21. What information from this patient's past medical history will be important to elicit at this time?

---

22. What is your interpretation of her ECG?

---

23. She tells you that she is taking digoxin, diltiazem, potassium, and furosemide. Could any of her home medicines be playing a role in her problem? If yes, which ones and why?

_____

_____

24. An older man is found unresponsive and bradycardic in a local park. A caretaker states that he complained of chest pain before collapsing. No one is available to give you any information regarding his history. Briefly outline specific findings you may encounter in your patient assessment if he has a cardiac history.

_____

_____

● ECG MONITORING

25. Place the positive (+) and negative (−) and electrodes for the four leads shown in Fig. 28-3.

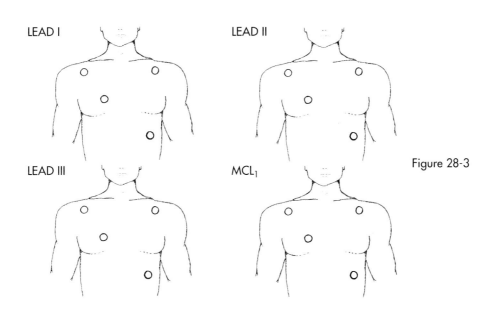

Figure 28-3

26. Describe the location of each of the 10 electrodes needed to record a 12-lead ECG.

a.   f.

b.   g.

c.   h.

d.   i.

e.   j.

27. List six problems that may interfere with a clear ECG recording. For each problem, discuss a possible solution.

  a.   **d.**

  b.   **e.**

  c.   **f.**

28. Label Fig. 28-4 with the appropriate measurement intervals.

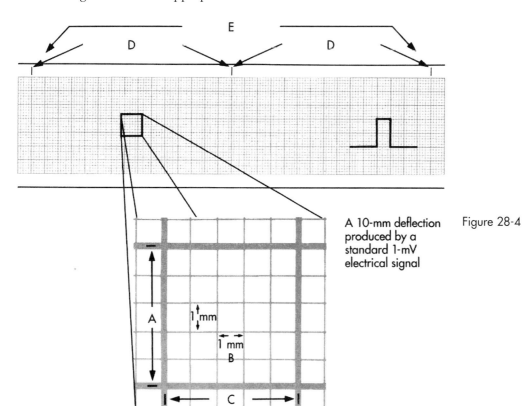

A 10-mm deflection produced by a standard 1-mV electrical signal

Figure 28-4

  a. _____ mm

  b. _____ sec

  c. _____ sec

  d. _____ sec

  e. _____ sec

29. Label the sample ECG tracing in Fig. 28-5.

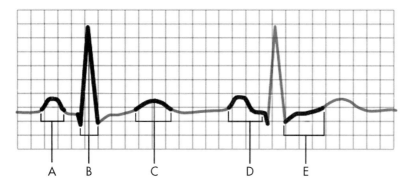

Figure 28-5

  a.

  b.

  c.

  d.

  e.

30. List five causes of artifact.

    a.

    b.

    c.

    d.

    e.

● ECG INTERPRETATION

31. List the five steps in ECG analysis.

    a.

    b.

    c.

    d.

    e.

32. Calculate the rate of the ECG in Fig. 28-6 using four different methods, describing the steps you use in each method.

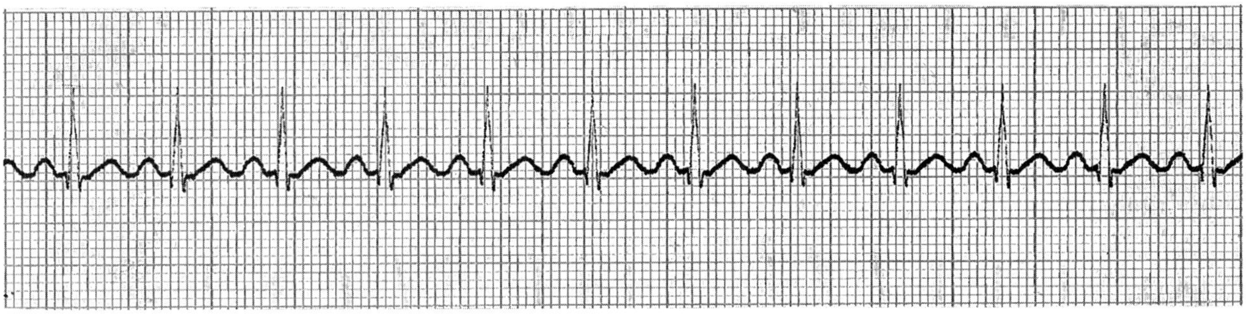

Figure 28-6

    a.

_____

_____

    b.

_____

_____

    c.

_____

_____

    d.

_____

_____

33. If the rate in Question 32 is within normal limits, can we assume the patient is stable in this situation?

_____

34. Which method of calculation would be *most* accurate if the rhythm in Question 32 was:

a. Regular:

_____

b. Irregularly irregular:

_____

35. What criterion must be met when analyzing the ECG rhythm to determine that the rhythm is regular?

_____

36. What analysis can be made about conduction in each of the following examples?

a. The QRS width is less than or equal to 0.12 second.

_____

b. The QRS width is greater than 0.12 second.

_____

37. List the four criteria that must be evaluated when analyzing the P waves.

a.

b.

c.

d.

38. Briefly describe the significance of each of the following PR-interval findings.

a. PR interval 0.08 sec:

_____

b. PR interval 0.16 sec:

_____

c. PR interval 0.24 sec:

_____

39. Analyze the ECG rhythm strip in Fig. 28-7 using the five steps described in Question 31, and give your interpretation.

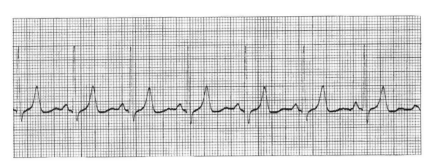

Figure 28-7

a. Step 1:

_____

b. Step 2:

_____

c. Step 3:

_____

d. Step 4:

_____

e. Step 5:

_____

Interpretation:

_____

● INTRODUCTION TO DYSRHYTHMIAS

40. When a dysrhythmia is noted on the monitor, what factors must be considered to determine whether any intervention is necessary?

_____

41. Dysrhythmias originating in the sinoatrial node frequently result from in-

creases or decreases in **(a)** _____

_____. ECG features common to all sinoatrial node
dysrhythmias are
b. QRS complex:

_____

c. P waves (lead II):

_____

d. PR interval:

_____

205

42. List two causes of each bradycardic and tachycardic dysrhythmia that originates in the sinus node.
    a. Sinus bradycardia:

_____

    b. Sinus tachycardia:

_____

    Complete the missing information on Flashcards 1 to 4 at the end of the text.
43. Complete Flashcard 1 (Fig. 28-8): Sinus bradycardia.

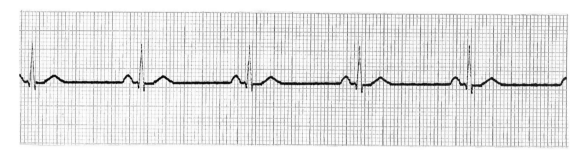

Figure 28-8

44. Complete Flashcard 2 (Fig. 28-9): Sinus tachycardia.

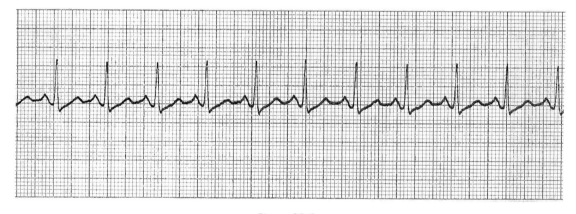

Figure 28-9

45. Complete Flashcard 3 (Fig. 28-10): Sinus dysrhythmia.

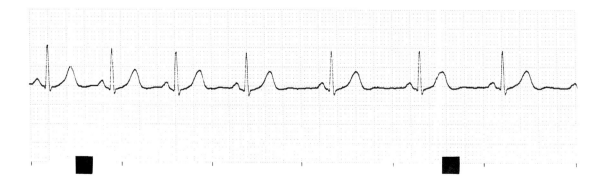

Figure 28-10

46. Complete Flashcard 4 (Fig. 28-11): Sinus arrest.

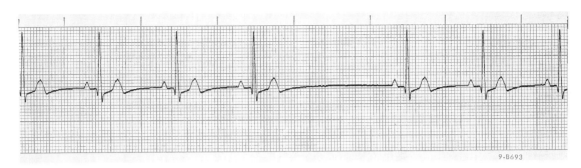

Figure 28-11

47. Atrial dysrhythmias originate in the **(a)** _____ of the

(b) _____ or in the **(c)** _____
pathways.

48. Common features of atrial dysrhythmias are:
  a. QRS complex:

_____

  b. P waves (if present):

_____

  c. PR intervals:

_____

49. List four causes of dysrhythmias that originate in the atria.
  a.

  b.

  c.

  d.

  Complete the missing information on Flashcards 5 to 9 showing dysrhythmias originating in the atria.
50. Complete Flashcard 5 (Fig. 28-12): Wandering atrial pacemaker.

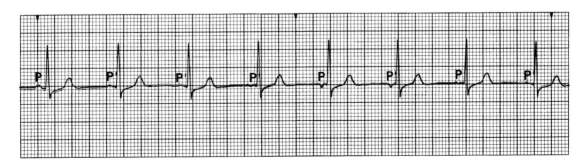

Figure 28-12

51. Complete Flashcard 6 (Fig. 28-13): Premature atrial contraction.

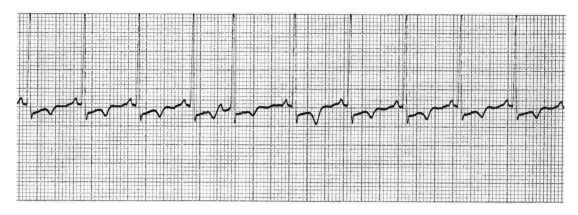

Figure 28-13

52. Complete Flashcard 7 (Fig. 28-14): Supraventricular tachycardia.

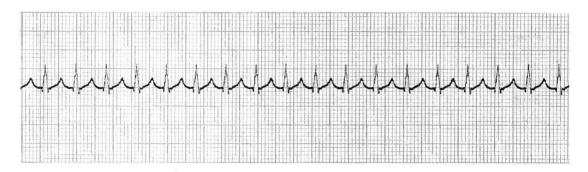

Figure 28-14

53. Complete Flashcard 8 (Fig. 28-15): Atrial flutter with 3:1 conduction.

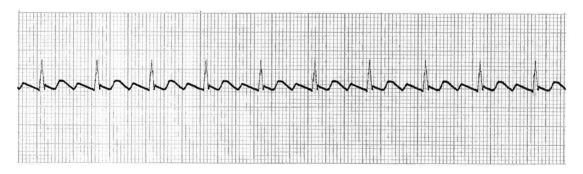

Figure 28-15

54. Complete Flashcard 9 (Fig. 28-16): Atrial fibrillation.

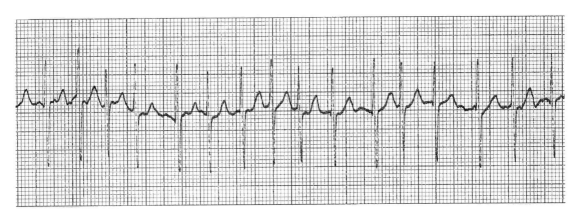

Figure 28-16

55. Rhythms that start in the atrioventricular node or junction are called

(a) _____ rhythms. These rhythms share the following common features:

b. QRS complex:

_____

c. P waves:

_____

d. PR interval:

_____

56. List four causes of dysrhythmias that start in the atrioventricular junction.
a.
b.
c.
d.

Complete the missing information on Flashcards 10 to 12 showing dysrhythmias originating in the atrioventricular junction.

57. Complete Flashcard 10 (Fig. 28-17): Sinus rhythm (borderline bradycardia) with two premature junctional contractions.

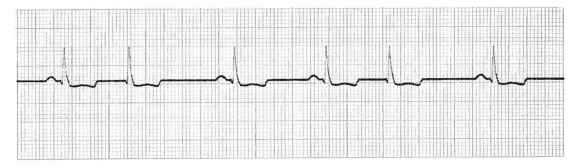

Figure 28-17

58. Complete Flashcard 11 (Fig. 28-18): Junctional escape rhythm.

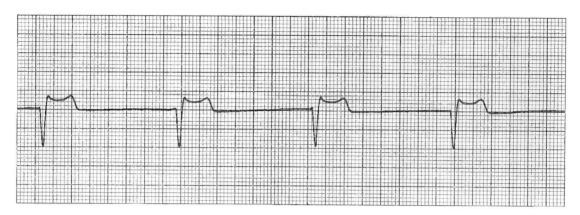

Figure 28-18

59. Complete Flashcard 12 (Fig. 28-19): Accelerated junctional rhythm.

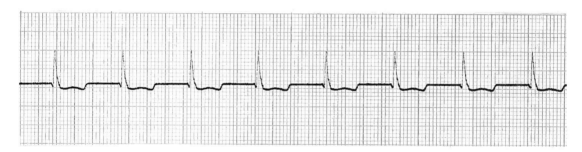

Figure 28-19

60. Rhythms originating from the ventricle have an intrinsic rate of **(a)**

_____ to _____ but can be ac-

celerated at rates up to **(b)** _____ or tachycardic

at rates greater than **(c)** _____.

61. List five causes of dysrhythmias that originate in the ventricles.
   a.
   b.
   c.
   d.
   e.

62. Identify five steps that can be used when evaluating a 12-lead ECG to distinguish between wide-complex tachycardias of ventricular versus supraventricular origin.
   a.
   b.
   c.
   d.
   e.

Complete the missing information on Flashcards 13 to 18 showing dysrhythmias originating in the ventricles.

63. Complete Flashcard 13 (Fig. 28-20): Ventricular escape rhythm.

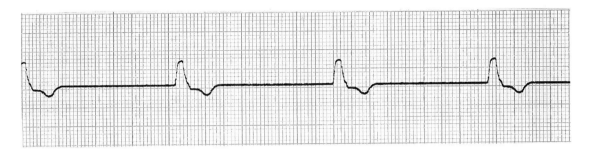

Figure 28-20

64. Complete Flashcard 14 (Fig. 28-21): Normal sinus rhythm with one premature ventricular contraction.

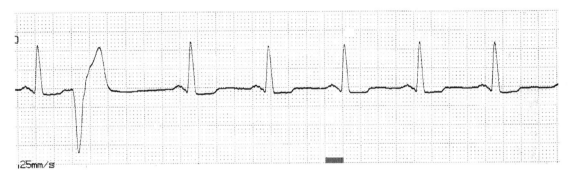

Figure 28-21

65. Complete Flashcard 15 (Fig. 28-22): Monomorphic ventricular tachycardia.

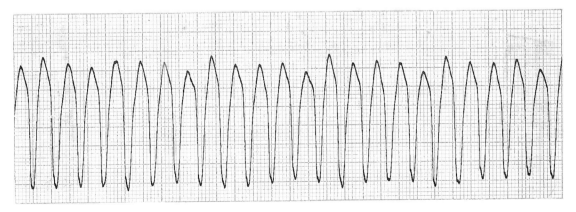

Figure 28-22

66. Complete Flashcard 16 (Fig. 28-23): Ventricular fibrillation.

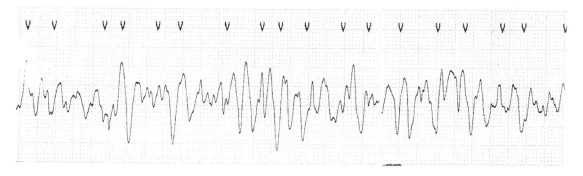

Figure 28-23

67. Complete Flashcard 17 (Fig. 28-24): Asystole.

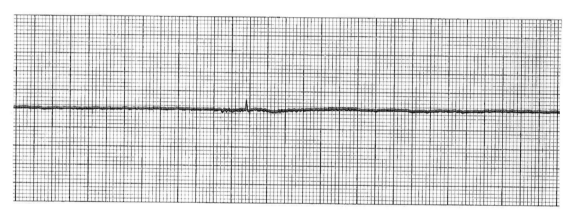

Figure 28-24

68. Complete Flashcard 18 (Fig. 28-25): Ventricular paced rhythm.

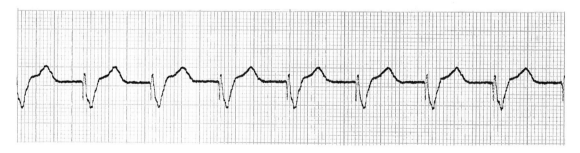

Figure 28-25

69. Delays or interruptions in cardiac electrical conduction are called

(a) _____ _____ . They may

be caused by disease of the **(b)** _____

_____ .

70. List five causes of dysrhythmias caused by delays in cardiac electrical conduction.

   a.

   b.

   c.

   d.

   e.

Complete the missing information on Flashcards 19 to 22 showing dysrhythmias originating from conduction disorders.

71. Complete Flashcard 19 (Fig. 28-26): Sinus rhythm with first-degree atrioventricular block.

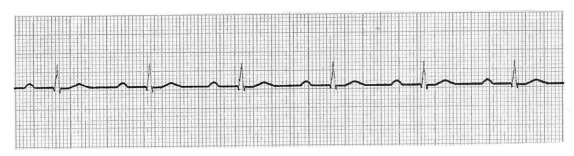

Figure 28-26

72. Complete Flashcard 20 (Fig. 28-27): Second-degree atrioventricular block (Mobitz type I or Wenckebach).

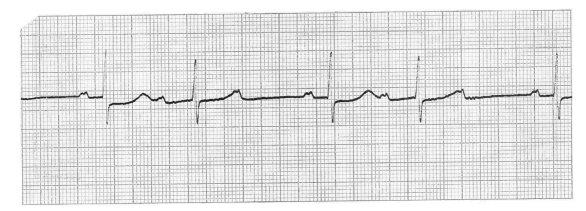

Figure 28-27

73. Complete Flashcard 21 (Fig. 28-28): Second-degree atrioventricular block (Mobitz type II).

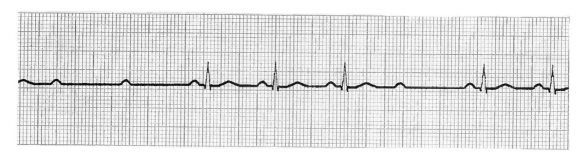

Figure 28-28

74. Complete Flashcard 22 (Fig. 28-29): Third-degree (complete) atrioventricular block.

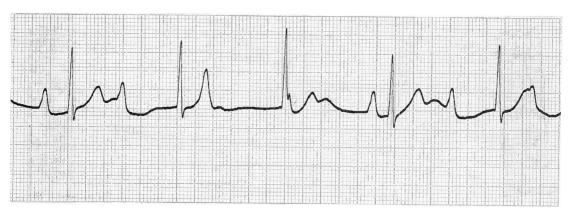

Figure 28-29

75. List the characteristics to identify:

   a. Right bundle branch block _____

   b. Left bundle branch block _____

   c. Anterior hemiblock _____

   d. Posterior hemiblock _____

76. Identify patients at risk for developing complete heart block if they are given procainamide, digoxin, verapamil, or diltiazem:

   a.

   b.

   c.

77. An approximately 50-year-old man is found unconscious in a parking lot downtown. He is pulseless and apneic. The attendant is certain he has been there fewer than 5 minutes but does not know what happened. The patient's ECG is shown in Fig. 28-30.

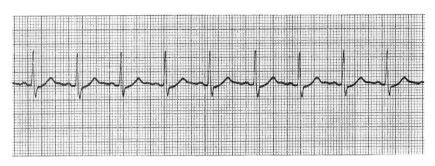

Figure 28-30

   a. You identify the rhythm as:

   _____

   b. Outline the appropriate interventions for this patient based on current treatment guidelines by the American Heart Association.

   _____

78. Outline the ECG features that may allow detection of a patient with Wolff-Parkinson-White syndrome (WPW):
   a. QRS complex:

   _____

   b. PR interval:

   _____

79. Why is it clinically important to recognize a patient with a history of WPW?

   _____

   _____

● SPECIFIC CARDIOVASCULAR DISEASES

80. Explain the pathophysiology of atherosclerotic effects on blood vessels.

   _____

   _____

81. List two triggers that may initiate an anginal attack in a susceptible patient:
   a.
   b.
82. Describe the following features of angina:
   a. Duration:

   _____

   b. Relieved by:

   _____

83. How can a paramedic distinguish between unstable angina and myocardial infarction in the prehospital environment?

_____

84. Briefly outline the sequence of pathophysiological events that occur from the time that a clot forms until cardiac tissue dies in acute myocardial infarction.

_____

_____

85. Complete the information regarding myocardial infarction that is missing in the following table:

Area of Heart Injured or Infarcted	Coronary Vessel Involved Most Often	Leads with Visible ST Segment Changes
Anterior		
Lateral		
Septal		
Inferior		

86. How much ST segment elevation must be present to be clinically significant?

_____

87. List six conditions other than myocardial infarction that can cause ST-segment elevation.
   a.
   b.
   c.
   d.
   e.
   f.

88. List the five-step analysis described in this text for infarct recognition.
   a.
   b.
   c.
   d.
   e.

89. Identify four complications secondary to myocardial infarction.
   a.
   b.
   c.
   d.

Questions 90-94 pertain to the following case study:

A 57-year-old, 80-kg man with a history of untreated hypertension complains of crushing midsternal chest pain that began 2 hours ago. He takes no medicines but admits to smoking two packs of cigarettes per day. His blood pressure is 162/102 mm Hg. His ECG strip is shown in Fig. 28-31.

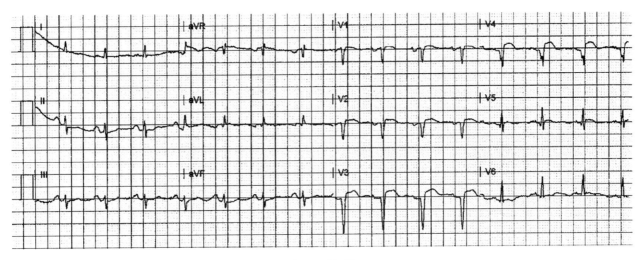

Figure 28-31

90. What other associated signs or symptoms may be present if the patient is experiencing a myocardial infarction?

_____

91. What is your interpretation of his ECG?

_____

92. Describe general treatment measures you will use for this patient.

_____

_____

93. List three drugs (excluding oxygen) with the appropriate dosage to administer to this patient.
    a.
    b.
    c.

94. You transmit the 12-lead to the hospital and are asked to determine whether the patient meets inclusion or exclusion criteria for thrombolytic therapy.
    a. List 5 inclusion criteria:

_____

    b. List 11 exclusion criteria:

_____

_____

_____

95. Interpret each of the following 12-lead ECGs.
   a. Fig. 28-32:

_____

_____

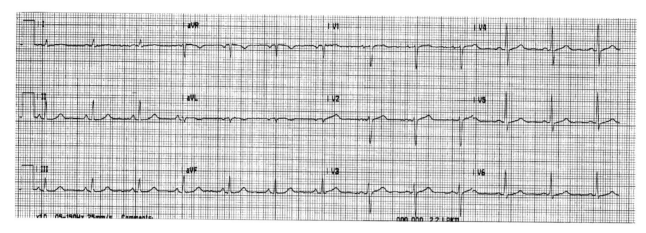

Figure 28-32

   b. Fig. 28-33:

_____

_____

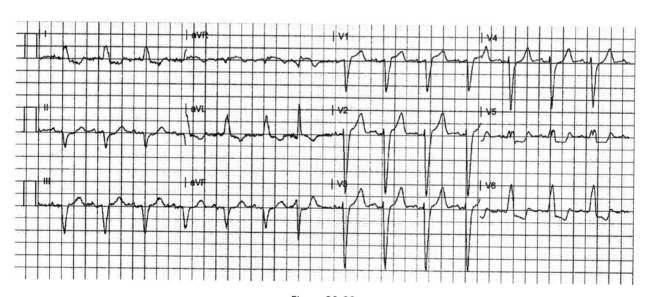

Figure 28-33

c. Fig. 28-34:

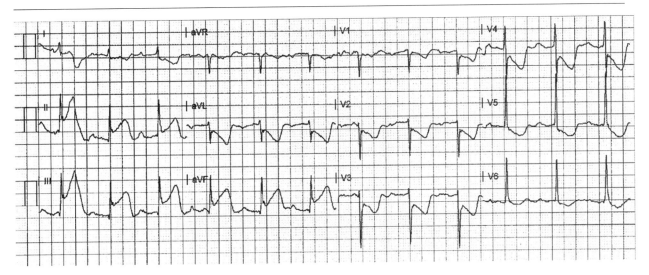

Figure 28-34

d. Fig. 28-35:

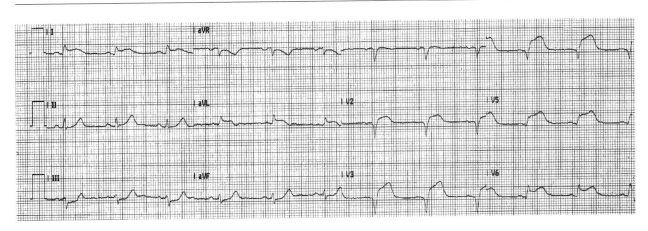

Figure 28-35

Questions 96-100 pertain to the following case study:

An 80-kg patient who had a syncopal episode and chest pain has the following ECG (Fig. 28-36).

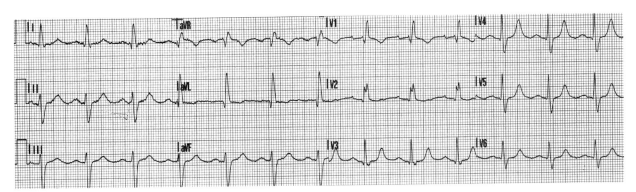

Figure 28-36

96. What is the axis of this ECG? _____

97. The QRS duration is 0.134 sec. Draw a triangle that begins at the J point in lead V1, and, working backward, ends at the first QRS deflection that is encountered. Does the triangle point up or down? _____

98. Based upon your determination of axis, the QRS duration, and the triangle you drew, identify the two blocks that are present in this ECG.

---

99. What is the significance of these blocks? _____

100. Based on the patient's chief complaint and your ECG findings, what interventions do you perform in addition to routine cardiac care?

Questions 101-105 pertain to the following case study:

A 72-year-old, 70-kg woman calls you to her home complaining of a sudden onset of severe dyspnea without chest pain. You find her anxious, sitting upright, with diaphoretic skin and circumoral cyanosis. Her only home medicine is a diuretic. Vital signs are blood pressure, 170/106 mm Hg; pulse, 124; and respirations, 28 and labored. Rales are audible to the level of the scapulae. SaO_2 is 86%. Her ECG is shown in Fig. 28-37.

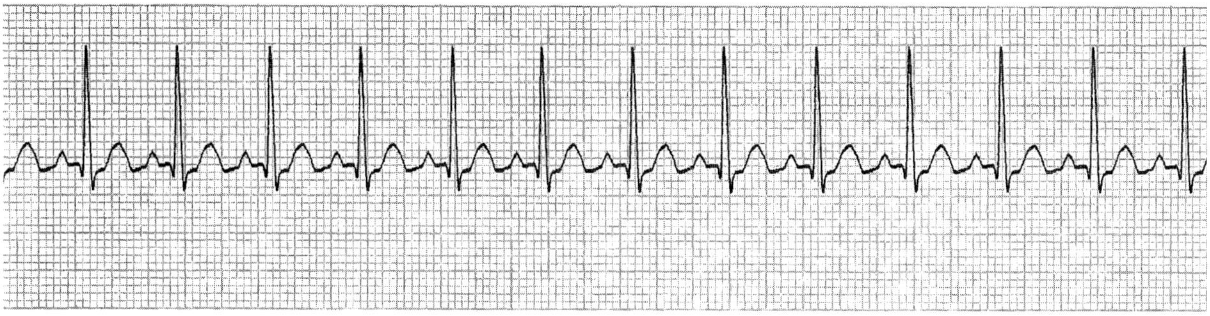

Figure 28-37

101. What medical condition or conditions do you suspect?

---

102. What other physical findings would help confirm this diagnosis?

---

103. What is your interpretation of her ECG?

---

104. You have placed the patient on oxygen and wish to administer other pharmacological agents to improve her oxygenation. List three drugs that you would consider and give the correct dose and desired effect of each.

   a. _____

   b. _____

   c. _____

105. You decide to administer furosemide 0.5 mg/kg. It is supplied in a 4-ml ampule that contains 40 mg of the drug. How many milliliters will you give? _____ ml

106. List causes and signs and symptoms of right-sided heart failure.

   a. Causes:

---

b. Signs and symptoms:

Questions 107-110 pertain to the following case study:

You are evaluating a 67-year-old man who has a history of two myocardial infarctions. His wife states he had chest pain that began 4 hours ago but he refused to let her call EMS and then passed out. He is conscious but confused and is pale and diaphoretic. His blood pressure is 80/50 mm Hg, his respiratory rate is 20/min, his SaO_2 is 90%, and his breath sounds are clear. His only home medicine is nitroglycerin paste, which he has on his left chest. This patient's ECG is shown in Fig. 28-38.

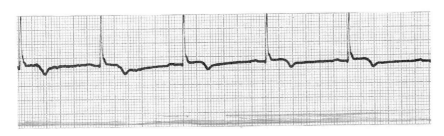

Figure 28-38

107. What is your interpretation of his ECG?

---

108. What drug and dosage will you administer in consultation with medical direction to correct this dysrhythmia?

After administering the first dose of this drug, the heart rate accelerates to 70/min; however, the patient's other physical findings remain unchanged.

109. What do you suspect this patient is suffering from?

---

110. List critical interventions, including drug therapy, that you should use, assuming that your estimated time of arrival to the hospital is 30 minutes.

Questions 111-114 pertain to the following case study:

A 70-year-old man experiences a sudden onset of a "tearing" abdominal pain at the area of the umbilicus that radiates to his back. He is pale and complains of the urge to defecate. His only history is hypertension, for which he takes captopril. Vital signs are blood pressure, 106/70 mm Hg; pulse, 100; and respirations, 20. On physical examination, you auscultate a bruit over the periumbilical area.

111. What illness do you suspect?

---

112. Should you palpate this patient's abdomen?

---

113. Should you allow this patient to go to the toilet and defecate?

---

114. Briefly outline your management of this patient.

_____

Questions 115-117 pertain to the following case study:

An older man complains of a severe "ripping" pain between his scapulae that extends down to his legs. He is pale and diaphoretic and has the following vital signs: blood pressure 170/110 mm Hg in the right arm and 130/80 mm Hg in the left arm.

115. What medical emergency do you suspect?

_____

116. Describe other physical findings that may confirm your suspicions.

_____

117. Outline your management of this patient in the prehospital phase.

_____

118. Differentiate between the following characteristics of embolic arterial occlusion and thrombotic arterial occlusion.

	Embolic	**Thrombotic**
Causes:		
Onset:		
Signs and symptoms:		

119. An older woman calls you to her home because she bumped her leg and a varicose vein is bleeding. What care should be rendered to this patient?

_____

120. List three signs or symptoms of acute deep vein thrombosis.
   a.
   b.
   c.

Questions 121-124 pertain to the following case study:

A 60-year-old man complains of a severe headache, blurred vision, and vomiting. He states that he has a history of hypertension but has not been taking his medicine because the cost is too high. His vital signs are blood pressure, 190/128 mm Hg; pulse, 88; and respirations, 20.

121. What medical emergency do you suspect?

_____

122. If this man is not treated promptly, what other signs and/or symptoms may result?

_____

123. Outline general management principles for this patient.

_____

124. If your transport time is delayed, list one drug (with the appropriate dose) that medical direction may order to lower this patient's blood pressure.

_____

● TECHNIQUES OF MANAGING CARDIAC EMERGENCIES

125. You are at a friend's home playing tennis. After retrieving the ball, you turn around see that your friend has collapsed on the court. Outline the steps you must take from this moment until EMS arrives if he has had a cardiac arrest. (Assume that no one else is nearby to help.)

_____

_____

_____

126. A basic life-support unit is caring for a patient who is in cardiac arrest when your advanced life-support unit arrives on the scene. An automated external defibrillator without a display is attached to the patient, and five shocks have already been delivered.
    a. When should you defibrillate this patient if you determine that ventricular fibrillation is present?

_____

    b. If a rescuer is in contact with the patient when the automated external defibrillator fires, will an injury occur?

_____

Questions 127-129 pertain to the following case study:

   You arrive on the scene to care for a patient who is pulseless and apneic. The monitor displays the rhythm shown in Fig. 28-39.

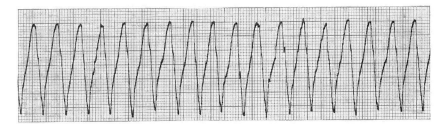

Figure 28-39

127. What is your interpretation of the ECG?

_____

128. What is your first intervention after rhythm determination and verification of pulselessness?

_____

129. List two factors that will improve the success rate of this treatment.
    a.
    b.

130. List the steps in performing this intervention.

_____

_____

_____

_____

131. You are at the home of a patient whose wife states that he was experiencing severe chest pain. Moments after you hook up the patient to your monitor, he loses consciousness, and the rhythm shown in Fig. 28-40 is displayed. Blood pressure is 60 mm Hg by palpation, and ventilations are adequate. Another paramedic applies oxygen by nonrebreather mask at 12 L/min. State the appropriate therapy for this patient up to and including administration of the first drug.

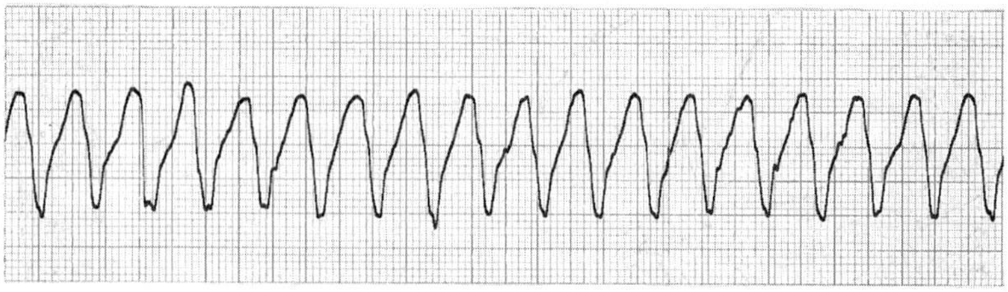

Figure 28-40

_____

_____

132. What is the advantage of synchronized cardioversion?

_____

133. Briefly outline the steps in synchronized cardioversion that are different from unsynchronized cardioversion.

_____

_____

224

134. A 69-year-old patient has a blood pressure of 76/50 mm Hg and the ECG shown in Fig. 28-41.

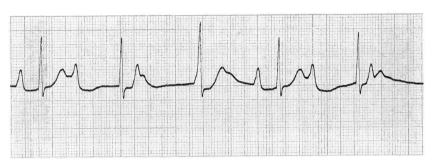

Figure 28-41

    a. What is your interpretation of the ECG?

_____

    b. Assuming that no drugs are readily available, list the steps you would take to initiate transcutaneous pacing on this patient.

_____

_____

_____

_____

_____

135. An older man is found unresponsive, apneic, and pulseless in the busy bathroom of a shopping mall. A quick examination reveals the monitor pattern shown in Fig. 28-42.

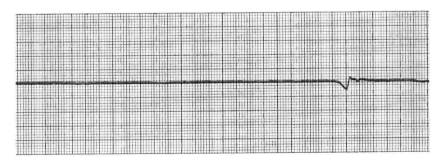

Figure 28-42

    a. What is your interpretation of the rhythm?

_____

    b. What drugs (with appropriate doses) should be administered?

_____

    c. What electrical therapy would be appropriate for this patient?

_____

136. You are en route to the hospital with a 55-year-old man whom you suspect is having an acute myocardial infarction. Suddenly, the patient gasps and becomes pulseless and apneic. As you look at the monitor, you note the ECG shown in Fig. 28-43.

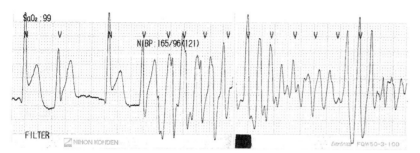

Figure 28-43

a. What is the rhythm?

_____

b. What single treatment modality is most likely to restore circulation in this patient?

_____

c. List the appropriate drugs (in the proper order) with correct doses that may be given to this patient if the answer in (b) is unsuccessful.

_____

_____

137. For each of the following situations, state whether criteria to stop resuscitation have been met. Explain your decision. Assume the patient is now in asystole.

a. The patient is 94 years old and was found in full arrest, having last been seen 30 minutes previously. You have intubated the patient, given epinephrine, and attempted pacing.

_____

_____

b. A 65-year-old patient collapses in a mall. You have been resuscitating for 20 minutes, although you have not been able to intubate. You have administered epinephrine (three doses), attempted pacing (unsuccessfully), and administered atropine sulfate (two doses).

_____

_____

c. A 16-year-old is in full arrest after falling from a fourth floor balcony. You initially got back a sinus rhythm with a pulse, but now asystole is on the monitor. The patient is intubated and you have two large-bore IVs infusing wide open and have given three doses of epinephrine, attempted pacing, and given two doses of atropine.

_____

d. A 70-year-old is in asystole. You have intubated and given epinephrine (three doses), attempted pacing (unsuccessfully), and administered the maximum dose of atropine with no success. You elect to terminate resuscitation, but the family is strongly objecting.

● STUDENT SELF-ASSESSMENT

138. Your patient is experiencing chest pain. He is 75 years of age, says his last cholesterol was 300 mg/dl, and takes Diabinese, Acupril, and indapamide. How many risk factors for cardiovascular disease did you identify in this patient?
   a. Two   **c.** Four
   b. Three   **d.** Five

139. Blood pressure is equal to which of the following?
   a. Heart rate × Stroke volume × Cardiac output
   b. Stroke volume × Peripheral vascular resistance
   c. Heart rate × Stroke volume × Peripheral vascular resistance
   d. Heart rate × Contractility × Stroke volume

140. Your patient is experiencing signs of a large infarct affecting the anterior portion of the left ventricle. Which coronary vessel is most likely involved?
   a. Circumflex artery   **c.** Left anterior descending
   b. Coronary sinus   **d.** Right coronary artery

141. Which valve separates the left atrium from the left ventricle?
   a. Aortic   **c.** Pulmonic
   b. Mitral   **d.** Tricuspid

142. The magnetic force that occurs when particles with opposite charges are separated across the cell membrane is known as which of the following?
   a. Action potential   **c.** Millivolts
   b. Depolarization   **d.** Potential energy

143. Which ions are critical to maintain the normal resting membrane potential?
   a. Chloride   **c.** Sodium
   b. Phosphate   **d.** Sulfate

144. Which drugs may affect the threshold level of cardiac conduction cells?
   a. Atropine   **c.** Nitroglycerin
   b. Morphine   **d.** Verapamil

145. Which phase of the cardiac action potential represents depolarization?
   a. Phase 1   **c.** Phase 3
   b. Phase 2   **d.** Phase 4

146. What is the purpose of the absolute refractory period in the heart?
   a. To allow electrolyte balance to be restored
   b. To initiate the next action potential
   c. To permit the muscle to relax so the heart can fill
   d. To stretch the cardiac fibers for more forceful contraction

147. Which are the smallest divisions of the HIS bundles?
   a. Anterior-superior fascicles
   b. Posterior-inferior fascicles
   c. Right and left bundle branches
   d. Purkinje fibers

148. Why do pacemaker cells fire repeatedly without external stimulation?
   a. Cerebral biorhythms cause intrinsic stimulation.
   b. Epinephrine initiates the action potential in regular cycles.
   c. Sympathetic nervous system causes hormonal stimulation.
   d. They have an unstable resting membrane potential.

149. Why is there a conduction delay in the AV node of the normal cardiac cycle?
   a. So ectopic rhythms do not have a chance to enter the cycle
   b. So simultaneous contraction of the atria can occur
   c. To allow for contraction of the atria before ventricular contraction
   d. To permit refilling of the coronary arteries before atrial systole

150. Which of the following may cause a decrease in SA node discharge, resulting in decreased heart rate?
   a. Acetylcholine   c. Norepinephrine
   b. Epinephrine   d. Parasympatholytic effects

151. Mechanisms that produce dysrhythmias secondary to reentry include which of the following?
   a. Atropine administration   c. Hypercapnia
   b. Digitalis toxicity   d. Hyperkalemia

152. Which of the following signs or symptoms would be atypical for a coronary event?
   a. Abdominal discomfort   c. Jaw pain
   b. Dyspnea   d. Syncope

153. Dyspnea associated with myocardial infarction is usually related to which of the following?
   a. Chronic obstructive pulmonary disease
   b. Drug administration
   c. Hypercarbia
   d. Pulmonary congestion

154. Syncope should be assumed to be caused by a dysrhythmia if which of the following is associated with it?
   a. Nausea preceded the event.
   b. The patient is older.
   c. There is a history of diabetes.
   d. It occurred when the patient was standing.

155. When evaluating a patient for jugular venous distention, the paramedic should do which of the following?
   a. Raise the head of the bed 90 degrees
   b. Raise the head of the bed 45 degrees
   c. Lay the patient in the supine position
   d. Have the patient stand with assistance

156. Why may it be helpful to find the point of maximum impulse on the patient's chest?
   a. For appropriate defibrillation or pacing patch placement
   b. For assessment of strength of myocardial contractions
   c. To identify a point to auscultate the mitral valve
   d. To place electrodes for monitoring a 12-lead ECG

157. What does the ECG tracing assess?
   a. Cardiac output   c. Myocardial contractility
   b. Electrical conduction   d. Stroke volume

158. Which of the following represents a bipolar lead?
   a. aVF   c. Lead II
   b. aVR   d. V1

159. In lead II the positive electrode is located on the left lower extremity. During normal conduction, which way should the QRS deflect?
   a. Biphasic   c. Isoelectric
   b. Downward   d. Upward

160. You are looking at leads II, III, and aVF. What part of the heart can you "view" in those leads?
   a. Anterior   c. Lateral
   b. Inferior   d. Septum

161. Modified chest leads mimic the view that can be obtained by looking at which of the following?
    a. Augmented leads
    c. Posterior leads
    b. Limb leads
    d. V leads

162. Where should the positive electrode be placed for MCL1?
    a. Below the lateral end of the left clavicle
    b. Below the lateral end of the right clavicle
    c. Fourth intercostal space to the right of the sternum
    d. Left axillary line at the level of the fifth intercostal space

163. Why are leads II and MCL1 preferred for routine monitoring for dysrhythmias?
    a. P waves can be easily visualized.
    b. The tallest QRS can be seen.
    c. Rates are more easily calculated.
    d. ST segment elevation or depression can be viewed.

164. Which precordial leads are septal leads?
    a. aVL
    c. V3 and V4
    b. V1 and V2
    d. V5 and V6

165. What represents the absence of electrical activity in the heart on the ECG strip?
    a. Isoelectric line
    c. QRS complex
    b. P wave
    d. ST segment

166. What is the normal duration of the QRS complex?
    a. 0.04-0.08 seconds
    c. 0.12-0.14 seconds
    b. 0.08-0.10 seconds
    d. 0.14-0.16 seconds

167. During what point does the absolute refractory period occur in the heart?
    a. P wave
    c. QT interval
    b. PR interval
    d. T wave

168. To accurately assess abnormal QRS width, the paramedic should do which of the following?
    a. Determine the J point and measure back from it.
    b. Identify the lead with the widest QRS and then measure it.
    c. Measure from the end of the P wave to the end of the S wave.
    d. Measure from R-R wave from left to right.

169. There are 10 small boxes between the R waves on the ECG tracing. What is the heart rate?
    a. 6/min
    c. 60/min
    b. 30/min
    d. 150/min

170. Identify the ECG tracing in Fig. 28-44.

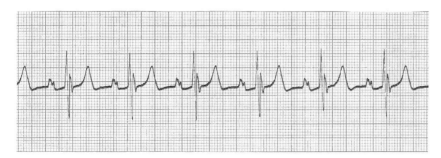

Figure 28-44

    a. Normal sinus rhythm
    b. Sinus rhythm with first-degree atrioventricular block
    c. Second-degree heart block type II
    d. Ventricular demand pacer with capture

229

171. Identify the ECG tracing in Fig. 28-45.

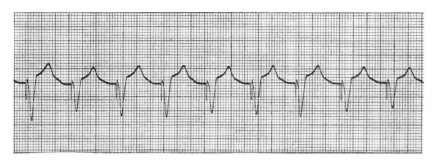

Figure 28-45

    a. Accelerated idioventricular rhythm
    b. Junctional tachycardia
    c. Ventricular pacemaker
    d. Ventricular tachycardia

172. Identify the ECG tracing in Fig. 28-46.

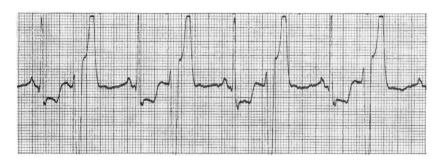

Figure 28-46

    a. Multifocal premature ventricular contractions
    b. Couplet of premature ventricular contractions
    c. Ventricular bigeminy
    d. Ventricular escape rhythm

173. Identify the ECG tracing in Fig. 28-47.

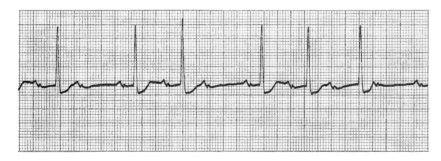

Figure 28-47

    a. Second-degree atrioventricular block type I
    b. Second-degree atrioventricular block type II
    c. Sinus arrest
    d. Sinus arrhythmia

174. Identify the ECG tracing in Fig. 28-48.

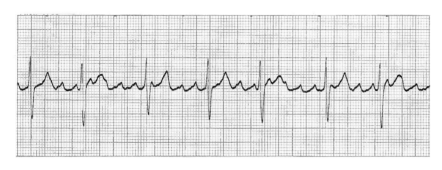

Figure 28-48

   a. Atrial fibrillation
   b. Atrial flutter
   c. Junctional tachycardia
   d. Third-degree atrioventricular block

175. Identify the ECG tracing in Fig. 28-49.

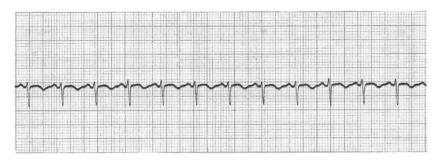

Figure 28-49

   a. Atrial fibrillation   **c.** Atrial tachycardia
   b. Atrial flutter   **d.** Sinus tachycardia

176. Identify the ECG tracing in Fig. 28-50.

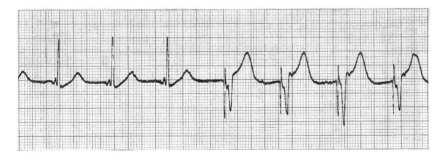

Figure 28-50

   a. Accelerated junctional rhythm followed by pacemaker
   b. Junctional rhythm followed by pacemaker
   c. Junctional rhythm followed by idioventricular
   d. Second-degree atrioventricular block type II followed by idioventricular

177. You are treating a 60-year-old woman with atrial fibrillation at a rate of 168/min. Her blood pressure is 80 by palpation, and she feels very faint. The appropriate intervention would be which of the following?
   a. Adenosine 6 mg via rapid intravenous administration
   b. Verapamil 2.5 mg intravenously over 2 min
   c. Procainamide 30 mg/min intravenously
   d. Synchronized cardioversion at 100 joules

178. Which of the following is an ectopic rhythm?
   a. Atrial tachycardia   c. Normal sinus rhythm
   b. Junctional tachycardia   d. Sinus bradycardia

179. Which of the following will *not* cause sinus bradycardia?
   a. Digoxin   c. Isoproterenol
   b. Increased vagal tone   d. Sleep

180. What is the most common cause of decreased cardiac output in atrial fibrillation or atrial flutter?
   a. Decreased ventricular contractility
   b. Development of blood clots
   c. Inadequate atrial filling
   d. Loss of atrial kick

181. What can result from atrial fibrillation?
   a. Congestive heart failure   c. Rheumatic heart disease
   b. Pericarditis   d. Vagal stimulation

182. If your patient presents with accelerated junctional rhythm, what medical history should you inquire about that is specifically associated with this rhythm?
   a. Chronic obstructive pulmonary disease
   b. Diabetes
   c. Marijuana use
   d. Treatment with digoxin

183. Which of the following mechanisms may cause ventricular dysrhythmias?
   a. Enhanced automaticity
   b. Reentry phenomena
   c. Both enhanced automaticity and reentry phenomena
   d. Neither enhanced authomaticity nor reentry phenomena

184. PVCs that occur every second complex are known as which of the following?
   a. Bigeminy   c. Idioventricular
   b. Couplets   d. Multifocal

185. Your patient has a wide complex tachycardia. Which of the following ECG findings would indicate ventricular tachycardia?
   a. All precordial leads (V leads) have a positive deflection.
   b. Negative QRS deflection with a single peak in MCL1 and MCL6.
   c. Positive QRS complex in leads I, II, and III.
   d. RS interval is less than 0.10 second in any V lead.

186. What type of pacemaker fires only when the patient's own heart rate drops below a predetermined rate?
   a. Asynchronous   c. Dual chamber
   b. Demand   d. Fixed rate

187. What rhythm occurs when a complete block develops at or below the AV node?
   a. Bundle branch block
   b. Fascicular block
   c. Second-degree AV block type II
   d. Third-degree AV block

188. Which of the following is true regarding left bundle branch block?
    a. It produces an initial R wave in MCL1 instead of the normal small Q wave.
    b. There is a shallow, narrow QS pattern and the QRS is less than 0.12 seconds.
    c. There is an RSR prime pattern seen in MCL1 with a QRS complex greater than 0.12 seconds.
    d. The fibers that usually fire the interventricular septum are blocked.
189. Which of the following has the greatest potential to deteriorate into complete heart block?
    a. Anterior hemiblock   c. Posterior hemiblock
    b. Bifascicular block   d. Right bundle branch block
190. Your patient has a history of Wolff-Parkinson-White syndrome. You note a wide-complex supraventricular tachycardia. Which drug is not appropriate for this patient?
    a. Adenosine   c. Procainamide
    b. Lidocaine   d. Verapamil
191. What distinguishes unstable angina from stable angina?
    a. It is caused by atherosclerotic disease of the coronary arteries.
    b. The pain lasts 1 to 5 minutes and is relieved by oxygen or nitroglycerin.
    c. The pain changes in its onset, frequency, duration, or quality.
    d. It is precipitated by physical exertion or emotional stress.
192. Death secondary to myocardial infarction is *most commonly* the result of which of the following?
    a. Dysrhythmias   c. Pulmonary embolism
    b. Low blood pressure   d. Cardiac rupture
193. Appropriate care for a stable patient with acute myocardial infarction would include all of the following except which one?
    a. Placing the patient in a semi-Fowler's position
    b. Administering lactated Ringer's solution at 500 ml/hr intravenously
    c. Administering oxygen by nasal cannula
    d. Documenting and reporting all intravenous sticks
194. Which of the following is *not* diagnostic of an acute myocardial infarction?
    a. Pathological Q waves   c. ST-segment depression
    b. Peaked tented T waves   d. ST-segment elevation
195. Medications that may help in the management of a patient with cardiac pulmonary edema include all of the following *except* which one?
    a. Epinephrine   c. Morphine
    b. Furosemide   d. Nitroglycerin
196. When a patient suffers from right-sided heart failure, blood backs up into which of the following?
    a. Aorta   c. Pulmonary veins
    b. Pulmonary arteries   d. Venae cavae
197. Cardiogenic shock is:
    a. Fatal in only 10% to 15% of patients
    b. Caused by extensive myocardial damage
    c. The result of an intravascular electrolyte imbalance
    d. Caused by obstruction of the renal vessels
198. Your patient has a history of cancer and is having chest pain and tachycardia. What is an early sign that may indicate the development of cardiac tamponade?
    a. Decreased systolic pressure   c. Pericardial friction rub
    b. Jugular venous distention   d. Tracheal deviation

199. Which is the most common presentation of dissection of the thoracic aorta?
  a. Chest heaviness of slow onset
  b. Intense back pain with sudden onset
  c. Neck pain that began suddenly
  d. Substernal dull pain that increased gradually

200. Acute arterial occlusion may result in which of the following?
  a. Absent distal pulses
  c. Pulmonary congestion
  b. Hypertension
  d. Torsades de pointes

201. You suspect that your patient has an arterial occlusion affecting the lower leg. Which of the following treatment measures would be appropriate?
  a. Initiate intravenous fluid therapy and administer a fluid challenge.
  b. Massage the affected extremity to encourage circulation.
  c. Immobilize the affected extremity and protect it from injury.
  d. Administer furosemide 40 mg intravenously to flush out the embolus.

202. Chronic, uncontrolled hypertension puts a patient at risk for all *except* which of the following?
  a. Cerebral hemorrhage
  c. Myocardial infarction
  b. Diabetes mellitus
  d. Renal failure

203. According to the American Heart Association, how soon should basic cardiac life support be initiated in the patient in cardiac arrest?
  a. 4 min   **c.** 8 min
  b. 6 min   **d.** 12 min

204. You work at a service that uses biphasic defibrillation. Which of the following is true regarding this device?
  a. It delivers lower energy shocks.
  b. The batteries are larger.
  c. The energy flows in one direction.
  d. Three patches are needed.

205. What principle should be followed when placing paddles or patches on the chest for defibrillation?
  a. Anterior-posterior placement may be used for patches.
  b. Never reverse the polarity or defibrillation will not occur.
  c. Place one paddle over the sternum directly over the heart.
  d. Use pediatric paddles for children up to 8 years of age.

206. What should you consider when caring for a patient who has an implantable cardioverter defibrillator?
  a. Apply a magnet to the chest to activate these devices if the patient is unresponsive.
  b. If defibrillation at 360 joules is unsuccessful, paddle placement should be changed.
  c. The complete sequence of up to three shocks may take as long as 1 minute.
  d. Touching the patient during ICD defibrillation is dangerous and should be avoided.

207. Which of the following statements is true with regard to synchronized cardioversion?
  a. It is faster than unsynchronized cardioversion.
  b. It is not as safe as unsynchronized cardioversion.
  c. It is indicated for pulseless ventricular tachycardia.
  d. It is indicated for unstable PSVT.

208. When attempting to initiate transcutaneous pacing on a conscious patient, set the current at which of the following?
  a. 70-80/min and increased until patient is stable
  b. 50 mA and increased until capture occurs
  c. 70-80/min and decreased until the patient becomes unstable
  d. Maximum mA and decreased until capture is lost

209. Which of the following drugs is used to treat asystole?
    a. Atropine   c. Calcium chloride
    b. Bretylium   d. Lidocaine
210. Which of the following is a side effect from bretylium tosylate?
    a. Drowsiness   c. Hypotension
    b. Headache   d. Hypothermia
211. Which of the following is an action of morphine sulfate?
    a. Dilation of peripheral vasculature
    b. Increase in cardiac preload
    c. Calming of the patient with a head injury
    d. Bronchodilation
212. Which of the following is true of digoxin?
    a. It increases the force of ventricular contraction.
    b. It is a first line drug in the management of bradycardia.
    c. It causes decreased cardiac output.
    d. It increases impulse conduction through the atrioventricular node.
213. Which of the following drugs stimulates the beta receptors?
    a. Amyl nitrite   c. Epinephrine
    b. Atropine   d. Propranolol
214. A 60-year-old, 100-kg woman has a blood pressure of 80/50 mm Hg. The ECG is shown in Fig. 28-51. Which of the following is not appropriate to correct this?

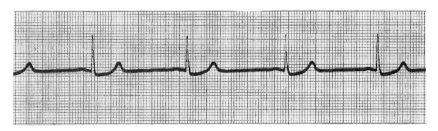

Figure 28-51

    a. Atropine 0.5-1.0 mg intravenously
    b. Dopamine 5-20 mcg/kg/min
    c. Epinephrine 2-10 mcg/kg/min
    d. Isoproterenol 2-10 mcg/min
215. Which of the following criteria should be considered to determine whether to terminate resuscitation of a patient?
    a. Family who objects to termination
    b. Presence of a nonofficial DNR order
    c. Quality of life judgments
    d. Time of collapse before EMS arrival

NEUROLOGY

● READING ASSIGNMENT

Chapter 29, pages 910-943, in *Mosby's Paramedic Textbook*, ed 2

● OBJECTIVES

As a paramedic, you should be able to:

1. Describe the anatomy and physiology of the nervous system.
2. Outline pathophysiological changes in the nervous system that may alter cerebral perfusion pressure.
3. Describe the assessment of a patient with a nervous system disorder.
4. Describe pathophysiology, signs and symptoms, and specific management techniques for each of the following neurological disorders: coma, stroke and intracranial hemorrhage, seizure disorders, headache, brain neoplasm and brain abscess, and degenerative neurological diseases.

● REVIEW QUESTIONS

For each of the etiologies listed in Column I, identify the appropriate general cause of coma in Column II. You may use each answer more than once.

	Column I	**Column II**
1. _____	The patient's blood pressure rose suddenly to 240/140 mm Hg.	**a.** Cardiovascular system
2. _____	The patient's chronic bronchitis is much worse.	**b.** Drugs
3. _____	The patient has missed dialysis for a week.	**c.** Infectious
4. _____	The patient's blood alcohol level is 400 mg/dl.	**d.** Metabolic system
5. _____	The patient's glucose is 30 mg/dl.	**e.** Respiratory system
6. _____	The teenage patient has meningitis.	**f.** Structural

Match the illness in Column II with the description in Column I. Use each illness only once.

	Column I	**Column II**
7. _____	Blurred vision and unsteady gait	**a.** Amytrophic lateral sclerosis
8. _____	Severe muscle spasms because of torticollis	**b.** Bell's palsy
9. _____	Burning sensation in the feet because of diabetes	**c.** Central pain syndrome
10. _____	Viral illness causing respiratory paralysis	**d.** Dystonia
11. _____	Muscle trembling because of decreased dopamine	**e.** Multiple sclerosis
12. _____	Male genetic disorder causing muscle wasting	**f.** Muscular dystrophy
13. _____	Intense facial pain activated by a trigger point	**g.** Myoclonus
14. _____	CNS degeneration in patients over	**h.** Parkinson's disease
		i. Peripheral neuropathy
		j. Polio
		k. Spina bifida

age 50 leading to severe muscle
deterioration

15. _____ Temporary facial paralysis because
of inflammation

16. _____ Genetic defect that leaves the spinal
cord exposed

17. Complete the following sentences. The cells of the nervous system that pro-

tect the neurons are called (a) _____. Each neuron
has three main parts. The area that contains the nucleus is the (b)

_____ _____; one or more
branching projections that receive impulses are known as the (c)

_____; and a single, elongated projection that trans-

mits impulses is called the (d) _____. In the peripheral nervous system, bundles of axons and their sheaths are called (e)

_____ _____. Neurons are
classified by the direction in which they transmit impulses. The neurons that
transmit impulses to the spinal cord and brain from the body are

(f) _____ neurons. Neurons that transmit im-

pulses away from the brain to muscle and glandular tissue are (g)

_____ neurons. Neurons that conduct im-
pulses from sensory neurons directly to motor neurons are (h)

_____. In its resting state the charge inside the neu-

ron is (i) _____ and the charge outside the neuron is

(j) _____. When the neuron is stimulated while the

outside is positively charged, (k) _____ ions rush

into the cell and begin a wave of (l) _____ that trav-
els down the cell. Myelinated axons have interruptions in the myelin

sheaths called (m) _____ _____

_____ that cause the action potential to be con-

ducted more (n) _____ than unmyelinated axons.
The space between the nerve endings of two adjacent neurons is known as

a (o) _____. Impulses are transmitted across

these spaces by neurotransmitters such as (p) _____,

_____, and _____.

237

18. List the basic anatomical components of a reflex.

_____

19. Name the two paired arteries that supply blood to the brain.
   a.
   b.
20. State whether the following factors will *increase, decrease,* or *not change* the cerebral blood flow:
   a. Intracranial pressure of 30 mm Hg:
   b. Mean arterial pressure of 40 mm Hg:
   c. Expanding tumor in the brain:
   d. Hypovolemic shock:
21. List at least two causes of coma for each of the following six general classifications:
   a. Structural:

_____

   b. Metabolic:

_____

   c. Drug induced:

_____

   d. Cardiovascular:

_____

   e. Respiratory:

_____

   f. Infection:

_____

22. You have been called to care for a patient who is suspected of suffering from a neurological disorder. He opens his eyes when you call his name but does not know what day it is. He is moving all extremities normally.
   a. List six specific questions that you should ask the family to elicit the nature of the neurologic problem.

_____

   b. What vital sign findings would suggest increased intracranial pressure?

_____

   c. Using the AVPU assessment, describe his level of consciousness.

_____

   d. What is his score on the Glasgow coma scale?

_____

   e. Describe your assessment of this patient's eyes.

_____

23. State whether the following symptoms of coma are most likely to be found in structural or toxic-metabolic coma:
   a. Asymmetrical neurological findings:
   b. Slow onset:
   c. Unilateral fixed dilated pupil:

238

24. You arrive at a private residence to evaluate a 65-year-old woman whose neighbors found her unresponsive. She has snoring respirations at a rate of 8/min, and an oral airway is easily placed. Carotid and radial pulses are present and rapid. Blood pressure is 110/70 mm Hg. She flexes to painful stimuli, no history is available, and her blood glucose is 60 mg/dl. Outline your assessment and management of this patient, including appropriate dose and route of drugs you would give.

_____

_____

_____

Questions 25-29 refer to the following case study:

You respond to a private residence where you find an elderly African-American man lying on the sofa. His family states, "he hasn't been acting right." On exam you find him awake and confused, with slurred speech. He follows commands appropriately and when you ask him to smile, he has an apparent facial droop on the right. Ongoing assessment reveals weakness in the left arm and leg. His vital signs are: BP 160/108, P 72, and R 16 and regular, his SaO$_2$ is 95%, and his blood glucose level is 94 mg/dl. History reveals no allergies, and his medications include diazide, nitroglycerin, and insulin. His family said that a similar incident occurred yesterday lasting about 5 minutes after he took a walk. He smokes one pack of cigarettes per day.

25. List eight risk factors for stroke that you can identify for this patient and note whether each is modifiable or nonmodifiable.

Risk Factor	**Modifiable (Yes or No)**
a.	
b.	
c.	
d.	
e.	
f.	
g.	
h.	

26. List at least six signs or symptoms of cerebrovascular accident that are common to embolic and thrombotic strokes. (Place a star beside the ones experienced by this patient.)

_____

27. List the physical findings that would indicate the probability of stroke for this patient based on:

a. The Cincinnati stroke scale

b. The Los Angeles Prehospital Stroke Screen

28. List the 7 D's of stroke management.

_____

_____

29. Outline your prehospital care of this patient.

_____

_____

_____

30. Although patients may have diverse presentations, describe the typical progression of signs and symptoms of hemorrhagic stroke.

_____

_____

31. List five causes of seizures:
   a.
   b.
   c.
   d.
   e.

32. State the type of seizure for each of the following signs and symptoms:
   a. Numbness of the body or unusual visual, auditory, or taste symptoms:

_____

   b. Brief loss of consciousness in a child without loss of posture lasting less than 15 seconds:

_____

   c. Partial seizure activity that spreads in an orderly fashion to surrounding areas:

_____

   d. Preceding aura followed by loss of consciousness and tonic-clonic motor activity followed by a postictal state:

_____

   e. Aura followed by automatisms such as lip-smacking and chewing, during which time the patient is amnesic:

_____

33. What history should be obtained from the family of a patient who has had a grand mal seizure?

_____

_____

34. List two findings suggesting that the seizure is hysterical versus grand mal.
   a.
   b.

35. State whether each of the following characteristics is more suggestive of seizure or syncope:

a. It starts in a standing position:

_____

b. It is preceded by lightheadedness:

_____

c. The patient remains unconscious for minutes to hours:

_____

d. Tachycardia occurs:

_____

36. List two anticonvulsants with the appropriate doses that may be given to the adult patient who is having a seizure.

a.

b.

37. Identify the type of headache (tension, migraine, cluster, or sinus) typically associated with each of the following case presentations.

a. You are dispatched at 0100 to care for a patient who is complaining of a severe headache that awoke him. He says the pain is most intense around his left eye, and you note that his eyes are tearing and his nose is running. _____

b. Your partner is recovering from an upper respiratory infection and complaining of a headache affecting her forehead and upper face. She describes an intense pressure sensation that increases when she bends over.

_____

c. Your patient is complaining of a dull, throbbing headache that started a week ago and will not stop. _____

d. A 24-year-old woman is complaining of a severe headache that began as an intense throbbing on the right side of her head and is now generalized. She has vomited three times. She indicates a history of this and takes a beta blocker. _____

● **STUDENT SELF-ASSESSMENT**

38. Which blood vessel or vessels supply the front lobes of the brain?
  a. Anterior cerebral arteries
  b. Midline basilar artery
  c. Posterior cerebral arteries
  d. Right and left vertebral arteries

39. An important function of the Circle of Willis is to maintain blood supply to the brain if which of the following occurs?
  a. The patient becomes hypoxic because of shock.
  b. The patient has a large hemorrhagic stroke.
  c. Intracranial pressure increases suddenly.
  d. The vertebral or internal carotid arteries are blocked.

40. Which of the following will cause a decrease in the cerebral blood flow?
  a. Blood pressure of 70/50 mm Hg
  b. Intracranial pressure of 15 mm Hg
  c. Decreased levels of intraocular fluid
  d. Body temperature of 102° F (38.9° C)

41. Respiratory patterns associated with neurological disorders include all of the following *except* which symptom?
    a. Ataxic respirations
    b. Cheyne-Stokes respirations
    c. Diaphragmatic breathing
    d. Kussmaul respirations
42. Posturing caused by structural impairment of the subcortical regions of the brain is known as which of the following?
    a. Extension rigidity
    b. Flexion rigidity
    c. Dysconjugate gaze
    d. Flaccidity
43. Your comatose patient's pupils are 2 mm and round and reactive to light. What does this suggest?
    a. Barbiturate overdose
    b. Medullary injury
    c. Opiate overdose
    d. Temporal herniation
44. Management of the postictal patient with a known seizure disorder who initially aroused to pain and then begins to moan and move spontaneously includes which of the following?
    a. Administration of naloxone 2 mg intravenously
    b. Administration of diazepam 5 mg intravenously
    c. Intravenous fluid therapy of normal saline 100 ml/hr
    d. Recumbent positioning of patient
45. Significant findings in the medical history of a patient you suspect is having a stroke include all of the following *except* which characteristic?
    a. Cigarette smoking
    b. Obesity
    c. Oral contraceptive use
    d. Sickle cell disease
46. Which of the following findings would indicate high probability of stroke based on the Cincinnati prehospital stroke scale?
    a. The patient has the worst headache ever felt.
    b. The patient cannot speak clearly to you.
    c. The patient experiences a new onset of seizures.
    d. The patient complains of double vision.
47. Your patient has continuous rapid muscle jerking that the family says is related to his neuromuscular disease. What are these movements called?
    a. Dystonia
    b. Inanition
    c. Myoclonus
    d. Palsy

ENDOCRINOLOGY

● READING ASSIGNMENT

Chapter 30, pages 944-965, in *Mosby's Paramedic Textbook,* ed 2

● OBJECTIVES

As a paramedic, you should be able to:

1. Describe how hormones secreted from endocrine glands function to assist the body to maintain homeostasis.
2. Describe the anatomy and physiology of the pancreas and how its hormones work to maintain normal glucose metabolism.
3. Discuss pathophysiology as a basis for key signs and symptoms, patient assessment, and patient management for diabetes and diabetic emergencies of hypoglycemia, diabetic ketoacidosis, and hyperosmolar hyperglycemic nonketotic coma.
4. Discuss pathophysiology as a basis for key signs and symptoms, patient assessment, and patient management of disorders of the thyroid gland.
5. Discuss pathophysiology as a basis for key signs and symptoms, patient assessment, and patient management of Cushing's syndrome and Addison's disease.

● REVIEW QUESTIONS

Match the signs or symptoms listed in Column II with the appropriate diabetic emergencies listed in Column I. You may use each answer more than once.

Column I	Column II
1. _____ Diabetic ketoacidosis	**a.** Abdominal pain
	b. Coma
	c. Cool, clammy skin
	d. Fruity breath odor
	e. Kussmaul respirations
2. _____ Hyperosmolar hyperglycemic nonketotic coma	**f.** Polyuria
	g. Psychotic behavior
	h. Seizures
	i. Tachycardia
	j. Warm, dry skin
3. _____ Hypoglycemia	**k.** Vomiting

4. Name the hormone secreted from each of these cells in the pancreas.
   a. Alpha cells:
   b. Beta cells:
   c. Delta cells:
5. When food is ingested, it is broken into smaller units and used or stored. Name the breakdown products and storage sites of the following food types.

Food	Breakdown Products	Storage
a. Carbohydrates		
b. Proteins		
c. Fats		

6. a. How is excess glucose stored in the liver?

_____

   b. How are glucose stores released from the liver?

_____

7. Briefly explain the role of glucagon in the metabolism of food.

_____

8. Why does a patient develop cerebral signs and symptoms of hypoglycemia rapidly?

_____

9. List at least three signs or symptoms that might lead you to suspect that a patient has undetected type 1 diabetes.

_____

_____

10. List at least three medical illnesses associated with long-term diabetes.

_____

_____

11. You arrive on the scene of a suspected diabetic emergency. You find a 35-year-old man whose wife says he took his insulin 2 hours ago and has not eaten. He arouses only to pain and has noisy, snoring respirations. He has no other medical history. Outline the steps in your patient management.

_____

_____

_____

Questions 12-16 refer to the following case study:

A 20-year-old diabetic patient calls you complaining of difficulty breathing. On arrival, the patient states he has had the flu for 2 days. You note that his respiratory rate is 40/min and his breath has a very sweet odor. You auscultate his lungs, and his breath sounds are clear bilaterally.

12. What do you suspect?

_____

13. What other specific questions will you ask about the history of this patient's illness?

_____

_____

14. What specific findings will you be looking for during your physical assessment of the patient?

_____

You perform a blood glucose analysis and your machine reads "high." The patient appears dehydrated.

15. What interventions should you perform for this patient in the prehospital setting?

_____

16. Should you be concerned about rapid transport for this patient? Why?

_____

17. List six factors that predispose a patient to the development of hyperosmolar hyperglycemic nonketotic coma.

a.

b.

c.

d.

e.

f.

18. Complete the missing information in the following table for each endocrine disorder.

Disorder	Endocrine gland and hormone affected	Excess or shortage of hormone?	Signs and symptoms	Potentially life threatening?
Graves' disease				
Thyroid storm				
Myxedema				
Cushing's syndrome				
Addison's disease				

● **STUDENT SELF-ASSESSMENT**

19. How do hormones achieve their desired actions?
   a. They travel by ducts to the specific organ to be stimulated.
   b. They stimulate nerves to send messages to their target tissue.
   c. They trigger cell-specific receptors to initiate specific functions.
   d. They activate the organ adjacent to the gland that produces them.

245

20. What is the primary action of insulin?
    a. To reduce the glucose needs of the cells
    b. To increase blood glucose levels
    c. To transport glucose into the cells
    d. To manufacture amino acids
21. Oral hypoglycemic agents include all of the following *except* which drug?
    a. Diabinese   c. Insulin
    b. Dymelor   d. Orinase
22. Type II diabetes mellitus most likely does which of the following?
    a. Requires insulin injections
    b. Develops after age 40
    c. Has a sudden onset of symptoms
    d. Results in life-threatening emergencies
23. What is the breakdown of glucose stores in the liver called?
    a. Glucagon   c. Gluconeogenesis
    b. Glucosuria   d. Glycogenolysis
24. Before administration of D50W in a lethargic patient with diabetes, you should do all of the following *except* which procedure?
    a. Initiate intravenous fluids   c. Draw a blood sample
    b. Administer glucagon   d. Determine blood glucose
25. Before giving D50W to a diabetic who is also a known alcoholic, what should you administer?
    a. Glucagon   c. Insulin
    b. Half the usual dose   d. Thiamine
26. What is an advantage of glucagon over D50W?
    a. Faster acting   c. Given IM
    b. Less expensive   d. More effective
27. What is the correct dose of glucagon for an adult?
    a. 0.5-1.0 mg IM   c. 12.5 g IV
    b. 1.0-2.0 mg IM   d. 25 g IV
28. Which of the following signs or symptoms would be *unlikely* in a patient who has hyperosmolar hyperglycemic nonketotic coma?
    a. Altered level of consciousness
    b. Dry mucous membranes
    c. Fruity breath odor
    d. Thirst
29. Your patient is very anxious and is complaining of abdominal pain and difficulty breathing. Her vital signs are BP 80/50 mm Hg, P 136, and R 24 and you note basilar rales in her lungs. What endocrine condition may cause this presentation?
    a. Cushing's syndrome
    b. Graves' disease
    c. Myxedema
    d. Thyroid storm

ALLERGIES AND ANAPHYLAXIS

● **READING ASSIGNMENT**

Chapter 31, pages 966-975, in *Mosby's Paramedic Textbook*, ed 2

● **OBJECTIVES**

As a paramedic, you should be able to:
1. Describe the antigen-antibody response in an allergic reaction.
2. Describe signs and symptoms and management of local allergic reactions based on an understanding of the pathophysiology associated with this condition.
3. Identify allergens associated with anaphylaxis.
4. Describe the pathophysiology, signs and symptoms, and management of anaphylaxis.

● **REVIEW QUESTIONS**

1. Complete the following sentences. Antigens can enter the body by (a)

_____, (b) _____,

(c) _____ or (d) _____. The allergic reaction is initiated when a circulating (e) _____

combines with a specific antigen, causing a (f) _____

reaction or to antibodies bound to (g) _____

_____ or (h) _____.

2. List agents in each of the following groups that can cause anaphylaxis.
   a. Drugs:

   _____

   b. Insects:

   _____

   c. Foods:

   _____

   d. Other:

   _____

3. List the signs and symptoms associated with each of the following chemical mediators released from basophils and mast cells in an anaphylactic reaction.

   a. Histamines:

   _____

   b. Leukotrienes:

   _____

   c. Eosinophil chemotactic factor:

   _____

4. You are called to a church picnic to care for a 30-year-old woman with wheezing and dyspnea. After a careful assessment, you determine that she is having an anaphylactic reaction.

   a. What other illness or injury may produce these symptoms?

   _____

   b. List 2 home medicines that may influence your care of this patient.

   _____

   Questions 5-7 refer to the following case study:

   You are at a Chinese restaurant caring for a 25-year-old patient experiencing an anaphylactic reaction. He is in acute respiratory distress with wheezing and has a blood pressure of 90/70 mm Hg.

5. What are some causative agents that may be found at this restaurant to trigger this man's anaphylaxis?

   _____

6. After a rapid primary survey and vital sign assessment, you determine that immediate pharmacological therapy is indicated. Identify two drugs, with appropriate dose and route, that may be indicated for this patient.

   a.

   b.

7. Describe other signs or symptoms that this patient may exhibit.

   _____

   _____

8. You arrive at a dental office, where you find a 35-year-old woman who rapidly developed hives, angioedema, and stridor after an injection of a local anesthetic. She is unconscious, with labored, stridorous respirations, no radial pulse, and a rapid, irregular, barely palpable carotid pulse. No medicines have been administered to treat her. Describe your priorities of care for this patient, including the appropriate drugs, doses, and routes.

   _____

   _____

   _____

   _____

9. What is any substance that causes the formation of antibodies in the body called?
    a. Anaphylactic   c. Basophil
    b. Antigen   d. Mast cell
10. Which immunoglobulin (antibody) is responsible for anaphylaxis?
    a. IgA   c. IgG
    b. IgE   d. IgM
11. Which of the following is a sign or symptom of a type IV (localized) allergic reaction?
    a. Angioedema   c. Vomiting
    b. Hoarseness   d. Wheezing
12. Your 20-year-old patient has hives, normal vital signs, clear breath sounds, and complains of severe itching. Which of the following drugs would be indicated in this situation?
    a. Diphenhydramine (Benadryl) 5 mg IV
    b. Diphenhydramine (Benadryl) 25 mg IM
    c. Epinephrine (Adrenalin) 0.1 mg (1:1000) IV
    d. Epinephrine (Adrenalin) 0.3 mg (1:1000) SQ
13. What are mediators that cause blood vessels to dilate called?
    a. Chemotactic substances   c. Opsonins
    b. Leukotactic substances   d. Vasoactive substances
14. Which of the following agents is *not* commonly associated with anaphylaxis?
    a. Acetaminophen   c. Fire ants
    b. Aspirin   d. Peanuts
15. What is the most likely cause of death in anaphylaxis?
    a. Upper airway obstruction
    b. Hypoxia resulting from bronchospasm
    c. Hypotension resulting from fluid leak
    d. Vasogenic shock resulting from histamines
16. Which of the following signs or symptoms is *not* associated with anaphylaxis?
    a. Abdominal cramps   c. Rhinorrhea
    b. Cool, pale skin   d. Urticaria
17. Diphenhydramine is considered which of the following?
    a. Anticholinergic   c. Bronchodilator
    b. Antihistamine   d. Sedative-hypnotic
18. Which of the following is a potential complication of IV epinephrine?
    a. Dysrhythmias   d. Vomiting
    b. Myocardial ischemia   e. All of the above
    c. Seizures

GASTROENTEROLOGY

● READING ASSIGNMENT
Chapter 32, pages 976-989, in *Mosby's Paramedic Textbook,* ed 2

● OBJECTIVES
As a paramedic, you should be able to:
1. Label a diagram of the abdominal organs.
2. Describe signs and symptoms, complications, and prehospital management of gastrointestinal disorders that primarily cause abdominal pain.
3. Describe signs and symptoms, complications, and prehospital management of gastrointestinal disorders that primarily cause bleeding.
4. Outline prehospital assessment of a patient who has abdominal pain.
5. Describe general prehospital management techniques for the patient with abdominal pain.

● REVIEW QUESTIONS
Match the gastrointestinal disorder in Column II with its description in Column I. Use each disorder only once.

Column I	Column II
1. _____ Occlusion of the intestinal lumen	a. Appendicitis
	b. Arteriovenous malformation
2. _____ Increased pain after ethyl alcohol ingestion; may have fever and signs of sepsis and shock	c. Cholecystitis
	d. Diverticulitis
3. _____ Protrusion of viscus from normal position through opening in groin or abdominal wall	e. Diverticulosis
	f. Esophageal varices
4. _____ Pain most intense at McBurney's point	g. Esophagitis
5. _____ Most common cause of massive rectal bleeding in older adults	h. Gastritis
	i. Hemorrhoids
6. _____ Open erosion wound in digestive system that may bleed	j. Hernia
	k. Intestinal obstruction
7. _____ Characterized by blood dripping into toilet after normal bowel movement	l. Pancreatitis
	m. Peptic ulcer
8. _____ Left lower quadrant abdominal pain resulting from a pouch in colon wall	
9. _____ Painless bleeding resulting from vascular abnormality in gastrointestinal tract	
10. _____ Bright red hematemesis caused by rupture of vessels distended by portal hypertension	
11. _____ Inflammation of the gallbladder	
12. _____ Inflammation of the gastric mucosa	

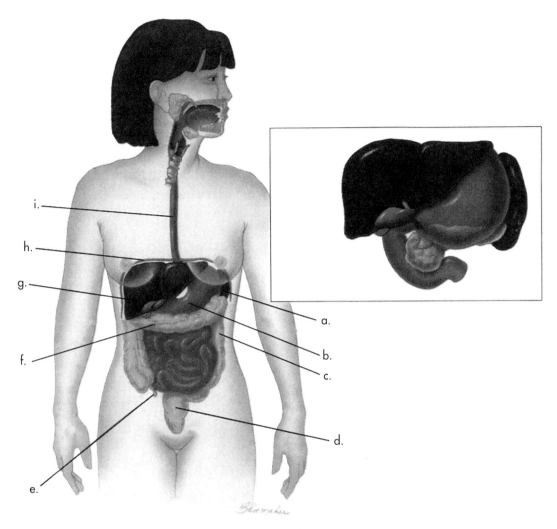

Figure 32-1

13. Label the abdominal organs in Fig. 32-1.
14. Your patient is a 72-year-old man complaining of left lower quadrant abdominal pain. State why you would or would not suspect each of the following illnesses as a cause of his pain.
    a. Pancreatitis:

    _____

    b. Cholecystitis:

    _____

    c. Diverticulitis:

    _____

    d. Peptic ulcer:

    _____

15. A 65-year-old man complains of severe epigastric pain.
   a. List specific questions you must ask of this patient to obtain a complete medical history and to determine whether this is a gastrointestinal problem.

_____

_____

_____

   b. What other significant medical problems must you try to rule out by asking these questions?

_____

16. Name the type of pain described in each of the following statements.
   a. Your patient is supine with his legs flexed and complains of a constant, sharp, stabbing pain:

_____

   b. A 40-year-old woman complains of a severe cramping pain at the umbilicus that peaks and then subsides. She is nauseated and has vomited twice:

_____

   c. A 30-year-old man complains of severe flank pain that goes into his groin:

_____

17. A 17-year-old boy states that he had severe right lower quadrant pain that diminished several hours ago and is now generalized.
   a. What signs and symptoms would indicate that this patient has an acute abdominal condition and may be developing peritonitis?

_____

   b. Describe the prehospital treatment for this patient.

_____

_____

_____

● **STUDENT SELF-ASSESSMENT**

18. Which of the following abdominal organs is located in the retroperitoneal space?
   a. Liver   c. Spleen
   b. Pancreas   d. Stomach

19. A 78-year-old man states that he has been unable to have a bowel movement for a week and has been vomiting profusely. What do you suspect?
   a. Appendicitis   c. Diverticulosis
   b. Bowel obstruction   d. Peptic ulcer

20. You are called at 1900 to care for a 40-year-old woman who is complaining of intermittent severe right upper quadrant abdominal pain. She is vomiting and has a low-grade fever. What do you suspect?
   a. Colitis   c. Esophagitis
   b. Cholecystitis   d. Hepatitis

21. Which of the following is most likely to cause life-threatening hemorrhage?
    a. Arteriovenous malformations   c. Esophagogastric varices
    b. Diverticulitis   d. Hemorrhoids
22. The cause of acute abdominal pain is most accurately assessed in the pre-hospital setting by which of the following?
    a. Abdominal examination   c. Secondary survey
    b. Patient history   d. Vital sign assessment
23. Which of the following is most suggestive of a hemorrhagic gastrointestinal problem?
    a. Anorexia   c. Melena
    b. Fever   d. Tachycardia
24. Prehospital management of the patient with severe right lower quadrant abdominal pain and nausea and vomiting will include which of the following?
    a. Meperidine 25 to 50 mg intramuscularly
    b. Morphine 2 to 5 mg intravenously
    c. Nitrous oxide self-administered
    d. Rapid and gentle transport for physician evaluation

UROLOGY/RENAL

● READING ASSIGNMENT

Chapter 33, pages 990-999, in *Mosby's Paramedic Textbook,* ed 2

● OBJECTIVES

As a paramedic, you should be able to:

1. Label a diagram of the urinary system.
2. Describe pathophysiology, signs and symptoms, assessment, and prehospital management of the patient with urinary retention, urinary tract infection, pyelonephritis, urinary calculus, epididymitis, and testicular torsion.
3. Outline the physical examination for patients with genitourinary disorders.
4. Discuss general prehospital management for the patient with a genitourinary disorder.
5. Distinguish between acute and chronic renal failure.
6. Describe the signs and symptoms of renal failure.
7. Describe dialysis and emergent conditions associated with renal failure, including prehospital management.

● REVIEW QUESTIONS

Match the genitourinary problem in Column II with the description in Column I. Use each disorder only once.

Column I	Column II
1. _____ Can cause vascular infarction and loss of function	**a.** Acute renal failure
2. _____ Inflammation of part of male reproduction system	**b.** Chronic renal failure
3. _____ Systemic disease linked with diabetes and hypertension	**c.** Epididymitis
4. _____ Infectious process causing dysuria and hematuria	**d.** Pyelonephritis
5. _____ Causes include large prostate and CNS dysfunction	**e.** Testicular torsion
6. _____ Caused by too much insoluble salts in urine	**f.** Urinary calculus
7. _____ Upper urinary infection treated with IV antibiotics	**g.** Urinary retention
	h. Urinary tract infection

8. Label the urinary system shown in Fig. 33-1.
   a.
   b.
   c.
   d.

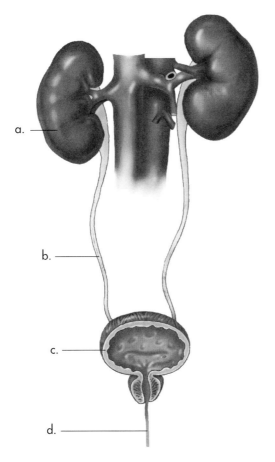

a. —————

b. —————

c. —————

d. —————

Figure 33-1

9. Identify the genitourinary disorder suspected and the prehospital care needed in each of the following situations.
   a. A 35-year-old afebrile man complains of a sudden onset of severe flank pain that radiates into his testicle.

   Condition: _____

   Care: _____
   b. Your 21-year-old patient complains of painful swelling in the scrotal sac, unrelieved by elevation. He is in acute distress and has vomited twice.
   Condition: _____

   Care: _____
   c. A 35-year-old woman with a recent history of recurrent urinary infections complains of fever, chills, and severe flank pain.

   Condition: _____

   Care: _____
   d. A 27-year-old woman complains of burning on urination and feels like she must urinate every 20 minutes.

   Condition: _____

   Care: _____

10. How can you minimize psychological discomfort for a patient with a urology problem when performing the physical examination?

_____

_____

11. Identify three causes of each of the following disorders:
   a. Acute renal failure:

_____

   b. Chronic renal failure:

_____

12. You are called to a dialysis center for a person in shock.
   a. What types of patient problems should you anticipate en route to this call?

_____

   b. If the patient is hypotensive and needs fluid resuscitation, describe how you will initiate fluid therapy and indicate the volume you will infuse.

_____

_____

13. Complete the information in the following table of dialysis emergencies.

Disorder	Cause	Affect on Patient	Interventions
Hemorrhage			
Hypotension			
Chest pain			
Hyperkalemia			
Disequilibrium syndrome			
Air embolism			

14. You are dispatched to a private residence for a patient in full arrest. On arrival, you find a 55-year-old man in asystolic cardiac arrest. The family reports that he lost consciousness about 5 minutes before your arrival. The patient's history includes renal failure. He missed hemodialysis this week and was feeling bad before cardiac arrest.
   a. You begin CPR and prepare to initiate transcutaneous pacing. List the first three drugs, including dose, you should consider administering to this patient.

b. How will the drug therapy help to correct some of the problems that may have caused his cardiac arrest?

c. What problem may occur if this combination of drugs is administered improperly?

● STUDENT SELF-ASSESSMENT

15. Which genitourinary emergency requires treatment within 4 hours to prevent irreversible damage?
    a. Epididymitis   **c.** Testicular torsion
    b. Pyelonephritis   **d.** Urinary calculus

16. Which of the following is a prerenal cause of acute renal failure?
    a. Kidney infection   **c.** Shock
    b. Prostatic enlargement **d.** Ureteral strictures

17. How is prehospital care affected when you care for a patient with a dialysis fistula or shunt?
    a. Check blood pressure in the arm opposite the shunt
    b. Elevate the arm where the shunt is placed
    c. Initiate vascular access in the fistula or shunt
    d. No special consideration is needed

18. You are caring for a patient with a temperature of 102.5° F (39.2° C) who is on continuous peritoneal dialysis. What is a common cause of fever for patients undergoing this treatment?
    a. Dehydration   **c.** Peritonitis
    b. Infected fistula **d.** Pneumonia

19. You are called to the home of an unconscious person in chronic renal failure. The ECG tracing is shown in Fig. 33-2. Which electrolyte imbalance do you suspect?
    a. Hyperkalemia **c.** Hypercalcemia
    b. Hypokalemia   **d.** Hypocalcemia

20. What drug may be ordered by medical direction to correct the underlying electrolyte imbalance illustrated in question 19?
    a. Atropine sulfate 1.0 mg intravenously
    b. Sodium bicarbonate 1.0 mEq/kg intravenously
    c. Magnesium sulfate 1.0 to 2.0 g intravenously
    d. Verapamil 2.5 mg intravenously

21. What physiological problem makes patients in renal failure more susceptible to hypoxia?
    a. Anemia   **c.** Pericarditis
    b. Glucose intolerance **d.** Uremia

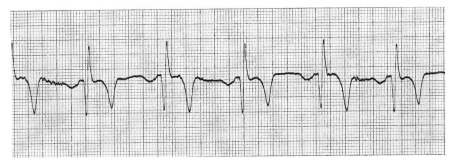

Figure 33-2

TOXICOLOGY

● **READING ASSIGNMENT**

Chapter 34, pages 1000-1061, in *Mosby's Paramedic Textbook,* ed 2

● **OBJECTIVES**

As a paramedic, you should be able to:

1. Define poisoning.
2. Identify general management principles for the four most common toxic syndromes based on a knowledge of the characteristic physical findings associated with each syndrome.
3. Describe general principles for assessment and management of the patient who has ingested poison.
4. Describe the causative agents and pathophysiology of selected ingested poisons and management of patients who have taken them.
5. Describe how physical and chemical properties influence the effects of inhaled toxins.
6. Distinguish between the three categories of inhaled toxins: simple asphyxiants, chemical asphyxiants and systemic poisons, and irritants or corrosives.
7. Describe general principles of managing the patient who has inhaled poison.
8. Describe the signs, symptoms, and management of patients who have inhaled ammonia or hydrocarbon.
9. Describe the signs, symptoms, and management of patients with organophosphate or carbamate poisoning.
10. Outline the general principles of managing patients with drug overdose.
11. Describe the effects, signs and symptoms, and specific management for selected drug overdose.
12. Describe the short- and long-term physiological effects of ethanol ingestion.
13. Describe the signs, symptoms, and management of alcohol-related emergencies.
14. Describe the signs, symptoms, and management of patients injected with poison by insects, reptiles, and hazardous aquatic creatures.

● **REVIEW QUESTIONS**

Match the illnesses in Column II with the toxic syndromes in Column I. You may use the signs and symptoms more than once.

Column I	Column II
1. _____ Anticholinergic syndrome	a. Bradycardia
2. _____ Cholinergic syndrome	b. Cardiac dysrhythmias
3. _____ Opiate/sedative/ethanol syndrome	c. Dry mouth
4. _____ Sympathomimetic syndrome	d. Hypertension
	e. Respiratory depression
	f. Salivation
	g. Tachycardia
	h. Urination

Match the poisons in Column II with their descriptions in Column I. Use each poison only once.

Column I

5. _____ Metabolizes to formic acid and causes toxic visual effects

6. _____ Ingestion of odorless, sweet liquid in antifreeze causes central nervous system depression

7. _____ Inhalation, ingestion, and absorption prevents oxygen from reaching cells

8. _____ Inhalation produces lacrimation, dyspnea, and inflammation of the airway

9. _____ Vomiting should not be induced for phenol and others in this group

10. _____ These chemicals include lye and cause immediate damage to the mucosa

11. _____ The long duration of action requires treatment with atropine and pralidoxime

Column II

a. Acid
b. Alkali
c. Ammonia
d. Carbamate
e. Cyanide
f. Ethylene glycol
g. Hydrocarbon
h. Isopropanol
i. Methanol
j. Organophosphate

12. You are called to the home of a young child whose family states that he ingested some liquid from a bottle in the garage. He is arousable only to painful stimulation. After a rapid assessment of the patient, you contact the regional poison control center.

   a. What information should you be prepared to give the center?

_____

_____

   b. What general care measures should you take when caring for this patient if the source of the poisoning is unknown?

_____

_____

13. You insert a 36 to 40 French orogastric tube into a patient.

   a. What position should the patient be in?

_____

   b. What precaution should be taken for the unconscious patient?

_____

   c. How should irrigation be performed?

_____

_____

14. Complete the information missing in the following table.

Ingested Poison	Charcoal (Yes/No)	Other Interventions
a. Bleach		
b. Ammonia		
c. Gasoline		
d. Methanol		
e. Ethylene glycol		
f. Isopropanol		
g. Cyanide		

15. A 65-year-old woman complains of food poisoning after eating at a local seafood restaurant 2 hours earlier.
   a. What is the typical time onset for signs of food poisoning?

   b. What treatment should be provided for the patient with food poisoning?

Questions 16-18 refer to the following case study:

A 21-year-old man calls 9-1-1 after becoming extremely ill from eating some wild mushrooms. The patient is awake and complaining of nausea, vomiting, and diarrhea. He has pinpoint pupils and the following vital signs: BP, 90/50; P, 48; and R, 24. His ECG rhythm shows a sinus bradycardia with occasional ventricular escape beats.

16. What type of toxic syndrome does this patient appear to be exhibiting?

17. How can you find out more about the specific poison involved in this case?

18. What treatment measures may be indicated for this patient in consultation with medical direction?

19. Complete the information missing in the following table.

Toxic Chemical	Class of Toxin	Signs and Symptoms	Treatment
Copper welding fumes			
Hydrogen sulfide			
Methane gas			
Chlorine gas			

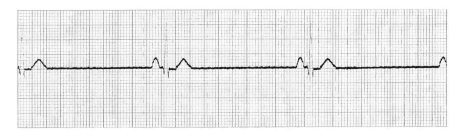

Figure 34-1

20. A worker in a chemical plant is exposed to ammonia gas and is dyspneic, choking, and wheezing. What treatment should be provided for this patient?

_____

_____

Questions 21-24 refer to the following case study:

A farmer calls you to his ranch after spraying pesticide on a windy day. On your arrival, he is coming out of the bathroom complaining of severe diarrhea and says he cannot stop urinating. Tears are running down his face, and he is coughing up large amounts of phlegm. His ECG is shown in Fig. 34-1.

21. What poisoning do you suspect?

_____

22. What other signs or symptoms might be present?

_____

23. What is your interpretation of the ECG?

_____

24. List specific interventions to be used in his care.

_____

_____

25. Interpret the following historical information presented to you at the scene of a potential drug overdose.
  a. "He main-lined some China white."

_____

  b. "She was space-basing angel dust and candy."

_____

  c. "They were freebasing a rock."

_____

  d. "He was skin-popping some M."

_____

  e. "She snorted some PCP before she went crazy."

_____

Match the drugs in Column II with the appropriate overdose description in Column I. Use each drug only once.

Column I	Column II
26. _____ Central nervous system stimulant and depressant properties can produce violent, unpredictable behavior.	a. Acetaminophen
	b. Cocaine
	c. Heroin
	d. Iron
27. _____ It causes visual disturbances, dry mouth, seizures, and tachycardia with wide QRS complex.	e. Phencyclidine
	f. Salicylate
	g. Tricyclic antidepressant
28. _____ It causes tachypnea, central nervous system depression, gastrointestinal irritation, and tinnitus.	
29. _____ Mild, influenza-like symptoms are followed by latent liver failure.	
30. _____ This stimulant can cause dysrhythmias, myocardial infarction, and hyperthermia	

Questions 31 and 32 refer to the following case study:

A 32-year-old woman has overdosed on sleeping pills. She is awake but drowsy.

31. What information regarding the poisoning is critical to the care of this patient?

_____

_____

32. What dose of activated charcoal should be given?

_____

33. Complete the information missing in the following table.

Ingested Poison	Charcoal (Yes/No)	Other Interventions
a. Aspirin		
b. Acetaminophen		
c. Iron		

34. Give two examples of drugs commonly abused in each of the following categories.
   a. Narcotics: _____

   b. Central nervous system depressants: _____

   c. Central nervous system stimulants: _____

   d. Hallucinogens: _____

Questions 35-37 refer to the following case study:

> Your patient injected heroin intravenously and arouses only to pain. He has pinpoint pupils and slow, snoring respirations.

35. What is the primary life threat that must be immediately managed in this patient?

_____

36. List the appropriate drug and dose used to improve this patient's condition.

_____

37. If this man is a chronic heroin abuser and the drug listed previously is administered, what signs and symptoms of narcotic withdrawal will you anticipate?

_____

Questions 38-40 refer to the following case study:

> A 17-year-old has taken approximately 50 tablets of chlordiazepoxide and is comatose, with slow, irregular respirations.

38. What is the pupil response likely to be in this patient?

_____

39. What drug may be given to this patient on arrival to the emergency department to antagonize the effects of this ingestion?

_____

40. Before you administer an antidote, careful history and scene assessment must be done to ensure that the patient has not taken which additional medication?

_____

41. Local college students call you to a party, where participants have been free-basing cocaine. One of the participants has lost consciousness. What life-threatening effects of this drug may have caused loss of consciousness in this patient?

_____

Questions 42-44 refer to the following case study:

> A popular group is playing at a local club. Security calls you to the parking lot to care for a patient who has reportedly taken PCP.

42. What should be your primary concern when caring for this patient?

_____

43. Describe the appropriate initial approach to this patient, who is alert and quiet.

_____

44. List signs and symptoms that may be displayed by this patient.

_____

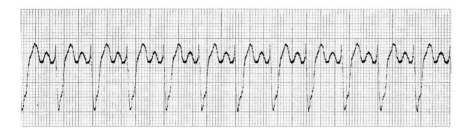

Figure 34-2

Questions 45-48 refer to the following case study:

An 18-year-old woman took approximately 20 tablets of amitriptyline approximately 1 hour before your arrival at her home. She is drowsy and confused, has a dry mouth, and complains of blurred vision. Her ECG is shown in Fig. 34-2.

45. Should you administer syrup of ipecac to this patient? Why or why not?

_____

_____

46. What is your interpretation of the ECG?

_____

47. What drug and appropriate dose may be given to prevent deterioration of this patient's cardiac status?

_____

48. What additional signs and symptoms do you anticipate as this patient's condition deteriorates?

_____

Questions 49 and 50 refer to the following case study:

Your unit is on the scene of a two-car accident. You are caring for a 47-year-old man who appears to be intoxicated. His friend says that he is an alcoholic. The patient states that he drank three beers in the past 5 hours.

49. Should you accept this history of the number of drinks as reliable?

_____

50. If the patient is an alcoholic, what *chronic* physiological changes in the following areas will make it more difficult to assess his condition and more likely for severe injury to occur?
a. Neurological changes:

_____

b. Nutritional problems:

_____

c. Fluid and electrolyte imbalances:

_____

d. Coagulation disorders:

_____

51. Describe the management of a comatose patient suspected to be severely intoxicated by alcohol.

_____

_____

_____

52. Describe the management of a patient experiencing alcohol withdrawal accompanied by severe seizures.

_____

_____

_____

53. List signs and symptoms of delirium tremens.

_____

_____

54. You are at the first aid station for a church picnic. A 16-year-old boy comes to the station complaining of a bee sting. No signs of anaphylaxis are present.
   a. List general care measures for this person.

_____

   b. Describe the method for removing the stinger.

_____

55. List two diseases produced by ticks and possible signs and symptoms for each.

   a.

   b.

56. Describe the proper technique for removing a tick.

_____

57. A hysterical 20-year-old man states that he has just been bitten by a copperhead snake while camping.
   a. List signs and symptoms that would be present if a moderate envenomation had occurred.

_____

   b. Describe the appropriate prehospital management of this patient.

_____

_____

58. For each of the following marine animal classifications, list one example and outline general management principles for envenomation:
   a. Coelenterates:

   _____

   _____

   b. Echinoderms:

   _____

   _____

   c. Stingrays:

   _____

   _____

   _____

● STUDENT SELF-ASSESSMENT

59. Any substance that produces harmful physiological or psychological effects is known as a(n):
   a. Overdose
   b. Poison
   c. Toxin
   d. Venom

60. Which toxic syndrome would present for the patient who has ingested cocaine?
   a. Anticholinergic syndrome
   b. Cholinergic syndrome
   c. Opiate/sedative/ethanol syndrome
   d. Sympathomimetic syndrome

61. What is the primary goal when assessing a poisoned patient?
   a. Begin decontamination of the poison as quickly as possible with activated charcoal
   b. Determine the exact nature of the poison so that appropriate treatment can be given
   c. Obtain a history to determine the exact time that the poisoning occurred
   d. Identify the effects on the respiratory, cardiovascular, and central nervous system

62. Charcoal is effective in treating specific overdoses because it does which of the following?
   a. Reverses the effects of the ingested drug
   b. Binds the drug and prevents absorption
   c. Causes severe nausea and vomiting
   d. Makes the drug speed through the intestine

63. Which is true regarding syrup of ipecac?
   a. It is indicated for use in petroleum distillate ingestion.
   b. It is not associated with life-threatening complications.
   c. It may interfere with other methods of decontamination.
   d. It should be given within the first 2 hours after ingestion.

64. What should be your primary concern when caring for a patient who has ingested hydrocarbon?
   a. Aspiration
   b. Central nervous system effects
   c. Dysrhythmias
   d. Hypotension

65. Medical direction may advise administration of sodium bicarbonate in all of the following *except* which poisoning and overdose situation?
    a. Ethylene glycol
    b. Methanol
    c. Isopropanol
    d. Tricyclic antidepressant

66. Which of the following is true regarding poison plant ingestions?
    a. Dialysis is an effective treatment for most plant poisons.
    b. Ingestion of poisonous plants is common in the United States.
    c. Most signs and symptoms are delayed several days.
    d. Specific treatment should not begin until the plant is identified.

67. Symptoms commonly associated with poisonous mushroom ingestion are likely to include which of the following?
    a. Bradycardia
    b. Dry mouth
    c. Hypertension
    d. Hyperthermia

68. Which of the following hydrocarbon properties is associated with the greatest risk?
    a. Low adhesion of molecules along a surface
    b. Low surface tension
    c. High viscosity
    d. High volatility

69. Toxic hydrocarbon inhalation is most often associated with which of the following?
    a. Childhood ingestions
    b. Industrial exposures
    c. Mixing chemicals
    d. Recreational huffing

70. Which of the following overdose or poisoning will typically lead to bradycardia?
    a. Carbamates
    b. Cocaine
    c. Isopropanol
    d. Methanol

71. What should your first priority be when evaluating a patient contaminated with organophosphates?
    a. Administer atropine
    b. Establish intravenous therapy
    c. Put on protective gear
    d. Suction excess secretions

72. Atropine is supplied in a 10-ml syringe that contains 1 mg of the drug. You wish to administer 2 mg to a patient who has organophosphate poisoning. How many milliliters will you give?
    a. 1 ml
    b. 2 ml
    c. 10 ml
    d. 20 ml

73. Naloxone will antagonize the effects of all of the following except which drug?
    a. Diazepam
    b. Meperidine
    c. Morphine
    d. Propoxyphene

74. What should your highest priority be when caring for a patient at a methamphetamine lab?
    a. Administration of diazepam to control tremors
    b. Decontamination of the patient
    c. Maintaining scene safety
    d. Talking down the paranoid patient

75. The patient who has taken an overdose of oil of wintergreen will most likely present with which of the following?
    a. Bradycardia, hyperglycemia, and nystagmus
    b. Seizures, hyperglycemia, and ventricular tachycardia
    c. Hypoglycemia, tachypnea, and tinnitus
    d. Hematemesis, metabolic alkalosis, and coma

76. What are the typical findings in patients within the first 24 hours of an overdose of acetaminophen?
    a. Dysrhythmias   **c.** No symptoms
    b. Hypoglycemia   **d.** Right upper quadrant abdominal pain
77. When ingestion of multivitamins is suspected in a child, it is critical to determine whether the preparation contains:
    a. Ascorbic acid   **c.** Iron
    b. Folic acid   **d.** Thiamine
78. Which of the following drugs will most likely produce tachycardia if a patient overdoses?
    a. Digoxin (Lanoxin)   **c.** Sertraline (Zoloft)
    b. Propranolol (Inderal)   **d.** Verapamil (Calan)
79. An alert 4-year-old child ingested approximately 10 of his grandmother's blood pressure tablets 20 minutes ago. He is awake and alert. What drug should be administered in this situation?
    a. Activated charcoal   **c.** Calcium chloride
    b. Atropine   **d.** Dopamine
80. Intravenous therapy in the alcoholic with depleted thiamine stores may lead to which of the following?
    a. Disulfiram-ethanol reaction   **c.** Mallory Weiss tears
    b. Guillain-Barré syndrome   **d.** Wernicke-Korsakoff syndrome
81. Which of the following is true regarding delirium tremens?
    a. It affects almost all alcoholics going through alcohol withdrawal.
    b. It is associated with a high mortality rate if untreated.
    c. It is characterized by bradycardia, hypotension, and hypothermia.
    d. It usually occurs 12 to 24 hours following cessation of alcohol.
82. Alcohol withdrawal seizures should be treated with which of the following?
    a. Dextrose 50%   **c.** Magnesium sulfate
    b. Diazepam   **d.** Thiamine
83. An 18-year-old man who attempts to extract honey from a beehive on a dare sustains approximately 20 to 30 stings. He has a headache, fever, and involuntary muscle spasms and reports a syncopal episode. What type of reaction do you suspect?
    a. Anaphylactic   **c.** Local
    b. Delayed   **d.** Toxic
84. A 52-year-old man states that he was bitten by a spider at a woodpile. He is now complaining of back, chest, and abdominal pain and has a severe headache. What type of spider envenomation would produce these symptoms?
    a. Black widow   **c.** Tarantula
    b. Brown recluse   **d.** Wolf
85. A hiker states that he was bitten by a red and yellow snake and is now complaining of slurred speech and dysphagia. His pupils are dilated. You suspect envenomation by what kind of snake?
    a. Copperhead   **c.** Coral
    b. Cottonmouth moccasin   **d.** Massasauga
86. Which treatment may be harmful for the patient who has sustained a venomous snake bite?
    a. Applying ice to wound on affected extremity
    b. Initiating an IV in an unaffected extremity
    c. Positioning extremity in dependent position
    d. Splinting the affected extremity in neutral position
87. For which overdose would isoproterenol be indicated to treat symptomatic bradycardia?
    a. Digoxin   **c.** Propranolol
    b. Nortriptyline   **d.** Verapamil

CHAPTER 35
HEMATOLOGY

● READING ASSIGNMENT
Chapter 35, pages 1062-1077, in *Mosby's Paramedic Textbook*, ed 2

● OBJECTIVES
As a paramedic, you should be able to:
1. Describe the physiology of blood and its components.
2. Discuss pathophysiology and signs and symptoms of specific blood disorders.
3. Outline general assessment and management of patients with hematological disorders.

● REVIEW QUESTIONS
Match the hematology terms in Column II with the description in Column I. Use each term only once.

Column I	Column II
1. _____ Include eosinophils, basophils, and neutrophils	a. Basophils
2. _____ Destroy red blood cells	b. Bilirubin
3. _____ Destroy invading organisms and include monophils	c. Erythrocytes
4. _____ Waste product after destruction of hemoglobin	d. Macrophages
5. _____ Activate chemicals that trigger inflammation	e. Phagocytes
6. _____ Contains albumin, globulins, and fibrinogen	f. Plasma
7. _____ Composed of water and hemoglobin	g. Platelets
	h. White blood cells

8. Complete the information in the following table.

Condition	Cause	Signs and Symptoms
Anemia		
Leukemia		
Lymphomas		
Polycythemia		

Disseminated intravascular
   coagulation

Hemophilia

Sickle cell disease

Multiple myeloma

9. You respond to a private residence and find a 21-year-old African-American woman who is complaining of pain in her abdomen, hands, and feet. She said she had the flu and vomited three times yesterday. She tells you that she suffers from sickle cell disease.
   a. What type of sickle cell crisis may present in this manner?

   _____

   b. What event may have triggered a crisis in this patient?

   _____

   c. What specific organ should you try to palpate on your physical examination of this patient?

   _____

   d. Outline the prehospital care of this patient.

   _____

   _____

   _____

● **STUDENT SELF-ASSESSMENT**
10. Which is true regarding red bone marrow?
    a. Only white blood cells are formed here.
    b. It is formed in the liver.
    c. It is composed mainly of connective tissue and fat.
    d. It is found in the vertebrae, pelvis, sternum, and ribs.
11. Which of the following is a normal value for hemoglobin?
    a. 10 g/100 ml   c. 35%
    b. 15 g/100 ml   d. 50%
12. Which type of anemia may be cured by splenectomy?
    a. Aplastic   c. Iron deficiency
    b. Hemolytic   d. Sickle cell
13. Which is true of acute myeloblastic leukemia?
    a. It affects mostly young children.
    b. Reed-Sternberg cells are present.
    c. Generalized itching may be present.
    d. It is difficult to cure.

14. Which hematological disorder is diagnosed using bone marrow biopsy?
    a. Disseminated intravascular coagulation
    b. Leukemia
    c. Hodgkin's disease
    d. Sickle cell anemia
15. Which of the following is a target organ in Hodgkin's lymphoma?
    a. Kidney   c. Spleen
    b. Liver   d. Testes
16. What can trigger secondary polycythemia?
    a. Blood loss   c. Hypoxia
    b. Hypothermia   d. Infection
17. Which of the following occurs when disseminated intravascular coagulation is present?
    a. Coagulation inhibition levels are increased.
    b. Fibrin is deposited in small vessels in multiple organs.
    c. Platelets and fibrinogen V, VIII, and XIII increase.
    d. Thrombin is destroyed.
18. What is needed to stop the bleeding that occurs during hemophilia?
    a. Factor VIII   c. Oxygen administration
    b. Intravenous fluids   d. Topical thrombin
19. Although all sickle cell disease emergencies can cause death, which one represents an immediate life-threatening situation?
    a. Aplastic crisis   c. Splenic sequestration
    b. Hemolytic crisis   d. Vasoocclusive crisis
20. In which hematological disorder of the bone marrow does the tumor destroy bone tissue?
    a. Hodgkin's disease   c. Lymphoma
    b. Leukemia   d. Multiple myeloma
21. Prehospital care for a conscious patient with a hematological problem should always include which of the following?
    a. Analgesics   c. Blood transfusion
    b. Antidysrhythmics   d. Emotional support

ENVIRONMENTAL CONDITIONS

● READING ASSIGNMENT

Chapter 36, pages 1078-1099, in *Mosby's Paramedic Textbook,* ed 2

● OBJECTIVES

As a paramedic, you should be able to:
1. Describe the physiology of thermoregulation.
2. Discuss the risk factors, pathophysiology, assessment findings, and management of specific hyperthermic conditions.
3. Discuss the risk factors, pathophysiology, assessment findings, and management of specific hypothermic conditions and frostbite.
4. Discuss the risk factors, pathophysiology, assessment findings, and management of drowning and near-drowning.
5. Identify mechanical effects on the body based on a knowledge of basic properties of gases.
6. Discuss the risk factors, pathophysiology, assessment findings, and management of diving emergencies and high-altitude illness.

● REVIEW QUESTIONS

Match the terms related to environmental conditions in Column II with the appropriate description in Column I. Use each term only once.

Column I	Column II
1. _____ Goose bumps	a. Afterdrop phenomenon
2. _____ Dissipation of heat in the body by various mechanisms	b. Boyle's law
	c. Cold diuresis
3. _____ Sudden return of cold blood and wastes to the core	d. Dalton's law
4. _____ Temperature difference between body and environment	e. Dysbarism
	f. Henry's law
5. _____ Gas volume inversely related to its pressure	g. Piloerection
	h. Rewarming shock
6. _____ Decompression sickness	i. Thermal gradient
7. _____ Heat immersion causing hypotension from vasodilation	j. Thermogenesis
	k. Thermolysis
8. _____ Total pressure of gases equaling the sum of partial pressure of component gases	
9. _____ Regulation of heat production in the body	
10. _____ Amount of gas dissolved in fluid volume is proportional to pressure of gas with which it is in equilibrium	

11. Briefly describe how each of the following contributes to heat production in the body.
    a. Chemical control:

    _____

    b. Musculoskeletal system:

    _____

    c. Endocrine system:

    _____

12. For each of the following situations, select the mechanisms of heat loss that apply (conduction, convection, evaporation, and radiation). You may use each answer more than once.
    a. On a windy autumn evening, you remove the clothing of a trauma patient to assess his injuries more accurately. On arrival to the emergency

       department, his temperature is 94° F (34.4° C). _____.
    b. During a multiple patient situation, you extricate a partially clothed patient onto a cold metal backboard. On arrival to the emergency depart-

       ment, her temperature is 96° F (35.6° C). _____.
    c. On a dry, cool spring evening you transport a wet patient who injured her neck after diving into a swimming pool. On arrival to the emergency

       department, her temperature is 94.6° F (34.8° C). _____.
    d. A patient with a 40% BSA burn is continuously cooled with normal saline en route to the hospital. On arrival to the emergency department,

       his temperature is 93.5° F (34.2° C). _____.
13. You are on the scene of a multiple-car collision on a hot July day. List four ways your body will compensate to prevent your temperature from rising.
    a.

    b.

    c.

    d.
14. You are assisting with a search-and-rescue effort after a hurricane. It is cold, wet, and windy. List four ways your body will attempt to maintain a normal temperature.
    a.

    b.

    c.

    d.

15. For each of the following examples, identify the type of heat illness and briefly describe the appropriate prehospital patient care.
    a. You are working at an amusement park on a 95° F (35° C) humid day. A hot, sweaty 45-year-old woman comes to your aid station complaining of severe cramping in her calves. Her vital signs are BP, 116/72 mm Hg; P, 116; and temperature, 98.6° F (37° C).
    Illness:

    _____

    Management:

    _____

    b. A 55-year-old man is complaining of dizziness, nausea, and vomiting while participating in a long-distance walk fund-raiser. His vital signs while lying down are BP, 104/70 mm Hg; P, 108. His vital signs while standing are BP, 86/50 mm Hg; P, 128; and his temperature is 101° F (38.3° C).
    Illness:

    _____

    Management:

    _____

    c. On a 100° F (37.8° C) day, an 80-year-old woman becomes confused and agitated and has a seizure in her apartment, which does not have air-conditioning. She is responsive to pain, has jugular venous distention, and is sweating profusely. Her vital signs are BP, 92/70 mm Hg; P, 120/minute; R, 24; and temperature, 106° F (41.1° C).
    Illness:

    _____

    Management:

    _____

16. Why is the increased metabolic rate that is produced in mild hypothermia undesirable for a patient who already has an injury or medical illness?

    _____

    _____

    Questions 17-19 refer to the following case study:

    You are caring for a snowmobiler whose rig broke through the ice 30 minutes ago. He pulled himself out of the water and collapsed before rescuers reached him 20 minutes later. He has been moved to a safe area.

17. Describe general measures of care to begin immediately on this patient.

    _____

    _____

18. You determine that he is apneic and pulseless. His ECG displays the rhythm shown in Fig. 36-1. What actions should be taken if the following occur?
    a. His core temperature is less than 86° F (30° C).

    _____

    _____

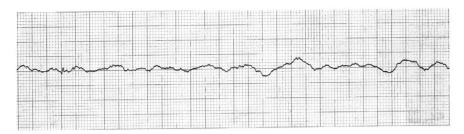

Figure 36-1

b. His core temperature is greater than 86° F (30° C).

_____

_____

19. When should resuscitation efforts be terminated?

_____

20. You are transporting a hiker who became lost on a trail. He is shivering and hungry and has a temperature of 97° F (36.1° C). How would you treat this patient?

_____

_____

21. A firefighter dives into an ice-covered pond to rescue a child who has fallen through the ice on a windy, cold January evening. On the 10-minute walk back to the firetruck, the firefighter develops slurred speech and ataxia and complains that his heart is pounding. At the ambulance, his temperature is 89.5° F (31.9° C). His ECG is shown in Fig. 36-2.

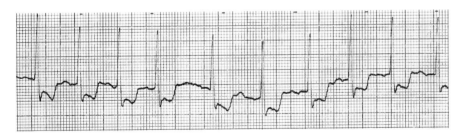

Figure 36-2

a. What is your interpretation of the ECG tracing?

_____

b. Describe your management of this patient.

_____

_____

_____

Questions 22-24 refer to the following case study:

> During a cross-country ski meet, a participant complains of coldness, numbness, and extreme pain in the fingers of his right hand.

22. Differentiate between the findings you would anticipate for superficial frostbite and deep frostbite.

_____

_____

23. List four factors that increase susceptibility to frostbite that you should look for in this patient.
    a.
    b.
    c.
    d.
24. How would you treat frostbite in this patient?

_____

_____

Questions 25-27 refer to the following case study:

> A 2-year-old child pulled from a backyard pool is apneic and pulseless.

25. Identify four factors that will influence this patient's clinical outcome.
    a.

    b.

    c.

    d.
26. What complications do you anticipate if the patient is resuscitated?

_____

_____

_____

27. Describe prehospital management of this child.

_____

_____

28. List five body areas on the patient where pain may occur resulting from SQUEEZE.
    a.   d.
    b.   e.
    c.

29. A diver experiences acute distress immediately after rapidly surfacing from a deep dive.
    a. List five signs or symptoms of air embolism.
       a.   d.
       b.   e.
       c.

b. Describe special considerations necessary for care of this patient while you are providing advanced life support and transport.

_____

_____

30. A tourist at a local resort complains of severe joint pain, fatigue, vertigo, and paraesthesia 12 hours after returning from his first dive.
    a. What diving injury do you suspect?

_____

    b. Describe prehospital management of this patient.

_____

_____

31. You respond to a mountain resort where a participant in a cycling event has become ill.
    a. List the three types of high-altitude illness.
       a.
       b.
       c.
    b. What single intervention is most critical to long-term improvement of the patient suffering from high-altitude illness after the ABCs have been managed?

_____

● STUDENT SELF-ASSESSMENT

32. What is the most important organ that regulates body temperature?
    a. Heart   **c.** Pituitary gland
    b. Lungs   **d.** Skin
33. You are assessing firefighters in the rehab area of a major fire on a summer day. Your patient is dizzy and nauseated and has orthostatic hypotension. What should you do?
    a. Administer medication for his nausea
    b. Ask him to rest for 15 minutes before returning to the fire
    c. Have him drink a fluid-replacement beverage
    d. Initiate an intravenous line and administer a fluid bolus
34. What causes shock to develop in the patient with heat stroke?
    a. Fluid loss   **c.** Peripheral vasodilation
    b. Myocardial depression   **d.** All of the above
35. What is the most critical intervention for heat stroke?
    a. Fluid resuscitation   **c.** Rapid cooling in transit
    b. Medication administration   **d.** Rapid transport to a hospital
36. When does shivering stop in a hypothermic patient?
    a. The body temperature drops to 90° F (32.2° C).
    b. Glucose or glycogen is depleted.
    c. Excessive amounts of insulin are excreted.
    d. P_{CO_2} increases to more than 50 mm Hg.
37. Prehospital care of a frostbitten extremity should include which of the following?
    a. Application of a tourniquet
    b. Elevation of the affected extremity
    c. Rapid rewarming in hot water
    d. Refreezing of the injured extremity

38. All drownings are characterized by which of the following?
   a. Hypovolemia, hypoxia, and acidosis
   b. Hypoxia, acidosis, and hypothermia
   c. Hypoxia, acidosis, and hypercapnia
   d. Hypovolemia, acidosis, and hypercapnia
39. Which of the following best describes the term *drowning?*
   a. Death from submersion up to 24 hours after arrival in the emergency department
   b. Death related to submersion that occurs at any time after the incident
   c. Swimming-related distress sufficient to require care in the emergency department
   d. Swimming-related distress sufficient to require support in the prehospital setting
40. What is the single most important factor in determining survival after submersion injury?
   a. Age of the patient
   b. Contaminants in the water
   c. Duration of submersion
   d. Water temperature
41. Which law of physics atates that the volume of gas is inversely related to its pressure at a constant temperature?
   a. Boyle's law
   b. Dalton's law
   c. Henry's law
   d. Newton's law
42. A diver is in respiratory distress after ascent. You palpate subcutaneous emphysema. He is probably suffering from which of the following?
   a. Barotrauma of descent
   b. Decompression sickness
   c. Pulmonary air embolus
   d. Pulmonary overpressurization syndrome
43. What is the primary danger of nitrogen narcosis?
   a. Hypoxemia
   b. Impaired judgment
   c. Respiratory acidosis
   d. Shock resulting from hypovolemia
44. What is the critical sign or symptom that indicates deterioration in a patient with acute mountain sickness?
   a. Ataxia
   b. Headache
   c. Irritability
   d. Vomiting

CHAPTER 37
INFECTIOUS AND COMMUNICABLE DISEASES

● READING ASSIGNMENT
Chapter 37, pages 1100-1143, in *Mosby's Paramedic Textbook*, ed 2

● OBJECTIVES
As a paramedic, you should be able to:
1. Identify general public health principles relative to infectious diseases.
2. Describe the chain of elements necessary for an infectious disease to occur.
3. Explain how internal and external barriers affect susceptibility to infection.
4. Distinguish among the four stages of infectious disease: the latent, incubation, communicable, and disease periods.
5. Describe the mode of transmission, pathophysiology, prehospital considerations, and personal protective measures taken for HIV, hepatitis, tuberculosis, meningococcal meningitis, and pneumonia.
6. Describe the mode of transmission, pathophysiology, signs and symptoms, and prehospital considerations taken for rabies or tetanus.
7. List the signs, symptoms, and potential secondary complications of selected childhood viral diseases.
8. List the signs, symptoms, and potential secondary complications of influenza and mononucleosis.
9. Describe the mode of transmission, pathophysiology, prehospital considerations, and personal protective measures taken for sexually transmitted diseases.
10. Identify signs, symptoms, and prehospital considerations of lice and scabies.
11. Outline the reporting process for exposure to infectious and communicable diseases.
12. Discuss your role in preventing disease transmission.

● REVIEW QUESTIONS
Match the infectious diseases listed in Column II with their descriptions in Column I. Use each disease only once.

Column I	Column II
1. _____ Infection that produces influenza-like symptoms, dark-colored urine, and light-colored stools	**a.** Chlamydia
2. _____ Macular rash that can cause severe birth defects if a susceptible mother is exposed in pregnancy	**b.** Gonorrhea **c.** Hepatitis **d.** Herpes simplex **e.** HIV infection
3. _____ Bacterial pulmonary infection spread by airborne droplets	**f.** Meningitis
4. _____ Viral infection that impairs the body's ability to fight other infectious disease	**g.** Rubella **h.** Syphilis
5. _____ Sexually transmitted disease characterized in the early stage by a painless chancre	**i.** Tuberculosis **j.** Varicella
6. _____ Inflammation of lining of the central nervous system that may produce headache, stiff neck, seizures, and coma	

7. _____ Bacterial infection that produces mucopurulent discharge but rarely causes septicemia

8. _____ Generalized illness accompanied by vesicular lesions, fever, and malaise

9. List the six components of the chain of elements that must be present for an infectious disease to occur.

a.   d.

b.   e.

c.   f.

10. Describe two situations that interfere with the body's external barriers to infection, thereby increasing the risk of infection.

a.

b.

11. Name two factors that can affect the ability of the body's internal barriers to fight infectious disease.

a.

b.

12. For each of the following patient care scenarios, describe the personal protective measures that you should take.

a. A 23-year-old woman is about to deliver her fourth child. The baby's head is crowning, and you are preparing for delivery.

_____

b. A 50-year-old man is complaining of severe substernal chest pain. You are preparing to initiate an intravenous line to administer medications.

_____

c. You are preparing to administer epinephrine subcutaneously to a 25-year-old patient with dyspnea because of anaphylaxis.

_____

d. A 17-year-old girl ingested a large amount of alcohol and barbiturates, vomited, and rapidly lost consciousness. You elect to intubate her trachea.

_____

e. A 55-year-old man attempted suicide by holding a shotgun under his chin and firing. He is combative and thrashes about as you try to control the large amount of bleeding and secure his airway.

_____

f. A butcher sustained a laceration to her hand at work. The wound is oozing a small amount of blood.

_____

Questions 13-16 refer to the following case study:

While caring for a 40-year-old man who had nausea, vomiting, right upper quadrant abdominal pain, and jaundice, you puncture your finger with a needle contaminated with the patient's blood. The hospital notifies you the next day that he tested positive for hepatitis.

13. What type or types of hepatitis can produce the symptoms experienced by this patient?

_____

14. What are the most effective measures you can take to prevent exposure to hepatitis at work?

_____

15. Describe the modes of transmission for hepatitis B.

_____

_____

16. Can you do anything now that you are exposed so that you will not get hepatitis?

_____

_____

17. What signs and symptoms may be evident on the prehospital examination of a patient in each of the following stages of infection from the human immunodeficiency virus?
   a. Acute retroviral infection:

_____

   b. Asymptomatic infection:

_____

   c. Early symptomatic infection:

_____

   d. Late symptomatic infection:

_____

18. You are transporting a patient with human immunodeficiency virus to the hospital after he sustained a sprained ankle at a volleyball game. No other injuries are evident.
   a. What personal protective measures should you take while caring for this patient?

_____

   b. How should the ambulance be cleaned before transport of the next patient?

_____

19. What is the best way for emergency care workers to monitor whether they have been exposed to a patient with tuberculosis?

_____

20. A 23-year-old man has a severe headache and a temperature of 102° F (38.9° C) and complained earlier of a stiff neck. Now he is limp and arouses only to a loud voice. You suspect meningitis.
   a. What personal protective measures should you use on this call? (You plan to initiate an intravenous line and apply oxygen by mask.)

_____

b. If the emergency department contacts you later to inform you that the patient has bacterial meningitis, should you report an exposure?

---

c. What is the likelihood that you will be given prophylaxis if you have used appropriate BSI from the beginning of this call?

---

21. List three chronic signs or symptoms that may develop if syphilis is untreated for a number of years.

a.

b.

c.

22. What personal protective measures should be taken when examining the mouth of a child with an outbreak of herpes simplex on the lips?

---

23. For each of the following ailments, list the signs and symptoms and site of infestation:
a. Pubic lice:

---

b. Head lice:

---

c. Scabies:

Questions 24-26 refer to the following case study:

> You transport a child who has a temperature of 101° F (38.3° C) and a generalized skin rash that began the previous day. Some lesions are flat and red, some are raised blisters, and others have scabbed. On arrival to the emergency department, the pediatrician confirms that the child has chickenpox.

24. Is this disease communicable at this stage?

---

25. If you have never had chickenpox, how long would you expect to wait before symptoms appear?

---

26. Are you contagious during this entire time?

Questions 27-35 refer to the following case study:

> During your care of a patient at the scene of a motor-vehicle crash, you had blood splash into your eyes while your partner was intubating the patient and you were holding inline immobilization of the C-spine. You had gloves on at the time.

27. Has a significant exposure to blood or body fluids occurred?

---

28. When should you report this exposure?

29. Besides evaluation for postexposure prophylaxis, what other emergency care will you need in this situation?

The patient refuses to give permission to test for HIV.

30. Can the emergency department ignore the patient's refusal and run an HIV test in this situation? Why?

31. What other questions should you ask the patient?

32. What are your options for postexposure prophylaxis if the patient refuses testing?

33. After counseling and examination by the emergency department staff, you are offered a course of medicine for postexposure prophylaxis. How will you decide whether to take the medicine?

34. Why do you think some paramedics might need psychological counseling after this incident?

35. How could this exposure have been prevented?

● STUDENT SELF-ASSESSMENT

36. Which agency is responsible for establishing the guidelines for body substance isolation and universal (standard) precautions?
   a. Centers for Disease Control (CDC)
   b. Department of Health (DOH)
   c. Department of Transportation (DOT)
   d. Occupational Safety and Health Administration (OSHA)

37. Which of the following could be used to interrupt the portal of entry in the chain of elements of an infectious disease?
   a. Administering antibiotics to kill a bacterium
   b. Cleaning a blood spill with an appropriate agent
   c. Receiving immunizations at appropriate intervals
   d. Using gloves as defined in the BSI guidelines

38. Which of the following is an internal barrier to infection?
   a. Flora
   b. Leukocytes
   c. Nasal hairs
   d. Prostatic fluid

39. The internal defense that provides antibodies to destroy invading organisms is produced by which of the following?
   a. Cell-mediated immunity
   b. Complement
   c. Humoral immunity
   d. Killer cells

40. The infectious disease phase that begins when the agent invades the body and ends when the disease process begins is which period?
   a. Communicability
   c. Incubation
   b. Disease
   d. Latent

41. Death secondary to hepatitis is most likely to occur from which strain of the virus?
   a. Hepatitis A
   c. Hepatitis C
   b. Hepatitis B
   d. Non-A, non-B hepatitis

42. What type of organism causes hepatitis?
   a. Bacteria
   c. Parasite
   b. Fungus
   d. Virus

43. Which sign or symptom can help to distinguish pneumonia from other respiratory illness?
   a. Fatigue and loss of appetite
   c. Shaking chills and chest pain
   b. Headache and muscle aches
   d. Yellow productive cough

44. Which of the following is a classic sign or symptom of tetanus?
   a. Flaccid paralysis
   c. Trismus
   b. Seizures
   d. Urticaria

45. What is the reaction causing muscle spasms that prevents a patient with rabies from drinking called?
   a. Hydropenia
   c. Polydipsia
   b. Hydrophobia
   d. Polyuria

46. What is the primary mode of transmission for rubella, mumps, and varicella?
   a. Blood-to-blood contact
   c. Lesion contact
   b. Fecal contamination
   d. Respiratory droplets

47. Complications of varicella may include all of the following *except* which disease?
   a. Bacterial infection
   c. Meningitis
   b. Croup
   d. Reye's syndrome

48. Which treatment measure is usually given to patients with chickenpox, influenza, or herpes simplex?
   a. Antibiotic therapy
   c. Comfort measures
   b. Aspirin for pain and fever
   d. Intravenous therapy

49. Which childhood disease is characterized by a violent cough that can persist for 1 to 2 months?
   a. Influenza
   c. Pertussis
   b. Mumps
   d. Pneumonia

50. What secondary complication of influenza is often associated with severe illness or death?
   a. Aspiration
   c. Meningitis
   b. Dehydration
   d. Pneumonia

51. Which sign or symptom associated with mononucleosis could produce a life-threatening condition if the patient is not maintained at rest?
   a. Fever
   c. Oral rash
   b. Lymphadenopathy
   d. Splenomegaly

52. A patient has a headache, malaise, fever, lymphadenopathy, and a symmetrical rash that involves the palms and soles. He states that an ulcerated sore on his penis healed spontaneously 3 weeks earlier. Which infectious disease do you suspect?
   a. Chlamydia
   c. Herpes
   b. Gonorrhea
   d. Syphilis

53. Which body system harbors the dormant herpes virus?
   a. Cardiovascular system
   c. Integumentary system
   b. Gastrointestinal system
   d. Nervous system

BEHAVIORAL AND PSYCHIATRIC DISORDERS

● READING ASSIGNMENT
Chapter 38, pages 1144-1165, in *Mosby's Paramedic Textbook*, ed 2

● OBJECTIVES
As a paramedic, you should be able to:
1. Define what constitutes a behavioral emergency.
2. Identify potential causes for behavioral and psychiatric illnesses.
3. List three critical principles that should be considered in the prehospital care of any patient with a behavioral emergency.
4. Outline key elements in the prehospital patient examination during a behavioral emergency.
5. Describe effective techniques for interviewing a patient during a behavioral emergency.
6. Distinguish between key symptoms and management techniques for selected behavioral and psychiatric disorders.
7. Identify factors that must be considered when assessing suicide risk.
8. Formulate appropriate interview questions to determine suicidal intent.
9. Explain prehospital management techniques for the patient who has attempted suicide.
10. Describe assessment of the potentially violent patient.
11. Outline measures that may be used in an attempt to safely diffuse a potentially violent patient situation.
12. List situations when patient restraints can be used.
13. Discuss key principles in patient restraint.
14. Describe safety measures taken when patient violence is anticipated.
15. Explain variations in approach to behavioral emergencies in children.

● REVIEW QUESTIONS
Match the psychiatric conditions in Column II with their descriptions in Column I. Use each condition only once.

Column I	Column II
1. _____ Feelings of worthlessness and guilt	a. Conversion hysteria
2. _____ Unfounded fear of situation or object	b. Depression
3. _____ Loss of touch with reality in this major mental disorder	c. Mania
4. _____ Loss of sensory or motor function without organic cause	d. Neurosis
5. _____ Excessive elation, irritability, talkativeness, and delusions	e. Panic attack
6. _____ Logical, highly developed delusions	f. Paranoia
	g. Phobia
	h. Psychosis

7. You arrive at the home of a 60-year-old man whose behavior is erratic. He alternates between hysterical bursts of laughter, irritability, sitting quietly, and crying. You find chlorpropamide (Diabinese), hydralazine, and thyroxin in the medicine chest and note an ecchymotic area on his left temple. His skin is hot and moist. Based on this patient's history, what are some likely organic causes of his behavior that must be ruled out before assuming that this is a behavioral emergency?

_____

_____

_____

8. **a.** List three psychosocial causes of mental illness.

_____

   b. List three sociocultural causes of mental illness.

_____

   Questions 9-11 refer to the following patient case study:

   You are called to a private residence to care for a behavioral emergency. Police report that the patient is "OBS." On arrival, you find a 34-year-old woman sitting quietly in a living room chair. She is complaining of depression.

9. What four general management principles should you consider on this and all behavioral calls?

   a.

   b.

   c.

   d.

10. What should your scene survey include?

_____

11. What minimum patient data should be obtained if possible?

_____

12. Should a detailed secondary survey be performed on a patient with a behavioral emergency?

_____

13. Complete the missing information in the following table.

Illness	Classification	Clinical Presentation	Treatment (Medical or EMS)
Dementia			
Schizophrenia			
Posttraumatic syndrome			
Bipolar disorder			
Somatization disorder			
Bulimia nervosa			

14. A patient with a phobia of heights must be rescued by ladder from a high bridge. What measures can you take to prevent a panic attack?

_____

15. A manic patient is being transported to the hospital for psychiatric evaluation. Describe effective patient management techniques in this situation.

_____

16. Family members call you to the home of a 25-year-old man who has become increasingly out of touch with reality. He feels that aliens are trying to kidnap him so that they can remove his brain. He tells you that they are trying to control his thoughts. He states, "They're here. Can't you hear them laughing?"
  a. What behavioral illness does this presentation suggest?

_____

  b. What approach will enable therapeutic communication with this patient?

_____

17. You are on the scene with a 25-year-old woman who cut her wrist with a razor blade. She is crying, "Let me go. Why didn't you let me do it?" She has a small laceration with controlled bleeding, minimal blood loss, and stable vital signs.
  a. How can you best assess the patient's suicidal risk?

_____

  b. What are your goals in caring for this patient during transport?

_____

Questions 18-22 refer to the following case study:

A distraught family calls you to take their son to the hospital for a court-ordered, involuntary psychiatric evaluation. They state that he has been breaking furniture for the past few hours and refuses to take his antipsychotic drugs.

18. What four factors should you rapidly assess to determine the potential for violence in this patient?
  a.
  b.
  c.
  d.

Your patient is pacing, verbally abusive, and threatening injury to those who approach. He is not armed.

19. You elect to restrain him. What help should you request?

_____

20. When approaching the patient to prepare for restraint, what should you note about the physical environment?

_____

21. Assuming that the patient meets the standard for involuntary detention in your state, how should he be restrained (including position and ways to secure extremities and torso)?

_____

_____

22. After restraints are applied, what should you monitor en route to the hospital?

_____

● **STUDENT SELF-ASSESSMENT**

23. What is a change in mood or behavior that cannot be tolerated by the involved person or others and needs immediate attention called?
  a. Behavioral emergency   **c.** Neurosis
  b. Delusion   **d.** Psychosis

24. What is the characteristic of abnormal (maladaptive) behavior?
  a. Deviates from the person's normal behavior
  b. Does not conform to your idea of normal behavior
  c. Interferes with a person's ability to function
  d. Violates a societal law

25. Which of the following questions would be most appropriate to begin a conversation with a mentally ill patient?
  a. Did you start feeling this way today?
  b. Are you feeling bad now?
  c. How did this all begin?
  d. Are you OK?

26. Which response by the paramedic is most likely to lead to an effective interview in the prehospital setting?
  a. Everything will be fine.   **c.** Yes, I see those scary bugs too.
  b. I know exactly how you feel.   **d.** You look very sad.

27. Which condition is a state of acute mental confusion commonly brought on by a physical illness?
  a. Delirium   **c.** Dementia
  b. Delusions   **d.** Depression

28. A middle-aged woman suddenly loses the ability to speak after catching her husband in an extramarital affair. What behavioral illness may have caused her problem?
  a. Conversion hysteria   **c.** Panic attack
  b. Depression   **d.** Phobia

29. Which of the following feelings commonly characterizes depression?
  a. Hopelessness   **c.** Increased libido
  b. Hunger   **d.** Restlessness

30. You are transporting a man who believes he is Elvis Presley. His wife states that he quit his job, keeps calling her Priscilla, and is preparing to move to Graceland. You suspect that he is suffering from which of the following?
    a. Delusions   c. Paranoia
    b. Neurosis   d. Phobia
31. A panic attack typically occurs with any of the following *except* which symptom?
    a. Chest pain and vertigo   c. Suicidal intent
    b. Hyperventilation   d. Trembling and sweating
32. What is the highest priority on a suicide call?
    a. Ensuring safety of crew members   c. Talking the person out of it
    b. Managing life threats   d. Listening empathetically
33. Which of the following statements regarding suicide is true?
    a. People who talk about killing themselves rarely do it.
    b. Men commit suicide more often than women.
    c. Suicide is an inherited tendency.
    d. When depression lifts, suicide risk disappears.
34. When should a violent patient be released from physical restraints?
    a. Immediately after administration of haloperidol intramuscularly
    b. As soon as the patient assures cooperation
    c. When the police have adequate personnel to control the patient
    d. When a physician at the hospital determines the patient is no longer dangerous
35. You are caring for a violent psychiatric patient. Which of the following drugs would *not* be appropriate for chemical restraint?
    a. Diazepam   c. Haloperidol
    b. Diphenhydramine   d. Lorazepam
36. Which strategy should be used to maintain EMS crew safety when on a behavioral emergency call?
    a. Be firm and tell the patient to behave or you will have to use restraints.
    b. Interview the patient privately while your partner waits outside of the room.
    c. Kneel and put your arm on the patient's shoulder to show you care.
    d. Stay closer to the exit than the patient, with furniture between you and the patient.
37. Which strategy will be helpful when caring for a child who is experiencing a behavioral emergency?
    a. Avoid having the parents present during care.
    b. Don't be concerned about the possibility of violence.
    c. Keep the interview questions brief.
    d. Lie if you need to gain cooperation.

GYNECOLOGY

● READING ASSIGNMENT
Chapter 39, pages 1166-1177, in *Mosby's Paramedic Textbook,* ed 2

● OBJECTIVES
As a paramedic, you should be able to:
1. Describe the physiological processes of menstruation and ovulation.
2. Describe the pathophysiology of the following nontraumatic causes of abdominal pain in women: pelvic inflammatory disease, ruptured ovarian cyst, cystitis, dysmenorrhea, Mittelschmerz, endometriosis, ectopic pregnancy, and vaginal bleeding.
3. Describe the pathophysiology of traumatic causes of abdominal pain in women, including vaginal bleeding and sexual assault.
4. Outline the prehospital assessment and management of the woman with abdominal pain.
5. Outline specific assessment and management for the patient who has experienced sexual assault.
6. Describe specific prehospital measures to preserve evidence in sexual assault cases.

● REVIEW QUESTIONS
Match the gynecological problems in Column II with their description in Column I. Use each term only once.

Column I	Column II
1. _____ Abdominal pain at ovulation	**a.** Dysmenorrhea
2. _____ Beginning of menses	**b.** Endometriosis
3. _____ Intraabdominal growth of the uterine lining	**c.** Endometritis
	d. Menarche
4. _____ Infection of the female pelvic organs	**e.** Mittelschmerz
	f. Pelvic inflammatory disease
5. _____ Menstrual cramps	
6. _____ Fluid sac that ruptures	**g.** Ruptured ovarian cyst

7. The normal menstrual cycle is about **(a)** _____ days.

The average menstrual flow is **(b)** _____

to _____ ml and usually lasts from

(c) _____ to _____ days.
During the menstrual cycle, some of the primary follicles become

(d) _____ _____. These
enlarge and form a lump on the surface of the ovary and when mature

are known as the **(e)** _____ or

_____ _____. The release of

the oocyte from the follicle is called **(f)** _____. After ovulation, the follicle turns into a glandular structure called the

(g) _____ _____, whose cells

secrete large amounts of **(h)** _____ and some

(i) _____. If pregnancy occurs, the fertilized oocyte

(j) (_____) begins releasing a hormonelike substance

called **(k)** _____ _____, which keeps the corpus from degenerating.

8. Other than pain, list three signs or symptoms that a woman may experience during menses.
   a.
   b.
   c.

Questions 9-12 refer to the following case study:

> You are called to a private residence to evaluate a 19-year-old woman who is complaining of severe pelvic pain. Her pain began yesterday and she says it is unbearable now. She has no allergies, takes no medicines, and has no significant medical history.

9. What specific questions related to her obstetric history should you ask her?
   a.

   b.

   c.

   d.

   e.

   f.

   g.

   h.

   i.

   j.

She tells you that she has never been pregnant, that she presently has her menstrual period, and that it is of normal color and amount. She denies vaginal discharge or the possibility of pregnancy because she uses birth control pills. She states that she has not had intercourse in 4 months. She denies other symptoms of pregnancy and any history of gynecological problems.

10. What should you specifically assess on the physical examination?

_____

_____

Her lower abdomen is diffusely tender. Vital signs are within normal limits and her skin is warm and dry.

11. What are some potential causes of her pain?

_____

_____

12. What prehospital interventions will you provide for this patient?

_____

_____

13. What measures can be taken in the prehospital environment to minimize the fear and stress experienced by a victim of sexual abuse?

_____

14. Describe five guidelines for evidence preservation on a sexual abuse call.
   a.
   b.
   c.
   d.
   e.

● **STUDENT SELF-ASSESSMENT**

15. How often does a typical woman have menstrual flow?
   a. Every 14 days   **c.** Every 28 days
   b. Every 21 days   **d.** Every 35 days
16. Which hormone initiates the ovarian cycle leading to ovulation?
   a. Estrogen   **c.** Luteinizing hormone
   b. Follicle-stimulating hormone   **d.** Progesterone
17. What is the most common cause of pelvic inflammatory disease?
   a. Gonorrhea
   b. Herpes virus
   c. Human immunodeficiency virus
   d. Syphilis
18. Which of the following factors increases the incidence of dysmenorrhea?
   a. Increased age   **c.** Childbirth
   b. Frequent exercise   **d.** Infection
19. A ruptured ovarian cyst may mimic all of the following *except* which disorder?
   a. Appendicitis   **c.** Ectopic pregnancy
   b. Cholecystitis   **d.** Salpingitis

20. Which of the following is a normal sign or symptom of cystitis?
    a. Blood in the urine
    c. Inability to urinate
    b. Flank pain
    d. Painless urination
21. Which of the following is true regarding endometriosis?
    a. It is an inflammation of the uterine lining.
    b. It is common in young women.
    c. It has no effect on fertility.
    d. Its pain may increase during menstruation.
22. Which of the following gynecological problems may cause severe internal hemorrhage?
    a. Dysmenorrhea
    c. Salpingitis
    b. Mittelschmerz
    d. Ruptured ovarian cyst
23. Which of the following is a traumatic cause of vaginal bleeding?
    a. Abortion attempts
    c. Onset of labor
    b. Disorders of the placenta
    d. Pelvic inflammatory disease
24. What is your most important role in caring for a victim of sexual abuse?
    a. Allow only a paramedic of the same gender to care for the patient.
    b. Provide a safe and secure environment for the patient.
    c. Preserve evidence exactly as outlined by protocol.
    d. Perform a complete history and thorough examination.
25. Which of the following should you do to preserve evidence on a sexual abuse call?
    a. Ask the patient to shower.
    c. Place the clothing in a paper bag.
    b. Thoroughly clean wounds.
    d. Search the scene for evidence.

OBSTETRICS

● **READING ASSIGNMENT**

Chapter 40, pages 1178-1209, in *Mosby's Paramedic Textbook,* ed 2

● **OBJECTIVES**

As a paramedic, you should be able to:
 1. Describe the structure and function of the specialized structures of pregnancy.
 2. Outline fetal development from ovulation through adaptations at birth.
 3. Explain normal maternal physiological changes during pregnancy and how they influence prehospital patient care and transport.
 4. Describe appropriate information to be elicited during the obstetrical patient history.
 5. Describe specific techniques for assessment of pregnant patients.
 6. Describe general prehospital care of the pregnant patient.
 7. Discuss the implications of prehospital care after trauma to the fetus and mother.
 8. Describe the assessment and management of patients with preeclampsia and eclampsia.
 9. Explain the pathophysiology, signs and symptoms, and management of the processes that cause vaginal bleeding in pregnancy.
10. Outline the physiological changes during the stages of labor.
11. Describe the role of the paramedic during normal labor and delivery.
12. Compute an Apgar score.
13. Describe assessment and management of postpartum hemorrhage.
14. Discuss the identification, implications, and prehospital management of complicated deliveries.

● **REVIEW QUESTIONS**

Match the types of abortion in Column II with their description in Column I. Use each term only once.

Column I	Column II
1. _____ Abortion before 12 weeks not externally induced	a. Complete abortion
2. _____ Legal termination of pregnancy to preserve the mother's health	b. Incomplete abortion
3. _____ All the products of conception passed before 12 weeks	c. Induced abortion
4. _____ Symptoms of impending abortion with a closed cervix	d. Missed abortion
5. _____ Failure to pass a fetus after 4 weeks of fetal death	e. Spontaneous abortion
6. _____ Intentional termination of pregnancy	f. Therapeutic abortion
	g. Threatened abortion

Match the problems of pregnancy in Column II with their description in Column I. Use each problem only once.

Column I

7. _____ Painless bleeding in third trimester of pregnancy
8. _____ Hypertension, proteinuria, and visual disturbance in the third trimester
9. _____ Severe abdominal pain, shock, and easily palpable fetal parts
10. _____ Painful third-trimester bleeding
11. _____ Third-trimester seizure after a new onset of hypertension
12. _____ Abdominal pain, scant vaginal bleeding, and shock in the first trimester

Column II

a. Abortion
b. Abruptio placentae
c. Eclampsia
d. Ectopic pregnancy
e. Placenta previa
f. Preeclampsia
g. Uterine rupture

13. In what lunar month do the following fetal development characteristics typically occur?
    a. Fetal movement felt by the mother:

    _____

    b. Fetal heart beat:

    _____

    c. Distinct fingers and toes:

    _____

    d. Eyebrows and fingernails:

    _____

    e. Possible viability if born:

    _____

14. What causes the arteriovenous shunts to close at birth?

    _____

    _____

15. What do the following pregnancy terms mean?
    a. A patient is gravida 6 para 5 (G6 P5).

    _____

    b. She is a multipara.

    _____

    c. The patient has postpartum bleeding.

    _____

    d. You are called to care for a nullipara who is term.

    _____

16. A woman in her 40th week of pregnancy complains of heartburn, dizziness, and frequency of urination. Her heart rate is 100; respirations are 20 and deep; and blood pressure is 90/60 mm Hg. (She says her normal is 100/70 mm Hg.) She has slight edema of the ankles and tortuous varicose veins. Explain how the physiological alterations of pregnancy cause each of the signs or symptoms she is experiencing.

    a. Heartburn:

    _____

    _____

    b. Dizziness:

    _____

    _____

    c. Frequency of urination:

    _____

    _____

    d. Hypotension:

    _____

    _____

    e. Pedal edema and varicose veins:

    _____

    _____

17. Briefly explain why each of the following historical findings would cause concern if delivery is imminent in the field:

    a. No prenatal care:

    _____

    _____

    b. Diabetic mother:

    _____

    _____

    c. Vaginal bleeding:

    _____

    _____

    d. Current heroin intoxication:

    _____

    _____

Questions 18-20 refer to the following case study:

A 28-year-old woman who is in her third trimester complains of abdominal pain after an automobile accident in which she was the unrestrained driver. She is pale, and her vital signs are blood pressure, 90/60 mm Hg; pulse, 134; and respirations, 28. Her abdomen is tender to palpation, and you note some vaginal bleeding.

18. What other subjective information do you need from the mother?

_____

_____

19. How can you determine whether the infant is in distress?

_____

_____

20. Describe prehospital care and transport of this patient.

_____

_____

_____

Questions 21-24 refer to the following case study:

A 30-year-old woman says she is 9 weeks pregnant and complains of severe cramping pain in the lower abdomen and vaginal bleeding. She states that she has saturated 6 sanitary napkins and passed some "white stringy stuff" that her husband shows you in the toilet.

21. What condition of pregnancy do you suspect?

_____

22. What actions should you take so that the physician can determine whether she has had a complete abortion?

_____

23. Estimate her blood loss if you feel the history was accurate.

_____

24. Why might this patient be exhibiting a grief reaction?

_____

_____

25. An obstetrician calls you to his office to transport a 28-year-old woman who has an ectopic pregnancy (determined by ultrasound). She complains of severe abdominal pain and has frank signs of shock.

   a. What other signs or symptoms might she experience?

   _____

   b. Describe interventions you will use on your 20-minute trip to the emergency department.

   _____

   _____

26. What general patient care measures should be taken for any patient who has third-trimester bleeding without shock?

   _____

   _____

Questions 27-31 refer to the following case study:

   A 40-year-old primipara in the third trimester complains of headache, dizziness, and nausea. Vital signs are blood pressure, 160/100 mm Hg; pulse, 110; and respirations, 20. Her hands and feet are markedly swollen, and you note intermittent facial twitching. She says her doctor was worried about protein in her urine.

27. What complication do you suspect?

   _____

28. In what position should you transport this patient?

   _____

29. List two drugs with appropriate doses that may be ordered by medical direction to stop seizure activity in these types of patients.

   _____

30. Besides medication, what EMS actions can minimize the risk of seizures?

   _____

31. What risks to the fetus exist with this condition?

   _____

   _____

Questions 32-36 refer to the following case study:

   You are called to a private residence 30 minutes from the nearest hospital to care for a woman in labor.

32. What information in the patient's past medical history is important to help gauge how quickly labor will progress?

   _____

   _____

33. What specific signs or symptoms during labor would lead you to believe that delivery is imminent?

_____

_____

34. As the baby's head delivers, what assessment and interventions should you perform?

_____

_____

35. Describe the procedure to clamp the umbilical cord.

_____

_____

36. When should the Apgar score be calculated?

_____

37. If necessary, when should oxytocin be administered and what is the proper dose and route?

_____

38. Labor fails to progress after a baby in breech position is delivered to the level of the chest. Describe the steps you should take in this situation.

_____

_____

_____

39. After the head of a baby with shoulder dystocia is delivered, what can you do to deliver the shoulders while minimizing fetal injury?

_____

_____

_____

40. A 35-year-old woman who is G6 P5 states that she is ready to deliver her baby at home. Her membranes have ruptured, her contractions are frequent, and she wants to push. When you examine her perineum, you see the umbilical cord protruding from the vagina.
   a. What actions should you take immediately to prevent fetal hypoxia?

_____

_____

_____

   b. Should you attempt to deliver this baby on the scene?

_____

41. Functions of the placenta include all except which of the following?
    a. Excretion of wastes   **c.** Metabolism of drugs
    b. Hormone production   **d.** Transfer of gases

42. The primary role of amniotic fluid is which of the following?
    a. Excretion   **c.** Nutrition
    b. Hydration   **d.** Protection

43. The fetal structure that allows blood to bypass the liver and go directly into the inferior vena cava is which of the following?
    a. Ductus arteriosus   **c.** Foramen ovale
    b. Ductus venosus   **d.** Umbilical vein

44. The umbilical cord carries which of the following?
    a. Deoxygenated blood by one umbilical artery and oxygenated blood by one umbilical vein
    b. Deoxygenated blood by two umbilical arteries and oxygenated blood by one umbilical vein
    c. Oxygenated blood by one umbilical artery and deoxygenated blood by one umbilical vein
    d. Oxygenated blood by two umbilical arteries and deoxygenated blood by one umbilical vein

45. Where should the uterus be palpable at week 20 of gestation?
    a. At the lower border of the umbilicus
    b. Between the symphysis pubis and umbilicus
    c. Halfway between the umbilicus and the xiphoid
    d. Just above the symphysis pubis

46. Which of the following is the normal fetal heart rate?
    a. 80 to 120/minute   **c.** 160 to 200/minute
    b. 120 to 160/minute   **d.** 200 to 240/minute

47. In which of the following positions should the hypotensive pregnant patient who is more than 4 months gestation be transported?
    a. High Fowler's   **c.** Prone
    b. Left lateral recumbent   **d.** Supine

48. Immediately after the delivery of a healthy baby, your patient's eyes roll back and she becomes pulseless. She has no previous medical history. Which of the following may have caused her cardiac arrest?
    a. Abruptio placentae   **c.** Aortic dissection
    b. Amniotic fluid embolism   **d.** Congestive cardiomyopathy

49. When attempting to resuscitate a patient in cardiac arrest who is 8 months pregnant, what special care measures should you employ to be most effective?
    a. Decrease ventilation volumes to minimize gastric distention
    b. Increase the dose of epinephrine to maximize vasoconstriction
    c. Perform chest compressions lower on the sternum
    d. Tilt her torso laterally to prevent compression of the vena cava

50. By which of the following signs is eclampsia distinguished from preeclampsia?
    a. Edema   **c.** Hypertension
    b. Glucosuria   **d.** Seizures

51. The primary complication from administration of magnesium sulfate is which of the following?
    a. Increased hypertension   **c.** Respiratory depression
    b. Precipitous delivery   **d.** Ventricular dysrhythmias

52. Excessive traction on the umbilical cord during placental delivery may cause which of the following?
    a. Fetal distress   **c.** Uterine inversion
    b. Placenta previa   **d.** Uterine rupture

53. Which of the following occurs in the second stage of labor?
    a. Cervical dilation
    c. Expulsion of the placenta
    b. Delivery of the infant
    d. Fetal descent into the birth canal

54. When delivering a baby's head, you note that the umbilical cord is wrapped around the baby's neck. Which of the following is the first action you should take?
    a. Cut the cord in two places, clamp, and proceed with delivery.
    b. Elevate the mother's hips and have her pant until you reach the hospital.
    c. Gently unloop the cord around and over the baby's head.
    d. No special action is needed; the cord will free itself as the shoulders deliver.

55. A minute after delivery, a baby has a weak cry, a pink body with blue extremities, and a pulse of 128; he actively moves about and sneezes when a catheter is introduced into his nose. The Apgar score is which of the following?
    a. 6
    c. 8
    b. 7
    d. 9

56. Hemorrhage control in the postpartum period may include all of the following *except* which?
    a. Elevation of the mother's hips
    b. Delivery of oxytocin intravenously
    c. Breastfeeding of the baby
    d. Vigorous uterine massage

57. For which of the following is the premature infant at risk?
    a. Gestational diabetes
    c. Placenta previa
    b. Hypothermia
    d. Prolapsed umbilical cord

58. Which of the following is a frequent complication of multiple gestation?
    a. Eclampsia
    c. Premature delivery
    b. Placenta previa
    d. Uterine rupture

59. Which of the following complications of pregnancy is most likely to require delivery by cesarean section?
    a. Breech presentation
    c. Shoulder distocia
    b. Cephalopelvic disproportion
    d. Vaginal bleeding

60. A 30-year-old woman develops dyspnea and severe chest pain 24 hours after delivery of her third child. She is hypotensive and in acute distress. Based on her history, you suspect which of the following?
    a. Eclampsia
    c. Pneumonia
    b. Myocardial infarction
    d. Pulmonary embolism

61. Which of the following is the primary danger to an infant delivered during a precipitous delivery?
    a. Abruptio placentae
    c. Nuchal cord
    b. Cerebral trauma
    d. Placenta previa

62. Which of the following describes chorioamnionitis?
    a. Amniotic fluid embolism
    b. Excessive amniotic fluid
    c. Infection of fetal membranes
    d. Premature rupture of the membranes

DIVISION SIX:
SPECIAL CONSIDERATIONS

NEONATOLOGY

● READING ASSIGNMENT
Chapter 41, pages 1212-1229, in *Mosby's Paramedic Textbook*, ed 2

● OBJECTIVES
As a paramedic, you should be able to:
1. Identify risk factors associated with the need for neonatal resuscitation.
2. Describe physiologic adaptations at birth.
3. Outline the prehospital assessment and management of the neonate.
4. Describe resuscitation of the distressed neonate.
5. Discuss postresuscitative management and transport.
6. Describe signs and symptoms and prehospital management of specific neonatal resuscitation situations.
7. Identify injuries associated with birth.
8. Describe appropriate interventions to manage the emotional needs of the neonate's family.

● REVIEW QUESTIONS
Match the structures described in Column I with the correct term in Column II.

Column I	Column II
1. _____ A vertical split in the lip	a. Choanal atresia
2. _____ Abnormalities that include a small mandible and defects of the eyes and ears	b. Cleft lip
	c. Diaphragmatic hernia
3. _____ Occlusion that blocks the passage between the nose and pharynx	d. Gastroesophageal reflux
4. _____ Protrusion of stomach through the diaphragm	e. Pierre Robin syndrome

5. List two risk factors that may indicate the need for neonatal resuscitation in each of the following categories:
   a. Antepartum risk factors

   b. Intrapartum risk factors

6. What three major adaptations are necessary for the survival of the neonate at birth?
   a.
   b.
   c.

7. List three actions that help maintain body warmth of the neonate.

    a.

    b.

    c.

8. Arrange the following steps in neonatal resuscitation (assuming you have a blue infant with slightly decreased respirations and a heart rate of 70 that does not improve at each step) in the correct order in the following table.

Incorrect Order	Correct Order
Administer epinephrine	
Obtain vascular access	
Oxygen at 5 L/min	
Ventilate with bag-mask device	
Perform chest compressions	
Warm, dry, suction, stimulate	

Questions 9-14 pertain to the following case study:

> A 3 kg baby is delivered, his airway has been suctioned, and he has been properly positioned. Tactile stimulation has been provided; however, he is still not breathing.

9. At what rate should you ventilate the neonate?

_____

After ventilations are initiated, you detect a pulse of 70/min.

10. Where should you palpate the pulse on a neonate?

_____

11. What steps should you take now?

_____

After you initiate chest compressions, there is no improvement. Your partner has intubated the baby.

12. What size endotracheal tube would be appropriate for this infant?

_____

13. What are your options to obtain vascular access?

_____

14. What drug/dose should you administer when vascular access has been established?

_____

15. List an intervention for each of the following neonatal postresuscitation complications:

    a. Endotracheal tube dislodgement

_____

    b. Endotracheal tube occlusion by mucus

_____

    c. Pneumothorax

_____

16. In which of the following situations will you anticipate the need for neonatal resuscitation?
    a. Contractions have been occurring for 6 hours
    b. Physician states the baby weighs 3600 g (7.5 lb.)
    c. Rupture of the membranes occurred 12 hours ago
    d. The baby is at 36 weeks gestation

17. What initiates respiration in the newborn?
    a. Chemical and temperature changes
    b. Chest compression
    c. Closure of the patent ductus
    d. Cutting the umbilical cord

18. What is a proper position to maximize the airway of a neonate?
    a. Prone with neck slightly extended
    b. Supine with neck slightly flexed
    c. Supine with towel under the shoulders
    d. Supine with towel under the head

19. Which neonatal suctioning technique is appropriate after delivery if no meconium has been observed?
    a. Cut the umbilical cord before suctioning.
    b. Suction the mouth first and then the nose.
    c. Suction the nose first and then the mouth.
    d. Suctioning is unnecessary if meconium is not observed.

20. Priorities of care for neonatal resuscitation are as follows:
    a. Prevent heat loss, administer intravenous fluids, and allow the infant to feed at the breast.
    b. Position the neonate, suction to clear the airway, minimize external stimulation, and initiate intravenous fluids.
    c. Prevent heat loss, position the neonate, suction to clear the airway, and provide stimulation.
    d. Position the infant, suction to clear the airway, administer intravenous fluids, and provide stimulation.

21. Deep suctioning of the posterior pharynx of the neonate may cause which of the following?
    a. Bradycardia
    b. Central nervous system depression
    c. Hypocarbia
    d. Tachypnea

22. After delivery the infant is warmed, dried, and stimulated. Respirations are 30 per minute and heart rate is 110, but the baby's lips and ears are still blue. What should you do?
    a. Administer oxygen at 5 L/min by holding the tubing ½ inch from the nose.
    b. Begin bag-mask ventilation with 100% oxygen until the color improves.
    c. Initiate bag-mask ventilation and chest compressions.
    d. No intervention is needed; this is a normal finding in the newborn.

23. Which of the following is an acceptable method of neonatal stimulation?
    a. Shouting loudly close to the baby's ear
    b. Holding the baby by the ankles and slapping the buttocks
    c. Slapping or flicking the soles of the feet or rubbing the back
    d. Vigorously shaking the baby by firmly grasping the shoulders

24. When should the paramedic consider intubation of the neonate?
    a. If the heart rate increases after bag-mask ventilation is performed
    b. If prolonged ventilation is likely to be needed
    c. Immediately after absent respirations are noted
    d. When the gestational age is less than 39 weeks

25. What is the normal heart rate of an infant?
    a. 60/min   c. 120/min
    b. 80/min   d. 160/min
26. Which finding may indicate a postresuscitation complication related to intubation in the neonate?
    a. Decreased resistance to ventilation
    b. Diminished breath sounds
    c. Increase in chest expansion
    d. Return of tachycardia
27. Apnea in infants may be related to which of the following?
    a. CNS disorders   c. Meconium aspiration
    b. Excessive stimulation   d. Use of stimulants
28. The most common factor for respiratory distress and cyanosis in a neonate is prematurity. Which of the following factors can also be responsible for this condition?
    a. Cleft lip congenital anomaly
    b. Mucus obstruction of the nasal passages
    c. Premature rupture of membranes
    d. Postterm delivery
29. What is the correct first drug and dose used for the treatment of neonatal bradycardia in the presence of adequate ventilation and oxygenation?
    a. Atropine 0.01 mg/kg IV
    b. Atropine 0.02 mg/kg IV
    c. Epinephrine 0.01 mg/kg (1:1,000) IV
    d. Epinephrine 0.01 mg/kg (1:10,000) IV
30. Which of the following is a risk factor associated with cardiac arrest in the newborn?
    a. Amniotic fluid aspiration
    b. Gestational diabetes
    c. Intrauterine asphyxia
    d. Premature cutting of the cord after birth
31. Which is true regarding vomiting in the neonate?
    a. An intravenous line should be established if this is observed.
    b. It is very unusual and associated with serious illness.
    c. It is a frequent occurrence and should be of no concern.
    d. Persistent bile-stained vomit may indicate a bowel obstruction.
32. What sign or symptom can be found secondary to phototherapy for hyper-bilirubinemia?
    a. Bradycardia   c. Seizures
    b. Diarrhea   d. Vomiting
33. You are called to evaluate a 4-day-old breastfed infant whose mother states the child has diarrhea. When asked, she says the child is having five or six "loose" yellow stools per day. What is your assessment of this situation?
    a. This number of stools is normal for a breastfed baby.
    b. This indicates a serious situation that requires immediate IV therapy.
    c. This indicates bowel obstruction secondary to a congenital defect.
    d. The yellow stools could indicate hepatitis, the mother should be assessed for risk.
34. A mother states that she has observed repetitive eye deviation and blinking and sucking and swimming movements of the 2-day-old infant's arms. This may indicate which of the following?
    a. Focal clonic seizures   c. Subtle seizures
    b. Multifocal seizures   d. Tonic seizures

35. What should be assessed in the prehospital setting when evaluating an infant with apparent seizures?
   a. Blood glucose level
   b. Blood pressure
   c. Child's ability to feed normally
   d. Glasgow coma scale

36. Which is true of a temperature of 100.4° F (38.0° C) in a neonate?
   a. It is a normal result of immature temperature control and does not require treatment.
   b. It may indicate a life-threatening infection and requires immediate transport.
   c. It often results in the development of febrile seizures that are difficult to control.
   d. Prehospital care should involve ice packs in the groin area to lower temperature.

37. A 3-kg infant delivered at home yesterday is limp and has irregular respirations. You assess the child, maintain warmth, assist ventilations, and initiate vascular access. The blood glucose drawn when the IV was started is 40 mg/dl. What should you administer?
   a. 3 g of a D10W solution
   b. 3 g of a D50W solution
   c. 6 g of a D10W solution
   d. 6 g of a D50W solution

38. Which of the following injuries may occur during childbirth?
   a. Clavicle or extremity fracture
   b. Liver or spleen injury
   c. Spine or spinal cord injury
   d. All of the above

39. Which of the following statements by the paramedic would be helpful when speaking to the parents of an infant that is being resuscitated in the prehospital setting:
   a. Everything's going to be OK.
   b. Everything possible is being done for your baby.
   c. I can't tell you anything at all about your baby.
   d. I think your baby's going to make it; this is a great crew.

CHAPTER 42

PEDIATRICS

● READING ASSIGNMENT

Chapter 42, pages 1230-1277, in *Mosby's Paramedic Textbook*, ed 2

● OBJECTIVES

As a paramedic, you should be able to:
1. Identify the role of emergency medical services for children.
2. Identify modifications in patient assessment techniques to assist in examination of patients at different developmental levels.
3. Identify common age-related illnesses and injuries in pediatric patients.
4. Outline general principles of assessment and management of pediatric patients.
5. Describe pathophysiology, signs and symptoms, and management of selected pediatric respiratory emergencies.
6. Describe pathophysiology, signs and symptoms, and management of shock in pediatric patients.
7. Describe pathophysiology, signs and symptoms, and management of selected pediatric dysrythmias.
8. Describe pathophysiology, signs and symptoms, and management of pediatric seizures.
9. Describe pathophysiology, signs and symptoms, and management of hypoglycemia and hyperglycemia in pediatric patients.
10. Describe pathophysiology, signs and symptoms, and management of infectious pediatric emergencies.
11. Identify common causes of poisoning and toxic exposure in pediatric patients.
12. Describe special considerations for assessment and management of specific injuries in children.
13. Outline pathophysiology and management of sudden infant death syndrome.
14. Describe risk factors, key signs and symptoms, and management of injuries or illness resulting from child abuse and neglect.
15. Identify prehospital considerations for the care of infants and children with special needs.

● REVIEW QUESTIONS

Match the drugs in Column II with their appropriate initial *pediatric* dose in Column I. Use each drug only once.

Column I		Column II
1. _____ 0.1 ml/kg		a. Adenosine
2. _____ 2 to 20 mcg/kg/min		b. Amiodarone
3. _____ 1 mEq/kg per dose		c. Atropine sulfate
4. _____ 0.1 to 0.2 mg/kg		d. Diazepam
5. _____ 1 mg/kg		e. Dopamine
6. _____ 0.02 mg/kg		hydrochloride
7. _____ 5 mg/kg		f. Epinephrine (1:10,000)
		g. Lidocaine
		h. Sodium bicarbonate

8. In what pediatric age group(s) are you most likely to see the following illness or injuries?
    a. Sepsis:

    _____

    b. Febrile seizures:

    _____

    c. Jaundice:

    _____

    d. Ingestions:

    _____

    e. Falls:

    _____

    f. Child abuse:

    _____

    g. Drowning or near-drowning:

    _____

    h. Suicidal gestures:

    _____

Questions 9-12 pertain to the following case study:

> A 7-year-old boy is in acute respiratory distress after visiting a friend's home. He gives a history of asthma and allergy to dogs (his friend has three). His home medicines include an Atrovent inhaler, montelukast sodium (Singulair) tabs, which he takes daily, and albuterol by nebulizer as necessary, which he has not used for a week. He has circumoral cyanosis, is working very hard to breathe, and has faint inspiratory and expiratory wheezes.

9. What interventions are appropriate for this child? Include two possible beta-agonist drugs you could administer (with appropriate doses).

    _____

    _____

10. What side effects do you anticipate from the administration of these drugs?

    _____

11. In 15 minutes, you see no clinical improvement and your estimated arrival time is still 20 minutes. What do you do?

    _____

12. What aspects of the physical examination will change when the patient improves?

    _____

    _____

13. List three characteristic signs or symptoms of epiglottitis.
    a.
    b.
    c.

14. A 20-month-old with croup is in mild respiratory distress on a cool October evening.
    a. What intervention should you use before entering the ambulance that may cause rapid improvement in the patient's signs and symptoms?

    b. When in the ambulance, how will you care for this child?

Questions 15-19 pertain to the following case study:

A limp, 11-month-old boy is carried into the ambulance base by his mother. She states that he has had a fever with vomiting and diarrhea for 3 days. His eyes are sunken, his tongue is furrowed, and his lips are cracked. Physical examination reveals rapid respirations; cold, mottled extremities; and the electrocardiogram in Fig. 42-1.

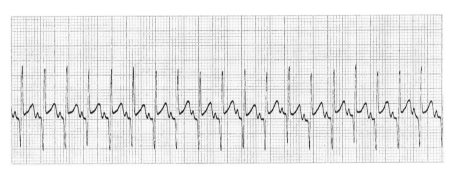

Figure 42-1

15. What is this child's problem?

16. Interpret the electrocardiogram.

17. Describe management of this child, assuming a 45-minute transport time.

18. What are the appropriate vital signs for this child?

19. What other clinical signs of improvement will you watch for besides an improvement in vital signs?

Questions 20-23 refer to the following case study:

A 3-year-old, 15-kg child is found unconscious after suffocation with a plastic bag. On arrival, you find a dusky, pale child who is unresponsive and apneic. Occasionally, you can palpate a faint pulse at the carotid artery, but you obtain no blood pressure reading. The electrocardiogram is shown in Fig. 42-2.

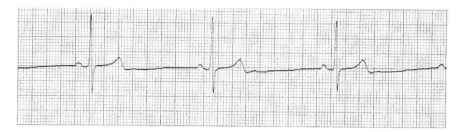

Figure 42-2

20. Interpret the electrocardiogram tracing.

_____

21. What actions will you take immediately up to and including the first drug (with appropriate dose)?

_____

_____

22. If an intravenous line cannot be immediately established, what two actions can be taken?
    a.
    b.
23. After your initial interventions result in no patient improvement, what is the next drug (and dose) that is indicated?

_____

24. A 3-week-old, 5-kg infant with a history of congenital heart defects suddenly becomes unconscious and stops breathing. On arrival, you find him pulseless and apneic. Cardiopulmonary resuscitation is initiated, the child's trachea is intubated, and lactated Ringer's solution is initiated intravenously. The electrocardiogram tracing in Fig. 42-3 is noted.

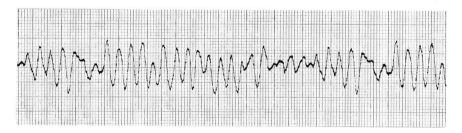

Figure 42-3

a. Outline your continued care of this patient up to and including the first two drugs (including dose).

_____

_____

_____

b. If a repeat dose of epinephrine is necessary, what is the correct dose and concentration?

_____

Questions 25-27 refer to the following case study:

A frightened mother tells you that when she put her 14-kg, 4-year-old child to bed he complained of a slight earache with a low-grade temperature. She heard a noise several hours later and found her child having a grand mal seizure, which stopped after approximately 1 minute. The child's temperature is 105.5° F (40.8° C). He appears to be postictal at this time.

25. After you have ensured that the child is stable, what history should you obtain from the mother?

_____

_____

26. What care should be provided en route to the hospital?

_____

_____

27. If the child has a seizure during transport, list two anticonvulsant drugs with the appropriate dose and route(s) that may be given.
   a.

   b.

28. You are called to an elementary school to care for a 6-year-old who is "acting funny." She is only responsive to pain. The nurse says the child has a history of diabetes. You check a fingerstick glucose level and determine that this child's blood sugar is 35 mg/dl.
   a. What drug should you administer (include dose and route)?

_____

   b. What other signs or symptoms may this child have exhibited before becoming this ill?

_____

_____

29. Your 3-year-old patient weighs 17 kg. He was involved in a head-on motor vehicle collision and was restrained only by a lap belt. He says his "tummy hurts." The physical examination reveals an anxious, pale child with a rigid, tender abdomen. Discuss the significance of the following physiologic differences in children and specific ways they will influence your care of this child.

    a. Children have a greater percentage of circulating blood volume than adults.

_____

_____

    b. Children have a large body surface area in proportion to body weight.

_____

_____

    c. Children's hearts function at near-maximal performance in a normal, healthy state.

_____

_____

    d. Volume replacement in children is weight related.

_____

_____

_____

_____

    e. Intravenous access is difficult to establish in children.

_____

_____

30. How do you determine that an intraosseous needle is properly placed?

_____

Questions 31-33 pertain to the following case study:

At 1 AM on a cool February night, you are dispatched for a "baby choking." On arrival, you find a well-nourished 4-month-old baby boy apneic and pulseless in his crib. There is frothy sputum in the nose and mouth, and his diaper is wet and full of stool. The child is cold, and dependent lividity is present. The hysterical mother states that he and his older sister have both had a slight cold, but otherwise he was healthy.

31. What characteristics of sudden infant death syndrome are consistent with this call?

_____

32. What other findings should you document in this situation?

_____

You spend some time at the scene comforting the family and making the appropriate notifications and then ride back quietly to the firehouse with your normally talkative partner. You ask if he is OK, and he says, "Of course, I'm fine." Then he immediately rushes to the phone, where you hear him awaken his wife and ask her to check on their 6-month-old daughter.

33. Should you ignore your partner's unusual behavior, since he told you he is OK? If not, what action(s) can you take?

_____

_____

Questions 34-36 pertain to the following case study:

A mother tells you that her 8-month-old son fell off his tricycle early in the day but seemed to be feeling fine. Later, she could not wake him from his nap. On physical examination, you find a dirty child who has agonal respirations, a slow pulse, and extension posturing. No visible signs of trauma are present on the head, although small bruises are noted on the shoulders.

34. What should your immediate interventions be for this child?

_____

_____

35. What findings might lead you to suspect child abuse?

_____

_____

36. After you deliver the child to the appropriate medical center, what are your responsibilities?

_____

_____

37. What history and physical examination should be performed on a child who is a victim of sexual abuse?

_____

_____

● STUDENT SELF-ASSESSMENT

38. Which of the following is a component of an effective EMSC system?
    a. Access to care
    b. Immunization programs
    c. Legislative committees
    d. Medical direction
39. Which examination strategy can help reduce anxiety in school-age children?
    a. Allow them to take part in decisions about their care.
    b. Assure them that they are not being punished.
    c. Let them play with equipment.
    d. Use deep-breathing and relaxation techniques.
40. Which age group fears bodily injury and mutilation and interprets words literally?
    a. Adolescents
    b. Preschoolers
    c. School-agers
    d. Toddlers

313

41. You are called to care for a 6-month-old child who has respiratory distress. Which of the following would be the most likely cause of this complaint in this age group?
    a. Asthma
    b. Bronchiolitis
    c. Epiglottitis
    d. Foreign body airway obstruction
42. A great deal of the child's physical examination can be done by which step?
    a. Assessing the skin temperature and moisture
    b. Auscultating the breath sounds
    c. Observing the child's behavior
    d. Palpating the central and distal pulses
43. Which of the following is a sign of respiratory distress in a child?
    a. Crying
    b. Elevated temperature
    c. Flushed skin
    d. Head bobbing
44. Which of the following is a bacterial infection of the upper airway and sub-glottic trachea that occurs during or after croup?
    a. Bronchiolitis
    b. Epiglottitis
    c. Pneumonia
    d. Tracheitis
45. Which of the following may be indicated for the management of severe respiratory distress associated with bronchiolitis?
    a. Albuterol 0.15 mg/kg by inhalation
    b. Atropine 0.01 mg/kg by inhalation
    c. Epinephrine 0.1 mg/kg subcutaneously
    d. Terbutaline 0.2 mg/kg subcutaneously
46. Which of the following is an appropriate intervention for a child in whom epiglottitis is suspected?
    a. Lay the child supine on the mother's lap.
    b. See if the epiglottis is swollen.
    c. Infuse intravenous normal saline fluids at 20 ml/kg.
    d. Give humidified oxygen by mask.
47. Which drug may be administered to relieve respiratory distress in the child with bronchiolitis?
    a. Albuterol
    b. Alupent
    c. Epinephrine
    d. Diphenhydramine
48. Which of the following findings would be your first indication that an infant is developing dehydration and needs a fluid bolus?
    a. Decreasing blood pressure and poor skin turgor
    b. Flat fontanelle and warm skin
    c. Loss of appetite and nausea
    d. Very dry mucous membranes and tachycardia
49. A 20-kg child is lethargic and tachycardic and has dry mucous membranes after a 3-day history of "flu." Medical direction asks for a fluid bolus of normal saline. How much will you administer initially?
    a. 20 ml
    b. 100 ml
    c. 200 ml
    d. 400 ml
50. You are caring for a child who has fatigue, difficulty breathing, and peripheral edema. Crackles are audible in the bases of both lungs. Which illness do you suspect?
    a. Anaphylaxis
    b. Asthma
    c. Cardiomyopathy
    d. Pneumonia
51. A 5-year-old, 44-lb child is in ventricular fibrillation. Which is the correct *initial* energy level for defibrillation?
    a. 20 joules
    b. 40 joules
    c. 80 joules
    d. 88 joules

52. What is the maximum single dose of atropine that should be given to a 6-year-old child?
    a. 0.05 mg   c. 0.1 mg
    b. 0.01 mg   d. 0.5 mg
53. What is the correct sequence of interventions for a bradycardic, hypotensive child after the airway has been secured, an intravenous line has been established, and cardiopulmonary resuscitation has been initiated?
    a. Atropine and epinephrine   c. Atropine only
    b. Epinephrine and atropine   d. Epinephrine only
54. An infant who "wasn't acting right" has a heart rate of 230. He is awake but somewhat lethargic, and his skin is pale with delayed capillary refill. You determine that he has SVT, and your partner has established vascular access. What is the initial treatment of choice for this child?
    a. Adenosine   c. Synchronized cardioversion
    b. Digoxin   d. Verapamil
55. Which of the following is *not* likely to cause seizures?
    a. Central nervous system infection   c. Prolonged dehydration
    b. Metabolic abnormalities   d. Serious head trauma
56. After intravenous administration of diazepam, you should monitor closely for which of the following?
    a. Decreased pulse   c. Respiratory depression
    b. Increased blood pressure   d. Vomiting or nausea
57. Your 7-year-old patient is lethargic and has a blood pressure of 70/50 mm Hg and a pulse of 138/min. Respirations are 40/min and smell fruity. His mother says he has been losing weight and has had increased urination and thirst for several weeks. What condition should you consider?
    a. Head injury   c. Hyperglycemia
    b. Hydrocarbon ingestion   d. Hyperthermia
58. What life-threatening condition may be found in a child after ingestion of alcohol?
    a. Hypoglycemia   c. Hypokalemia
    b. Hypothermia   d. Hypocalcemia
59. What clinical finding may be present in the child who has ingested a large amount of aspirin?
    a. Bradycardia   c. Hypothermia
    b. Hiccoughs   d. Tachypnea
60. You are caring for a teenager who was "huffing" some toluene. What effects could this produce?
    a. Pulmonary edema   c. Uncontrolled bleeding
    b. Renal failure   d. Visual disturbances
61. A 14-year-old is experiencing anxiety, tremors, and chest pain after smoking crack cocaine. His vital signs are: BP 180/100 mm Hg, P 130/min, and R 20/min. Which of the following drugs would *not* be indicated in the initial care of this child?
    a. Aspirin   c. Lorazepam
    b. Epinephrine   d. Nitroglycerin
62. A 4-year-old has taken 10 tricyclic antidepressant tablets. Her BP is 60 mm Hg by palpation, P is 130/min, and she is drowsy. Which intervention would be indicated to improve her cardiac output?
    a. Lidocaine 1 mg/kg   c. Oxygen at 2 l per minute
    b. Normal saline 30 ml/kg bolus   d. Sodium bicarbonate 1 mEq/kg
63. Glucagon may be helpful as an antidote to an overdose of:
    a. Beta blockers   c. Cocaine
    b. Calcium channel blockers   d. Tricyclic antidepressant drugs

64. Which mechanism of injury accounts for the largest number of trauma deaths in children?
   a. Drowning
   c. Fire
   b. Falls
   d. Motor vehicle crashes

65. Which is a sign of increasing intracranial pressure unique to an infant?
   a. Bulging fontanelle
   c. Hypotension
   b. Cheyne-Stokes respirations
   d. Tachycardia

66. Why is the child more vulnerable to liver and splenic injuries?
   a. Those organs are larger in a children under the age of 8 years.
   b. Mechanisms of injury in children are more likely to affect these areas.
   c. The abdominal musculature is minimal and does not protect these organs.
   d. These organs are more fragile in a child and injure more easily.

67. Which is a risk factor associated with a higher incidence of SIDS?
   a. High maternal or paternal age
   b. Rank of first in the birth order
   c. Premature birth and low birth weight
   d. Higher socioeconomic groups

68. Which of the following injuries should be considered as the result of possible abuse?
   a. Any fractures of a child less than 5 years of age
   b. Injuries localized to one area of the body
   c. Bruises or burns in unusual patterns
   d. Lacerations on the forehead of a toddler

69. You are called to care for a 10-month old child who "didn't wake up from his nap." He is unconscious and has vomited. What other physical findings may indicate abuse?
   a. Dirty diaper
   c. Other children in the room
   b. Increased respiratory rate
   d. Retinal hemorrhage

70. Respiratory distress is reported in a child who has a tracheostomy. The tube appears to be partially obstructed. Which of the following should be your first intervention?
   a. Intubate the child orally.
   b. Insert a tracheal dilator to enlarge the hole.
   c. Remove and replace the tracheostomy.
   d. Suction the tracheostomy.

71. A child is experiencing signs and symptoms of hypoxia while on a home ventilator. On arrival, you should immediately perform which of the following?
   a. Begin ventilation with a bag-valve device.
   b. Check the connections on the machine and oxygen.
   c. Contact medical direction to help trouble-shoot.
   d. Request that the home health agency repair the ventilator.

72. A frantic mother calls you to check her son's central venous catheter because it is leaking. On arrival, you note that the catheter is cracked and leaking. The child's condition is stable. What action should you take?
   a. Clamp the line.
   c. Remove the line.
   b. Flush the line.
   d. Tape around the crack.

73. A child with a gastric feeding tube develops respiratory distress. What complication should you assess for?
   a. Allergic reaction
   c. Hypoglycemia
   b. Aspiration
   d. Pulmonary embolism

CHAPTER 43

GERIATRICS

● READING ASSIGNMENT

Chapter 43, pages 1278-1303, in *Mosby's Paramedic Textbook*, ed 2

● OBJECTIVES

As a paramedic, you should be able to:

1. Explain the physiology of the aging process as it relates to major body systems and homeostasis.
2. Describe general principles of assessment specific to older adults.
3. Describe the pathophysiology, assessment, and management of specific illnesses that affect selected body systems in the geriatric patient.
4. Identify specific problems with sensation experienced by some geriatric patients.
5. Discuss effects of drug toxicity and alcoholism in the older adult.
6. Identify factors that contribute to environmental emergencies in the geriatric patient.
7. Discuss prehospital assessment and management of depression and suicide in the older adult.
8. Describe epidemiology, assessment, and management of trauma in the geriatric patient.
9. Identify characteristics of elder abuse.

● REVIEW QUESTIONS

1. An 85-year-old woman fell down an escalator at a department store. Explain how age-related changes in each of the following areas increase her risk of sustaining trauma or influence her body's response to a major injury.

   a. Respiratory system:

   _____

   _____

   b. Cardiovascular system:

   _____

   _____

   c. Renal system:

   _____

   _____

   d. Musculoskeletal system:

   _____

   _____

   e. Thermoregulation:

   _____

   _____

2. A woman calls you to the home of her 70-year-old father, who has fallen. He says he is just fine. On your arrival, she states that he has a history of diabetes, a heart attack, heart failure, and lung disease. His home medications include Lanoxin, insulin, Dyazide, Slow-K, Theo-Dur, and a number of vitamins and laxatives. He is on oxygen at 2 L/min by nasal cannula.

   a. What factors will make it difficult to assess and determine the nature of his acute problem?

   _____

   _____

   _____

   b. List eight possible causes of his fall.

a.	e.
b.	f.
c.	g.
d.	h.

   Questions 3-5 pertain to the following case study:

   > A 70-year-old man calls you to his home complaining of dyspnea and weakness. He has no underlying pulmonary problems. His ECG is shown in Fig. 43-1.

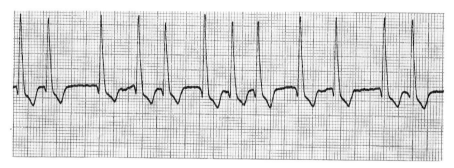

Figure 43-1

3. Why should you assess the appropriate history and physical examination for myocardial infarction and pulmonary embolism on this patient?

   _____

4. What is your interpretation of the ECG rhythm?

   _____

5. List two complications associated with this dysrhythmia.

   a.

   b.

6. A 76-year-old woman complains of diffuse abdominal pain. Identify four conditions that can cause this symptom.
   a.
   b.
   c.
   d.

7. Briefly describe the following characteristics of delirium.
   a. Onset:

   _____

   b. Duration:

   _____

   c. Metabolic causes:

   _____

8. List four reversible causes of dementia.

   a.   c.

   b.   d.

   Questions 9-11 pertain to the following case study:

   An 80-year-old man experiences a syncopal episode in church. He is conscious but pale and diaphoretic. His blood pressure is 80/50 mm Hg, and his ECG is shown in Fig. 43-2.

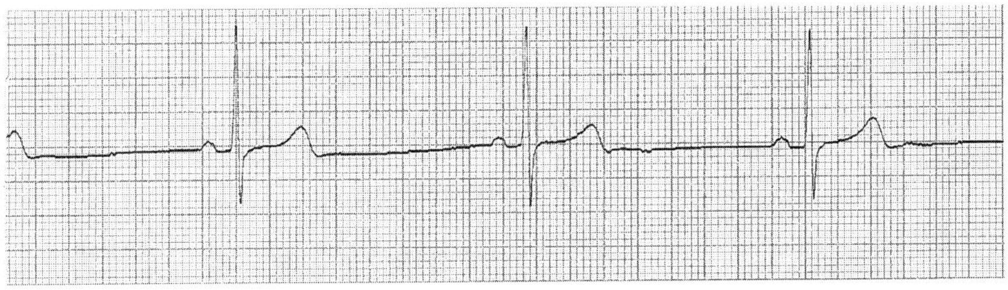

   Figure 43-2

9. What is your interpretation of the rhythm?

   _____

10. a. State the dose and route of administration of the drug to treat this rhythm.

   _____

   b. What other intervention should be considered if drug therapy is unsuccessful?

   _____

11. List two possible causes of the signs and symptoms this patient is experiencing.
   a.
   b.

Questions 12-15 pertain to the following case study:

On arrival at a call for "difficulty breathing," you find a 69-year-old woman complaining of dyspnea and chills. She states that she has been ill with a mild cough and weakness for approximately 1 week. Her skin is cold and clammy, and vital signs are blood pressure, 108/70 mm Hg; pulse, 135; and respirations, 30. Breath sounds in the right base are diminished with scattered crackles and her ECG is shown in Fig. 43-3.

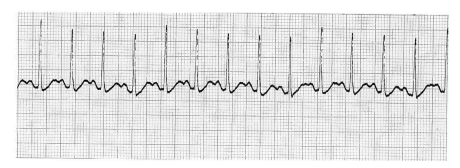

Figure 43-3

12. Identify the rhythm.

_____

13. What illness do you suspect?

_____

14. Should you use synchronized cardioversion or adenosine to treat the rhythm?

_____

15. What other interventions would be indicated for this patient?

_____

_____

16. An older man with a history of chronic lung disease is being transferred to another hospital. He has applied a Venturi mask that supplies oxygen at 24%. His vital signs are within normal limits, and his ECG tracing is shown in Fig. 43-4.

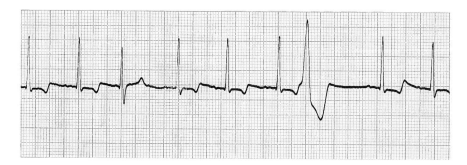

Figure 43-4

320

a. Identify the rhythm strip.

b. What interventions are indicated in the presence of this rhythm?

c. What signs and symptoms of acute decompensation of COPD will you observe for?

17. An older patient who had a syncopal episode is now awake and has the following vital signs: blood pressure, 108/70 mm Hg; pulse, 50; and respirations, 18 and unlabored. The lungs are clear, and the ECG is shown in Fig. 43-5.

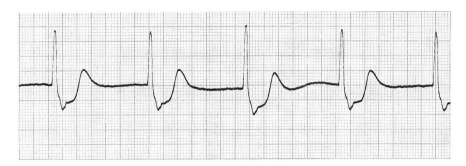

Figure 43-5

a. Identify the rhythm strip.

b. After oxygen is applied and intravenous therapy is initiated, what interventions should be performed en route to the medical center?

c. What age-related changes predispose this patient to developing this rhythm?

Questions 18-21 refer to the following case study:

A 72-year-old man's family states that he suddenly became confused and disoriented to time and place over the past few hours. His vital signs are as follows: blood pressure, 168/110 mm Hg; pulse, 100; and respirations, 20. His ECG is shown in Fig. 43-6.

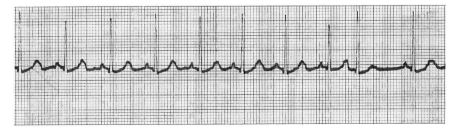

Figure 43-6

18. Is he likely experiencing dementia or delirium?

_____

19. Identify the rhythm strip.

_____

20. Are his symptoms related to his ECG tracing?

_____

21. List two factors that could cause this change in behavior.
   a.
   b.

   Questions 22 and 23 refer to the following case study:

   An 80-year-old woman complains of dizziness and shortness of breath. Vital signs are as follows: blood pressure, 82/50 mm Hg; pulse, 50; and respirations, 24. Her ECG tracing is shown in Fig. 43-7.

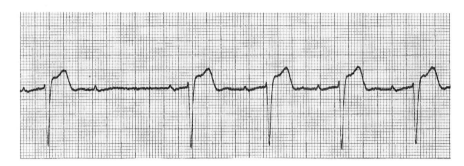

Figure 43-7

22. Identify the rhythm strip.

_____

23. a. What illness may be causing her signs and symptoms?

_____

   b. List prehospital interventions that you will consider for this patient.

_____

24. A 94-year-old woman who was found in her apartment is confused and difficult to arouse. You note that it feels very cold inside, and her temperature is 95° F.
   List at least nine reasons (physiological, social, or medical) that she is at risk for hypothermia.

_____

_____

25. Adverse drug reactions are common in the older adult. For each of the following drugs or drug groups, list two signs or symptoms associated with overdose or adverse effects:
   a. Anticoagulants:

_____

   b. Diuretics:

_____

c. Digitalis:

_____

d. Tricyclic antidepressants:

_____

e. Sedative-hypnotic drugs:

_____

f. Propranolol:

_____

g. Theophylline:

_____

h. Quinidine:

_____

Questions 26-29 refer to the following case study:

You are on the scene of a single-car collision in which a compact car struck a bridge abutment at high speed. The driver is an anxious 75-year-old man complaining of mild abdominal discomfort. His blood pressure is 90/70 mm Hg, his pulse is 70, and his respirations are 24 and somewhat labored. His skin is pale and clammy, and his nailbeds are dusky.

26. What vital sign assessment does *not* fit with this man's clinical picture?

_____

27. What aspect of his history may explain this discrepancy?

_____

28. Because he has just mild abdominal pain, should you be concerned?

_____

29. What prehospital treatment should be given after the cervical spine is appropriately immobilized?

_____

_____

30. You are at the home of an older patient who appears dehydrated and very dirty. You note large ecchymotic areas on the back and hips that the daughter, who lives with the patient, says were caused by a fall.
   a. If you suspect elder abuse, what should you do?

_____

b. Does the caregiver have any characteristics of an elder abuser?

_____

31. Alterations in lung and chest wall compliance in the older adult result in a decrease in which of the following?
    - **a.** Alveolar diameter
    - **c.** Total lung capacity
    - **b.** Residual volume
    - **d.** Vital capacity

32. Humpback posture that develops as a result of osteoporosis is known by which of the following terms?
    - **a.** Kyphosis
    - **c.** Osteoarthritis
    - **b.** Lordosis
    - **d.** Scoliosis

33. An elderly patient presents with a sudden onset of dyspnea. The patient has crackles and wheezes. He had an MI 3 years ago and has no other history. Blood pressure is 170/94 mm Hg; P, 124; R, 28; and Sao_2, 90% on room air. You apply oxygen. What drug is indicated next?
    - **a.** Albuterol
    - **c.** Epinephrine
    - **b.** Aspirin
    - **d.** Furosemide

34. An elderly patient, whose only past medical history is metastatic breast cancer, has been on bedrest. She suddenly develops dyspnea and tachycardia. Which of the following would be the *least* likely cause of her symptoms?
    - **a.** Chronic obstructive pulmonary disease
    - **b.** Myocardial infarction
    - **c.** Pneumonia
    - **d.** Pulmonary embolus

35. Which of the following are possible causes of dementia?
    - **a.** Alzheimer's disease
    - **c.** Hyperglycemia
    - **b.** Epilepsy
    - **d.** Pneumonia

36. Which illness causes trembling, a rigid posture, slow movement, and a shuffling, unbalanced walk?
    - **a.** Alzheimer's disease
    - **c.** Dementia
    - **b.** Delirium
    - **d.** Parkinson's disease

37. Administration of which of the following would be a critical prehospital intervention for the unconscious diabetic patient suffering from hyperglycemic hyperosmolar nonketotic coma?
    - **a.** Dextrose
    - **c.** IV fluids
    - **b.** Glucagon
    - **d.** Sodium bicarbonate

38. Which of the following is a consequence of thyroid dysfunction that might lead to a call for EMS?
    - **a.** Altered mental status
    - **c.** Diarrhea
    - **b.** Bradycardia
    - **d.** Weight gain

39. Your elderly male patient complains that he is unable to urinate. What condition should you inquire about specifically when obtaining his history?
    - **a.** Constipation
    - **c.** Kidney stones
    - **b.** Epididymitis
    - **d.** Prostate enlargement

40. Pressure ulcers are caused by which of the following?
    - **a.** Burns
    - **c.** Infection
    - **b.** Hypoxia
    - **d.** Tears of the tissue

41. Which eye condition causes damage to the optic nerve and can result in blindness if untreated?
    - **a.** Cataracts
    - **c.** Corneal abrasion
    - **b.** Conjunctivitis
    - **d.** Glaucoma

42. A patient is being treated for Parkinson's disease. What sign, if present, might you attribute to drug toxicity?
    - **a.** Altered vision
    - **c.** Paresthesias
    - **b.** Hypokalemia
    - **d.** Tardive dyskinesia

43. Which of the following medications may increase the elderly patient's risk of hyperthermia?
    a. Amitriptylline (Elavil)
    c. Cimetidine (Tagamet)
    b. Aspirin
    d. Coumadin
44. Which of the following may be a physiological cause of depression in an elderly patient?
    a. Hyperglycemia
    c. Hyponatremia
    b. Hypertension
    d. Hypothermia
45. Which is the most common psychiatric disorder in older adults?
    a. Bipolar disorder
    c. Hysteria
    b. Depression
    d. Schizophrenia
46. Why might the symptoms of increased intracranial pressure be delayed in an older patient?
    a. Altered blood brain barrier
    c. Decreased cerebral blood flow
    b. Cerebral atrophy
    d. Fragile bridging veins
47. Which is the most frequent fracture sustained from falls in the older adult?
    a. Ankle
    c. Hip
    b. Clavicle
    d. Wrist
48. Which of the following home medications increases the older person's risk of falling?
    a. Alprazolam
    c. Hydrochlorothiazide
    b. Digoxin
    d. Dipyridamole

ABUSE AND NEGLECT

● READING ASSIGNMENT
Chapter 44, pages 1304-1317, in *Mosby's Paramedic Textbook,* ed 2

● OBJECTIVES
As a paramedic, you should be able to:
1. Define battering.
2. Describe the characteristics of abusive relationships.
3. Outline findings that indicate a battered patient.
4. Describe prehospital considerations when responding to and caring for battered patients.
5. Identify types of elder abuse.
6. Discuss legal considerations related to elder abuse.
7. Describe characteristics of abused children and their abusers.
8. Outline the physical examination of the abused child.
9. Describe the characteristics of sexual assault.
10. Outline prehospital patient care considerations for the patient who has been sexually assaulted.

● REVIEW QUESTIONS
Questions 1-5 pertain to the following case study:

> You are called to a private residence by a woman who says her husband "beat her up." On arrival, you hear loud shouting coming from the house.

1. What measures should be taken before entering the home?

_____

2. When you begin your examination, what measures should you take to enhance safety and allow for a better history and examination?

_____

> The patient's vital signs are stable, and she has several bruises around her face. She is alert and oriented and does not wish to have further care. You contact medical direction, and despite both your and their recommendation, the patient refuses transport.

3. What reasons might someone have for staying with an abusive partner?

_____

4. If you tell her to move out immediately, would that be the safest course of action without planning on her part? Why?

_____

5. What advice and resources can you offer her before you leave the scene?

_____

Questions 6-8 refer to the following case study:

> You are dispatched to a residence in a middle-class neighborhood for an "accidental injury." On arrival, you find an 80-year-old widow with a tender, swollen, ecchymotic left upper arm. She is awake and alert but very withdrawn. You note multiple other bruises on both arms and her back that are yellow, brown, and green. Her 60-year-old daughter lives with her and says that her mother tripped and fell. When you ask the patient to confirm this, she nods slowly; when you ask about the old bruises, she just shrugs. She has a history of heart disease, emphysema, and adult onset diabetes. Vital signs are normal.

6. What characteristics typical of an "average" victim of elder abuse does this woman have?

_____

7. What physical findings suggest possible abuse?

_____

8. What action should you take if you suspect abuse on this call?

_____

Questions 9-12 refer to the following case study:

> You are dispatched to an address in your district that is well-known to you and your partner. Both the woman that lives at this address and her boyfriend are heavy drinkers, and you have responded to multiple calls at their home. When you arrive, you find a 2-year-old girl with bilateral circumferential second-degree burns to her feet, lower legs, and buttocks. The mother says that when she was filling the tub to bathe the child after she dirtied her pants, the child stepped into the tub and got burned. You take the child to the ambulance to provide care and notice that she does not cry for her mother to be with her. She shudders when you touch her to begin your assessment and jumps every time someone approaches or opens a door.

9. What characteristics of an abusive family situation are present in this situation?

_____

10. What specific characteristics of the injuries increase your suspicion of possible abuse?

_____

11. How does the child's behavior suggest the possibility of an abusive family situation?

_____

12. What are your legal responsibilities related to this situation?

_____

13. List five measures to help preserve evidence on a sexual assault call.
    a.
    b.
    c.
    d.
    e.

14. List at least four injuries that may accompany sexual assault.

a.

b.

c.

d.

● STUDENT SELF-ASSESSMENT

15. The establishment of control and fear in a relationship through violence and other forms of abuse is known by which of the following terms?

a. Assault
c. Intimidation
b. Battering
d. Terrorism

16. What typically occurs in the third phase of the domestic violence cycle?

a. An argument occurs, and the situation escalates.

b. Threats of violence and harm are made to the victim.

c. Physical or sexual abuse occurs.

d. The abuser apologizes for what has happened.

17. What does the victim of domestic violence often fear most?

a. That her children will be harmed or taken away

b. That she will be humiliated in front of their friends

c. That she will not be able to achieve financial independence

d. That the abuser will hurt himself if the victim leaves

18. Which of the following characteristics may an abuser or victim of domestic violence have?

a. Alcohol or drug dependence
c. Fear of love and affection
b. Dislike of discipline
d. Rigid personal boundaries

19. Which of the following injury patterns is more suggestive of domestic abuse?

a. Contusions of the breast
c. Laceration of the finger
b. Fracture of the ankle
d. Scald burn of the hand

20. What is an effective way to treat a patient who you suspect has been injured in a domestic violence situation?

a. Ask the police to speak to her partner so that you can examine her privately.

b. Don't pry if she doesn't volunteer any information about abuse.

c. If she won't talk, ask her, "you've been abused, haven't you?"

d. Force her to go to the hospital even if she doesn't want to.

21. Which is an example of psychological abuse of an elder?

a. Sexual molestation
c. Verbal threats
b. Theft of property
d. Withholding food

22. What action should the paramedic take if elder abuse is suspected?

a. Confront the suspected abuser about the abusive behavior and threaten to report it.

b. Report your suspicions to medical direction and the appropriate state agency.

c. Discuss the patient's rights and ways to follow-up with authorities.

d. Wait to see whether it happens again before you take action so that you can be sure.

23. Which of the following descriptions is most characteristic of a child abuser?

a. 20-year-old mother
c. 50-year-old father
b. 45-year-old female neighbor
d. 70-year-old uncle

24. What is helpful in most cases in assessing whether a child's injury is accidental or inflicted by an adult?
    a. Assessing the family for the characteristics of abusers
    b. Checking with the police to see whether a record of abuse exists
    c. Matching the description of the event to the injury
    d. Performing a careful, detailed physical examination
25. Which of the following statements about sexual assault is true?
    a. All victims of sexual assault are women.
    b. Rape is motivated by sexual desire.
    c. Threats of harm or use of weapons during the attack is rare.
    d. Victims often know their attackers.
26. What statement by the paramedic may be most helpful to a child who has been sexually assaulted?
    a. Don't worry about anything; you are OK.
    b. They'll probably get the person that did this.
    c. You didn't do anything wrong; this wasn't your fault.
    d. You're really lucky; it could have been a lot worse.

CHAPTER 45
PATIENTS WITH SPECIAL CHALLENGES

● READING ASSIGNMENT

Chapter 45, pages 1318-1335, in *Mosby's Paramedic Textbook,* ed 2

● OBJECTIVES

As a paramedic, you should be able to:

1. Identify considerations in prehospital management related to physical challenges, such as hearing, visual, and speech impairments; obesity; and paraplegia or quadriplegia.
2. Identify considerations in prehospital management of patients who have mental illness or are developmentally disabled or emotionally or mentally impaired.
3. Describe special considerations for prehospital management of patients with selected pathological challenges.
4. Outline considerations in the management of culturally diverse patients.
5. Describe special considerations in the prehospital management of terminally ill patients.
6. Identify special considerations in the management of patients with communicable diseases.
7. Describe special considerations in the prehospital management of patients with financial challenges.

● REVIEW QUESTIONS

Match the pathological condition in Column II with the appropriate description in Column I. Use each condition just once.

	Column I		Column II
1. _____	Nonprogressive disorders of movement and posture	**a.**	Arthritis
2. _____	Inherited disorder that causes slow muscle deterioration	**b.**	Cerebral palsy
3. _____	Congenital defect exposing part of spinal cord	**c.**	Cystic fibrosis
4. _____	Autoimmune disorder weakening muscles of head and extremities	**d.**	Multiple sclerosis
5. _____	Inflammation of the joints	**e.**	Muscular dystrophy
6. _____	Inherited disease of lungs and digestive tract	**f.**	Myasthenia gravis
7. _____	Autoimmune disease affecting the CNS	**g.**	Poliomyelitis
		h.	Spina bifida

For the patient situations in Questions 8-20, identify which of the following special prehospital considerations may be necessary to accommodate their special needs.

a. Provide communication aids
b. Allow additional time for history and management
c. Obtain detailed information about the preexisting condition
d. Determine baseline level of functioning
e. Obtain additional resources and manpower to prepare for transport

8. _____ The patient had a stroke 6 months ago, has weakness on the right side, and speaks slowly and with a stutter. He called you today complaining of inability to urinate.

9. _____ Your patient complains of crushing chest pain. He weighs approximately 375 lb.

10. _____ You are providing an interfacility transfer for a quadriplegic patient who is in halo traction.

11. _____ A man with a history of schizophrenia is having difficulty breathing related to his asthma.

12. _____ A 12-year-old girl with Down syndrome is having extreme weakness after chemotherapy for her leukemia.

13. _____ A moderately retarded man lacerated his finger at his job in the cafeteria.

14. _____ A severely arthritic patient was involved in a motor vehicle crash.

15. _____ A 14-year-old patient with quadriplegic spastic paralysis and mental retardation caused by cerebral palsy is febrile and congested.

16. _____ A child with cystic fibrosis has vomiting and diarrhea.

17. _____ A 43-year-old woman with multiple sclerosis complains of severe vertigo.

18. _____ An 8-year-old boy with Duchenne muscular dystrophy says he can't breathe.

19. _____ A 45-year-old patient who suffered a head injury 5 years ago is confused and pale.

20. _____ A 65-year-old man tells you he is being treated for tuberculosis.

● STUDENT SELF-ASSESSMENT

21. Which of the following accommodations might be helpful to many patients with hearing impairment?
    a. No accommodation is necessary.
    b. Speak very loudly into the patient's ear.
    c. Speak very slowly, with very exaggerated lip movements.
    d. Write key questions or instructions on a piece of paper.

22. Which of the following fits the definition of obesity?
    a. A person who is impaired as a result of excessive weight
    b. A person who weighs 20% or more than the maximum desirable weight relative to height
    c. A person who weighs 50 pounds more than the average weight for someone of that age
    d. A person who weighs more than 250 pounds

23. During the initial examination of a patient with a mental illness, what is your priority?
    a. To determine whether the patient is aware of the mental illness
    b. To determine whether the patient is dangerous
    c. To determine the patient's specific form of mental illness
    d. To determine the type of medications that the patient is taking

24. What challenge exists when caring for a patient who is emotionally impaired?
    a. Determining whether symptoms are produced by stress or medical illness
    b. Determining whether the patient is lying or telling the truth
    c. Obtaining an accurate medical history from caregivers
    d. Obtaining the patient's trust so that you can perform the examination

25. A patient with severe arthritis of the spine falls down some steps. What is likely to be the largest challenge in caring for this patient?
    a. Communicating so that you can understand the patient
    b. Determining whether the patient has any serious injuries
    c. Obtaining a reliable patient history and medication list
    d. Securing the patient to a spine board to minimize pain

26. Which of the following terms describes the involuntary writhing movements found in some patients with cerebral palsy?
    a. Ataxia
    c. Diplegia
    b. Athetosis
    d. Mucoviscidosis
27. During transport of the patient with severe cystic fibrosis, you should anticipate the need for which of the following?
    a. Antidysrhythmic treatment
    c. Nitrous oxide inhalation
    b. Blood glucose monitoring
    d. Suctioning
28. Which is true regarding cultural diversity in prehospital patient care?
    a. All generations within a culture share the same beliefs.
    b. Personal prejudices and belief systems should not interfere with patient care.
    c. People must accept your explanation of the cause of their illness.
    d. You should agree with every aspect of a patient's cultural beliefs.
29. What is a primary consideration during transport of a terminally ill patient?
    a. The family should be encouraged to deal with the imminent death.
    b. Talking to the family may interfere with their grieving process.
    c. Pain management is usually the priority of care.
    d. Rapid transport is essential for definitive care.
30. How can you show respect for the dignity of a patient with AIDS during transport?
    a. Don't discuss their disease process.
    b. To keep the patient from feeling ashamed, don't use BSI.
    c. Encourage the patient to express feelings related to the disease.
    d. Respecting the patient's dignity should not be a primary concern during prehospital care.
31. What statement may be helpful when transporting a patient who has serious financial concerns?
    a. "Don't worry; the ambulance bill won't come for a couple of months."
    b. "I don't see why you are worried; you are sick now—worry about the money later."
    c. "I'll ask the nurse to contact social services to see whether there is a program to help you."
    d. "We have people who never pay a dime for our service, and they abuse us all the time."

ACUTE INTERVENTIONS FOR THE HOME HEALTH CARE PATIENT

● **READING ASSIGNMENT**

Chapter 46, pages 1336-1359, in *Mosby's Paramedic Textbook*, ed 2

● **OBJECTIVES**

As a paramedic, you should be able to:

1. Discuss general issues related to home care patients.
2. Outline general principles of assessment and management of the home health patient.
3. Describe medical equipment, assessment, and management of the home health patient with inadequate respiratory support.
4. Identify assessment findings and acute interventions for problems related to vascular access devices in the home health setting.
5. Describe medical equipment and assessment and management of the patient with a GI or GU crisis in the home health setting.
6. Identify key assessments and principles of wound care management in the home care patient.
7. Outline maternal/child problems that may be encountered early in the post-partum period in the home care setting.
8. Describe medical therapy associated with hospice and comfort care in the home health setting.

● **REVIEW QUESTIONS**

Questions 1-4 refer to the following case study:

> You are called to care for a patient who has difficulty breathing. When you arrive at his home, you find a man who has a tracheostomy and is on a ventilator. The low pressure alarm is sounding.

1. What signs and symptoms might the patient exhibit if hypoxic?

_____

_____

2. What should your first action be?

_____

_____

3. What will you check on the ventilator to assess the problem?

_____

_____

_____

4. How can you calm the patient before placing him back on the ventilator?

_____

_____

_____

Questions 5-7 refer to the following case study:

An elderly patient has a home IV infusion. You are called to treat her for difficulty breathing. She has a history of multiple myeloma. Her husband thinks the pump hasn't been working correctly and too much has run in.

5. What specifically would you assess to check for fluid overload?

_____

_____

She has crackles bilaterally in the bases of her lungs. Her neck veins are slightly distended, and her vital signs are as follows: BP, 160/84; P, 100; and R, 24. Her SaO_2 is 93% on room air.

6. What interventions should you perform in cooperation with medical direction?

_____

_____

_____

7. Should you transport her for a physician evaluation?

_____

Questions 8 through 13 pertain to the following case study:

You are called to a home for an "assist invalid" call. An elderly woman greets you, and after you help her husband to bed (he couldn't get off the commode), she asks you to check his arm. She says that he burned it 4 days ago. When you remove the dressing, you note a green wound bed, surrounded by black tissue. The drainage is green and foul smelling.

8. What does the appearance of this wound suggest?

_____

9. How would it look if it were healing normally?

_____

10. What should you look for in the surrounding skin?

_____

The skin around the wound is reddened and warm to the touch.

11. What does this assessment suggest?

_____

_____

12. What systemic assessment should you perform on this patient?

_____

His vital signs are as follows: BP, 150/80 mm Hg; P, 110/min; and R, 16. His skin feels hot to the touch. The rest of the exam is normal.

13. What action should you take?

_____

_____

Questions 14-17 refer to the following case study:

You respond to a call for "baby not breathing." On arrival, you find a woman sobbing while holding her 4-day-old infant in her arms. The baby is awake, lying quietly in her mother's arms. The parents state that they had just put her down for a nap, when they noticed she wasn't breathing and her color looked bad. They state the episode lasted about 15 to 20 seconds.

14. What assessments should you perform?

_____

_____

_____

The baby's examination looks normal. While you are on the phone with medical direction, your partner shouts at you. She states that the baby stopped breathing for approximately 15 seconds and was very pale, and the heart rate dropped to 80/min on the monitor. Now she is breathing normally.

15. What are some possible causes of infantile apnea?

_____

_____

16. What interventions should you perform?

_____

_____

17. What equipment should you have prepared and made easily accessible during transport?

_____

_____

● **STUDENT SELF-ASSESSMENT**

18. What was the historical focus of home health care?
   a. To benefit the rich
   b. To care for rural patients
   c. To provide wider physician care
   d. To provide preventative care

19. Home health care services in America include which of the following?
   a. Diagnostic radiology
   b. Minor surgical procedures
   c. IV antibiotic therapy
   d. Physician visits for acute illness

20. Haddon's matrix states that any injury or disease can be broken into three component factors. Which is correct?
    a. Agent, host, environment
    b. Agent, host, mechanical force
    c. Patient, host, environment
    d. Agent, disease, environment
21. What type of infection control standards should be practiced in the home health setting?
    a. No precautions are needed.
    b. Use precautions only for HIV patients.
    c. Wear reusable rubber gloves.
    d. Observe universal precautions.
22. Assessment of the milieu in home care includes evaluation to ensure which of the following?
    a. Infectious waste is disposed of properly.
    b. Dogs and other pets are contained.
    c. No hazards are present in the home.
    d. The home has heat, water, and electricity.
23. When arriving at a call in which home care is being provided, your priority, after ensuring that the scene is safe, is to assess for the presence of which of the following?
    a. Abusive caregivers
    b. Equipment failure
    c. Life-threatening illness or injury
    d. Medical device malfunction
24. Which of the following systems will not work during a power failure?
    a. Demand valve
    b. Liquid oxygen
    c. Oxygen concentrators
    d. Oxygen cylinders
25. You are called because the high pressure alarm keeps sounding on a home care ventilator. What might this indicate?
    a. Cuff leak
    b. Disconnected tubing
    c. Insufficient oxygen
    d. Water in tubing
26. Which of the following is a peripheral vascular access device?
    a. Groshon
    b. Hickman
    c. Intracath
    d. Mediport
27. Which of the following complications of vascular access devices does not pose an immediate life threat?
    a. Circulatory overload
    b. Embolus
    c. Hemorrhage
    d. Site infection
28. Which of the following is a sign of air embolus that may occur if air enters a vascular access device?
    a. Distended neck veins
    b. Fever
    c. Hypotension
    d. Pulmonary congestion
29. How much heparin should be used when flushing a peripheral vascular device?
    a. 2.5 to 3.0 ml (10 U/ml)
    b. 2.5 to 3.0 ml (100 U/ml)
    c. 3.0 to 5.0 ml (10 U/ml)
    d. 3.0 to 5.0 ml (100 U/ml)
30. What complication can result from an untreated urinary tract infection in a patient with a urinary catheter?
    a. Kidney stones
    b. Prostatic hypertrophy
    c. Sepsis
    d. Urinary retention
31. Which complication of tube feedings can cause serious skin breakdown and fluid and electrolyte imbalances?
    a. Bowel obstruction
    b. Choking
    c. Diarrhea
    d. Irritable bowel syndrome
32. What is a critical step in the insertion of a urinary catheter?
    a. Do not retract the foreskin (if present).
    b. Inflate the balloon with 10 to 15 ml of sterile saline after insertion.
    c. Use aseptic technique until the catheter is inserted and the balloon inflated.
    d. Use significant force to overcome resistance during catheter insertion.

33. Which of the following enhances wound repair?
    a. Environmental contamination
    c. Moisture
    b. Eschar
    d. Necrotic tissue

34. Your patient delivered a baby 3 days ago. She is complaining of severe abdominal pain, weakness, and shaking chills. What postpartum complication should be anticipated?
    a. Appendicitis
    c. Hemorrhage
    b. Endometritis
    d. Pulmonary embolism

35. You are called to the home of a woman who appears to have signs and symptoms of postpartum depression. Your priority should be to assess for which of the following?
    a. Depressive psychosis
    c. Severe sleep disturbances
    b. Forgetfulness or memory loss
    d. The well-being of the baby

36. A mother calls you to evaluate her 11-day-old infant. She says she has been nursing him, but he doesn't "seem right." He is difficult to awaken and pale, and he has dry mucous membranes and a sunken fontanelle. She thinks he hasn't wet a diaper in about 18 hours. What do you suspect?
    a. Apnea
    c. Jaundice
    b. Dehydration
    d. Sepsis

37. Which of the following terms describes abnormal retardation of the growth and development of an infant resulting from maternal deprivation or malnutrition?
    a. Cerebral palsy
    c. Failure to thrive
    b. Cystic fibrosis
    d. Muscular dystrophy

38. What is the primary goal of palliative care?
    a. To ensure that optimal nutritional requirements are met
    b. To help families accept the reality of impending death
    c. To improve the quality of a person's life as death approaches
    d. To provide complete relief of any pain or discomfort

DIVISION SEVEN
ASSESSMENT-BASED MANAGEMENT

ASSESSMENT-BASED MANAGEMENT

● READING ASSIGNMENT
Chapter 47, pages 1362-1371, in *Mosby's Paramedic Textbook,* ed 2

● OBJECTIVES
As a paramedic, you should be able to:
1. Discuss the ways assessment-based management contributes to effective patient and scene assessment.
2. Describe factors that affect assessment and decision making in the prehospital setting.
3. Outline effective techniques for scene and patient assessment and choreography.
4. Identify essential take-in equipment for general and selected patient situations.
5. Outline strategies for patient approach that promote an effective patient encounter.
6. Describe techniques to permit efficient, accurate presentation of the patient.

● REVIEW QUESTIONS
For Questions 1-5, what is your "field impression" based on the "patterns" described in each of the following scenarios (knowing that further assessment is necessary to confirm each). Describe the key differences in each pair that distinguish the pattern.

1. **a.** A 24-year-old patient with a history of diabetes is found confused and diaphoretic with right-sided weakness.

_____

  b. An 80-year-old patient with a history of hypertension is found confused and diaphoretic with right-sided weakness.

_____

  c. Key differences in patterns:

_____

2. **a.** A 20-year-old woman whose last menstrual period was 8 weeks ago has severe right lower quadrant abdominal pain and signs of shock.

_____

  b. A 12-year-old boy has severe right lower quadrant abdominal pain, fever, and vomiting.

_____

    c. Key differences in patterns:

---

3. a. A 38-year-old man has severe left lower back pain that radiates down into his testicle and hematuria.

---

    b. A 70-year-old man had a sudden onset of lower back pain described as "ripping." He is pale, wants to have a bowel movement, and has a cool left foot.

---

    c. Key differences in patterns:

---

4. a. A healthy 4-month-old infant is found pulseless, with rigor mortis, and in bed with no obvious signs of trauma.

---

    b. A healthy 16-year-old patient is found pulseless, with rigor mortis, and in bed with no obvious signs of trauma.

---

    c. Key differences in patterns:

---

5. a. A 70-year-old man complains of crushing substernal chest pain. He is diaphoretic and having multifocal PVCs. His history includes hypertension, smoking, and diabetes.

---

    b. A 25-year old woman complains of crushing substernal chest pain. She is diaphoretic and having multifocal PVCs. Her chest struck the steering wheel in a motor vehicle crash 10 minutes ago.

---

    c. Key differences in patterns:

Questions 6 and 7 refer to the following case study:

> You are dispatched to an address where the resident is an alcoholic who calls often for minor problems. She curses at you for taking so long to respond, then says she fell out of bed yesterday, hit her head, and now has a headache. You note a large bruise on the temporal area of her head but no other injuries. Her speech is slurred, and she has a staggering gait. Her vitals are BP, 160/100; P, 64; and R, 16. You advise her that she'll be OK, and she declines transport. The next day she is found unconscious and is diagnosed with a large subdural hematoma that resulted in her death.

6. List factors that may have contributed to your decision in this case.

---

7. Why is this patient at increased risk for intracerebral bleeding?

Questions 8-12 refer to the following case study:

> You are dispatched to a call for a stabbing. Your patient is a 17-year-old man who was stabbed at a street party. It's dark, and the police are trying to control a large, loud, belligerent crowd that has gathered at the scene. Your patient says he can't breathe, and when you pull his shirt off, you note a stab wound above the right nipple. Breath sounds are equal. An occlusive dressing is applied, and you elect to move the patient to the ambulance for further assessment and care.

8. During the initial contact with this patient, what are the responsibilities for each of the following team members?
   a. Team leader

   b. Patient care person (as described in this textbook)

9. Should you carry your drug box with you on a call like this? Why?

10. Explain why either the contemplative or the resuscitative approach would be appropriate for this call.

> When you get in the ambulance, you talk to the patient, assess his airway and breathing, and apply oxygen. Your partner begins transport. As you begin to initiate an IV, you note blood dripping off the side of the ambulance cot. You cut the patient's clothing off and find a wound in the groin spurting blood.

11. List two factors that you think delayed detection of the patient's bleeding.
    a.
    b.
12. What pertinent positives should be included in your patient care report?

● STUDENT SELF-ASSESSMENT

13. Which of the following terms describes the process of gathering, evaluating, and synthesizing information; making appropriate decisions based on available information; and taking the appropriate actions required for patient care?
    a. Assessment-based management
    b. Initial assessment
    c. Ongoing assessment
    d. Patient-focused care

14. Field impression of any given situation is based on which of the following factors?
    a. Information gathered before any physical examination
    b. Advice of medical direction and perception of the call
    c. The paramedic's "gut instinct" and pattern recognition
    d. The patient's chief complaint and assessment of the problem
15. What should you rule out if you encounter an uncooperative patient?
    a. Chest pain or dyspnea
    b. Hypoxia or hypoglycemia
    c. Neuromuscular disorder
    d. Personality disorder
16. Why is it important to predesignate roles for EMS calls?
    a. To identify who is at fault if a problem occurs on a call
    b. To allow all paramedics to perform the skills at which they excel
    c. To ensure appropriate skills acquisition
    d. To promote coherent, efficient patient care delivery
17. What is the advantage of taking notes while obtaining the patient history?
    a. To obtain adequate billing information
    b. To provide evidence that may be used in court
    c. To prevent the need for repetitive questioning of the patient
    d. To reassure the patient that you are listening
18. In which of the following patient situations would the contemplative approach to patient care be appropriate?
    a. A large bleeding laceration
    b. Cramping abdominal pain
    c. Decreased level of consciousness
    d. Dyspnea and diaphoresis
19. You respond to a call in which you find a 24-year-old woman who is hyperventilating. What is the *last* condition you should assess for while performing your history and physical exam?
    a. Anxiety attack
    b. Asthma
    c. Diabetic ketoacidosis
    d. Pulmonary embolus
20. You are caring for a patient who is seriously injured after a fall. What is a serious consequence of inadequately presenting your patient during your report to the hospital?
    a. Appropriate resources may not be ready.
    b. The nursing staff will be angry with you.
    c. The patient may misunderstand you.
    d. You may have an increased time out of service.
21. Which of the following is a characteristic of an effective patient presentation?
    a. Every assessment finding is described.
    b. It should last no longer than 5 minutes.
    c. It should include the name of the patient and the doctor.
    d. It should follow a standard format and be consise.

DIVISION EIGHT
OPERATIONS

CHAPTER 48
AMBULANCE OPERATIONS

● **READING ASSIGNMENT**

Chapter 48, pages 1374-1385, in *Mosby's Paramedic Textbook,* ed 2

● **OBJECTIVES**

As a paramedic, you should be able to:
1. List standards that govern ambulance performance and specifications.
2. Discuss the tracking of equipment, supplies, and maintenance on an ambulance.
3. Outline the considerations for appropriate stationing of ambulances.
4. Describe measures that can influence safe operation of an ambulance.
5. Identify air medical crew members and training.
6. Describe appropriate use of air medical services from the prehospital setting.

● **REVIEW QUESTIONS**

1. Cite two standards that define ambulance design or performance.
   a.
   b.
2. List three types of prehospital care supplies that should be routinely checked on an ambulance.
   a.
   b.
   c.
3. What would be a consequence of the following supply/equipment problems?
   a. The batteries aren't charged on the portable suction unit, and your patient is trapped in a car with a mouth full of blood and vomit.

   _____

   b. The defibrillator doesn't work, and the patient is in ventricular fibrillation.

   _____

   c. You run out of strips to check blood glucose levels on a call with an elderly man who has an altered level of consciousness and no available history.

   _____

   d. Someone forgot to replace the OB (delivery kit) after the last delivery.

   _____

e. You run out of oxygen while on a call for pulmonary edema.

4. EMS and community planners must consider a number of factors when determining ambulance placement to provide acceptable availability and response times. List four of these factors.

   a.

   b.

   c.

   d.

5. Explain how you can decrease the risk of vehicle accidents in each of the following situations:

   a. You are being followed by a police escort.

   b. It's 0500, and there is a light rain and heavy fog.

   c. The lights and sirens are on, and you are preparing to proceed through a red light at an intersection.

Questions 6-10 refer to the following case study:

> You respond to a rollover MVC with a patient ejected at 0800. On arrival, you find a 4-year-old who was thrown 20 feet from the vehicle. She is unconscious; has rapid, shallow respirations; and exhibits signs of shock. The nearest hospital is 40 minutes away, and a pediatric trauma center is 45 minutes away by ground, 20 minutes by air. Air medical ETA to your location would be 10 minutes.

6. List two reasons that this is an appropriate situation for use of air medical transport.

   a.
   b.

7. What information should you give the dispatcher when you call to activate the air medical transport?

8. Describe landing zone selection and preparation for this air medical response.

343

The crash occurred across from a baseball diamond that is easily accessible, and the LZ is set up there.

9. What patient management procedures should be performed before arrival of the helicopter?

_____

_____

10. List three safety measures that should be taken as you approach the helicopter to load the patient when it lands.

_____

_____

● STUDENT SELF-ASSESSMENT

11. Which of the following is true of the KKK A-1822 standards?
    a. They contradict the AMD 001-009 performance standards.
    b. They designate design standards for Types I, II, and III ambulances.
    c. They define performance specifications for air ambulances.
    d. They outline ambulance driving standards and qualifications.
12. Why are routine ambulance equipment checks essential?
    a. So that accurate patient billing and reimbursement can occur in a timely manner
    b. So that disciplinary action will not be necessary if an equipment failure occurs
    c. So that essential equipment is available and in working order during patient care
    d. So that state laws and regulations can be met and licensure can be maintained
13. Emergency vehicle placement in a community should be determined by which of the following?
    a. Average response times that meet national standards
    b. The number of receiving hospitals in the region
    c. The projected revenue flow from reimbursement
    d. Where the citizens would like to have ambulances
14. Which of the following help promote safety when driving an ambulance?
    a. Drive no faster than 20 miles per hour over the speed limit on routine calls.
    b. Ensure that only the driver and the patient are always restrained.
    c. Use extreme caution at intersections, especially when using lights and sirens.
    d. Use lights and sirens often so that other drivers will yield the right of way.
15. How can the paramedic promote safety when responding to a vehicle crash on the highway?
    a. Park 100 feet past the crash.
    b. Park downhill from hazardous materials.
    c. Park on the opposite side of the road.
    d. Turn off emergency lights.

16. All air medical crew members should receive specialized training in which of the following areas?
    a. Airway management techniques
    b. Flight physiology
    c. Medication administration
    d. Vascular access techniques
17. Which of the following situations would justify the use of air medical transport by an advanced life support unit with a 40 minute ETA?
    a. Possible fractured tibia with good pulses
    b. Possible aneurysm with absent pedal pulses
    c. Home delivery with both patients stable
    d. Asthma patient with pulse 100/min, R 20/min
18. Which of the following safety measures should be used when approaching the helicopter to load patients?
    a. Approach the aircraft as soon as it lands.
    b. At least six people should help load the aircraft.
    c. Long objects should be carried vertically to maintain control.
    d. The aircraft should be approached from the front.

MEDICAL INCIDENT COMMAND

● **READING ASSIGNMENT**

Chapter 49, pages 1386-1403, in *Mosby's Paramedic Textbook*, ed 2

● **OBJECTIVES**

As a paramedic, you should be able to:
1. Identify the components of an effective incident command system.
2. Outline the activities in the preplanning, scene management, and postdisaster follow-up phases of an incident.
3. Identify the five major components of FEMA's incident command system (ICS).
4. List command responsibilities during a major incident response.
5. Describe the section responsibilities in FEMA's ICS.
6. Identify situations that may be classified as major incidents.
7. Describe the steps necessary to establish and operate the incident command system.
8. Given a major incident, describe sectors that would need to be established and the responsibilities of each.
9. List common problems related to the ICS and mass casualty situations.
10. Outline principles and technology of triage.
11. Identify resources for management of critical incident stress.

● **REVIEW QUESTIONS**

Match the terms in Column II with their definitions in Column I. Use each term only once.

	Column I	Column II
1. _____	Contracts agreeing to interagency exchange of resources when necessary	**a.** Apparatus
2. _____	Pumpers, ladder trucks, rescue trucks	**b.** Command
3. _____	Rendezvous location for all arriving EMS, fire, and rescue equipment	**c.** Command post
4. _____	Responsible for coordination of major incident situation	**d.** Communication center
		e. Mutual aid
		f. Sector
		g. Staging area

Questions 5-13 refer to the following case study:

Dispatch radios your crew to respond to a local sports stadium for a bleacher collapse at a college football game. During your initial size-up, you determine that 50 to 100 people are injured, with a substantial number of victims still trapped under the fallen concrete seats. It is rush hour, and traffic conditions will be heavy for at least 2 more hours.

5. List three actions that should be taken by the first unit arriving at the scene.

_____

_____

6. a. How will command be determined?

_____

_____

b. Will there be single or unified command?

_____

_____

7. List nine command responsibilities during this incident.
  a.
  b.
  c.
  d.
  e.
  f.
  g.
  h.
  i.

8. Fill in Fig. 49-1 with the appropriate positions needed in this incident command situation.

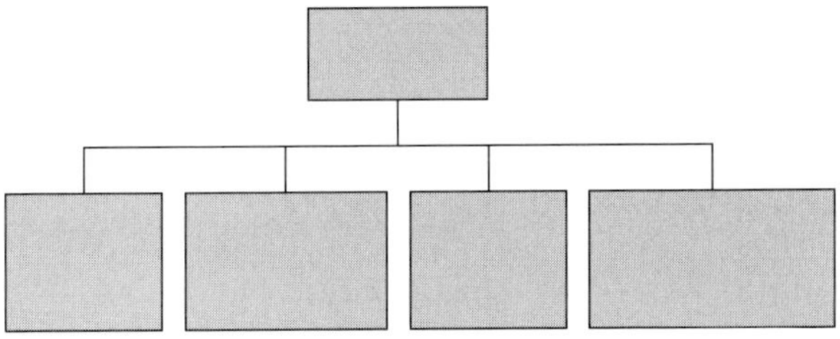

Figure 49-1

9. Briefly describe the responsibilities of each of the following sectors that command has established for this incident.
  a. Support:

_____

_____

  b. Staging:

_____

_____

  c. Extrication:

_____

_____

d. Treatment:

_____

_____

e. Transportation:

_____

_____

_____

10. Explain how communications can be initiated in an effective manner in this situation.

_____

_____

_____

11. a. What special resources will be necessary during this incident?

_____

_____

   b. How will command know where to obtain those resources?

12. Triage each of the following patients injured at this scene using START triage and METTAG categories.
   a. A man walks over to you, complaining of chest pain.

_____

   b. A woman has a respiratory rate of 20 and no radial pulse, but a carotid pulse is present.

_____

   c. A man is lying under a bleacher. His respiratory rate is 24, a radial pulse is present, he can't touch his nose with his index finger, and he knows his name but not the date or year.

_____

   d. A woman is leaning against a bleacher, unable to walk. Her respiratory rate is 16, a radial pulse is present, she can stick out her tongue and touch her nose with her index finger, and she knows her name, the date, and the year.

_____

   e. A man has a respiratory rate of 8. He has no radial pulse, but a carotid pulse is present.

_____

   f. A woman is trapped under a post. She is not breathing and has no pulse.

_____

13. During triage, what care should be provided to the patients in Question 12?

_____

14. An ideal incident command system should have which of the following characteristics?
    a. It should be able to expand to a larger incident in a logical manner.
    b. It should be used only for large or complex mass casualty situations.
    c. It should provide for just single jurisdiction involvement.
    d. It should respond to one specific incident or situation.

15. Which phase of major incident planning involves establishing an inventory of community resources needed for selected disasters?
    a. Logistics operations
    b. Postdisaster follow-up
    c. Scene management
    d. The preplan

16. What are the five major components of FEMA's ICS organization?
    a. Communications, logistics, operations, staging, support
    b. Communications, finance, staging, support, treatment
    c. Command, finance, logistics, operations, planning
    d. Command, operations, planning, transportation, treatment

17. Which of the following should have the highest priority when the incident commander is considering whether to expand the ICS organization during an incident?
    a. Cost
    b. Incident stability
    c. Life safety
    d. Property conservation

18. What is the primary responsibility of the section chiefs in an MCI situation?
    a. To assume overall accountability for the MCI situation
    b. To ensure section members are working toward a common goal
    c. To operate rescue equipment and supervise staff in the sector
    d. To provide patient care and stabilization within a defined area

19. Which section has overall responsibility for the areas that provide care to medical staff?
    a. Finance
    b. Logistics
    c. Operations
    d. Planning

20. Which of the following situations would be *least* likely to be declared a major incident?
    a. Rural EMS service, motor vehicle collision requiring four EMS units
    b. City EMS service, train derailment, possible hazardous materials leak
    c. Rural EMS service, two-patient incident with high-angle rescue
    d. City EMS service, two-person motor vehicle collision, no patient trapped

21. Except in unusual circumstances, patient care and stabilization should be provided by the _____ sector.
    a. Extrication
    b. Support
    c. Treatment
    d. Triage

22. What is an appropriate role for a physician brought to the scene from a local hospital?
    a. Incident commander
    b. Extrication sector resource
    c. Staging sector resource
    d. Transport sector resource

23. The most appropriate *radio* communication during a mass casualty incident would be between which of the following crew members?
    a. Command and sector officers
    b. Individuals within each sector
    c. Treatment sector and hospital
    d. Public information officer and press

24. Which of the following may create a problem at an MCI?
    a. Organizing patients rapidly at a treatment area
    b. Prematurely transporting patients
    c. Performing rapid "initial" stabilization of patients
    d. Wearing sector identification vests

25. Patient classification during mass casualty incidents should be based on which of the following?
    a. Physiological signs, mechanism of injury, and anatomical injury
    b. Mechanism of injury, anatomical injury, and patient age
    c. Chief complaint, physiological signs, and anatomical injury
    d. Physiological signs, anatomical injury, and concurrent disease
26. Your patient has a gunshot wound to the chest, is conscious, and has a respiratory rate of 36. Which of the following would be the appropriate triage category, using the triage systems discussed in the text?
    a. Urgent, yellow   c. Dead/dying, black
    b. Critical, red   d. Delayed, green
27. Mental status examination during START triage should include which of the following?
    a. Asking the patient to touch his nose
    b. AVPU
    c. Glasgow coma scale
    d. Observing for arm drift
28. What information should be included on the patient tracking log?
    a. Patient's age   c. Patient's next of kin
    b. Patient's injuries   d. Patient's priority
29. Which of the following is *not* typically provided in a critical incident stress management program?
    a. Advice to command during large scale incidents
    b. Defusing services immediately after a large-scale incident
    c. Long-term psychiatric counseling
    d. On-scene support for distressed personnel

CHAPTER 50
RESCUE AWARENESS AND OPERATIONS

● READING ASSIGNMENT
Chapter 50, pages 1404-1429, in *Mosby's Paramedic Textbook,* ed 2

● OBJECTIVES
As a paramedic, you should be able to:
1. Describe factors that must be considered to ensure appropriate timing of medical and mechanical skills during rescue.
2. Outline each phase of a rescue operation.
3. Identify appropriate personal protective equipment that should be used during rescue situations.
4. Describe considerations during EMS response to surface water rescue situations.
5. Discuss considerations during EMS response to situations associated with hazardous atmospheres, including confined space and trench/cave-in rescues.
6. Describe hazards that may be present during EMS operations on the highway.
7. Describe considerations during EMS response over hazardous terrain.
8. Outline special considerations needed for prehospital assessment and management during rescue.

● REVIEW QUESTIONS
Questions 1 and 2 refer to the following case study:

> A woman who is kayaking on a winter day is swept under the ice. You can see her about 3 feet from the edge of the ice where the water is rolling up over a large rock. Her team is frantically screaming at you to do something.

1. What hazards do you face if you enter the water to attempt a rescue?

_____

> Additional equipment is called, and a cut is made in the ice to retrieve the woman, but she does not survive the 90-minute submersion.

2. What services of the local CISM team might your crew need after this incident?

_____

Questions 3-8 refer to the following case study:

> A party-goer falls into an open sewer standpipe. You estimate that he is approximately 30 feet down the 48-inch pipe. Bystanders report that he was talking to them when they arrived, but you hear him moaning only occasionally at this time.

3. What additional assistance will you request?

_____

4. What potential injuries should you worry about regarding this patient?

_____

5. Why must the rescue team test the air quality at several levels in the pipe?

_____

6. Why might the rescuer who enters the pipe wear an SABA instead of an SCBA during this rescue?

_____

7. What can cause problems when using an SABA?

_____

8. Aside from a confined space rescue, what other hazardous rescue situation exists here?

_____

_____

Questions 9-18 refer to the following case study:

> You are called to the scene of a motor vehicle collision at a busy urban shopping center. On arrival at the scene, you find that a large sedan has hit the side of a compact car, wedging it between the sedan and a storefront. A large crowd of spectators has gathered and is impeding your access to the patient. You note a trickle of gasoline coming from one of the vehicles. No other equipment or law enforcement personnel have been dispatched.

9. What should you be looking for as you do your scene size-up?

_____

10. What information/assistance did you receive on your response?

_____

_____

11. What steps should you take to gain control of the crowd?

_____

_____

_____

> One patient was pulled from the sedan by bystanders before your arrival. He is pale and complains of abdominal pain. Your partner begins care. A second patient in the compact car is unconscious. He is trapped and inaccessible.

12. List the additional equipment and other resources you should request at this time.

_____

13. What hazards have you identified that should be reported to incoming crews?

_____

14. What actions can be taken to decrease the risks associated with the hazards you identified?

_____

_____

A rescue truck arrives and breaks a window, which provides limited access to the patient while rescue operations proceed.

15. What can you do for your patient at this time?

_____

16. How can you ensure patient safety during the rescue?

_____

_____

A brief primary survey reveals an unconscious patient with gurgling respirations and a strong radial pulse of 70 beats/min. You observe a large ecchymotic area on the temporal region of the patient's head.

17. You have limited time and access to the patient. What are your priorities of care?

_____

_____

18. Describe the disentanglement and packaging and removal segments of the rescue operation and your responsibilities to the patient during these phases.

_____

_____

_____

_____

_____

_____

_____

19. Discuss safety measures that should be taken at the scene of an accident in which an energized wire is in contact with an involved auto.
   a. The rescuers

_____

_____

   b. The persons trapped in the involved automobile

_____

_____

20. Give two examples of equipment that may be used to disentangle a person who is trapped inside a vehicle.
   a.
   b.

353

21. Aside from ensuring safety, the rescue operations should be guided by which of the following?
    a. Performance of techniques in the standardized manner
    b. The desire of the rescue team to complete the task
    c. The medical and physical needs of the patient
    d. The number of bystanders observing the scene
22. What is the responsibility of the paramedic in any rescue situation?
    a. To coordinate overall scene safety
    b. To direct scene and tactical operations
    c. To know when it is safe to attempt rescue
    d. To operate all rescue and extrication equipment
23. Safety of the _____ should be the *first* priority at the scene of any rescue.
    a. Bystanders   c. Injured
    b. Crew   d. Trapped
24. When does scene size-up begin on a call for rescue?
    a. On arrival to the scene   c. When the call is received
    b. When specialized teams arrive d. When the patient is visible
25. Which is true regarding medical treatment during a rescue situation for a safely accessible patient?
    a. All standardized procedures should be followed.
    b. Medical treatment should be directed by the rescue commander.
    c. No treatment should be attempted until the patient is freed.
    d. Rapid assessment and basic stabilization should be attempted.
26. What routine safety measures should be employed to protect the patient's safety during a vehicle rescue that does not involve fire or hazardous materials?
    a. A blanket   c. A surgical mask
    b. Air bags   d. An SCBA
27. According to NFPA and OSHA standards, EMS rescue personnel should have access to all the following personal protective equipment *except:*
    a. Ear plugs   c. Rubber boots
    b. Protective helmet   d. Waterproof gloves
28. Which is true when responding to a rescue in swift water?
    a. A foot trapped in water should be freed the opposite way it went in.
    b. Do not walk through fast-moving water that is over knee depth.
    c. Flat water does not create any serious hazard.
    d. Higher dams create more dangerous situations than low dams.
29. What factors contribute to drowning?
    a. Cool water temperature   c. PFDs that are worn properly
    b. Increased patient age   d. Swimming after eating
30. What factor would be an acceptable reason *not* to resuscitate a person who has drowned?
    a. More than 5 minutes of submersion was documented by witnesses.
    b. Evidence of activation of the mammalian diving reflex exists.
    c. Patient is cold, and temperature can't be detected on a regular thermometer.
    d. Rigor mortis or dependent lividity is present.
31. What is the first measure that should be employed to attempt rescue for a person in the water?
    a. Go   c. Row
    b. Reach   d. Throw
32. Which of the following oxygen levels is considered hazardous?
    a. Greater than 19.5%   c. Greater than 21%
    b. Greater than 22%   d. Less than 21%

33. Which is a clue to help identify an oxygen-limiting silo?
    a. An audible tone will sound.
    b. The color is usually blue.
    c. The placard states this information.
    d. The smell will be sweet.
34. You arrive at the scene of a trench collapse. When do you enter the trench to rescue the patient without specialized rescue equipment?
    a. The patient is unconscious.
    b. The patient is completely covered.
    c. The trench is less than waist deep.
    d. The trench is more than 3 feet wide.
35. Which of the following techniques may be used to increase safety at the scene of a vehicle accident with a gasoline leak at night?
    a. Put flares adjacent to the involved vehicles to alert motorists.
    b. Stage all apparatus on the highway and not on sideroads.
    c. Use all warning lights and headlights to increase visibility.
    d. Wear high-visibility clothing, such as orange highway vests.
36. To decrease the risk of fire at the scene of a motor vehicle collision in which gasoline is leaking, a paramedic should *always* perform which of the following?
    a. Disconnect the battery cable.
    b. Douse the vehicle with foam.
    c. Place a tarp over the spilled fuel.
    d. Turn off the automobile ignition.
37. Which type of extinguisher can be used to suppress a combustible metal fire?
    a. Class A   c. Class C
    b. Class B   d. Class D
38. What type of equipment is helpful for vehicle stabilization during rescue?
    a. Chain saws   c. Hurst tools
    b. Cribbing   d. Pry bars
39. You respond to a vehicle crash with an undeployed airbag. What measure may create a hazard for rescuers?
    a. Using tools that generate sparks
    b. Cutting the steering column to disable the system
    c. Disconnecting or cutting both battery cables
    d. Cutting into the airbag module
40. What is the primary risk associated with hazardous terrain rescue?
    a. Avalanche of debris   c. Injury from falls
    b. Dropping the patient   d. Injury from projectiles
41. Which term describes rescue on steep terrain that is capable of being walked on without the use of hands?
    a. Graded terrain rescue
    b. High-angle rescue
    c. Low-angle rescue
    d. Rescue on flat terrain with obstructions
42. Which of the following factors that can interfere with the paramedic's ability to adequately assess and treat a patient is unique during a rescue situation?
    a. Cumbersome personal protective equipment
    b. Lack of cooperation among your team members
    c. Hostile, uncommunicative patient
    d. Unstable vital signs and neurological status
43. Which is a complication of crush syndrome?
    a. Hypertension   c. Myoglobinemia
    b. Metabolic alkalosis   d. Sepsis

HAZARDOUS MATERIALS INCIDENTS

● READING ASSIGNMENT

Chapter 51, pages 1430-1453, in *Mosby's Paramedic Textbook*, ed 2

● OBJECTIVES

As a paramedic, you should be able to:
1. Define hazardous materials terminology.
2. Identify legislation regarding hazardous materials that influences emergency health care workers.
3. Describe resources to assist in identification and management of hazardous materials incidents.
4. Identify protective clothing and equipment necessary to respond to selected hazardous materials incidents.
5. Describe pathophysiology and signs and symptoms of internal damage caused by exposure to selected hazardous materials.
6. Identify pathophysiology, signs and symptoms, and prehospital management of selected hazardous materials that produce external damage.
7. Outline the prehospital response to a hazardous materials emergency.
8. Describe medical monitoring and rehabilitation of rescue workers who respond to a hazardous materials emergency.
9. Describe the emergency decontamination and management of patients who have been contaminated by hazardous materials.
10. Outline the steps to decontaminate rescue personnel and equipment at a hazardous materials incident.

● REVIEW QUESTIONS

Match the haz-mat terms in Column II with the appropriate definition in Column I. Use each term *only* once.

Column I	Column II
1. _____ The weight of pure vapor compared with weight of equal volume of dry air	a. Flammable/ exposure limits
2. _____ Dose of chemical that will kill 50% of animals	b. Flash point
3. _____ Exposure limit of 15 minutes	c. IDLH
4. _____ Gas or vapor concentration that will burn or explode with ignition source	d. Ignition temperature
5. _____ Safe exposure for a 40-hour work week	e. LD50
6. _____ Minimum temperature to ignite gas without spark or flame	f. PEL
7. _____ Atmosphere that causes immediate harm	g. TLV-C
8. _____ Vapor's ability to mix with water	h. TLV-STEL
9. _____ Maximum concentration not to be exceeded even for a moment	i. Vapor density
10. _____ Temperature at which liquid produces enough vapor to ignite and flash over but not continue to burn without more heat	j. Vapor pressure
	k. Vapor solubility

Match each of the hazardous chemicals listed in Column I with *all* the health hazards in Column II with which they are associated. You may use answers *more* than once.

Column I

11. _____ Arsenic
12. _____ Halogenated hydrocarbons
13. _____ Hydrochloric acid
14. _____ Hydrogen cyanide
15. _____ Lead
16. _____ Malathion
17. _____ Mercury

Column II

a. Asphyxiant
b. Anesthetic
c. Carcinogen
d. Cardiotoxin
e. Hemotoxin
f. Hepatotoxin
g. Irritant
h. Nephrotoxin
i. Nerve poison
j. Neurotoxin

18. Briefly describe each of the five categories of emergency response personnel who may respond to a hazardous materials situation:

a. First responder awareness:

_____

_____

b. First responder operations:

_____

_____

c. Hazardous material technician:

_____

_____

d. Hazardous material specialist:

_____

_____

e. On-scene incident commander:

_____

_____

19. You arrive on the scene of a motor vehicle collision involving an overturned tanker truck. You note a cloud of white vapor escaping from a relief valve on top of the truck. Describe the formal and informal means of identifying hazardous materials that may be involved in this situation.

a. Formal:

_____

_____

b. Informal:

_____

_____

20. After a hazardous material has been identified, what other resources can help the emergency response crew in determining hazards and management of the scene?

_____

_____

21. Describe the protective clothing that will be necessary in the following hazardous materials response situations:

  a. The hazardous materials crew provides emergency care to a seriously injured worker who is lying in an area contaminated with a liquid acidic chemical. No contaminated gas is present from the spill.

_____

_____

  b. Your fire rescue team must enter a burning building to extricate trapped victims. No known hazardous materials are reported on the scene.

_____

_____

  c. An equipment malfunction inside a chemical manufacturing plant has resulted in the release of toxic gases. Hazardous materials specialists must enter to attempt to locate a victim known to be just inside the hot zone.

_____

_____

22. Describe the health problems that can be encountered when an individual sustains exposure to the following agents:

  a. Irritants:

_____

  b. Asphyxiants:

_____

  c. Nerve poisons, anesthetics, and narcotics:

_____

  d. Hepatotoxins:

_____

  e. Cardiotoxins:

_____

  f. Neurotoxins:

_____

  g. Hemotoxins:

_____

  h. Carcinogens:

_____

23. You respond to the scene of a fire in which hazardous materials of unknown origin are involved. Describe signs and symptoms exhibited by scene workers that may cause you to suspect exposure to hazardous materials.

24. Your crew arrives at an industrial chemical manufacturing plant where a worker has sustained a splash exposure of a corrosive chemical to the eyes. Describe patient management in this situation.

25. Label Fig. 51-1, and briefly describe each of the three safety zones for a hazardous materials situation response that has been established by hazardous materials specialists.

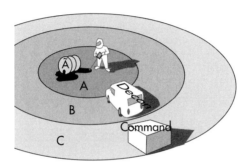

Figure 51-1

A.

B.

C.

Questions 26-28 refer to the following case study:

You are the first team dispatched to the scene of a train derailment where three victims remain trapped. The bystanders who called in the incident report that placards indicating the presence of hazardous materials are present on several of the involved train cars.

26. Describe any actions you should take during your initial response to this situation.

_____

_____

_____

_____

_____

27. Describe special considerations in the prehospital management of contaminated patients.

_____

_____

_____

_____

_____

28. The incident commander on this scene delegates your EMS crew to establish a medical monitoring station. Describe the responsibilities of this role.

_____

_____

29. What steps should rescuers take as they leave the "hot zone" at a haz-mat scene?

_____

_____

● **STUDENT SELF-ASSESSMENT**

30. What is the term for substances and materials capable of posing an unreasonable risk to health, safety, and property?
   a. External hazards
   b. Hazardous materials
   c. Immediately dangerous to life and health
   d. Internal hazards

31. What term describes the legislation, enacted in 1986, that established requirements for federal, state, and local governments and industry regarding emergency planning and the reporting of hazardous materials?
    a. Hazardous Materials Control Act
    b. Occupational Health and Safety Law
    c. Ryan White Law
    d. Superfund Amendments and Reauthorization Act
32. According to the HAZWOPER rules, the five categories of individuals who may respond to an emergency involving hazardous materials include all of the following *except:*
    a. First responder operations   c. Hazardous material specialist
    b. Hazardous material technician   d. Rescue operation technician
33. Which of the following is a formal means of identifying hazardous products?
    a. Container characteristics   c. Patient signs and symptoms
    b. Incident location   d. United Nations Labeling System
34. Which agency requires Material Safety Data Sheets when chemicals are stored, handled, or used in the workplace?
    a. International Air Transport Association
    b. National Fire Protection Association
    c. Occupational Safety and Health Administration
    d. U.S. Department of Transportation
35. General signs or symptoms of inhalation exposure to a hazardous material may include which of the following?
    a. Hemiplegia   c. Seizure
    b. Hematemesis   d. Urticaria
36. External exposure to corrosive chemicals generally causes which of the following?
    a. Acidosis   c. Coughing
    b. Burns   d. Systemic effects
37. Which of the following signs or symptoms should prompt a rescuer to seek immediate medical attention at the site of a hazardous materials incident?
    a. Confusion and lightheadedness
    b. Shortness of breath and coughing
    c. Tingling of the extremities
    d. Nausea and vomiting
    e. Any of the above
38. When responding to the scene of a hazardous material incident, the EMS crew should approach from which direction?
    a. Downhill and downwind   c. Uphill and downwind
    b. Downhill and upwind   d. Uphill and upwind
39. The "pre-suit" medical monitoring of an individual who will be entering a hazardous material situation should include all of the following *except* which one?
    a. Heart rate   c. Temperature
    b. Reflexes   d. Weight
40. General recommendations for emergency management of contaminated patients include all of the following *except* which one?
    a. Emergency patient care overrides all safety considerations.
    b. All patients in the hot zone are considered contaminated.
    c. Intravenous therapy should be initiated only with a physician's order.
    d. The patient's clothing should be completely cut off.
41. Which is an appropriate step in the decontamination of a rescue person who is leaving a haz-mat site?
    a. Shave all body hair.
    b. Shake clothing vigorously before reapplying.
    c. Take haz-mat suit to the ambulance to be used later.
    d. Shower and cleanse with soap and water.

CRIME SCENE AWARENESS

● READING ASSIGNMENT

Chapter 52, pages 1454-1467, in *Mosby's Paramedic Textbook*, ed 2

● OBJECTIVES

As a paramedic, you should be able to:
1. Describe general techniques for detection of and response to a violent scene.
2. Outline techniques for recognizing and responding to potentially dangerous residential calls.
3. Outline techniques for recognizing and responding to potentially dangerous calls on the highway.
4. Describe signs of danger and EMS response to violent street incidents.
5. Identify characteristics of and EMS response to situations involving gangs, clandestine drug labs, and domestic violence situations.
6. Outline general safety tactics that EMS personnel may use when a dangerous situation is encountered.
7. Describe special EMS considerations when providing tactical patient care.
8. Discuss EMS documentation and evidence preservation considerations at a crime scene.

● REVIEW QUESTIONS

Questions 1 and 2 apply to the following case study:

You are responding to a routine call in a residential neighborhood.

1. When should your scene size-up begin?

_____

2. List six warning signs of danger that you should look for on this call.

a.

b.

c.

d.

e.

f.

3. List strategies to increase safety as you approach each of the following:
   a. A darkened residence:

_____

   b. A vehicle stopped on the side of the highway:

_____

4. For each of the following situations, describe which tactic is indicated to increase your safety and how you would use it. (Avoidance, tactical retreat, cover and concealment, or distraction and evasive maneuvers.)
   a. You respond to a school shooting. En route, you determine that several shots fired in a school classroom have been reported; however, there is no confirmation that the perpetrator has been apprehended.

   _____

   b. You are providing care to an injured fan at a large soccer match when irate fans begin to hurl bottles at you and your partner.

   _____

   _____

   _____

   c. You are on bike patrol at a community picnic. You respond to a call for a "person injured." You find a teenager dressed in known gang attire who was punched in the face. As you begin your care, you hear the sound of gunfire in close vicinity.

   _____

   _____

   d. During assessment of a patient who has an altered level of consciousness in the living room of a small home, his behavior escalates suddenly and he starts yelling and threatening to hurt you as he lunges toward you.

   _____

   _____

5. List six types of physical evidence that may be found on a crime scene.
   a.
   b.
   c.
   d.
   e.
   f.

● STUDENT SELF-ASSESSMENT

6. When should assessment of the potential for violence at the scene begin?
   a. If the patient threatens the crew
   b. On arrival to the scene
   c. When the patient is encountered
   d. En route to the call
7. Which of the following may indicate that the residence you are about to enter is potentially dangerous?
   a. Darkened residence
   b. History of multiple calls
   c. No car in the driveway
   d. Person waving you in
8. Which represents the safest approach to a single vehicle stopped on the highway?
   a. Approach from the passenger side of the vehicle
   b. Simultaneous approach by both crew members
   c. Ambulance lights turned off to eliminate glare
   d. Walking between the ambulance and the other vehicle

9. Which of the following is most likely to protect the paramedic from danger during a violent street scene?
   a. Allow police to control the scene and proceed as usual.
   b. Attempt to disperse the crowd while providing care.
   c. Retreat immediately from the scene with the patient.
   d. There is no danger; crowds will not attack paramedics.
10. How can you learn about gang-related activity in your EMS response area?
    a. Police
    b. School officials
    c. Social service agencies
    d. All of the above
11. Which of the following drugs are commonly produced or altered in drug labs?
    a. Codeine
    b. Marijuana
    c. Methamphetamine
    d. Morphine
12. Which of the following may signal a situation that includes domestic violence?
    a. Darkened rooms
    b. Excessive nervous talking
    c. Inaccurate medical history
    d. Inconsistent injuries
13. Which of the following is a common EMS safety strategy in a dangerous situation?
    a. Avoidance
    b. Contact
    c. Negotiation
    d. Use of weapons
14. Which is an appropriate location for cover during gunfire?
    a. Bushes
    b. Car door
    c. Large tree
    d. Wooden sign
15. Which of the following provides a clue that a patient may become violent?
    a. Crossed legs
    b. Hands on hips
    c. Quiet dialogue
    d. Verbal abuse
16. Body armor is least effective against which of the following weapons?
    a. Air guns
    b. Handguns
    c. Ice picks
    d. Knives
17. Which of the following does tactical paramedic training usually include?
    a. Haz-mat decontamination
    b. Minor surgical techniques
    c. Radiographic interpretation
    d. Suturing and advanced wound care
18. Which of the following is an appropriate way to approach a crime scene?
    a. Document any suspicions you may have.
    b. Follow the same path to and from the victim.
    c. Move visible evidence so that police can find it.
    d. Save patient items in a plastic bag.

EMERGENCY DRUG INDEX

1. List the actions, indications, and side effects of steroids.

_____

_____

_____

2. For each of the following two drugs, list the time of onset, duration, and dose:

   a. Methylprednisolone:

   _____

   b. Dexamethasone:

   _____

For each of the scenarios in Questions 3 through 28, complete the corresponding flashcard (after the ECG flashcards at the end of this workbook) with the appropriate drug information, including trade name, class, descriptions, indications, contraindications, adverse reactions, onset, duration, dosage (adult and pediatric, if appropriate), and special considerations. Verify your drug choice before completing the flashcard by looking at the generic drug name on the back.

3. Your patient is experiencing urticaria and severe itching resulting from an allergic reaction. His vital signs are stable, and no wheezes are audible on auscultation of his lungs. You administer _____. (Complete Flashcard 23.)

4. After delivering three shocks to your patient who is in ventricular fibrillation cardiac arrest, you wish to give a potent vasoconstrictor with a long duration of action. What do you administer? _____. (Complete Flashcard 24.)

5. Your crew is unable to initiate an intravenous line on an unconscious diabetic patient who is known to be hypoglycemic. Transport time is 45 minutes. The drug of choice to increase the blood glucose level is _____. (Complete Flashcard 25.)

6. Your patient is in ventricular fibrillation cardiac arrest. After you defibrillate three times and administer epinephrine, medical direction asks you to administer an antidysrhythmic drug. List two specific antidysrhythmic drugs other than lidocaine that you may administer. _____. (Complete Flashcards 26 and 27.)

7. A 65-year-old woman calls you complaining of shortness of breath and chest pain radiating down her left arm. Her blood pressure is 110/70 mm Hg. The initial drug of choice to relieve her pain is _____. (Complete Flashcard 28.)

8. You place a 22-year-old patient with a pounding sensation in her chest on a monitor and discover ventricular tachycardia. The patient's blood pressure is normal, she has no chest pain, and the rest of the history and physical examination are unremarkable. The appropriate drug to use to suppress ventricular dysrhythmia in this situation is _____. (Complete Flashcard 29.)

9. Your 30-year-old patient fell while rollerblading and has obvious deformity of the right wrist with significant pain. What nonnarcotic analgesic can you give him either IM or IV? _____ (Complete Flashcard 30.)

10. You are called to an outpatient surgery center to evaluate a nurse who is unconscious. Co-workers confide that they have suspected drug abuse for some time, and an empty meperidine (Demerol) tubex is found in her pocket. All other available medical history is negative. Pupils are pinpoint, and respirations are 12 and shallow. What drug do you administer first if an overdose is suspected? _____ (Complete Flashcard 31.)

11. You are performing transcutaneous pacing on a conscious patient who is complaining of severe discomfort related to the procedure. What short-acting IV medicine can you administer to reduce anxiety, relax skeletal muscles, and provide amnesia? _____ (Complete Flashcard 32.)

12. You are called to a nursing home to care for an 88-year-old woman who has fainted. The patient is extremely bradycardic (pulse 40) and has a blood pressure of 80 systolic by palpation. Her only history is hypertension. What emergency care drug is indicated initially to correct her sinus bradycardia? _____ (Complete Flashcard 33.)

13. Initial electrical countershocks do not convert successfully your cardiac arrest patient from ventricular fibrillation. An adrenergic drug that should be repeated every 3 to 5 min is: _____. (Complete Flashcard 34.)

14. A 32-year-old patient fell while playing softball and has an apparent dislocation of the left shoulder, which is very painful. Medical direction wishes to administer a short-acting analgesic so that accurate emergency department evaluation will be possible. What is an appropriate, self-administered analgesic agent in this situation? _____ (Complete Flashcard 35.)

15. You have been trying without success to resuscitate a 73-year-old woman who is in cardiac arrest. Tricyclic antidepressant overdose is suspected. What drug may be considered at this point? _____ (Complete Flashcard 36.)

16. The police call you to evaluate an unconscious person. The patient is a known alcoholic, and friends say that he has not eaten for several days. Dextrostix analysis reveals a blood glucose level of 40 mg/dl (normal range 80 to 120 mg/dl). No drug use is suspected. The two drugs indicated for this patient are _____ and _____. (Complete Flashcards 37 and 38.)

17. A frantic husband calls you to evaluate his wife, who has been having seizures for 10 minutes. You find that she is experiencing repetitive grand mal seizures. The husband tells you that she is a known epileptic who has not taken any phenytoin (Dilantin) for 2 days. What is your drug of choice under these circumstances? _____ (Complete Flashcard 39.)

18. Your 24-year-old patient is a known asthmatic who is experiencing an acute attack. Inspiratory and expiratory wheezes are audible throughout the chest, and the patient is tachypneic. What drug would you initially administer by inhalation? _____ (Complete Flashcard 40.)

19. A 56-year-old woman has severe crushing substernal chest pain and diaphoresis. You administer vasodilators and a narcotic analgesic to relieve pain. What antiplatelet drug should you administer en route? _____ (Complete Flashcard 41.)

20. You are called to treat a 32-year-old woman with a sudden onset of palpitations. The electrocardiogram reveals a rapid supraventricular tachycardia. The patient states that she has Wolff-Parkinson-White syndrome. What is the safest drug to use to convert this rhythm to sinus rhythm? _____ (Complete Flashcard 42.)

21. Airport authorities call you to care for a mechanic whose arm is trapped in the landing gear of a small aircraft. Extrication time is lengthy, and the patient is in extreme distress because of pain. Vital signs are stable, and no other injuries are noted. List two narcotic analgesics that may be administered to this patient. _____ and _____ (Complete Flashcards 43 ands 44.)

22. Your 67-year-old patient is experiencing a severe headache and blurred vision resulting from his blood pressure, which is now 230/160 mm Hg. He is awake and cooperative. Which α- and β-adrenegic blocker drug may improve this potentially disastrous situation by lowering the blood pressure? _____ (Complete Flashcard 45.)

23. A 21-year-old took an overdose of an antidepressant 10 minutes ago and is awake and alert. What drug may be used to prevent absorption of the antidepressant in the gastrointestinal tract? _____ (Complete Flashcard 46.)

24. Your patient is 8 months pregnant and has been diagnosed with preeclampsia. Co-workers found her experiencing a grand mal seizure in the restroom. The patient appears to be in a postictal state. Blood pressure is 160/116 mm Hg. What drug may be given if she has a recurrence of seizure activity? _____ (Complete Flashcard 47.)

25. You have a 30-minute estimated time of arrival to the hospital with an 86-year-old patient from a nursing home whose vital signs are blood pressure, 80/50 mm Hg; pulse, 124; and respirations, 24. The urine in her Foley catheter bag is milky green and foul smelling. Cardiac history is negative, and no reason exists to suspect blood or fluid volume loss. What is the drug of choice to acutely treat her hypotension after fluid resuscitation in this situation? _____ (Complete Flashcard 48.)

26. The 65-year-old patient you are called to evaluate has the following vital signs: blood pressure, 130/90 mm Hg; pulse, 160; and respirations, 24. The electrocardiogram monitor shows atrial fibrillation with a rapid ventricular response. She has mild signs of congestive heart failure, but all other physical findings are negative. What class IV antidysrhythmic drug is indicated for this patient? _____ (Complete Flashcard 49.)

27. Your 72-year-old patient is experiencing severe dyspnea that began suddenly during the night. She is in obvious distress, with cyanosis of the nail beds and lips. Lung sounds reveal rales and wheezes throughout, and she has a cough that produces frothy, pink sputum. History reveals two previous myocardial infarctions. Vital signs are blood pressure, 170/108 mm Hg; pulse, 132; and respirations, 32. Identify the diuretic to administer in an attempt to improve this patient's condition. _____ (Complete Flashcard 50.)

28. You have just delivered a healthy baby boy, followed minutes later by a complete placenta. Despite vigorous massage, the patient's uterus is very soft, and she is experiencing profuse vaginal bleeding. What pharmacological agent can you administer to help control this bleeding? _____ (Complete Flashcard 51.)

Complete the remaining flashcards with drugs not included in the previous questions that are administered within your EMS system.

29. When is the use of dopamine most clearly indicated?
    a. Cardiac arrest
    c. Head injury
    b. Cardiogenic shock
    d. Internal bleeding
30. Which of the following is the appropriate drug to administer to a patient who was in a motor vehicle collision and is complaining of severe abdominal pain?
    a. Meperidine
    c. Nitrous oxide
    b. Morphine
    d. None of the above
31. Which of the following is an indication for administration of epinephrine 1:1000 subcutaneously?
    a. Anaphylaxis
    c. Electromechanical dissociation
    b. Asystole
    d. Ventricular fibrillation
32. Which drug is recommended to control atrial fibrillation with a rate of 170/minute when the patient has Wolff-Parkinson-White syndrome?
    a. Adenosine
    c. Atenolol
    b. Amiodarone
    d. Diltiazem
33. Which of the following is *not* true regarding use of atropine?
    a. It is indicated for management of bradycardia.
    b. The initial dose in bradycardia is 0.5 mg intravenously.
    c. It should be given in asystole.
    d. It is an antidote for verapamil.
34. Dopamine, when administered at low doses (1.0 to 2.0 mcg/kg/min), has which of the following effects?
    a. Renal and mesenteric vessel dilation
    b. Profound arteriolar constriction
    c. Decreased cerebral edema
    d. Ventricular dysrhythmias
35. Your patient has severe chest pain and is nauseated and diaphoretic. His 12-lead ECG shows ST segment elevation in leads II, III, and AVF. His breath sounds are clear and his BP is 86/50 mm Hg, P 64/min, and R 20/min. Which of the following drugs would be indicated during your 10 minute transport to the ED?
    a. Aspirin
    c. Nitroglycerin
    b. Morphine
    d. Verapamil
36. Your patient is in ventricular fibrillation and has been shocked three times. An intravenous infusion has been started. Your first choice for drug therapy is which of the following?
    a. Epinephrine
    c. Morphine
    b. Hydralazine
    d. Nifedipine
37. Which of the following drugs does *not* cause bronchodilation?
    a. Albuterol
    c. Diphenhydramine
    b. Epinephrine
    d. Isoproterenol
38. Verapamil is contraindicated if the patient can be described as which of the following?
    a. Complaining of palpitations
    c. Tachycardic
    b. Hypotensive
    d. Under 45
39. Which of the following drugs is self-administered by mask for relief of pain?
    a. Albuterol
    c. Nitroglycerin
    b. Morphine sulfate
    d. Nitrous oxide:oxygen
40. Which of the following is a drug indicated for the management of hypertension?
    a. Dobutamine
    c. Phenytoin
    b. Hydralazine
    d. Procainamide
41. Which of the following drugs affects blood clotting by inhibition of platelets?
    a. Aspirin
    c. Streptokinase
    b. Reteplase
    d. Tissue plasminogen activator

42. Pharmacological management of the patient suffering from coma of unknown origin includes which of the following?
    a. Naloxone, glucagon, and D50W
    b. Butorphanol (Stadol), glucagon, and thiamine
    c. Naloxone, thiamine, and D50W
    d. Dexamethasone, glucagon, and D50W
43. In which of the following situations is mannitol indicated?
    a. Myocardial infarction   c. Digoxin toxicity
    b. Acute cerebral edema   d. Shock
44. Which of the following pharmacological agents is useful in status epilepticus, as an antianxiety agent, and as a skeletal muscle relaxant?
    a. Diazepam   c. Naloxone
    b. Morphine   d. Phenytoin
45. Which of the following drugs is indicated for management of postpartum bleeding?
    a. Dopamine   c. Magnesium sulfate
    b. Insulin   d. Oxytocin
46. Diphenhydramine is contraindicated in which of the following situations?
    a. Anaphylactic shock   c. Allergic reactions
    b. An acute asthma attack   d. Patients over 35 years of age
47. Syrup of ipecac may be given to which of the following patients?
    a. Those without a gag reflex
    b. Those who have ingested prochlorperazine (Compazine)
    c. Those who have ingested phenytoin (Dilantin)
    d. Those who have ingested gasoline
48. Naloxone is an antagonist to all of the following, except which?
    a. Propoxyphene   c. Meperidine
    b. Heroin   d. Phenobarbital
49. Which of the following medications may cause respiratory depression?
    a. Atropine   c. Magnesium sulfate
    b. Dexamethasone   d. Thiamine
50. A patient has monomorphic ventricular tachycardia at 160/min (normal QT interval). Her BP is 100 mm Hg, and the patient has crackles in both lung bases. Which drug is indicated initially to manage this rhythm?
    a. Lidocaine   c. Metoprolol
    b. Magnesium sulfate   d. Procainamide
51. Which of the following side effects may occur after nitroglycerin ingestion?
    a. Headache   c. Burning under the tongue
    b. Hypotension   d. All of the above
52. Which of the following drugs exerts a positive chronotropic effect?
    a. Adenosine   c. Haloperidol
    b. Epinephrine   d. Propranolol
53. Furosemide is indicated in the management of which of the following?
    a. Angina   c. Hypotension
    b. Dysrhythmias   d. Pulmonary edema
54. Which of the following is a calcium channel blocker that slows conduction and is useful to slow the heart rate in atrial flutter?
    a. Adenosine   c. Dobutamine
    b. Albuterol   d. Diltiazem
55. All of the following drugs are indicated to manage pulmonary edema that develops secondary to left-sided heart failure, except which?
    a. Atropine   c. Morphine
    b. Furosemide   d. Nitroglycerin

56. When meperidine is given alone, which of the following side effects should be anticipated?

    a. Increased heart rate   **c.** Vasoconstriction

    b. Nausea and vomiting   **d.** Hyperactivity

57. Your patient is a 35-year-old man who is psychotic and violent. Which of the following is the drug of choice for his care?

    a. Haloperidol   **c.** Meperidine

    b. Hydroxyzine   **d.** Nifedipine

58. Dexamethasone and methylprednisolone belong to which of the following classes of drugs?

    a. Analgesics   **c.** Sympathomimetics

    b. Inotropics   **d.** Steroids

PARAMEDIC CAREER OPPORTUNITIES

Since its inception in 1967, EMS has developed into a sophisticated profession with various levels of care that result in improved care of the sick and injured. With the evolution of EMS has come career opportunities for EMTs, paramedics, nurses, and physicians. Although specific job opportunities depend on geographical locations, in general, opportunities for prehospital emergency responders have emerged from volunteer to paid career positions. For a certified EMT-Paramedic, many options are available.

● OTHER AREAS OF INTEREST

Aside from traditional prehospital roles, some paramedics have taken on expanded duties. Although much controversy has surrounded the use of paramedics within the emergency department, some hospitals in the United States employ paramedics to use their full skills and knowledge. Others may hire them as orderlies, pathology assistants, intravenous team members, phlebotomists, suture technicians, and respiratory therapists.

Some hospitals also have extended emergency departments in which paramedics have an expanded function. These facilities offer treatment for minor illnesses or injuries, physical examinations, and health screenings. They often are located within industrial settings, universities, or stand-alone buildings not part of hospitals.

Finally, paramedics who pursue advanced education can find additional opportunities. Many universities offer credit hours toward a bachelor's degree for any individual with a paramedic certification. For a field paramedic with experience, other advanced opportunities may include training as a nurse or physician's assistant.

● POSITION

A **field paramedic**—requires current certification as an EMT-Paramedic. Some states and organizations also require National Registry certification.

A **paramedic supervisor**—usually requires substantial experience as a field provider and supervisory experience.

A **flight paramedic**—usually requires substantial experience as a field provider and the ability to work under pressure. Additional certifications or training may be required by the individual service.

An **interhospital transport medic**—usually requires certification/licensure as a paramedic. Additional specialized training may be required or provided by the employer.

An **EMS administrator**—in addition to paramedic certification/licensure, often requires advanced degrees in EMS, business, or health-care administration.

An **EMS educator**—usually requires paramedic certification and experience as an instructor.

Specialized training in education to meet the minimum requirements set forth by each state usually is needed. Advanced-degree certification often is desired for high-level training programs.

● DESCRIPTION

Many paramedics enjoy the day-to-day operations of a field provider, administering emergency care to the sick and injured. Roles and responsibilities of paramedics undoubtedly will grow as the emergency department extends into the community through advanced life support (ALS) personnel.

An ALS supervisor is usually an experienced paramedic with administrative or management skills. Responsibilities for this position generally include recruitment, scheduling, discipline, and supervision of emergency care personnel.

Flight paramedics use their knowledge and skills to care for victims who require air medical evacuation and rapid transport to hospitals. A flight crew usually is composed of a pilot, a flight medic, and a flight nurse. Some organizations hire paramedics to assist with the interhospital, intercontinental, or international transfer of patients requiring monitored transportation. Responsibilities for this position generally include monitoring of patients during transport and initiation of emergency care when necessary. Additional training for specialty skills often is necessary in this role to meet the needs of high-risk infants, children, or other patients who are critically ill or injured.

Experienced paramedics with backgrounds in management can act in administrative capacities within various organizations. Although advanced training often is necessary, administrative positions in hospitals, government emergency services organizations, and independent companies are all possibilities.

Many colleges and universities offer programs in EMS, including paramedic certification programs, associate's degrees, bachelor's degrees, and even master's degrees. Paramedics with experience in education can obtain positions as instructors for such programs.

ANSWERS

1. a. Dispatcher; b. Advanced life support; c. Hospital delivery; d. Patient rehabilitation and education (Objective 2)

2. a. Physical preparation for the job (exercise program)
   b. Having appropriate equipment and supplies
   c. Responding to the scene in a safe manner
   d. Performing a quick patient assessment to form priorities for care
   e. Contacting medical direction for assistance with the care plan
   f. Managing the emergency in the appropriate manner
   g. Stabilizing the patient in the field
   h. Providing transport by the appropriate means to the correct facility
   i. Reporting to the staff regarding the patients condition on arrival
   j. Replacing equipment and debriefing the call (Objective 7)

3. a. Advocating citizens' role in the EMS system by teaching community programs such as CPR.
   b. Continuing personal professional development by attending continuing education programs (Objective 7)

4. c

5. f

6. g

7. d

8. b

9. a

10. e

11. h (Questions 4-11
    Objective 1)

12. a

13. c

14. b (Questions 12-14
    Objective 3)

15. a, b, c, d

16. c

17. a, b, c

18. b, c, d

19. a, b, c, d

20. c, d

21. c, d

22. b, c

23. b, c

24. b, c, d

25. c, d

26. a, c, d
    (Questions 15-26, Objectives 4, 5, 8, 9)

27. To determine the efficacy of IV midazolam to aid in prehospital intubations that failed conventional methods

28. No. There is no hypothesis stated. The hypothesis could have been that the use of midazolam will facilitate intubation in patients who could not be intubated by conventional means.

29. The study population are the 154 ETIs that occurred within the study period.

30. The sample were the patients who could not be intubated by conventional means (20 patients).

31. No. Random sampling was not done. All patients who met the criterion (failed intubation) were included.

32. There were descriptive statistics used to report the findings in this quantitative paper.

33. This means that about 65% of the patients received 3.6 mg $\pm$ 1.1 mg of midazolam in the successful ETI group.

34. There are many other things to consider. Here are just a few other questions that could be asked. Did the age of the patients affect the success? Were the missed patients trauma or medical and did that influence success rates? Is 20 a large enough sample size to make a broad generalization to all EMS patients? What was the experience level of the paramedics in the "success" group versus the "fail" group?

35. The use of any drug is associated with potential risks and complications. Objective data supporting the effectiveness of drugs, especially in the unique prehospital environment, support the standards and practice of paramedic care. (Questions 27-35 (Objective 10)

36. d. This act, passed in 1966, mandated states to develop effective EMS programs or lose federal construction funds. It enabled large amounts of money to be spent for development of EMS and ALS pilot programs. Accidental Death and Disability: the Neglected Disease of Modern Society (the "white" paper) was not an act but a report published by the National Academy of Science– National Research Council's Committee on Trauma and Shock. Its recommendations paved the way for the Highway Safety Act of 1966. The EMSS act of 1973 developed regional EMS organizations. It identified 15 required components of the EMS System. The Consolidated Omnibus Reconciliation Act (COBRA) eliminated federal funds for EMS and redistributed them under state block grants.
    (Objective 1)

37. b. Although insurance reimbursement is necessary for many EMS systems to operate, the insurance providers are not considered a part of the system. (Objective 2)

38. b. Patients' health plans now often restrict their choice of hospitals. Except in life-threatening emergencies, patients must seek care at their preferred provider or lose reimbursement. In some areas, this has resulted in expanded transport

areas for some EMS agencies to meet the needs for the health care consumers they serve. Generally, the health care changes have resulted in decreases rather than increases in reimbursement. (Objective 2)

39. c. Certification authorizes a person who has met specific qualifications to participate in an activity. Licensure grants a license to practice a profession. Registration is the act of enrolling a person's name in a book of record. (Objective 6)

40. b. Although this role may fall to the paramedic in some systems, it is not defined by the government as an integral role. (Objective 3)

41. b. Other personnel should assume patient care and administrative and maintenance duties. The primary role of the EMS physician medical director is to ensure quality patient care. (Objective 8)

42. a. Online medical direction should be contacted to attempt to arbitrate the situation. If this is not possible, police intervention may be recommended. Written policies addressing this issue should be prepared by the medical director so that the actions to take in this situation are clearly defined. (Objective 8)

43. a. The continuing education program can be offered to introduce new material, concepts, or skills so that appropriate patient care will be delivered when that knowledge or skill is needed. This is proactively done to ensure quality before a problem occurs. Direct observation of care is a concurrent method of CQI and review of records and tapes is done after the actual care is delivered (retrospectively). (Objective 9)

44. b. Alternative time sampling selects participants based on a predetermined time interval (day of week, month, and so on). Sampling using a statistical table involves selection of patients based on a table that predetermines which patient will be following a selected protocol. Systemic sampling enrolls patients in the order in which they are encountered. For example, it may be established that every other patient encountered gets the test intervention. (Objective 10)

45. a. 4 is the number that occurs most frequently. The mean, or average of the sum of the times is 5, as is the median, or middle of the group. (Objective 10)

46. a. Although traditional informed consent is not always possible, an acceptable alternative must be demonstrated to the IRB before approval of your project. The purpose of the research is to either prove or disprove the hypothesis; this answer will only be known after completion of the study. If there are risks associated with the research, you must demonstrate that the potential benefit of the study warrants the risk. The primary responsibility of the IRB is to consider ethical, not procedural, issues with the research. (Objective 11)

● CHAPTER 2
THE WELL-BEING OF THE PARAMEDIC

1. h
(Objective 8)
2. e
(Objective 8)
3. i
(Objective 8)
4. b
(Objective 8)
5. d
(Objective 8)
6. g
(Objective 8)
7. a. To reduce the risk of acquiring infectious disease, the paramedic should obtain appropriate immunizations, maintain good personal health and hygiene, use universal precautions during patient care (in this case, gloves and goggles/mask and gown if there is risk of splash or spray), not resheath needles, dispose of contaminated sharps in an appropriate container, wash hands thoroughly after patient care is concluded, and appropriately dispose of soiled linens, equipment, and trash.

b. To reduce the risk of injury during moving and lifting of this patient, the paramedic should maintain good physical conditioning, obtain assistance to move the patient if the size is too great for the paramedic and a partner, pay attention when walking, move forward when possible, take short steps, bend at the knees and hips, lift with the legs, keep the load close to the body, keep the patient's body in-line when moving, and use the appropriate device for the situation (for example, stair chair versus long back board).

c. To decrease the risk of injury when providing care in a hostile environment, the paramedic should coordinate activities with law enforcement, scan the area for the fastest escape route, stay alert and move the patient out of the hostile area as quickly as possible, and leave the area if the situation becomes too dangerous. The best policy is to avoid entering the situation until the police have controlled the scene.

d. To ensure maximal safety while departing this scene and transporting the patient to the hospital, the paramedic should use lights and sirens as dictated by local policy, proceed carefully through in-

tersections, and maintain due regard for the safety of others.
(Objectives 5, 11)

8. a. The pituitary gland releases adrenocorticotropic hormone, stimulating the sympathetic nervous system. b. Adrenal glands release epinephrine and norepinephrine, which c. cause a rise in blood pressure by increasing systemic vascular resistance; d. slow the digestive tract; e. dilate bronchioles, allowing deeper breathing; f. stimulate glucose production in the liver; g. dilate the pupils; and h. increase the rate and strength of the heart's contractions.
(Objective 7)

9. Good physical conditioning will permit rapid movement of the patient out of this hostile situation with decreased risk of injury to the paramedic. Good emotional health practices will facilitate use of healthy coping mechanisms to cope with the personal stressors involved on this call.
(Objective 2)

10. Situations that pose a threat to the rescuers' lives may be perceived as stressful depending on the situation and the individuals involved. Having a critically injured patient that is a close relative or acquaintance often produces a very stressful situation.
(Objective 10)

11. Individual consultation may be necessary if only one person was overwhelmed by the call. If this was perceived as very stressful by the whole group, defusing immediately after the incident, critical incident stress debriefing 24 to 72 hours after a stressful call, and follow-up services after a debriefing may be needed.
(Objective 9)

12. a. Working in hazardous situations; dealing with injured or dying children; working in an uncontrolled, unpredictable environment; dealing with emotionally upset, unpredictable clients; needing to make rapid life-and-death decisions. b. Physical illness of the self or a close family member; loss of job or a new job; personal financial troubles; death of a loved one; marital troubles, among others.
(Objective 7)

13. Irritability, apathy, chronic fatigue, feelings of not being appreciated, difficulty sleeping, drinking or drug abuse, decreased social activities, appetite changes, desire to quit work, and physical complaints.
(Objective 7)

14. Early recognition of signs and symptoms of stress, awareness of personal limitations, peer counseling, group discussions, proper diet, sleep, exercise, and pursuit of positive activities outside of EMS.
(Objective 8)

15. a. Bargaining: The mother is bargaining her life for her son's. b. Denial: The wife is denying the sever-

ity of the problem. c. Anger: The brother's anger is directed at the EMS personnel.
(Objective 10).

16. You should tell the family that the patient is critically ill and that you are going to do everything possible to help him. Remain calm and try to let the family remain close if patient care is not compromised. Assign tasks to the angry brother (for example, to stay with his mother and care for her).
(Objective 10)

17. Paramedics should be encouraged to talk about particularly distressing situations with other crew members and avail themselves of resources available through medical direction and employee assistance programs.
(Objective 8)

18. a. Yes. Use accessible sharps containers and lancet holders.
b. Yes. Wear mask, eye protection, and gown when there is a risk of splash or spray.
c. No.
d. Yes. Do not place objects in your mouth when biohazards are present.
(Objective 11)

19. a. Wash the area thoroughly.
b. Document the exposure.
c. Immediately report to the appropriate personnel.
d. Complete the medical follow-up.
(Objective 12)

20. d. Cellular function depends on a fluid environment. Amino acids are essential for body growth and cellular life and are not produced by the body. Polyunsaturated fats can help decrease high blood cholesterol levels if part of a low-fat diet.
(Objective 1)

21. b. An increase in muscle mass, metabolism, and resistance to injury should be anticipated with a carefully planned fitness program. Fitness programs can be tailored to accommodate the needs of individuals with preexisting medical conditions (e.g., arthritis, heart disease) and are encouraged.
(Objective 1)

22. b. Cigarette smoking should be eliminated to decrease the risk of heart disease. The triglyceride levels should not exceed 200 to 300 mg/dL and the LDL cholesterol should be lower than 160 mg/dL.
(Objective 4)

23. a. The other signs listed by the American Cancer Society are a sore throat, unusual bleeding or discharge, thickening or lump in the breast or elsewhere, obvious change in a wart or mole, and nagging cough or hoarseness.
(Objective 4)

24. b. Annual skin testing is an excellent measure to detect an exposure to tuberculosis so it can be appropriately treated, but it does not prevent infec-

tion. Needle recapping is never advised because this greatly increases the risk of injury and exposure. Body substance isolation measures should be used for all patients, not just those feared as high-risk.
(Objective 5)

25. a. To minimize injury risk, you should also hold the load close to your body, lift with your legs (not your back), and move forward rather than backward when possible.
(Objective 5)

26. b. Lying about using the substance indicates guilt about using the substance and is a warning sign.
(Objective 6)

27. d. Environmental stress results from factors such as siren noise and weather. Personality stress relates to the way individuals feel about themselves. Managerial stress is not a distinct entity.
(Objective 7)

28. a. *Phobias* are unrealistic fears. *Reaction formation* is a defense mechanism in which unacceptable desires are suppressed by accentuating opposite behaviors. *Stress* is a generalized response to certain situations.
(Objective 7)

29. b. *Projection* occurs when one's own undesirable feelings are attributed to someone else. *Regression* is a return to an earlier stage of emotional adjustment. *Sublimation* occurs when unacceptable urges are modified to become socially acceptable.
(Objective 7)

30. d. New paramedics may be at increased risk for high stress levels after a critical call; however, veterans are always still vulnerable to unusually stressful calls. Multiple patient situations may not always trigger stress responses in rescuers; it depends on the individual situation. A high-risk employee with psychological problems will likely require care outside of the critical incident stress debriefing program.
(Objective 9)

31. c. If the family raises the issue of death, a realistic description of the seriousness of the patient's condition should be briefly given. Direct eye contact and touch, if appropriate, may be used to convey concern and caring.
(Objective 10)

32. a. The family should watch for behavioral changes at home and at school and difficulty eating or sleeping and should encourage the child to express his or her feelings.
(Objective 10)

33. b. School-age children have begun to understand the concept of the finality of death; however, they still feel that it happens only to others.
(Objective 10)

34. c. All needle stick injuries should be reported im-

mediately so appropriate source testing and follow-up can be completed in a timely manner.
(Objective 12)

● **CHAPTER 3**
INJURY PREVENTION

1. About 42% of ED visits relate to injury.
(Objective 2)

2. In addition to the initial ED visit, other costs related to injury include lost quality of life, loss of income, and long-term hospitalizations/care.
(Objective 2)

3. EMS providers are ideally suited for educating elderly people in their community because they are welcomed into the home, viewed as experts, medically educated, considered to have the customers' best interests at heart, and may be the first to identify situations that pose a risk.
(Objectives 1, 3)

4. Injury prevention material specific to falls in the elderly would need to be obtained.
(Objective 4)

5. You will need financial support, endorsement of your agency, and possibly assistance from your boss to identify other community resources.
(Objective 4)

6. Census data should reflect the number of elderly; the area health department should have statistics on mortality and injury frequency and type; your own EMS system could provide information about the number of elderly patients transported due to fall-related injuries; and national agencies such as the CDC or National Safety Council can provide cost data and are accessible either through the Internet or the library.
(Objective 7)

7. Host: poor eyesight, impaired balance secondary to medication use, decreased sensation.
Environmental: poor lighting, loose area rugs, absence of or poorly maintained railings, icy walkways.
(Objective 8)

8. This is a primary intervention if you are conducting it on patients who have not had injuries from a fall.
(Objective 8)

9. You will need to consider the following: the cost of the materials (who will pay for it); whether someone in the community already has materials you could use (a hospital, health department); the reading level(s) of the audience: whether you need to prepare bilingual materials if you have a large group that does not read English; and the type size of the material (to accommodate clients with poor vision).
(Objective 10)

10. Host. Fatigue may cause deceased attention span in a person, which may lead to an injury.

11. Environment. The firefighter is placed into hostile environments at work, increasing his or her susceptibility to injury/illness.

12. Agent. Carbon monoxide is a poisonous gas that can cause illness/death.

13. Host. Certain diseases are more prevalent in one sex than another (e.g., rheumatoid arthritis).

14. Agent. Hepatitis is a virus that causes disease.

15. Host. Malnutrition deprives the body of essential nutrients necessary to maintain health.

16. Host. Poor personal hygiene predisposes an individual to infection.

17. Environmental. Floods may cause water contamination and an increased risk of epidemic spread of disease.

18. Agent. Excess cholesterol is associated with increased risk of heart disease.
(Questions 10-18, Objective 8)

19. c. Unintentional injuries are the top cause of death for persons between 1 and 38 years of age and the fifth leading cause of death overall.
(Objective 2)

20. b. The community usually has a high level of trust in EMS providers and will usually let them in to speak about these issues. The amount of time paramedics have in any given EMS system will depend on call volume and other commitments such as training or other departmental duties. EMS agencies do not always have financial resources but may have a community partner to fund the support materials for the program. EMS providers often have baseline knowledge about injury prevention but can be educated on specific injury prevention materials.
(Objective 3)

21. a. Ticketing people who fail to yield may be helpful but will only capture those who may have caused injury to EMS providers and/or their patients. Education is more desirable.
(Objective 4)

22. d. Penalizing personnel or forcing them to participate in an activity may be necessary but will not promote maximal participation in activities. Rewards and incentives are helpful.
(Objective 4)

23. c. Situations involving domestic violence are volatile and complicated. Measures to diffuse, rather than escalate, the situation should be employed unless there is an immediate danger to your crew, your patient, or the police.
(Objective 5)

24. b. This patient is calm and cooperative but is probably attentive to the fact that her injury could have been more serious. A few words about appropriate lighting and specific recommendations about how to accomplish that would likely be taken quite seriously at that moment. In the situation where the child was struck, calming may be a greater priority, and there is no evidence of a need to teach anything specific for him to relate to this incident. In both other answers, the patient/parent is not in an appropriate mental state to be taught.
(Objective 6)

25. a. Census data, which may be obtained over the Internet or through your library, will provide information about population demographics, including age and income levels. Your local health department can give you specific information about deaths in your community and their causes. The local paper may refer you to information sources but won't likely have specifics. The fire service has very specific call data related to fire and whether they also provide EMS and illness/injury information. The local chamber of commerce has economic data and information about industry, religious organizations, and cultural opportunities within a community.
(Objective 7)

26. a. The icy conditions undoubtedly are playing the greatest influence on the situation. The ice prevented the host from controlling the speed or direction of the sled, and it caused the crash.
(Objective 8)

27. c. The drunk-u-drama will attempt to educate students about how to prevent injuries from ever occurring. You are performing secondary interventions on the hypertensive group and the smokers—both are already known to have a condition that you are attempting to control or stop. Tertiary activities, designed to rehabilitate, would include the support group activities.
(Objective 9)

28. d. Although there are brief opportunities for teaching during an EMS call, a formal education plan wouldn't be appropriate. Your crew members may think the program is great, but the target audience may not relate to it at all. Slides are appropriate, but depending on your audience and your message, they may not be desirable or possible. For example, if your program is designed to be delivered to youth groups on a street corner, an alternative method would have to be selected.
(Objective 10)

● CHAPTER 4
MEDICAL/LEGAL ISSUES

1. c. Physical force against individuals against their will and without legal justification is battery.

2. h. Making statements about a person with malicious intent is slander.

3. f. You released information about the nurse that could cause ridicule, embarrassment, or notoriety.

4. d. Forcible restraint and confinement against one's will is false imprisonment.

5. f. Making false written statements about a person with malicious intent is libel.

6. a. Failure to appropriately turn over care of the patient to a qualified individual may be considered abandonment.
(Questions 1-6, Objective 7, 8, 14)

7. False. If a criminal law is violated, a paramedic could be charged under that statute as well. For example, EMS personnel have in the past been charged with manslaughter when someone died as a result of a vehicular collision involving the ambulance.
(Objective 2)

8. True.
(Objective 4)

9. False. The lawsuit may be filed regardless of the presence of insurance. The insurance may, however, protect the paramedic's personal assets. This is controversial; some sources will advise against carrying insurance.
(Objective 6)

10. Child abuse or neglect; elder abuse or neglect; rape; animal bites; gunshot or stab wounds.
(Objective 3)

11. Duty to act; breach of duty; damage to the patient; and proximate cause are the four elements that must be proven to win a negligence suit.
(Objective 5)

12. Duty to act: The unit was on duty and was called to care for this patient.
Breach of duty: The standard of care would have indicated immobilizing and transporting this patient; the crew failed to act as the standard of care dictated.
Damage to the patient: The patient lost movement, stopped breathing, and died after being abandoned by the paramedic crew.
Proximate cause: The patient apparently died from spinal cord damage; the paramedic crew did not immobilize and protect the C-spine, which may have prevented death.
(Objective 5)

13. The paramedic may reduce the risk of liability claims by obtaining appropriate training, delivering competent patient care, and performing thorough documentation.
(Objective 6)

14. a. Informed
b. Expressed
c. Implied
(Question 14, Objective 8)

15. You must document the following: the patient's level of consciousness (awake and alert); that you explained to the patient the risks of refusing care, including paralysis or death; that you had the patient sign a refusal form and note any witnesses; any follow-up instructions that you gave the patient; and that you told the patient to call EMS again if his condition worsens or if he changes his mind.
(Objective 9)

16. Implied consent is assumed because the patient is unconscious.
(Objective 8)

17. The absence of heart rate (ECG) strip in several leads; absence of respirations, pulse, and spontanous movement; fixed and dilated pupils; and condition of the body (specifically wounds) should be documented. Additionally, the known time that the patient was breathless and pulseless before your arrival with no care should be documented. (Objective 11)

18. a. You should take care not to cut the clothing through the bullet hole. If the clothes are removed, you should not shake them. If removed on the scene, clothes should only be given to the police. If removed in the ambulance, the clothes should be placed in a paper bag and then given to a police officer at the hospital (if possible). b. You should not touch the weapon unless it poses a danger to your crew. c. If possible, try not to step in blood on the floor. d. Carefully and objectively document your findings on the scene. Note the specific location and position of both patients and the location of the weapon. Any other unusual scene findings should also be listed. e. Your ambulance should be parked away from any obvious evidence if it does not interfere with scene safety.
(Objective 12)

19. Typically, you may override a family's wishes for specific cases where state protocols indicate that patients may be taken to specialty centers such as trauma centers, which are known to improve survival for specific injuries.
(Objective 10)

20. Unless you have proof that the bag contains drugs, you should instead note only what you specifically observed (e.g., a bag containing a white powder substance and a syringe with needle were found to the right of the patient).
(Objective 13)

21. a. Yes.
b. No. Not unless (s)he has a legitimate medical or legal reason to know the information.
c. No. Specific department regulations about information to be released to the press should be followed—they would not include all of the personal details about the case.
d. Yes. Medical direction will need to know the facts of the case for quality improvement reasons.

e. No. Only hospital staff directly involved in the patient's care should be informed of the details of the case.
(Objective 7)

22. b. Administrative law refers to regulations that are developed by a government agency to provide details about the process of the law. Criminal laws are enacted by federal, state, or local government to protect society. Legislative laws are made by legislative branches of government and are determined by statutes and constitutions.
(Objective 1)

23. a. A patient who needs continuing advanced care should not be released by a paramedic to someone with lesser training.
(Objective 2)

24. d. Criminal law violations need not involve injury or criminal intent. The patient sues for damages in civil suits. A criminal law violation is based on proof that a statute has been violated.
(Objective 1)

25. d. If you have any suspicion of elder abuse or neglect, you are obligated to report it. You should remove clothing if necessary for care. Implied consent will be indicated on this call.
(Objective 3)

26. c. The Ryan White Comprehensive AIDS Resources Emergency Act of 1990 (PL 101-381) describes reporting requirements for hospitals to EMS providers who have been exposed to certain communicable diseases and lists other organizational responsibilities for infectious disease reporting.
(Objective 4)

27. c. The patient suffered damage as evidenced by the long hospitalization. This could result in loss of income if the person was employed. This was more likely a breach of duty or nonfeasance (failure to perform a required act or duty) than malfeasance (performing a wrongful or unlawful act). Although the potential exists that the paramedic's actions violated EMS law, the failure to provide standard of care is usually not legislated.
(Objective 5)

28. c. Privileged patient information should never be given to personnel with no legal right to know it.
(Objective 7)

29. a. Implied consent permits a paramedic to render lifesaving care if the patient is unable to agree because of a lack of mental competence. Informed consent means that the patient has been told the implications of the injury and illness, the treatment needed, and potential complications. Referred consent does not exist.
(Objective 8)

30. b. You should ask the patient to sign a refusal of care form; however, if he refuses, document his refusal and witness it. Be sure to advise the patient about further care for his condition. If he is awake and alert now, he may legally refuse transport.
(Objective 9)

31. d. EMS agencies are typically permitted to travel moderately faster (often 10 mph) than regular traffic; however, excessive speed is hazardous. Crews should slow down or stop until certain that traffic has stopped, and proceed cautiously though intersections. Traffic officers' instructions should be followed. If a dispute occurs, chief officers should be contacted immediately.
(Objective 10)

32. a. In most cases, a written rather than verbal do-not-resuscitate order is required to stop resuscitation. If airway or IV access can't be established, resuscitation efforts should not be terminated in the field. In some cases, specific time limitations on stopping resuscitation may be made—these should be done cooperatively with medical direction and are usually used only with very long transports. (Objective 11)

33. d. Do not cut through the stab hole. Do not give clothing to bystanders except authorized law enforcement. Do not move the knife unless it is essential for crew safety.
(Objective 12)

34. d. The patient care report should be as detailed as possible to paint a picture of the clinical findings and care given.
(Objective 13)

● **CHAPTER 5**
ETHICS

1. b
(Objective 4)
2. e
(Objective 1)
3. f
(Objective 4)
4. a
(Objective 4)
5. c
(Objective 4)
6. d
(Objective 1)
7. a. You can disclose nothing specific about the patient's injuries, except what is permitted by departmental policy (usually a condition report).
   b. Your feelings about whether this is ethical will be personal.
8. Your legal obligation would not change, regardless of your decision.
9. Your legal obligation will prevent you from disclosing information.
(Questions 7-9, Objective 2)

10. a. Legal (theft), professional, and moral conflicts may come into play here.
b. Professional and moral conflicts may be involved as you make a decision about how to respond to this situation.
c. Legal (working/driving while under the influence), professional, and moral standards are involved in the paramedic's actions and in your response to them.
d. Professional and moral issues are involved in this situation.
e. Legal (theft of equipment), professional (actions without medical direction), and moral (allocation of resources) issues are involved in this situation.
(Objective 2)

11. The answers to each of these questions are personal. Discuss your answers with a fellow student. How do your views compare?
(Objective 3)

12. a. Physician extender: possible actions: Clarify and repeat request for orders. Ask for a call review/critique to discuss the issue.
b. Consent: possible actions: Have on-line medical direction speak to the patient. Talk to the family to see if they can convince the patient. If not, provide detailed follow-up instructions, and try to leave the patient in the supervised care of family or friends.
c. Allocation of resources: possible actions: Reevaluate the resources to determine if resuscitation should proceed; ask for change of assignment if possible.
d. Decisions surrounding resuscitation: possible actions: Contact medical direction. Remove the family from the area and calmly explain the wishes of their loved one.
(Objectives 3, 4, 5)

13. b. Certification is a professional standard. Laws are legal standards. Morals are social standards.
(Objective 1)

14. b. Laws and regulations relate to legal accountability. Professional licensure and standards relate to education, and skills relate to professional accountability.
(Objective 2)

15. b. This is known as the impartiality test.
(Objective 3)

16. b. This is known as the universalizability test.
(Objective 3)

17. a. The impartiality test can correct partiality or personal bias. The second test, the universalizability test, helps eliminate moral decision difficulty. The third test, the interpersonal justifiability test, requires reasons for your actions and approval from others of those reasons.
(Objective 4)

18. c. If the family concurs and the living will is legal, there is no ethical question. If the patient has obvious signs of death, there is no ethical dilemma. If the living will document cannot be produced, legally it cannot be recognized.
(Objective 5)

19. d. Allocation of resources is an issue when the health care needs of the patient can't be met because of inadequate resources. Autonomy is a person's ability to make decisions. Care in futile situations arises when the care you are about to give serves no purpose.
(Objective 6)

● CHAPTER 6
OVERVIEW OF HUMAN SYSTEMS

1. d
(Objective 8)

2. c
(Objective 8)

3. f
(Objective 8)

4. b
(Objective 8)

5. e
(Objective 8)

6. h
(Objective 8)

7. i
(Objective 8)

8. g
(Objective 8)

9. a. centrioles b. ribosomes c. Golgi apparatus d. nucleus e. endoplasmic reticulum f. lysosome g. mitochondrion
(Objective 8)

10. False. Some cells, such as those of the nervous system, divide only until birth.
(Objective 9)

11. Person standing erect with palms and feet facing the examiner
(Objective 2)

12. a. Distal; b. lateral; c. superior; d. ventral
(Objective 3)

13. a. Extremities and their girdles; b. head, neck, thorax, and abdomen
(Objective 4)

14. Horizontally through the umbilicus and vertically from the xiphoid process through the symphysis pubis
(Objective 5)

15. You initially found the patient in the right lateral recumbent position.
(Objective 3)

16. a. Burn 1 is inferior and lateral to the left eye
b. Burn 2 is inferior to the mouth

c. Burn 3 is superior and lateral to the right nipple

d. Burn 4 is on the dorsal aspect (or palmar surface) of the hand

e. Burn 5 is inferior to the axilla

f. Burns 6 and 7 are on the medial aspect of both thighs

17. Burn 5 encroaches on the left upper quadrant of the abdomen.
(Objective 5)

18. a. Burn 3 overlies the thoracic cavity.
b. Burn 5 overlies the thoracic and abdominal cavities.

19. The wounds affect both axial and appendicular regions of the body.
(Objective 4)

20. Conduction of action potentials

Subgroup	Type	Body Area	Function
Striated voluntary	Muscle	Skeletal muscle	Movement of bones
Bone	Connective	Bones of body	Support and protection
Epithelium	Epithelial	Skin, glands	Protection, lining of body cavities
Adipose	Connective	Subcutaneous tissue	Insulation, protection, storage of energy
Hemopoietic	Connective	Marrow cavities, spleen, tonsils	Formation of blood and lymph cells
Striated involuntary	Muscle	Cardiac muscle	Contraction of heart
Neurons	Nervous	Nervous system	Conduction of action potentials
Cartilage	Connective	Articulating surface	Smooth movement of bones, ear, nose
Areolar	Connective	Around organs, under skin	Cushioning and affixing
Nonstriated involuntary	Muscle	Smooth muscle of viscera	Vegetative muscle functions
Neuroglia	Nervous	Nervous system	Support cells, nourishment, protection, insulation

(Objective 10)

21. Integumentary, skeletal, muscular, nervous, endocrine, circulatory, lymphatic, respiratory, digestive, urinary, and reproductive
(Objective 11)

22.

Structure	Function
Epidermis	Barrier against infection, protection, prevention of fluid loss
Dermis	Sense organ containing sweat glands
Subcutaneous	Insulation, storage of energy, shock layer, absorption

(Objective 11)

23. Lubrication to prevent drying, excretion of water and wastes, and temperature regulation
(Objective 11)

24. Decreased ability to perceive pain, decreased ability to regulate temperature, and decreased ability to preserve body fluids
(Objective 11)

25. a. Parietal; b. temporal; c. frontal; d. occipital; e. sphenoid; f. ethmoid; g. maxilla; h. mandible; i. zygomatic; j. nasal; k. lacrimal (Objective 11)

26. a. Cervical (7); b. thoracic (12); c. lumbar (5); d. sacrum (1 fused); e. coccyx (1 fused)
(Objective 11)

27. Protection for the organs of the thorax (and some abdominal organs) and maintenance of lung inflation
(Objective 11)

28. a. Manubrium; b. body; c. sternum; d. xiphoid process; e. jugular notch; f. sternal angle
(Objective 11)

29. Injury to underlying organs, impaired ventilation, and blood loss
(Objective 11)

30. a. Scapula; b. clavicle; c. attach the upper extremity to the axial skeleton; d. sternoclavicular joint
(Objective 11)

31. a. Humerus; b. head; c. greater tubercule; d. radius; e. ulna; f. trochlea; g. medial epicondyle; h. lateral epicondyle; i. olecranon; j. styloid process; k. radial tuberosity; l. carpals; m. metacarpals
(Objective 11)

32. a. Obturator foramen; b. ilium; c. ischium; d. pubis; e. anterior superior iliac spine
(Objective 11)

33. Protection of the pelvic organs and point of attachment for the lower extremity to axial skeleton
(Objective 11)

34. a. Neck; b. head; c. shaft; d. greater trochanter; e. lesser trochanter; f. medial condyle; g. lateral condyle; h. medial epicondyle; i. lateral epicondyle; j. tibia; k. fibula; l. tibial tuberosity; m.

head of fibula; n. lateral malleolus; o. tarsal bones; p. metatarsals; q. phalanges
(Objective 11)

35. a. Fibrous, cartilaginous, synovial; b. little or no; c. skull; d. radius, ulna; e. teeth, mandible (or maxilla); f. sternum; g. sternal angle; h. symphysis pubis; i. intervertebral disks; j. synovial fluid; k. plane (or gliding); l. saddle joints; m. hinge; n. pivot; o. ball and socket; p. ellipsoid
(Objective 11)

36. a. Supinate (supination) or pronate (pronation); b. opposition; c. flexion and extension; d. rotation; e. abduction; f. adduction; g. inversion or eversion; h. excursion; i. depression
(Objective 11)

37. Movement, muscle tone, and heat production
(Objective 11)

38. a. Muscle fibers; b. myofilaments; c. actin, myosin; d. sarcomere; e. ATP
(Objective 11)

39. a. Isometric muscle contraction maintains constant length of the muscles in the body. b. During an isotonic contraction, the amount of muscle tension is constant, but the length of the muscle changes, causing movement of a body part. c. Muscle tone is the constant tension of muscles responsible for posture and balance.
(Objective 11)

40. Excess energy from adenosine triphosphate in a muscle contraction is released as heat. If the body temperature falls below a certain level, muscles begin shivering, which can increase heat production up to 18 times the normal resting level.
(Objective 11)

41. Regulation and coordination of the body to maintain homeostasis
(Objective 11)

42. a. Brain and spinal cord; b. nerves and ganglia
(Objective 11)

43. The somatic division transmits impulses from the central nervous system to skeletal muscle, and the autonomic division transmits impulses from the central nervous system to smooth muscle, cardiac muscle, and certain glands.
(Objective 11)

44. a. Cerebral cortex; b. midbrain; c. pons; d. cerebellum; e. medulla; f. thalamus; g. hypothalamus
(Objective 11)

45. a. Is conduction pathway for ascending and descending nerve tracts; regulates heart rate, blood vessel diameter, breathing, swallowing, vomiting, coughing, and sneezing. b. Ascending and descending nerve tracts pass through and relay information from cerebrum to cerebellum and sleep and respiratory center. c. Involved in hearing and visual reflexes, regulates some automatic

functions such as muscle tone. d. Important for arousal and consciousness, sleep/wake cycle. e. Temperature regulation, water balance, sleep-cycle control, appetite, sexual arousal. f. Relays information from sense organs to cerebral cortex, influences mood.
(Objective 11)

46. a. Frontal lobe: voluntary motor function; motivation, aggression, and mood. b. Temporal lobe: olfactory and auditory input; memory. c. Parietal lobe: reception and evaluation of sensory information (except smell, hearing, and vision). d. Occipital lobe: reception and integration of visual input.
(Objective 11)

47. Coordination; balance; and smooth, flowing movement
(Objective 11)

48. Reflex center and transmits impulses to and from the brain and the rest of the body
(Objective 11)

49. a. Brain, spinal cord; b. choroid plexus
(Objective 11)

50. Sensory, somatomotor and proprioception, and parasympathetic
(Objective 11)

51. Affected

Affected Organ	Sympathetic	Parasympathetic
Heart	Increased rate, contractility, and electrical conduction speed	Decreased rate and contractility
Lungs	Bronchodilation	Bronchoconstriction
Pupils	Dilation	Constriction
Intestine	Decreased peristalsis	Increased peristalsis
Blood vessels	Constriction	No effect

(Objective 11)

52. Coordinates with the nervous system to regulate and control multiple body functions, including metabolic activities and body chemistry
(Objective 11)

53.

Hormone	Target Tissue	Action
Epinephrine	Heart, blood vessels, liver	Increased heart rate, contractility, increased blood to heart, release of glucose and fatty acids into blood
	Lungs	Bronchodilation
Aldosterone	Kidneys	Regulates water and electrolyte balance

Antidiuretic	Kidney	Stimulates water retention by kidneys
Parathyroid	Bone, kidney	Increases bone breakdown, helps maintain blood Ca^{++} levels
Calcitonin	Bone	Decreased breakdown of bone, maintenance of blood calcium levels
Insulin	Liver	Promotes glucose entry into cells
Glucagon	Liver	Increases blood glucose by glycogenolysis
Testosterone	Most cells	Male sex characteristics, behavior, spermatogenesis
Thymosin	Immune tissues	Development of immune system
Oxytocin	Uterus, mammary gland	Uterine contractions, milk expulsion from breasts
Thyroid	Most cells	Increased metabolic rate

(Objective 11)

54. Hormones are secreted into blood and travel to all tissues of the body but only act on the target tissues. (Objective 11)

55. Transports nutrients, carries hormones, transports wastes, regulates temperature and fluid balance, and provides protection from bacteria (Objective 11)

56. a. erythrocytes; b. hemoglobin; c. oxygen; d. carbon dioxide; e. leukocytes; f. thrombocytes; g. defense; h. clots; i. plasma (Objective 11)

57. a. septum; b. right atrium; c. tricuspid valve; d. right ventricle; e. pulmonic valve; f. pulmonary arteries; g. pulmonary veins; h. left atrium; i. mitral or bicuspid valve; j. left ventricle; k. aortic valve; l. aorta (Objective 11)

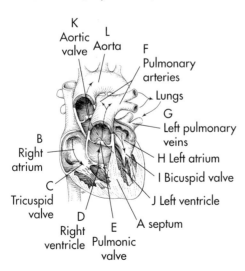

58. Aorta, smaller arteries, arterioles, capillaries, venules, veins, venae cavae, and right atrium (Objective 11)

59. Blood vessels have smooth muscle walls that give them the ability to dilate, which increases their diameter; or to constrict, which decreases their diameter. This allows blood flow to be directed away from less vital organs to the heart and brain during emergencies. (Objective 11)

60. Many veins, especially in the lower extremities, have valves that prevent the backflow of blood in this low-pressure system. (Objective 11)

61. The arteriovenous shunt can selectively allow blood to bypass the capillaries. This is useful to help maintain body temperature. (Objective 11)

62. Maintains tissue fluid balance, absorbs fats and other substances from the digestive tract, and enhances the body's defense system. (Objective 11)

63. Lymph is gathered from the tissues by lymph capillaries that have one-way valves to prevent the backflow of lymph into tissues. It flows to larger lymph capillaries that resemble veins. Then it passes through the lymph nodes (in the groin, axilla, and neck), where microorganisms and foreign substances are removed. The lymph vessels meet to enter the right or left subclavian vein, where the lymph reenters the blood. (Objective 11)

64. a. Epiglottis: protection of lower airway; b. conchae and turbinates: warming and filtering of air; c. eustachian and auditory tube: joining of nasopharynx to ear; d. sinuses: production of sound and mucus; e. hard palate: separation of oropharynx from sinuses; f. soft palate: prevents food from entering nasal cavities. (Objective 11)

65. a. Epiglottis; b. thyroid cartilage or Adam's apple; c. cricoid cartilage; d. hyoid bone; e. vocal folds. (Objective 11)

66. a. Trachea; b. bronchi; c. alveoli; d. carina (Objective 11)

67. Cartilage rings maintain patency of the airway. Goblet cells in the ciliated epithelium of the trachea sweep mucus, bacteria, and other small particles toward the larynx. (Objective 11)

68. The small bronchioles are surrounded by smooth muscle. Irritants cause constriction of that muscle, the airway size decreases, and a wheeze is produced as air is forced through a very tight airway. (Objective 11)

69. a. Alveoli are only one cell thick, which easily permits diffusion of gases from within them into the pulmonary capillaries. b. Pulmonary surfactant decreases the surface tension within the alveoli, which inhibits collapse of the alveoli. (Objective 11)

70. The base of the lungs rests on the diaphragm; the apex extends to a point 2.5 cm superior to the clavicles. (Objective 11)

71. a. Three lobes further divided into 10 lobules; b. Two lobes further divided into 9 lobules. (Objective 11)

72. a. A potential space that forms a vacuum and causes the lung to adhere to the chest wall and remain expanded. b. A lubricant that allows the pleural membranes to slide across one another and helps the visceral and parietal pleurae to adhere to one another. (Objective 11)

73. Provides the body with water, nutrients, and electrolytes (Objective 11)

74.

Digestive Juice	Function
Salivary amylase	Begins digestion of carbohydrates
Hydrochloric acid, mucus	Produces chyme (intrinsic factor, gastrin, semisolid mixture), pepsinogen
Amylase, sodium bicarbonate	Neutralizes stomach acid, continues digestion
Bile	Dilutes stomach acid, emulsifies fat
Mucus	Aids movement of feces

(Objective 11)

75. Removes wastes from the body and helps maintain normal body fluid volume and composition (Objective 11)

76. Control of red blood cell production and vitamin D metabolism (Objective 11)

77. a. Nephron; b. filtration; c. reabsorption; d. secretion (Objective 11)

78. a. Decreases; b. increases; c. increases; d. decreases (Objective 11)

79. a. Testis; b. epididymis; c. ductus deferens and vas deferens; d. urethra; e. seminal vesicles; f. prostate gland; g. bulbourethral glands; h. scrotum; i. penis (Objective 11)

80. a. Ovary; b. fallopian tube; c. uterine body; d. fundus; e. cervix; f. vagina (Objective 11)

81. a. Vagina; b. urethra; c. labia minora; d. labia majora; e. clitoris; f. clinical perineum; g. anus (Objective 11)

82. a. Nasal; b. olfactory tract; c. thalamic; d. olfactory (Objective 12)

83. a. Taste buds; b. tongue; c. palate, lips, throat; d. sweet, sour, bitter, salt (Objective 12)

84. a. Optic ; b. oculomotor; c. cornea; d. iris; e. rods; f. cones; g. aqueous; h. vitreous; i. intraocular pressure (Objective 12)

85. a. Shade eyes from direct sun and prevent perspiration from entering eyes; b. protect against foreign objects; c. moisten the eye, lubricate the eyelids, and wash away foreign objects (Objective 12)

86. a. Hearing; b. hearing, balance; c. vestibulocochlear; d. pinna; e. auditory; f. tympanic membrane; g. incus, stapes, malleus; h. organ of Corti; i. vestibule; j. semicircular canals (Objective 12)

87. d. The anatomical position is standing erect with palms forward. A person lying in the lateral recumbent position is reclining on the right or left side. The prone position refers to a patient who is lying on the stomach. (Objective 2)

88. d. The liver and gallbladder are located in the right upper quadrant, and the appendix is in the right lower quadrant. (Objective 5)

89. d. The lungs are found in the thoracic cavity, and the diaphragm separates the thoracic cavity from the abdominal cavity. The thyroid gland is found in the neck. (Objective 7)

90. b. Striated voluntary muscle is skeletal muscle, and nonstriated involuntary muscles are found in the viscera. Nonstriated muscles are always involuntary. (Objective 10)

91. c. A dendrite is a component of the neuron. Neuroglia are types of nerve cells that support the cells in the nervous system. Synapses are the gaps or spaces between nerve cells or effector tissues. (Objective 10)

92. d. Lymph is collected by the lymphatic system and drains into the circulatory system. Movement is a function of the musculoskeletal system. Vitamin C is ingested by food sources. A form of vitamin D is produced in the skin when exposed to light. (Objective 11)

93. a (Objective 4)

94. b. The lateral malleolus is on the outside of the ankle, the olecranon is at the elbow, and the patella is over the knee. (Objective 3)

95. b. Actin and myosin are the actual myofilaments (thin, threadlike structures) that pull together to cause movement. A sarcomere is the contractile unit that contains actin and myosin. (Objective 10)

96. d. The other actions described are attributed to the occipital lobe (a), temporal lobe (b), and parietal lobe (c). (Objective 11)

97. b. (Objective 11)

98. d. The layers from innermost to outermost are

pia, arachnoid, and dura. The choroid plexus is where the cerebral spinal fluid is manufactured. (Objective 11)

99. b. (Objective 11)
100. a. Immunoglobulins are antibodies, leukocytes are white blood cells, and platelets are cell fragments that aid in hemostasis. (Objective 11)
101. a. Pulmonary arteries carry deoxygenated blood from the heart to the lungs. Pulmonary veins carry oxygenated blood from the lungs to the heart, and the vena cava carries blood from the systemic circulation to the heart. (Objective 11)
102. d. Sinoatrial node impulses travel to the atrioventricular node, the bundle of His, and then to the Purkinje fibers. (Objective 11)
103. d. (Objective 11)
104. a. (Objective 11)
105. a. The trachea and bronchus convey air to the alveoli. The capillary is not part of the respiratory system. (Objective 11)
106. d. Absorption occurs in the other areas of the small intestine (duodenum and ileum) and to a much lesser extent in the colon; however, the primary site of absorption is the jejunum. (Objective 11)
107. c. (Objective 11)
108. c. Roughly 180 L/day is filtered from the glomerulus; however, all but approximately 2 L/day is reabsorbed into the blood. Potassium and ammonia are secreted from the blood into the urine. (Objective 11)
109. a. Glucagon promotes conversion of glycogen stored in the liver back to glucose. Oxytocin is a female sex hormone that stimulates uterine contractions and plays a role in lactation. Testosterone is the male sex hormone responsible for male sexual characteristics. (Objective 11)
110. d. Final maturation (but not production) of the sperm occurs in the epididymis. The prostate and seminal vesicle produce seminal fluid. (Objective 11)
111. d. (Objective 12)
112. b. The organ of Corti lies within the cochlea. The semicircular canals and vestibule are involved in balance. (Objective 12)

● CHAPTER 7
GENERAL PRINCIPLES OF
PATHOPHYSIOLOGY

1. a
2. g
3. f
4. e
5. c
6. d
(Questions 1-6, Objective 7)

7. a. Extracellular; b. interstitial; c. intracellular (Objective 1)
8. PO_4, phosphate, anion, intracellular; K+, potassium, cation, intracellular; Na+, sodium, cation, extracellular; HCO_3^-, bicarbonate, anion, extracellular; Mg++, magnesium, cation, intracellular; Cl−, chloride, anion, extracellular (Objective 1)
9. a. The property of a cell membrane that freely permits the passage of water but selectively allows the passage of solute particles. This permits the cell to maintain a relatively constant internal environment. b. A passive process that allows molecules or ions to move from an area of higher concentration to an area of lower concentration in an attempt to achieve a state of equilibrium. c. A situation in which the solute concentration is greater at one point than another in a solvent. Solutes diffuse from the area of high concentration to the area of lower concentration until equilibrium is achieved. d. The diffusion of water across a selectively permeable membrane from an area of higher water concentration to an area of lower water concentration. e. A rapid, carrier-mediated process that can move a substance across a selectively permeable membrane from an area of low concentration to an area of high concentration. This process requires energy. f. A carrier-mediated process (faster than diffusion) that can move a substance from an area of higher concentration to an area of lower concentration. This process does not require energy. (Objective 1)
10. a. Overhydration: fluid restriction, intravenous normal saline to keep the vein open
b. Hypokalemia: lactated Ringer's solution intravenously to keep the vein open, preparation to assist ventilations, and high-flow oxygen. In-hospital treatment may include administration of oral or IV potassium.
c. Hypocalcemia: possible calcium ions (calcium chloride) intravenously, airway management, seizure precautions, anticonvulsant therapy intravenously.
d. Isotonic dehydration: evaluation of the airway, breathing, and circulation; assessment for shock, intravenous therapy with an isotonic solution.
e. Hyponatremic dehydration: evaluation of the effectiveness of ventilations, high-flow oxygen, intravenous therapy with lactated Ringer's solution or normal saline, and evaluation of vital signs. Occasionally hypertonic saline may be adminstered.
f. Hypermagnesemia: open airway, assistance with ventilations as necessary, high-flow oxygen, evaluation of vital signs, intravenous line with normal saline to keep the vein open, possible in-

travenous administration of calcium salts. The most effective treatment is hemodialysis.
(Objective 2)

11. a. Buffers produce an immediate response to changes in pH. They represent the body's ability to adjust the concentration of bicarbonate and carbon dioxide in the blood to maintain a relationship of 1 mEq of carbonic acid to 20 mEq of base bicarbonate. If this relationship can be maintained, hydrogen ion concentration will be within normal limits.

b. The respiratory system can increase alveolar ventilation within minutes in response to an increase in hydrogen ion concentration. Hydrogen ions combine with bicarbonate to form carbonic acid, which in turn breaks down into carbon dioxide and water. Therefore by increasing the amount of carbon dioxide that the body eliminates, the process can be accelerated and hydrogen ion concentration reduced.

c. The renal system takes hours to days to act. It restores normal pH by reabsorbing or excreting bicarbonate or hydrogen ions.
(Objective 4)

12. a. Respiratory alkalosis: Treat cause of underlying hyperventilation.

b. Metabolic alkalosis: Initiate intravenous lactated Ringer's solution or normal saline.

c. Metabolic acidosis: Initiate intravenous administration of normal saline.

d. Respiratory acidosis: Assist ventilations.
(Objectives 5, 6)

13. a. Abnormal: Acidosis due to increased P_{CO_2}: Increase ventilations. b. Abnormal: Increase amount of oxygen delivery to patient. c. Abnormal: Increase rate of ventilations.
(Objective 6)

14.

Adaptation	Cause	Effect on Cells	Example
Atrophy	Diminished function, inadequate hormonal or nervous stimulation, reduced blood supply	Decrease or shrinkage in cellular size	Muscle size shrinks in a cast or from neuro-muscular disease; brain atrophy in old age
Dysplasia	Chronic irritation or inflamma-tion	Abnormal changes of mature cells	Precancer-ous changes of the cervix or lungs
Hyperplasia	Response to an increase in demand	Increase in the number of cells in a tissue or organ	Callus or endome-trial hyperpla-sia
Hypertrophy	Results from an increased demand for work by a cell	Increase in the size (not number) of cells	Large muscles of a body builder or enlarged heart or kidneys
Metaplasia	Cellular adaptation to adverse conditions	Conversion or replace-ment of normal cells by other cells	Bronchial metapla-sia secondary to cigarette smoke

(Objective 7)

15.

Disease	Factor	Environmental or Genetic
Stroke	Hypertension, high cholesterol, smoking	Environmental
Cervical cancer	Infection with gonorrhea	Environmental
Oral cancer	Chewing smokeless tobacco	Environmental
Melanoma (skin cancer)	Excessive exposure to sun	Environmental
Depression	Familial tendency	Genetic
	Metabolic disturbance, drug reaction, nutritional disorder, situational crisis	Environmental

(Objective 9)

16. a. Muscle is lost; therefore contractility and stroke volume decrease, lowering the cardiac output.

b. The additional fluid volume improves the preload, thereby increasing stroke volume and cardiac output.

c. A sudden drop in the heart rate results in a decrease in cardiac output.

d. Fear and anxiety cause the heart rate and stroke volume to accelerate, increasing cardiac output.
(Objective 10)

17. a. The vasoconstrictor center of the medulla is inhibited, and the vagal center is excited, resulting in peripheral vasodilation and a decrease in heart rate and the strength of contraction. This results in a decrease in blood pressure.

b. Vagal stimulation is reduced, resulting in a sympathetic response that causes increased peripheral vasoconstriction, heart rate, and strength of contraction. This results in an increase in blood pressure.

(Objective 10)

18. a. The low pressure results in a decrease in oxygen to the chemoreceptor cells, which in turn stimulates the vasomotor center of the medulla. This results in peripheral vasoconstriction.

b. Chemoreceptors are also stimulated by an increase in P_{CO_2}, which causes vasoconstriction and increased blood flow to the lungs, enhancing their ability to eliminate carbon dioxide.

(Objective 10)

19. The central nervous system ischemic response is initiated when the blood pressure drops below 50 mm Hg and causes intense vasoconstriction in an attempt to improve perfusion to the brain. If the ischemia lasts longer than 10 minutes, the vagal center may be activated, resulting in peripheral vasodilation and bradycardia.

(Objective 10)

20. a. Increased sympathetic stimulation causes the adrenal medulla to release epinephrine and norepinephrine, which results in increased heart rate, stroke volume, and vasoconstriction.

b. Low flow to the kidneys results in a release of renin, which by a series of chemical reactions causes plasma proteins to synthesize angiotensin II. Angiotensin II causes vasoconstriction and initiates the release of aldosterone. Aldosterone causes increased retention of sodium and water by the kidneys.

c. The hypothalamic neurons are stimulated by a drop in blood pressure or an increase in plasma solutes, and the secretion of antidiuretic hormone (vasopressin) is increased. This results in vasoconstriction and a decrease in the rate of urine production.

(Objective 10)

21. a. Vascular endothelial

b. Endotoxins, inflammatory mediators

c. Endothelium

d. Permeable

e. Interstitial

f. Hypotension, hypoperfusion

g. Complement, coagulation, kallikrein/kinin

h. Coagulation

i. Thrombus

j. Systemic vascular resistance

k. Edema

l. Cardiovascular instability

m. Clotting abnormalities

n. Cellular acidosis, impaired cellular function

o. Organ

(Objective 10)

22.

Sign or Symptom	Local or Systemic Response	Cause
Edematous throat	Local	Cellular accumulation of sodium causes edema. Also, hyperemia increases filtration pressure and capillary permeability, causing fluid to leak into interstitial spaces.
Purulent drainage	Local	Bacteria is destroyed by phagocytosis. Then macrophages clear and destroy tissues of dead cells. Destruction of leukocytes is initiated by phagocytosis. Dead tissues plus dead leukocytes plus fluid leaking in area form pus.
Fever	Systemic	Mast cell degranulation, increased metabolic rate due to inflammatory process.
Red throat	Local	Dilatation of arterioles, venules, and capillaries in area of cellular injury.
Difficulty swallowing	Local	Secondary to the edema described above.

(Objective 11)

23. a. O positive, O negative, A positive, A negative; b. O negative; c. O positive, O negative, A positive, A negative, B positive, B negative, AB positive, AB negative; d. O negative, B negative

(Objective 11)

24. a. Isoimmunity. The body is reacting to beneficial foreign cells.

b. Allergy. The body is responding to the introduction of a foreign protein (antigen) that it recognizes as harmful.

c. Isoimmunity. The body rejects helpful foreign tissue that it "sees" as harmful.

d. Allergy. The body may be reacting to the protein (antigen) in the latex.

e. Autoimmunity. It is thought that systemic lupus erythematosus and other diseases such as dermatomyositis, periarteritis nodosa, scleroderma, and rheumatoid arthritis may be caused by an autoimmune response.[1]

(Objective 12)

25. b. Prolonged emotional or psychological stress can result in physical illness.

[1]Glanze WD, Anderson KN, Anderson LE: *Mosby's medical nursing and allied health dictionary*, ed 3, St Louis, 1990, Mosby.

389

26. d. Patients undergoing chemotherapy or radiation therapy for cancer may experience significant suppression of the immune system.
27. e. Severe deficits in calorie or protein intake can seriously impair the immune system.
28. a. The human immunodeficiency virus (HIV) attacks the immune system, making the body easy prey for opportunistic infections and malignancies. (Questions 25-28, Objective 12)
29. a. Cortisol
    b. Vasoconstriction
    c. Heart
    d. Beta-2 receptors
30. a. Diffusion is a passive process involving the movement of molecules from an area of high concentration to an area of lower concentration. Facilitated diffusion uses a carrier molecule to move molecules rapidly down a concentration gradient. Osmosis is a process that causes the movement of fluid from an area of low solute concentration to an area of high solute concentration.
    (Objective 1)
31. c. All others are found chiefly in the extracellular fluid.
    (Objective 1)
32. d. *Atonic* means without tone. A hypertonic solution has a greater solute concentration than the cells, whereas a hypotonic solution is less concentrated than the cells.
    (Objective 1)
33. c. The capillary hydrostatic pressure filters fluid from the blood through the capillary wall. Oncotic pressure exerted by blood plasma proteins attracts fluid from the interstitial space into the blood. The lymph channels open and collect some of the fluid forced out of the capillaries by hydrostatic pressure and return it to the circulation.
    (Objective 2)
34. c. Hypernatremic dehydration is associated with excessive intake of sodium exceeding sodium losses. Hyponatremia dehydration typically presents with cramps; seizures; rapid, thready pulse; diaphoresis; and/or cyanosis. There is no classification of osmotic dehydration.
    (Objective 3)
35. b. A patient in renal failure is frequently hypocalcemic, not hypercalcemic.
    (Objective 2)
36. d.
    (Objective 2)
37. c. Both hydrogen and carbon dioxide bind to hemoglobin, which then carries them to the lungs for exhalation.
    (Objective 4)
38. c. Ventilation (due to decreased tidal volume) is frequently severely decreased in these patients. This inhibits the excretion of carbon dioxide from the lungs, causing increased carbonic acid levels and a decreased pH.
    (Objective 5)
39. b. Lactic acid decreases the peripheral response to catecholamines and can cause severe hypotension.
    (Objective 5)
40. c. A decreased pH and increased P_{CO_2} are signs of respiratory acidosis. An increased pH and decreased P_{CO_2} are signs of respiratory alkalosis. An increased pH and increased P_{CO_2} are signs of metabolic alkalosis.
    (Objective 6)
41. a. The decrease in cell size secondary to atrophy of brain cells causes the size of the brain to decrease. *Dysplasia* is an abnormal change of a mature cell. *Metaplasia* is the substitution of one cell type for another. *Hypertrophy* is an increase in cell size that results in an increase in organ size.
    (Objective 7)
42. a. *MODS* is the progressive failure of two or more organ systems secondary to severe illness or injury. *Necrosis* refers to the cellular changes that occur after local cell death. *Osmosis* is the movement of water across a semipermeable membrane.
    (Objective 7)
43. d. Sodium rushes into the injured cells, increasing the osmotic pressure, which draws more water into the cell.
    (Objective 8)
44. d. Tachycardia and pupil dilation are sympathetic responses but are not secondary to vasoconstriction. The container size should decrease because of vasoconstriction.
    (Objective 10)
45. d. When blood flow to the vasomotor center of the medulla is reduced to the point of ischemia, this response initiates profound vasoconstriction.
    (Objective 10)
46. b. All other mechanisms decrease urinary output to conserve blood volume.
    (Objective 10)
47. b. If sufficient cardiac muscle is destroyed in myocardial infarction, the stroke volume and therefore the cardiac output can be markedly decreased. Anaphylactic shock occurs secondary to exposure of a sensitized individual to an allergen, resulting in dyspnea, wheezing, shock, urticaria, erythema, angioedema, and other dramatic signs and symptoms. Septic shock occurs secondary to a bacterial infection that releases harmful endotoxins.
    (Objective 10)
48. a. Feline leukemia virus is a disease to which humans have a natural immunity. Acquired immunity will occur after immunization for measles and after having chicken pox (for most patients). Temporary acquired immunity will be conferred if

hepatitis B immune globulin is administered, but the vaccination is needed to ensure acquired long-term immunity.
(Objective 11)

49. c. Hypersensitivity may occur secondary to foreign antigens (allergy, isoimmune reactions) or in the case of autoimmunity, when the body attacks its own tissues. The response may be immediate or delayed up to several days. Hypersensitivity represents an abnormal immune response.
(Objective 12)

50. a. Dopamine exerts effects on the blood vessels. It causes renal and mesenteric dilation at low levels, beta effects at mid-range levels, and strong alpha stimulation at high levels. Epinephrine stimulates alpha and beta cells, causing increased heart rate and contractility and bronchiolar dilation; it also increases blood glucose by glycogenolysis. It does not suppress white blood cells as cortisol does. Norepinephrine exerts similar effects of epinephrine; however, its alpha effects predominate.
(Objective 13)

● **CHAPTER 8**
PHARMACOLOGY

1. h
2. b
3. j
4. i
5. k
6. l
7. a
8. c
9. g
(Questions 1-9, Objective 5)

10. a. Chemical; b. generic or nonproprietary; c. trade or proprietary; d. official
(Objective 2)

11. a. Protected the public from mislabeled drugs, prohibited the use of false and misleading claims for medications, and restricted sales of drugs with abuse potential. b. Prevented marketing of drugs until they were tested and required names of all ingredients and directions on labels. c. Controlled the sale of narcotics and established narcotic as a legal term.
(Objective 3)

12. a. Federal Trade Commission; b. Food and Drug Administration; c. Drug Enforcement Administration; d. Public Health Service
(Objective 3)

13. a. For chronic control of bronchial asthma; b. contraindicated in the treatment of acute episodes of asthma or status asthmaticus or if a known hypersensitivity exists (PDR)
(Objective 13)

14. A paramedic's responsibilities relative to drug ad-

ministration include the following: using correct techniques; observing and documenting effects of drugs; maintaining current knowledge regarding pharmacology; maintaining professional relationships; understanding pharmacology; evaluating drug indications and contraindications; using drug reference materials; taking a patient history; and consulting with medical direction.
(Objective 4)

15. The patient is demonstrating signs and symptoms of a type I hypersensitivity reaction.
(Objective 4)

16. The chemicals histamine and slow-reacting substance of anaphylaxis are released during an anaphylactic reaction.
(Objective 4)

17. Sometimes patients may have an allergic reaction to a drug they have never taken that is chemically similar to another drug they are allergic to.
(Objective 4)

18. a. Idiosyncrasy; b. stimulant; c. drug allergy; d. antagonism; e. potentiation; f. side effect; g. synergism; h. drug dependence; i. depressant; j. therapeutic action; k. contraindications; l. drug interaction; m. tolerance; n. cumulative action.
(Objective 6)

19. The nature of the absorbing surface through which the drug must travel, the blood flow to the site of administration, the solubility of the drug, the pH of the drug environment, the drug concentration, and the drug dosage form.
(Objective 7)

20. Drug-drug interactions are commonly associated with blood thinners, tricyclic antidepressants, amphetamines, digitalis glycosides, diuretics, alcohol, antihypertensives, and cigarette smoking.
(Objective 10)

21. Rectal
(Objective 8)

22. Subcutaneous
(Objective 8)

23. Intravenous
(Objective 8)

24. Intraosseous
(Objective 8)

25. Faster (Objective 8)

26. Placenta and blood-brain barrier
(Objective 8)

27. a. Less, more; b. decreased, more
(Objective 11)

28. Decreased renal function, altered nutrition habits, greater consumption of nonprescription drugs, reduced gastric acid, slowed gastric motility, decreased serum albumin, congestive heart failure, and decreased blood flow to the liver
(Objective 11)

29. Inability to pay for new drugs, forgetfulness or

confusion, lack of symptoms (causing patient to become noncompliant), and other physical disabilities not mentioned
(Objective 11)

30. a. Benzodiazepines: alprazolam (Xanax), chlordiazepoxide (Librium), clorazepate (Tranxene), diazepam (Valium), flurazepam (Dalmane), lorazepam (Ativan), prazepam (Centrax), triazolam (Halcion)

b. Thrombolytic agents: anisoylated plasminogen streptokinase activator (Eminase), streptokinase (Streptase), Reteplase (Retavase)

c. Antiemetics/antihistamines: diphenhydramine hydrochloride (Benadryl), hydroxyzine pamoate (Vistaril), meclizine hydrochloride (Antivert), promethazine hydrochloride (Phenergan)

d. Adrenergics: dobutamine (Dobutrex), dopamine (Intropin), isoproterenol (Isuprel), norepinephrine (Levophed)

e. Antihypertensives (arteriolar dilator drugs): diazoxide (Hyperstat), hydralazine (Apresoline); diuretics: furosemide (Lasix), spironolactone (Aldactone)

f. Cardiac glycosides: digitoxin (Crystodigin), digoxin (Lanoxin)

g. Anticonvulsants, barbiturate: mephobarbital (Gemonil)

h. Narcotic analgesics, opioid analgesics-agonists: codeine (Methylmorphine), meperidine (Demerol), methadone (Dolophine, Methadose), morphine sulfate (Astromorph and others), oxycodone (Percodan, Tylox, Percocet), propoxyphene (Darvon, Dolene)

i. Class IV antidysrhythmics: verapamil (Isoptin)

j. Antiplatelet agents: aspirin, sulfinpyrazone (Anturane)

k. Bronchodilators: albuterol (Proventil, Ventolin), bitolterol (Tornalate), aminophylline (Amoline, Somophyllin, Aminophyllin), ephedrine (Ephed II), dyphylline (Dilor, Droxine, Lufyllin), epinephrine (Adrenalin, Asmolin, and others), epinephrine hydrochloride (Adrenalin Chloride 1:1000), epinephrine inhalation aerosol (Bronkaid Mist, Primatene Mist), epinephrine inhalation solution (Adrenalin), ethylnorepinephrine (Bronkephrine), epinephrine suspension (Sus-Phrine 1:200), isoproterenol hydrochloride inhalation aerosol (Isuprel Mistometer, Norisodrine Aerotrol), isoproterenol inhalation solution (Aerolone, Vapo-Iso, Isuprel), racemic epinephrine inhalation solution (Asthma Nefrin, Micro-Nephrin, and others), terbutaline sulfate (Brethine, Bricanyl)

l. Non-barbiturate anesthetic agents: fentanyl (Sublimaze), sufentanil (Sufenta), alfentanil (Alfenta)

m. Anticoagulants: heparin sodium (Liquaemin)

n. Opioid agonist-antagonist agents: butorphanol tartrate (Stadol), nalbuphine hydrochloride (Nubain)

o. Other drugs used to treat respiratory emergencies: dexamethasone sodium phosphate (Decadron Phosphate), glycopyrrolate (Robinul)

p. Anticonvulsants (Succinamides): methsuximide (Celontin), phensuximide (Milontin)

q. Anorexiants: phenmetrazine (Preludin, Endurets), mazindol (Mazanor, Sanorex), dexfenfluramine (Redux)

r. Antipsychotic agents: chlorpromazine (Thorazine), thioridazine (Mellaril), fluphenazine (Prolixin), molindone (Lidone), loxapine (Loxitane), olanzapine, resperidol

s. Tricyclic antidepressants: imipramine (Tofranil), bupropion (Wellbutrin), fluoxetine (Prozac), trazodone (Desyrel), sertraline (Zoloft)

t. Cholinergic blocking agents: glycopyrrolate (Robinul), atropine (atropine [not used to manage ulcers])

u. Antihyperlipidemic drugs: cholestyramine (Questran), dextrothyroxine (Choloxin), niacin (Nicobid), lovastatin (Mevacor)

v. Immunosuppressants: azathioprine and corticosteroids (dexamethasone)

w. H_2-receptor antagonists: cimetidine (Tagamet), famotidine (Pepcid)
(Objective 12)

31.

Group	Drug Name	Actions
I-A	Quinidine, procainamide	Decrease conduction velocity; prolong electrical potential of cardiac tissue
I-B	Lidocaine, phenytoin	Increase or have no effect on conduction velocity
I-C	Flecainide, encainide	Profoundly slow conduction
II	Propranolol	Beta blockers
III	Bretylium, amiodarone	Antiadrenergic agents; positive inotropic action; terminate reentry dysrhythmias
IV	Verapamil, diltiazem	Block flow of calcium into cardiac and smooth muscle cells. Decrease automaticity

(Objective 12)

32.

Classification	Generic Name	Actions
Diuretics	Furosemide, hydrochlorothiazide, Aldactazide	Increase renal excretion of salt and water; decrease blood volume direct effect on arterioles

Beta-blocking agents	Propranolol, acebutolol, atenolol, metoprolol, labetalol, nadolol	Decrease cardiac output; inhibit renin secretion from kidneys; beta blockers compete with epinephrine for beta-receptor sites, inhibit tissue/organ response to beta stimulation
Adrenergic inhibiting agents	Clonidine (central acting), guanethidine, reserpine (peripheral inhibitors) prazosin hydrochloride, phentolamine, phenoxybenzamine (alpha1 & alpha2 blocking agents, nonselective)	Block sympathetic stimulation; have multiple sites of action
Vasodilator drugs	Diazoxide, hydralazine, minoxidil, (arteriolar dilator), sodium nitroprusside, amyl nitrite, isosorbide dinitrate, nitroglycerin (arteriolar and venous dilator drugs)	Act directly on smooth muscle walls of arterioles, veins, or both. Lower peripheral resistance and blood pressure.
ACE inhibitors	Captopril, enalapril, lisinopril	Inhibit the conversion of angiotensin I to angiotensin II. Angiotensin II is a powerful vasoconstrictor. Suppresses renin-angiotensin-aldosterone system.
Calcium channel blockers	Verapamil, nifedipine, diltiazem	Decrease peripheral resistance by inhibiting blockers the contractility of vascular smooth muscle.

(Objective 12)

33. b, a, e, g, f, d, c
(Objective 12)

34. b. An *antidote* is a specific drug taken to minimize the adverse effects of an ingested drug or poison. *Parenteral* refers to a drug route. A *vaccine* is an injection of drug given to prevent disease.
(Objective 1)

35. b
(Objective 3)

36. b. Only selected antibiotics pass through these barriers.
(Objective 8)

37. a. Antagonists block receptor sites and inhibit action.
(Objective 8)

38. d. LD 50 is the lethal dose for 50% of animals who took it. ED 50 is the effective dose for 50% of animals who took it. Biological half-life is the time required to excrete half of the total amount of drug introduced into the body.
(Objective 8)

39. d. Atropine, lidocaine, and epinephrine may also be given by this route.
(Objective 8)

40. d. Then intramuscular, subcutaneous, and oral.
(Objective 8)

41. b. All of the other routes listed give unpredictable, slow absorption because of poor perfusion in shock.
(Objective 8)

42. b. Butorphanol tartrate and pentazocine are opioid agonist-antagonists, and oxycodone hydrochloride is an opioid analgesic-agonist.
(Objective 12)

43. c. Nalbuphine is an opioid agonist-antagonist.
(Objective 12)

44. a. Ritalin and Cylert are used to manage patients with ADD and hyperactivity. Phenmetrazine is an anorexiant.
(Objective 12)

45. d. Depression is usually treated with a tricyclic antidepressant. Hypotension is treated based on the cause. Occasionally intravenous dopamine will be used, but it acts in a different manner than the drugs that affect brain dopamine levels. Drugs used to treat myasthenia gravis elevate acetylcholine at the myoneural junctions.
(Objective 12)

46. d. Tegretol is used to treat seizure disorders. Librium and Thorazine are both antipsychotic drugs. Baclofen (Lioresal) and diazepam (Valium) are also antispasmodics that may be used to manage muscle spasms.
(Objective 12)

47. c. These drugs paralyze muscles and are usually given concurrently with other drugs that decrease the intracranial pressure during intubation (lidocaine) and sedatives and/or pain relievers.
(Objective 12)

48. c. Physostigmine is used to manage poisonings. Glucagon is a pancreatic hormone that increases blood glucose, lorazepam is a minor tranquilizer, and verapamil is an antidysrhythmic drug.
(Objective 12)

49. a. Norepinephrine is the primary neurotransmittor for the sympathetic nervous system. *Adrenalin* is a trade name for epinephrine, and *Aramine* is the trade name for metaraminol.
(Objective 7)

50. c.
(Objective 12)

51. c.
(Objective 7)

52. d. Chronotropes increase heart rate; dromotropes increase conduction velocity. Cholinergic drugs increase parasympathetic effects.
(Objective 7)

53. a. Influenza-like symptoms and a variety of dysrhythmias are associated with digoxin toxicity. Tricyclic antidepressant or isoproterenol overdose would likely produce tachyarrhythmias. Verapamil overdose may cause bradycardias and severe hypotension.
(Objective 12)

54. d. Bretylium tosylate is a group III, lidocaine is a group IB, and procainamide is a group IA antidysrhythmic agent.
(Objective 12)

55. d. Some also decrease heart rate and contractility; however, the majority achieve their effects by decreasing vascular resistance.
(Objective 12)

56. d. All of the others prevent clot formation.
(Objective 12)

57. a. Ephedrine and isoproterenol are nonspecific beta agonists, and aminophylline is a xanthine derivative.
(Objective 12)

58. b. Antihistamines may worsen an acute asthma attack by thickening bronchial secretions.
(Objective 12)

59. b. Antiinfective and antiinflammatory agents are used to treat conjunctivitis or keratitis. Topical anesthetic agents are used to treat pain.
(Objective 12)

60. d. Insulin is continually secreted in amounts determined by the body's needs.
(Objective 12)

61. d. Amoxicillin and dicloxacillin are both penicillin drugs. A percentage of people who are allergic to penicillin have cross-reactivity to cephalosporins like cefazolin.
(Objective 12)

62. d. Acyclovir (Zovirax) is typically prescribed for herpes infection (some HIV patients may also take this to treat opportunistic herpes infections). Pyrimethamine (Daraprim) and quinine (Quinamm) are both antimalarial drugs.
(Objective 12)

63. d.
(Objective 12)

CHAPTER 9
VENOUS ACCESS AND MEDICATION ADMINISTRATION

1. a. 7 is the numerator, 8 is the denominator; b. 6 is the numerator, 13 is the denominator.
2. a. $\frac{1}{4}$; b. $\frac{3}{4}$; c. $\frac{1}{2}$; d. $\frac{1}{6}$; e. $\frac{1}{5}$; f. $\frac{1}{4}$; g. $\frac{1}{5}$; h. $\frac{9}{25}$; i. $\frac{1}{10}$; j. $\frac{2}{5}$; k. $\frac{17}{23}$; l. $\frac{2}{3}$
3. a. 15; b. 2; c. 3; d. $2\frac{1}{2}$
4. a. $\frac{43}{8}$; b. $\frac{7}{4}$; c. $\frac{37}{12}$; d. $\frac{47}{3}$
5. a. $\frac{18}{24}$; b. $\frac{48}{60}$; c. $\frac{79,000}{100,000}$
6. a. 45; b. 12; c. 24
7. a. Equal to; b. greater than; c. less than
8. a. $1\frac{3}{8}$; b. $3\frac{11}{12}$
9. a. 1; b. $1\frac{11}{12}$
10. a. $\frac{55}{208}$; b. $25\frac{1}{2}$; c. $13\frac{3}{4}$; d. $\frac{7}{24}$
11. a. $1\frac{1}{4}$; b. $3\frac{13}{14}$
12. a. 3.4; b. 5.35; c. 0.062
13. a. 0.25; b. 0.28; c. 0.02
14. a. $\frac{1}{2}$; b. $3\frac{6}{25}$; c. $6\frac{7}{1000}$
15. a. 0.47; b. 1.02
16. a. 29; b. 13.58
17. a. 0.0724; b. 1.08; c. 0.2175; d. 425.6; e. 29; f. 7052
18. a. 0.05; b. 2.58; c. 8; d. 4.0; e. 0.14237; f. 0.017
19. a. 7.6; b. 0.1; c. 0.9
20. a. 0.10; b. 5.63; c. 892.03
21. a. 5000:60 (5000 ml:60 seconds); b. 6000:60 (6000 ml:60 seconds); c. 100:30 (100 ml:30 minutes); d. 100:10 (100 mg:10 ml)
22. a. 83 ml/sec; b. 100 ml/sec; c. 3 ml/min; d. 10 mg/ml
23. a. True; b. not true; c. true
24. a. x = 3; b. x = 4; c. x = 9; d. x = 15; e. x = 27; f. x = 36; g. x = 28; h. x = 9
25. a. $x = \frac{10 \times 150}{50} = \frac{\cancel{10} \times \overset{30}{\cancel{150}}}{\cancel{50}} = 30$

b. $x = \frac{25 \times 2}{50} = \frac{{}^{1}\cancel{25} \times \cancel{2}^{1}}{\cancel{50}^{1}} = 1$

c. $x = \frac{2500 \times 500}{20,000} = \frac{25\cancel{00} \times 5\cancel{00}}{2\cancel{0,000}} = \frac{125}{2} = 62.5$

d. $x = \frac{1\text{ g} \times 1\text{ L}}{1\text{ g}} = \frac{1\cancel{\text{g}} \times 1\text{ L}}{1\cancel{\text{g}}} = 1\text{L}$

e. $x = \frac{2\text{ mg} \times 1\text{ cc}}{10\text{ mg}} = \frac{\cancel{2\text{ mg}} \times 1\text{ cc}}{{}^{5}\cancel{10\text{ mg}}} = \frac{1\text{ cc}}{5} = 0.2\text{cc}$

f. $x = \frac{10\text{ mg} \times 10\text{ml}}{100\text{ mg}} = \frac{\cancel{10\text{ mg}} \times 1\cancel{0}\text{ ml}}{\cancel{100\text{ mg}}} = 1\text{ ml}$

26. a. 0. 25; b. 1.1; c. 0.005
27. a. 34%; b. 229%; c. 7%
28. a. 68%; b. 20%; c. 43%
29.

Fraction	Ratio	Decimal	Percentage
a. $\frac{5}{6}$	5:6 or 5 to 6	0.83	83%
b. $\frac{1}{20}$	1:20 or 1 to 20	0.05	5%
c. $\frac{7}{33}$	7:33 or 7 to 33	0.21	21%

30. a. 11.25; b. 1.25
31. a. Liter; b. gram; c. meter
    (Objective 1)
32. Kilogram (kg), gram (g), milligram (mg), and microgram (mcg)
    (Objective 1)
33. 1000
    (Objective 1)
34. Right
    (Objective 1)
35. Left
    (Objective 1)
36. a. 2000 g; b. 4000 mcg; c. 2000 mg; d. 0.0006 kg; e. 0.4 mg; f. 0.35 g; g. 250 mcg; h. 12500 mg
    (Objective 1)
37. a. 1; b. 10; c. 0.25; d. 330
    (Objective 1)
38. Grain (gr)
    (Objective 1)
39. Minim
    (Objective 1)
40. 600 mg
    (Objective 1)
41. a. 0.4 mg; b. 0.3 mg
    (Objective 1)
42. a. 3; b. 16; c. 16; d. 4; e. 2; f. 8
    (Objective 1)
43. a. 5; b. 15: c. 30; d. 960; e. 10; f. 50
    (Objective 1)
44. a. 240; b. 960; c. 30; 480; d. 58; e. 5.2; f. 480; g. 0.9 and 900
    (Objective 1)
45. a. Magnesium sulfate; b. Aug. 1, 1995; c. 10 ml; d. 5g; e. 500 mg/ml (4mEq/ml)
    (Objective 2)
46. a. 10; b. 1; c. 10; d. 1; e. 0.4; f. 25; g. 50
    (Objective 2)
47. a. 40 mg/4 ml = 10 mg/ml; b. 1 mg/10 ml = 0.1 mg/ml; c. 25 g/50 ml = 25,000 mg/50 ml = 500 mg/ml; d. 50 mg/2 ml = 25 mg/ml; e. 1 g/250 ml = 1000 mg/250 ml = 4 mg/ml
    (Objective 2)
48. a. 100; b. 1020; c. 80; d. 250; e. 0.05 (don't forget to convert to kilograms); f. 80
    (Objective 2)

49. a. $x = \dfrac{20 \text{ mg} \times 4 \text{ ml}}{40 \text{ mg}} = 2$ ml

    b. $x = \dfrac{3 \text{ mg} \times 1 \text{ ml}}{10 \text{ mg}} = 0.3$ ml

    c. $x = \dfrac{300 \text{ mg} \times 3 \text{ ml}}{150 \text{ mg}} = 6$ ml

    d. $x = \dfrac{2.5 \text{ mg} \times 2 \text{ ml}}{10 \text{ mg}} = 0.5$ ml

    e. $x = \dfrac{12.5 \text{ mg} \times 1 \text{ ml}}{50 \text{ mg}} = 0.25$ ml

    f. $x = \dfrac{0.3 \text{ mg} \times 1 \text{ ml}}{1 \text{ mg}} = 0.3$ ml

    g. $x = \dfrac{0.5 \text{ mg} \times 500 \text{ ml}}{400 \text{ mg}} = 0.625$ ml
    (Objective 3)

50. a. 6 mg:x: :6 mg:2 ml

    $x \times 6 \text{ mg} = 6 \text{ mg} \times 2 \text{ ml}$

    $\dfrac{x \times 6 \text{ mg}}{6 \text{ mg}} = \dfrac{6 \text{ mg} \times 2 \text{ ml}}{6 \text{ mg}}$

    x = 2 ml
    b. 1 ml; c. 1 ml; d. 1 g:x: :20 g:100 ml, x = 5 ml
    (Objective 3)
51. a. 30; b. 100; c. 50; d. 19; e. 23; f. 30 g. 33; h. 500; i. 130; j. 60; k. 45
    (Objective 4)
52. a. 7.5 ml; b. 1.2 ml; c. 0.5 ml; d. 7.7 ml; e. 350 ml; f. 0.5 ml; g. 0.625 ml and 38 gtt/min; h. 0.5 ml and 30 gtt/min
    (Objectives 3, 4)
53. a. 5; b. 0.3; c. 2.0
    (Objective 3)
54.

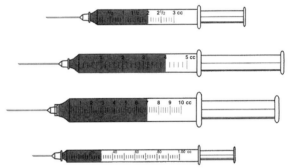

(Objective 3)
55. Avoid distractions; repeat orders to medical direction; verify that you are giving the right patient the right dose of the right drug at the right time by the right route; verify the correct drug on the label at least three times; verify the route of administration; ensure that the labeling information is correct for the drug you want to give; never give drugs from an unlabeled container; verify difficult calculations on paper, with a co-worker, or both; label the syringe immediately after withdrawing a drug that will not be completely administered immediately; do not give unlabeled drugs prepared by another person; do not give medications that are outdated or appear discolored, cloudy, or unusual; if the patient or a co-worker questions the drug or dose, dou-

395

blecheck it; monitor the patient for adverse effects after administration; and document carefully. (Objective 5)

56. a. Stop the infusion.

b. Evaluate the patient's response to the drug. Perform an assessment that includes level of consciousness, vital signs, and ECG rhythm.

c. Advise medical direction and the receiving physician of the amount of drug infused and ask for their treatment advice if you have not yet arrived at the receiving facility.

d. Document the amount of drug administered on the patient care report objectively. Document all facts surrounding the error on the appropriate confidential departmental quality improvement (incident) form.

e. Critique the situation with your crew (if appropriate) and identify measures that can be taken to prevent a similar error in the future. (Objective 6)

57. a. Wash hands before initiating the procedure.

b. Cleanse the area with an antiseptic solution before puncturing the skin. (Objective 7)

58. a. Upright (sitting); b. 4 to 8 ounces; c. stomach; d. tongue; e. dissolve; f. swallowed; g., h., and i. infection, lipodystrophy, abscesses, necrosis, skin slough, nerve injuries, prolonged pain, and periostitis; j. ½ or ⅝; k. 23 or 25 ; l. 1½ to 2; m. 19 or 21; n. prohibited; o. an appropriate sharp container; p. air; q. filter; r. 45 ; s. upper arm, abdomen, thigh, and back ; t. 90 ; u. deltoid muscle, dorsogluteal site, vastus lateralis muscle, rectus femoris muscle, and ventrogluteal muscle; v. gloves; w. 10; x. rapid onset and side effects (Objectives 8, 12, 15)

59. a. Hematoma, cellulitis, thrombosis, phlebitis, sepsis, pulmonary thromboembolism, catheter embolism, fiber embolism, infiltration. b. All complications in (a), plus air embolism, hematoma, damage to arteries or nerves, pneumothorax, hemothorax, and infiltration of fluid into the pleural space or mediastinum. c. All complications in (a), plus hematoma, thrombosis extending to deep veins, and an inability to use the saphenous vein. (Objective 10)

60. a. One to two fingerbreadths below the tubercle on the anteromedial surface of the tibia

b. Boring or screwing

c. Decreased resistance is felt (trapdoor effect)

d. Saline

e. Intravenous fluid infusion

f. Secure (Objective 11)

61. c. To convert °C to °F. $\dfrac{38.5 \times 9}{5} + 32 = 101.3°$ F.

(Objective 1)

62. a. Multiply pounds by 0.45 to convert to kg. 144 × 0.45 = 64.8. Round to 65 lb. (Objective 1)

63. d. $\dfrac{50 \text{ gm} \times 100 \text{ ml}}{10 \text{ gm}} = 500$ ml

(Objective 3)

64. c. $\dfrac{0.06 \times 10}{1} = 0.6$

(Objective 3)

65. a. The 1-ml syringe will permit the most accurate measurements. (Objective 8)

66. d. Many dose calculations can be done in your head; however, you should always write down any calculation that is difficult or that you question. Do not set down an unlabeled syringe with drug in it. Label the syringe or tape the medicine vial to it. The drug label should be verified at least three times before administration. (Objective 5)

67. c. On the patient care report, only the actual action taken (the incorrect route) should be documented. The circumstances surrounding the error, including the actual correct route ordered, should be recorded in the appropriate confidential incident (quality improvement) reports. (Objective 6)

68. a. Slower absorption and fewer systemic effects are achieved in this manner. (Objective 8)

69. d. The other muscles are not developed adequately in the young child. (Objective 13)

70. a. The 14 gauge, 1¼ inch needle has the widest diameter and is the shortest. Both of these properties will allow rapid fluid administration. (Objective 9)

71. a. The goal is to cause the air to stay in the right side of the heart and away from the cardiac valves. (Objective 10)

72. b. $\dfrac{30 \times 60}{60} = 30$

(Objective 4)

73. c. $\dfrac{200 \times 10}{15} = 133$

(Objective 4)

74. d. Intraosseous (IO) infusion is generally recommended for children who are 6 years of age or younger. Complications include infiltration of fluid, fat embolism, osteomyelitis, periostitis at the site, infection, or fracture. Absorption of drugs

and fluids from a properly placed IO needle is very rapid.
(Objective 11)

75. c. The patient is instructed to bite and swallow a nifedipine capsule. Swallowing a sublingual medicine will decrease its effectiveness; therefore water should not be given.
(Objective 8)

76. a. The angle of the ear canal will promote faster absorption if this technique is used.
(Objectives 12, 13)

77. d. Recognize the child's fear and allow them to express it in appropriate ways such as crying or yelling. Use mild restraint if necessary and firmly stabilize injection sites. Give injections quickly.
(Objective 13)

78. d. Blood should not be drawn from an IV catheter if IV fluids have already been infusing (except under special circumstances and with the authorization of medical direction). Typically a large 19- or 21-gauge needle should be used; however, in neonates, a smaller needle should be used.
(Objective 14)

● **CHAPTER 10**
THERAPEUTIC COMMUNICATIONS

1. e
2. f
3. g
4. h
5. a
6. d
7. b
8. a. You (the paramedic) are the source.
   b. You did the encoding.
   c. No, the patient did not interpret the message in an appropriate manner.
   d. The patient was the receiver of the first message.
   e. Feedback was needed to clarify the message.
   (Objective 2)
9. a. Face the patient when he or she speaks.
   b. Maintain eye contact.
   c. Avoid crossing your legs or arms.
   d. Avoid distracting body movements.
   e. Nod in acknowledgment at appropriate times.
   f. Lean toward the patient.
   (Objective 3)
10. Move the patient into the ambulance as quickly as possible for more privacy. Try to avoid interruptions until the interview is finished.
    (Objective 4)
11. a. How do you feel?
    b. Describe (or show me) where your chest hurts.
    c. Tell me when this problem began.
    d. What medicines do you take on a daily basis?
    (Objective 5)

12. a. You shouldn't offer false reassurance.
    b. Showing disapproval and offering unsolicited advice impairs effective communication.
    c. Using professional jargon impairs the patient's ability to understand you.
    d. "Why" questions may be viewed as accusations.
    (Objective 5)
13. a. Her resistance may be related to personal pride, fear of loss of self-esteem, or fear of retribution.
    b. Shifting the focus temporarily to her injuries, and making statements such as, "I've seen this pattern of injuries before in women who have been hurt by their husbands or boyfriends," may allow her to respond to your comments.
    c. Explain that you recognize she is in a dangerous situation and that you are worried about her, and then give her some information about social service agencies that can provide support or help if she changes her mind later. Report your observations to the hospital staff.
    (Objective 6)
14. a. Observe the patient's appearance, level of consciousness, and gait. Note how he or she is dressed and groomed. Look for any defensive or aggressive postures.
    b. Talk to the patient to see if he or she is oriented to person, place, and time. Note the quality of speech and the ability to think clearly, maintain a normal attention span, and concentrate on the discussion.
    (Objective 7)
15. a. Consider whether the patient's present illness or a preexisting condition may prevent him from speaking. Tell him that you are there to help. Question family members. See whether the patient can nod to questions if he is unable to respond verbally.
    b. Ensure that you are positioned close to an exit. Ensure that law enforcement officers are close by. Attempt to use normal interviewing techniques. Set limits. Follow protocols for restraint if the patient's behavior becomes violent.
    (Objective 8)
16. Ask the father questions first. Offer a distraction to the child and gradually approach and start talking to him. Speak at eye level in a calm, quiet voice. Use short sentences with concrete explanations.
    (Objective 8)
17. Inform the patient of your professional role and the inappropriate nature of the comments. Document the situation; if possible, have another caregiver ride in the patient compartment with you.
    (Objective 8)
18. b. Each of the other answers describes communication. Therapeutic communication is a planned, deliberate act that uses specific techniques to build

a positive relationship and share information to achieve goals for the patient.
(Objective 1)

19. b. Decoding involves interpretation of a message.
(Objective 2)

20. b. *Cultural imposition* means to impose your beliefs or values on people from other cultures. *Ethnocentrism* occurs when you view your own life as the most acceptable, the best, or superior to others. *Sympathy* is the expression of your feelings about another person's predicament.
(Objective 3)

21. c. Folding your arms may indicate a closed, defensive feeling. Although you need to be aware of a patient's personal space, in the prehospital setting, you need to make close contact on most calls to perform an effective examination.
(Objective 5)

22. a. Demonstrating personal bias that leads the patient in an unwanted direction can hamper communications. Interruptions occasionally may be necessary if a life-threatening condition exists, but a more appropriate action is to allow the patient to proceed uninterrupted. Excessive use of medical terminology with patients may impair their ability to understand you.
(Objective 5)

23. b. This observation is just one clue in the examination. All other choices reflect possible abnormal mental status exams.
(Objective 7)

24. c. The paramedic's abilities (regarding sign language) and circumstances of the call determine which method can be used. Whenever possible, the method that the patient chooses should be used.
(Objective 8)

● CHAPTER 11
AIRWAY MANAGEMENT AND VENTILATION

1. e
(Objective 5)
2. f
(Objective 5)
3. c
(Objective 5)
4. d
(Objective 5)
5. a
(Objective 5)
6. True
(Objective 1)
7. True
(Objective 3)
8. False. The pressure regulator reduces the pressure in the oxygen cylinder to 30 to 70 psi to permit safe

administration. The flowmeter regulates the amount of oxygen delivered.
(Objective 10)

9. During inspiration the dome of the diaphragm is flattened when it contracts. This causes an increase in the superior-inferior distance of the chest cavity. The intercostal muscles contract, resulting in an increase in the anteroposterior and lateral diameter of the chest cavity. This increase in the size of the chest cavity results in a pressure drop in the chest approximately 1 mm Hg below atmospheric pressure. This negative pressure causes gas to move into the lungs. During expiration the relaxation of the diaphragm and other breathing muscles results in a decrease in the size of the chest wall and an increase in pressure in the chest approximately 1mm Hg above atmospheric pressure. This positive pressure in the chest forces the gas out of the lungs.
(Objective 2)

10. a. 760 mm Hg; b. intrapulmonic; c. thoracic; d. decrease; e. increase; f. compliance; g. asthma, emphysema, bronchitis, pulmonary edema, and lung cancer.
(Objectives 2 and 3)

11. a. pulmonary arteries; b. pulmonary veins
(Objective 4)

12. Head: Inspect for cyanosis around lips and "puffing" of the cheeks; neck: inspect for the use of accessory muscles or tracheal tugging; chest: inspect for intercostal muscle use and an increased anteroposterior diameter of the chest, auscultate lung sounds; abdomen: inspect for the use of abdominal muscles when breathing.
(Objective 9)

13. a. 79; b. 760; c. 600.2; d. 21; e. 760; f. 160
(Objective 3)

14. Loss of pulmonary surfactant, increase in airway resistance, and decrease in pulmonary compliance
(Objective 2)

15. a. The lungs are coated with visceral pleura that adhere to the parietal pleura that line the chest wall. In the potential space between these two membranes, negative pressure "holds" the lungs to the chest wall. Disruption of this potential space causes collapse of the lung.

b. Surfactant reduces the surface tension in the alveoli. In other words it reduces the tendency of the alveolar walls to "stick" together. In the newborn with insufficient surfactant production, extremely high airway pressures must be used to maintain inflation of the alveoli so that effective ventilation can occur.

c. The bronchioles are surrounded by smooth muscle. During an asthma attack the smooth muscle contracts forcefully and decreases the diameter

of the bronchioles, which impairs the exchange of gases.
(Objectives 2 and 15)

16. a. right; b. not at all
(Objective 5)

17.

Alveolar Gas	Direction of Movement of Gas	Venous Blood (Pulmonary Capillaries)
P_{CO_2} <u>0</u> torr	←	P_{CO_2} <u>46</u> torr
P_{O_2} <u>100</u> torr	→	P_{O_2} <u>40</u> torr

(Objectives 3 & 5)

18. a. hemoglobin; b. plasma; c. metabolism; d. plasma, blood proteins, and bicarbonate ions.
(Objective 5)

19. a. Loss of function of respiratory muscles prevents ventilation from occurring without mechanical assistance. b. There will be decreased compliance of the lungs and decreased surface area for gas exchange. c. There will be increased resistance in the airways, which will decrease the flow of gases to and from the lungs. d. The respiratory centers may be damaged, resulting in abnormal or absent breathing. The airway may not be patent.
(Objective 15)

20.

Mechanism	Origin or Stimulus	Location of Effect	Action
Inspiratory centers	Medulla	Send impulses to spinal cord to phrenic and intercostal nerves	Stimulates muscles of respiration
Expiratory centers	Medulla	Send impulses to spinal cord to phrenic and intercostal nerves	Stimulates muscles of respiration to increase force of exhalation
Hering-Bruer reflex	Vagus nerve	Medulla discharges inhibitory impulses	Causes inspiration to cease so lungs do not overinflate
Pneumotaxic center	Pons	Inspiratory center	Inhibits inspiratory center during labored breathing
Apneustic center	Lower pons	Inspiratory center	Baseline stimulation of inspiratory neurons

(Objective 6)

21. a. The respirations increase or resume because of the increased P_{CO_2}, which stimulates the respiratory centers. b. The respiratory rate decreases as the respiratory centers of the brain are depressed by the morphine. c. Pain causes an increased respiratory rate. d. The fear involved in such a situation causes an increased respiratory rate. e. The respiratory rate slows because of the decreased metabolic rate during sleep. f. The history of chronic lung disease may mean that the patient is

operating on a hypoxic drive. If this is the case the chemoreceptors will sense an increase in the P_{O_2} and respond by decreasing the respiratory rate. g. During hypothermia the metabolic rate decreases, as does the respiratory rate.
(Objective 15)

22. a. The cough reflex is designed to expel foreign matter from the respiratory passages. b. Sneezing is caused by nasal irritation and also rids the respiratory tract of unwanted irritants. c. Hiccoughs serve no known useful purpose but may signal pathologic conditions. d. Sighing provides intermittent hyperinflation of the lungs to help maintain expansion of the alveoli.
(Objective 2)

23. a. Obstructed airway: The patient will initially be apneic, will lose consciousness, and finally will suffer cardiac arrest if untreated. b. Aspiration of food and possibly gastric juices: Initially the patient may experience a cough, mucus production, decreased breath sounds, or wheezes. c. Fractured larynx: The patient may experience localized pain, edema, or hemoptysis. Dysphagia and subcutaneous emphysema may be present if airway obstruction is imminent. d. Croup with potential for laryngeal spasm: The patient may be anxious and have crowing respirations (stridor) because of airway tissue swelling. e. Decreased level of consciousness may result in partial airway obstruction and aspiration of vomit.
(Objective 7)

24. The pulse oximeter permits monitoring of the effectiveness of interventions by observing the oxygen saturation and pulse rate. If the oxygen saturation does not improve, additional interventions may be needed.
(Objective 13)

25. a. Venturi mask at 24% oxygen: A nasal cannula would be ineffective because the patient has a nosebleed. b. Bag-valve-mask with reservoir device at 15 L/min oxygen: The patient is clearly not ventilating properly and needs ventilatory assistance in addition to the highest flow of oxygen possible. c. Nasal cannula at 4 L/min oxygen: The simple face mask should never be used with an oxygen flow set at less than 6 L/min. d. Complete nonrebreather mask at 10 L/min oxygen: The patient is demonstrating signs of shock and decreased oxygenation, so the highest amount of oxygen possible should be administered.
(Objective 10)

26. a. Percutaneous tracheal ventilation: All other less invasive airway maneuvers have been unsuccessful, possibly because of a laryngeal injury. The patient's airway is not patent, so needle access should be attempted. b. Oral airway: If this is an isolated seizure, the patient's level of conscious-

ness should be gradually improving, and a more invasive airway maneuver can probably be avoided. c. Nasal intubation: Because of the patient's spontaneous respirations, this would be selected over oral intubation because of the high probability of cervical spine injury. d. Nasal airway: This should quickly secure the airway while glucose is administered, which should arouse the patient. e. Oral endotracheal intubation (using manual in-line stabilization of the cervical spine): This would be chosen because of the possibility of cervical spine injury. Nasal intubation would not be an option until basilar skull fracture could be ruled out. f. Oral intubation: This is the airway of choice in the unconscious apneic patient with no potential for cervical spine injury.
(Objective 12)

27. a. This indicates that the tube is in the correct position. The tube should be secured. b. The endotracheal tube is in the correct position, so the tube may be secured. c. If breath sounds are absent, the cuff should be deflated and the tube quickly removed. After hyperventilation of the patient's lungs with a bag-valve-mask and 100% oxygen, another attempt at intubation may be made. d. The cuff should be deflated and the tube withdrawn 1 to 2 cm. The cuff should be reinflated and correct placement verified by auscultation of breath sounds bilaterally. e. The tube is probably in the esophagus. Auscultate for breath sounds, and if they are absent or diminished, deflate the cuff and remove the tube immediately. Hyperventilate the patient's lungs with a bag-valve-mask with a reservoir at 100% oxygen. f. The tube is probably not in the trachea. Placement should be confirmed by auscultation of lung and epigastric sounds and by direct visualization of the vocal cords and use of an end-tidal CO_2 detector.
(Objective 13)

28. a. EGTA; b. PtL; c. EOA, EGTA, and PtL; d. none; e. none; f. EOA and EGTA
(Objective 12)

29. a. Hyperventilate the patient's lungs with 100% oxygen for at least 2 minutes. b. With the laryngoscope in the left hand, insert the blade in the right corner of the mouth, displacing the tongue to the left. c. Advance the endotracheal (ET) tube through the right corner of the mouth and, under direct vision, through the vocal cords. d. Inflate the cuff with 5 to 8 cc of air and ventilate the patient's lungs with a mechanical airway device. e. Confirm ET tube placement by auscultation of the abdomen and chest during ventilation. f. Secure the ET tube to the patient's head and face and provide ventilatory support with supplemental oxygen. Continue to monitor correct placement of ET tube using end-tidal CO_2 detection and other methods.
(Objective 12)

30.

Adjunct	Advantage	Disadvantage
a. Mouth to mouth	Easy to perform	Risk of infectious disease
	No equipment necessary	No supplemental oxygen
b. Mouth to mask	Easy to apply	Not possible to deliver 100% oxygen
	Can give supplemental oxygen	
c. Bag-valve-mask	Can give 100% oxygen	Mask seal difficult to maintain
	Can vary volume	Frequently requires two people

(Objective 11)

31. Vomiting with inadequate ability to expel emesis, facial trauma with bleeding in mouth, and epistaxis (nose bleed) where blood is accumulating in the oral cavity.
(Objectives 8 and 12)

32. Place the patient on a cardiac monitor; hyperoxygenate the lungs with 100% oxygen for 5 minutes before the procedure, and apply suction for no longer than 10 seconds.
(Objective 12)

33. a. The tongue is disproportionately large in a child, and the oral airway can easily occlude the airway if it is inserted by rotation. b. A child younger than 8 years has a circular narrowing at the level of the cricoid cartilage that serves as a functional cuff. c. The vocal cords slope from front to back, necessitating rotation of the tube or performance of the Sellick maneuver to facilitate intubation.
Objective 14)

34. In many older patients there is increased thoracic rigidity, decreased elastic recoil of the lungs, and diminished Po_2. In addition, the chemoreceptors do not function as well, which results in a decreased ventilatory response because of compromise of the respiratory system. Therefore the patient who experiences a significant chest injury may lack the physiological capability to compensate for the injury and will need aggressive intervention by the paramedic.
(Objective 15)

35. b. External respiration is the transfer of O_2 and CO_2 between the inspired air and pulmonary capillaries. Pulmonary ventilation refers to the movement of air into and out of the lungs. Respiration

is the exchange of O_2 and CO_2 between an organism and the environment.
(Objective 1)

36. c. Pressure within the lungs (including the alveolar sacs) drops approximately 1 mm Hg during inspiration to permit the entry of air but is equal to atmospheric pressure at the end of quiet exhalation. The mediastinum does not maintain inflation of the lungs. Integrity of the thoracic cage is necessary to maintain negative pressure within the pleural space.
(Objective 2)

37. c. Only 3 ml of oxgyen can be dissolved in 1 L of blood at the normal arterial P_{O_2} of 100 mm Hg. Oxygen saturation measures the amount of hemoglobin that is saturated with oxygen. Normal oxygenation for a healthy 18-year-old is indicated by a P_{O_2} of 80 to 100 or greater. Venous P_{O_2} is typically in the area of 40 mm Hg.
(Objective 3)

38. a. Without pulmonary surfactant, alveoli tend to collapse, making the work of breathing more difficult. All other factors listed decrease the work of breathing.
(Objective 15)

39. b. Minute volume = tidal volume × respiratory rate. Anything that decreases one of these variables without a reciprocal increase in the other decreases the minute volume.
(Objective 15)

40. c. It means that all hemoglobin is saturated with oxygen. When oxygen saturation is 100%, the oxygen is typically between 80% and 100% but may vary under certain pathological conditions.
(Objective 13)

41. b. Oxygenation is impaired in all these examples by different mechanisms.
(Objective 15)

42. c.
(Objectives 5 and 15)

43. a. Only if the changes in respiratory rate alter the oxygen or carbon dioxide level or the pH will chemical receptors be triggered.
(Objective 6)

44. d. If the patient's physiological signs deteriorate, the rescuer should intervene.
(Objective 7)

45. c.
(Objective 7)

46. b. Because the tongue is the most frequent cause of airway obstruction, repositioning the airway may be the only maneuver necessary to permit air exchange.
(Objective 7)

47. a. Cricoid pressure (Sellick maneuver), if done properly, can greatly minimize the risk of aspiration during artificial ventilation until the airway is secured with an ET tube. Suctioning will reduce but not eliminate the risk of aspiration. A nasogastric tube will decrease the risk of aspiration by minimizing the gastric content, but an oropharyngeal airway may stimulate the gag reflex and cause aspiration. The most appropriate position to minimize the risk of aspiration is the left lateral recumbent position.
(Objective 8)

48. a. The mechanism of injury and signs are consistent with this life-threatening emergency, which necessitates aggressive airway management.
(Objective 7)

49. a. It is a frequently underused adjunct usually well tolerated by a semiconscious patient with a gag reflex.
(Objective 12)

50. b. The tube should be in the esophagus of a patient more than 5 feet tall, and no sounds should be audible over the gastric area when the patient's lungs are ventilated.
(Objective 12)

51. d. The tube is designed to function correctly in the trachea or esophagus.
(Objective 12)

52. a. Repeat attempts should be performed after hyperventilation.
(Objective 12)

53. d. Percutaneous transtracheal ventilation is a short-term (less than 45 minutes) airway device used when other measures to secure the airway are unsuccessful. The demand valve does not provide sufficient pressure to ventilate by this method. It offers no protection from aspiration.
(Objective 11)

54. c.
(Objective 11)

55. d.
(Objective 11)

56. a. Suction should be applied for no longer than 10 seconds. A cough is stimulated frequently and may increase intracranial pressure. Suction should be set between 80 and 120 mm Hg.
(Objective 12)

57. d.
(Objective 10)

58. b. A patient with this mechanism and symptoms of hypoxia clearly needs the highest percentage of oxygen available.
(Objective 10)

59. c. Ideally this should be done 3 minutes before intubation.
(Objective 12)

60. b. If the tube passes into tissue outside of the trachea, ventilation will not be possible. Aspiration, vocal cord injury, and perforation of great vessels also are complications but may still allow delivery of ventilation.
(Objective 12)

● CHAPTER 12
HISTORY TAKING

1. a. Does anything make the pain better or worse? What does the pain feel like? Show me where the pain is. Does it go anywhere else? On a scale of 1 to 10, with 1 being the least and 10 being the worst, where do you rate your pain? When did you first notice your pain? b. How is your health in general? Have you been hospitalized for any major illness or injury? Are you having any other signs or symptoms today (difficulty breathing, nausea, vomiting, dizziness, or palpitations)? Do you have any allergies? What medicines do you take? Have you taken anything today? What significant past medical history do you have (heart disease, lung disease, high blood pressure, diabetes)? When did you last eat? Was it anything unusual? What were you doing when you first noticed this pain? c. Do you smoke? Do you use alcohol or any other drugs? d. Are your parents living? Do (did) they have any heart disease or other major medical problems?
(Objective 3)

2. Chest pain
(Objective 2)

3. S—Does the patient have any associated signs or symptoms that may suggest a cardiac reason for the fall?

A—Allergies or allergic reactions are unlikely to explain a fall unless the patient becomes hypotensive secondary to anaphylaxis, loses consciousness, and then falls.

M—Some daily medicines can cause hypotension (especially orthostatic hypotension) that could lead to a fall. Other sedative, hypnotic, and psychotropic drugs may impair judgment or level of consciousness and predispose a person to a fall. Medications also can suggest preexisting medical conditions such as diabetes, heart disease, or neurological illness that may cause a fall.

P—Pertinent past medical history may include factors such as heart disease (dysrhythmias), neurologic disease (stroke with neurological deficit), diabetes (hypoglycemia), recent surgery, and other conditions that could alter balance, judgment, or consciousness and cause a fall.

L—If the last meal was not timed correctly and the patient is diabetic or hypoglycemic, a fall could result.

E—Did the patient have chest pain, visual disturbances, dizziness, palpitations, or any medical reason that could have caused the fall?
(Objective 3)

4. You should ask about: a. immunizations; b. tobacco use, alcohol use, screening tests (for tuberculosis), immunizations, home situation, exposure to contagious diseases, travel to other countries; c. alcohol or other drugs, use of safety measures (restraint devices); d. diet, exercise, sexual history (possibly physical abuse); e. alcohol and other drugs; f. alcohol and other drug use, sleep patterns, home situation, significant other (abuse or violence), sexual history, daily life, patient outlook, and economic condition; g. alcohol, drugs, and related substances, exercise and leisure activities; h. tobacco use, alcohol, other drugs and related substances, diet, home situation and significant other, physical abuse or violence, daily life, housing, and economic condition; i. tobacco use, alcohol, other drugs and related substances, sleep patterns, diet and exercise, and leisure activities.
(Objective 3)

5. a. Remain attentive and listen. Reflect on some of the emotions you sense the patient may be experiencing. b. Let the patient talk for a few minutes. Summarize his comments. c. Summarize the comments and ask the patient to select the most pressing ones to focus on in your examination. d. Remain calm and caring and reassure the patient. e. Reassure the patient that you are listening to her fears, that you are there to care for her, and that you understand her condition. f. Remain calm and set limits about ways he can express his feelings in an appropriate manner. Be alert for signs of escalation so you can maintain the safety of the patient, yourself, and your crew. g. Be clear that you are in a caring role and you feel the behavior is unacceptable. If it persists, consider trading roles with your partner if appropriate. h. Determine whether a family member can translate or use a translating resource if available.
(Objective 4)

6. c. The history can provide structure and guidance during the physical examination, where you hope to find signs of the illness or injury.
(Objective 1)

7. a. Vital signs are part of the physical assessment.
(Objective 2)

8. b. The patient often states the chief complaint but may not be able to if he or she is unconscious. Past medical history is obtained after the chief complaint. It may change during the call if the patient's condition changes.
(Objective 3)

9. d. Did the difficulty start today? is not an open-ended question. A better way to ask about time of

onset is "Tell me when you noticed that you were having trouble breathing." Answer b. also is not an open-ended question. Asking about location is inappropriate with this chief complaint.
(Objective 3)

10. d. Lung function and laboratory values can be affected by smoking and are important information for this patient.
(Objective 3)

11. b. Allergy to other nonsteroidal antiinflammatory drugs also is a contraindication.
(Objective 3)

12. c. Lack of food intake could lead to hypoglycemia and dizziness.
(Objective 3)

13. d. Tuberculosis may be found in family members because of transmission by close contact.
(Objective 3)

14. d. Offering false reassurances does not benefit the patient.
(Objective 3)

15. b. Establish limits for acceptable behavior.
(Objective 4)

16. a. Use phrases and words that can be easily understood.
(Objective 4)

● CHAPTER 13
PHYSICAL EXAMINATION

1. b.
(Objective 10)
2. g.
(Objective 10)
3. e.
(Objective 10)
4. f.
(Objective 10)
5. c.
(Objective 0)
6. a.
(Objective 10)
7. d.
(Objective 10)
8. h.
(Objective 10)
9. k.
(Objective 10)
10. e.
(Objective 10)
11. m.
(Objective 10)
12. g.
(Objective 10)
13. c.
(Objective 10)

14. l.
(Objective 10)
15. h.
(Objective 10)
16. b.
(Objective 10)
17. f.
(Objective 10)
18. d.
(Objective 10)

19. a. Observe the environment (scene), general patient appearance, and specific body regions to gather data. b. Use the palmar surface of the hands and fingers to feel for texture, mass, fluid, temperature, and crepitus in various body regions. c. Use a stethoscope or the unaided ear to assess sounds generated by the movement of air or gases within the body.
(Objective 1)

20.

Abnormality	Cause
a. Dilated/unresponsive	Cardiac arrest, hypoxia, drug use or misuse
b. Constricted/ unresponsive	Injury or disease of the central nervous system, narcotic drug use, use of eye medications
c. Unequal/one dilated and unresponsive	Cerebrovascular accident, accident, direct trauma to the eye, use of eye medications, use of an ocular prosthesis
d. Dull/lackluster	Shock or comatose states

(Objective 6)

21. a.
1. Mental status; 2. general survey; 3. vital signs; 4. skin; 5. head, eyes, ears, nose, and throat (HEENT); 6. chest; 7. abdomen; 8. posterior body; 9. extremities; 10. neurologic examination.
(Objective 7)
b. Assess whether the patient is alert and responsive to touch and verbal and painful stimuli. Assess the patient's general appearance and behavior. Note verbal and motor responses. If the patient is ambulatory when you arrive, note posture, gait, and motor activity. Observe dress and hygiene and note any body odors such as alcohol. Note facial expression and determine whether it is appropriate for the situation. Is the patient's affect appropriate for the situation? Is the speech understandable and moderately paced? Assess the quality, rate, loudness, and fluency of the patient's speech. Determine whether the patient has organized thoughts. Determine whether the patient is oriented to person, place, and time. Assess remote and recent memory.
(Objective 5)

c. Inspect for shape and symmetry of the skull and facial bones. Note bleeding, trauma, deformity, or drainage around the face or from the ears or nose. Inspect the mouth for bleeding and loose or missing teeth. Observe for pupil response to light and assess to see whether the patient's vision is intact. Examine the conjunctiva and sclera by asking the patient to look up while both lower lids are depressed with the thumbs. Palpate the lower orbital rims to determine structural integrity. Use the ophthalmoscope to check the cornea for lacerations, abrasions, or foreign bodies; to check for hyphema in the anterior chamber; to assess the fundus to see retinal vessels, the optic nerve, and retina; and to assess the vitreous. Palpate the scalp and face for deformities, swelling, indentations, or bleeding, noting pain or tenderness. Inspect the external ear for signs of bruising, deformity, or discoloration. Look for bleeding in the ear canal. Palpate the bones around the ear to see whether the patient feels discomfort. Look for discoloration on the mastoid process. Assess gross auditory acuity by covering one ear at a time and asking the patient to repeat short test words spoken in soft and loud tones. Pull the auricle up and back to perform the otoscopic examination and look at the eardrum. Before applying the cervical collar but while still maintaining cervical immobilization, inspect to ensure that the trachea is midline and note tracheal tugging or obvious symptoms of trauma. Palpate the anterior and posterior neck, noting pain, deformity, malalignment, or subcutaneous emphysema. (Objective 9)

22. Inspect for chest shape, symmetry, expansion, and the use of accessory muscles. Note the rate, depth, and pattern of respirations. Palpate for tenderness, bulges, depressions, unusual movement, crepitus, and chest expansion. Place both thumbs on the xiphoid process with palms lying flat on the chest wall and palpate for symmetry. Assess the posterior chest wall by placing the thumbs along the spinous processes at the level of the tenth rib. Percuss the chest to detect resonance (normal), hyperresonance (hyperinflation), or dullness or flatness (fluid or pulmonary congestion). Auscultate bilaterally (anterior and posterior) with the patient upright if possible and ask the patient to breathe in and out slowly through the open mouth, noting diminished or adventitious sounds. Palpate the apical impulse. Auscultate the heart at the fifth intercostal space to note frequency, intensity, duration, and timing as well as abnormal sounds such as murmurs. (Objective 9)

23. Inspect for symmetry, jaundice, or distention and look for surgical scars. Look for smooth movement of the abdomen during respiration. Auscultate all four quadrants for rumblings. Palpate for tenderness, masses, skin temperature, and rigidity and observe for guarding. Percuss all four quadrants of the abdomen to assess for tympany (normal over stomach and intestines) and dullness (over organs and solid masses). Percuss the liver by beginning just above the umbilicus in the right midclavicular line in an area of tympany. Continue in an upward direction until the change from tympany to dullness occurs (usually slightly below the costal margin, which indicates the upper border of the liver). During palpation of the liver the patient should be supine and relaxed. Stand on the patient's right side and place the left hand under the patient in the area of the eleventh and twelfth ribs. Place your right hand on the abdomen, with the fingers pointing toward the patient's head, resting just below the edge of the costal margin. As the patient exhales press the hand under the patient upward, while pushing your right hand gently in and up. If you can feel the liver, it should be firm and nontender. (A healthy adult liver usually cannot be palpated.) (Objective 9)

24. Inspect for obvious trauma, deformity, symmetry, or bleeding, especially from the urethra. Place the hands on each anterior iliac crest and press down and out, noting movement or crepitus. Place the heel of the hand on the symphysis pubis and press down to determine stability. Palpate the femoral pulses. (Objective 9)

25. For each extremity inspect for position, deformity, and obvious signs of trauma and compare the right extremity with the left. Palpate for structural integrity. Assess grips, have the patient push and pull the paramedic's hands against force, and have the patient push the feet against the opposing force of the paramedic's hands bilaterally to note muscle strength and tone. Assess distal pulse and sensation in all extremities. (Objective 9)

26. Log roll patient with cervical immobilization. Inspect the neck for midline position. Inspect the back for signs of injury, swelling, discoloration, and open wounds. Palpate the spine, beginning at the neck and proceeding to the sacrum, noting point tenderness or deformity. Place the palm of your hand over the costovertebral angle and strike the hand with your fist, noting painful reaction. (Objective 9)

27.

Cranial Nerve Number(s)	Cranial Nerve Name(s)	Assessment Technique
I	Olfactory	Test smell with ammonia inhalants

II	Optic	Test for visual acuity
II	Optic	Inspect the size and shape of the pupils; assess the pupil's response to light
III	Oculomotor	Test EOMs by asking the patient to look up and down, to the left and right, and diagonally up and down to the left and right
IV	Trochlear	
VI	Abducens	
V	Trigeminal	Ask the patient to clench the teeth while you palpate the temporal and masseter muscles; touch the forehead, cheeks, and jaw to determine sensation
VII	Facial	Note facial symmetry, tics, or abnormal movement; have patient raise eyebrows, frown, show upper and lower teeth, smile, and puff out cheeks; have patient close eyes tightly and resist while you try to open lids
VIII	Acoustic	Assess hearing acuity
IX	Glossopharyngeal	See whether the patient can swallow easily and produce saliva and normal voice sounds; ask patient to hold breath and then assess for slowing of the heart rate; test for gag reflex
X	Vagus	
XI	Spinal accessory	Ask patient to raise and lower shoulders and turn the head
XII	Hypoglossal	Ask the patient to stick out the tongue and move it in several directions

28. Remain calm and confident; do not separate the parents and child unless absolutely necessary; establish rapport with the parents and child; be honest with the child and parents; if possible, assign one caregiver to stay with the child; observe the patient before the physical examination. (Objective 11)

29. a. The child is not frightened, the child needs care to maintain body temperature, the child is in constant motion, the child is an abdominal breather, and the paramedic can use fontanelles to assess overhydration and underhydration. b. Separation anxiety occurs, the child has a fear of strangers, and the paramedic should explain procedures in short sentences. c. The child has a capacity for rational thought, the child can provide limited history, the paramedic should allow participation in care, the child has a limited understanding of the body, the child fears intrusion into private areas, and the paramedic must explain everything completely. d. The teenager is concerned about body image and privacy is a major concern, the paramedic should treat the teenager like an adult, and the paramedic must consider sexually transmitted diseases, pregnancy, and drug and alcohol use. (Objective 11)

30. The patient may have sensory loss that impairs communication, may experience memory loss and confusion, often has numerous health problems that require him or her to take a number of home medications, may have decreased sensory function that can conceal symptoms, and may have fears regarding hospitalization. (Objective 12)

31. a. Inspection involves looking, palpating involves feeling the body, and selected body areas are tapped during percussion. (Objective 1)

32. a. The otoscope is used for examining the ears, the penlight can be used to evaluate pupil response, and the sphygmomanometer is used to measure blood pressure. (Objective 2)

33. a. Blood pressure cuffs that are too wide give a false low reading and those that are too narrow give a false high reading. (Objective 2)

34. c. Although all the other information is important, the chief complaint and history of present illness guides the physical examination and permits you to focus on key areas. (Objective 3)

35. d. Chief complaint and history of present illness are historical findings. Vascular access is an intervention. (Objective 4)

36. c. (Objective 5)

37. d. The other terms are vague and may be interpreted in a variety of ways. (Objective 3)

38. b. Ask the patient to count from 1 to 10 using only odd numbers. Asking the patient to count by serial sevens or spell a word backward also can be used. (Objective 5)

39. a. Ataxia is a staggering gait and postural imbalance is associated with central nervous system lesions. Cranial nerve palsy does not cause a limp. (Objective 6)

40. c. Diabetic ketoacidosis is associated with an odor of acetone on the breath.
(Objective 6)

41. a.
(Objective 6)

42. c. Tachycardia, not bradycardia, is a common trait for all three. Cough is not present in pain or anxiety. Wincing is not associated with cardiorespiratory insufficiency.
(Objective 8)

43. d. This area has less pigmentation and pallor or cyanosis is easier to see in that area.
(Objective 7)

44. d. Oral thermometers should be left in place for 4 to 6 minutes and rectal thermometers for 5 to 8 minutes.
(Objective 7)

45. c. Palpation of the abdomen may create sounds that falsely indicate normal bowel function when none exists.
(Objective 10)

46. b. Beau's lines are transverse depressions in the nail that inhibit growth and are associated with systemic illness, severe infection, and nail injury. Paronychia is an inflammation of the skin at the base of the nail that may result from local infection or trauma. Terry's nails are transverse white bands that cover the nail except for a narrow zone at the distal tip and are associated with cirrhosis.
(Objective 10)

47. b. Pupil response and corneal touch test the cranial nerves. Palpation of the globe is used to assess for dehydration.
(Objective 9)

48. c. For the adult examination the auricle should be pulled gently up and backward.
(Objective 9)

49. a. This also may be noted if the patient is going through puberty.
(Objective 9)

50. c. This barrel-shaped appearance develops because of air trapping.
(Objective 10)

51. d. Dullness or flatness is heard when fluid is present or pulmonary congestion has occurred. Resonance is usually heard over normal lungs.
(Objective 10)

52. c. Normal breath sounds are louder on inspiration. The diaphragm is used to auscultate the lungs. Ideally the patient should be sitting if the condition permits.
(Objective 9)

53. b. Ideally the patient should be sitting up and leaning slightly forward or in a left lateral recumbent position.
(Objective 9)

54. b. Mean arterial pressure is diastolic pressure plus one third pulse pressure. Pulsus paradoxus is a fluctuation in systolic blood pressure with respiration. Pulse pressure is systolic blood pressure minus diastolic blood pressure.
(Objective 10)

55. d.
Objective 10)

56. c. Murmurs are prolonged extra sounds auscultated with a stethoscope. A bruit is an abnormal sound audible over the carotid artery or an organ or gland. A thrill may feel like a tremor or vibration.
(Objective 9)

57. b. The brachial pulse is on the arm, the popliteal pulse is behind the knee, and the posterior tibial pulse is on the medial aspect of the ankle, behind the tibia.
(Objective 9)

58. b. Pelvic fractures are often accompanied by substantial hemorrhage.
(Objective 10)

59. d.
(Objective 9)

60. a. Point-to-point movements are evaluated using the heel-to-shin and finger-to-nose tests. Stance and balance are tested with the Romberg test.
(Objective 9)

61. b. Anxiety is usually minimized while the child is in the parent's arms. This can minimize respiratory effort and distress and allow for a more effective assessment.
(Objective 11)

62. b. Anxiety can usually be decreased and cooperation increased if the parent and child remain together.
(Objective 11)

63. c.
(Objective 11)

64. c. These numerous illnesses can confuse the clinical picture and complicate the paramedic's examination of the patient.
(Objective 12)

● **CHAPTER 14**
PATIENT ASSESSMENT

1. a. Determine the mechanism of injury.
b. Find out the number of people injured.
c. Determine the need for rescue or hazardous materials resources and request from dispatch if needed.
d. Determine the best access for responders you request.
e. Secure the area, clearing unnecessary people from the scene.
(Objective 1)

2. a. Form a general impression of the patient.
b. Assess for life-threatening conditions.

c. Identify him as a patient who needs immediate care and transport.
(Objective 2)

3. The patient is male; has been ejected from a vehicle (a mechanism which is associated with severe injuries); and is not moving, which may indicate severe injury with altered mental status (or death).
(Objective 3)

4. AVPU (alert, responds to verbal, responds to pain, or unresponsive).
(Objective 3)

5. Facial or oral bleeding, vomiting, partial obstruction with the tongue and mucus, facial fractures, soft-tissue trauma to the face.
(Objective 4)

6. Goggles, mask, gloves, and possibly a gown.
(Objective 1)
Open the airway with a modified jaw thrust, suction, and insert an oral airway if the patient has no gag reflex.
(Objective 5)

8. Assess the rate, depth, and symmetry of chest movement. Expose the chest wall, inspect for accessory muscle use, and palpate for structural integrity, tenderness, and crepitus. Auscultate for bilateral breath sounds.
(Objective 4)

9. Begin to assist ventilation with bag-valve device and supplemental oxygen. Hyperventilate and intubate while maintaining in-line cervical immobilization.
(Objective 5)

10. Assess radial and carotid pulse. Determine skin color, temperature moisture, and capillary refill (although this determination is not likely be reliable because of cold environmental conditions).
(Objective 3)

11. He has a poor general impression and decreased level of consciousness, is unresponsive, has difficulty breathing, and is in shock (likely because of numerous injuries and mechanism of injury [ejection]).
(Objectives 4 and 7)

12. Continue spinal immobilization and perform a mental status assessment. Inspect and palpate for injuries or signs of injuries of the head, neck, chest, abdomen, pelvis, and extremities. Log roll and inspect and palpate the posterior surfaces of the body. Obtain baseline vital signs. Determine a brief patient history if anyone is on the scene to provide it.
(Objective 7)

13. Airway control, ventilation, and spinal immobilization (for spine and fracture immobilization); intravenous therapy can be initiated during transport.
(Objective 10)

14. 10 minutes
(Objective 10)

15. Because the patient is unstable (a priority patient), mental status, airway, breathing, and circulation should be reevaluated at least every 5 minutes during care and transport of this patient.
(Objective 9)

16. You will assess the patient's approximate age, sex, and race; look for obvious injury or indications of medical conditions; note the patient's general level of distress; and ask for the chief complaint.
(Objectives 2 and 3)

17. a. Ask the patient to speak and listen for stridor or gurgling. b. Evaluate the rate, depth, and symmetry of chest movement. Expose the chest and palpate, observing for respiratory use of the accessory muscles of the neck, chest, and abdomen. Auscultate for breath sounds. Observe for cyanosis, respiratory distress, and distended neck veins. Determine the need to assist ventilations. c. Assess the patient's skin color, moisture, and temperature and evaluate the pulse for quality, rate, and regularity.
(Objective 3)

18. a. Poor general impression; b. difficulty breathing
(Objective 4)

19. a. Chief complaint; b. history of present illness; c. past medical history; d. current health status
(Objective 6)

20. The priority with the trauma patient is to secure the airway while maintaining spinal immobilization, ventilate with high-flow oxygen, and initiate rapid transport for definitive care. This patient has a patent airway but needs oxygenation and possibly assisted ventilation if the condition deteriorates. Emergency vascular access and drug administration may rapidly improve her condition and may be initiated before transport.
(Objective 10)

21. d. Patient care activities will typically begin after the initial size-up. Medical direction should be contacted later. An MCI is unlikely in this setting.
(Objective 1)

22. c. The vital signs should be reassessed during the ongoing assessment.
(Objective 2)

23. a. The other components of the neurological examination are performed later in the assessment.
(Objective 3)

24. c. All other findings are identified later in the examination.
(Objective 4)

25. c. The life threat must be addressed before the examination can proceed.
(Objective 4)

26. a. The speed and focus of the examination is determined rapidly by the condition of the patient as noted in the initial assessment.
(Objective 6)

27. a. Detailed examination can be performed later if no life threats are identified. Otoscopic examination of the eyes is not indicated in this phase of the examination.
(Objective 6)

28. c. In each of the other patients care in the prehospital setting is generally directed to correction of the life threats.
(Objective 8)

29. c. This should be done every 15 minutes for stable (nonpriority) patients and at least every 5 minutes for unstable (priority) patients.
(Objective 9)

30. b. Intravenous fluid therapy should only be initiated on the scene if it will not delay transport. More often intravenous therapy can be started during transport.
(Objective 10)

● CHAPTER 15
CLINICAL DECISION MAKING

1. a. Gather, evaluate, and synthesize information. b. Develop and implement appropriate patient management plans. c. Apply judgment and exercise independent decision making. d. Think and work effectively under pressure.
(Objective 1)

2. a. The language barrier makes it impossible to explain properly to the patient what needs to be done, yet you cannot forcibly treat the patient. b. Wheezing caused by chronic obstructive pulmonary disease is treated with a beta agonist such as albuterol; however, treatment for congestive heart failure involves furosemide, nitroglycerin, and morphine. Critical thinking is required to identify subtle findings and point you to the correct treatment path for this patient. c. The correct treatment for this patient is to place him on a spine board (because of the mechanism of injury and age); however, this increases his pain and perhaps his injury because of his altered anatomy so critical thinking is required to determine an acceptable compromise to meet this patient's needs. d. Standard of care requires you to perform a patient assessment on this child; however, when you attempt to do this, her condition worsens. You must determine a compromise that will not harm her.
(Objectives 2 and 5)

3. a. Concept formation occurred when the patient assessment was done; b. data interpretation included interpretation of the vital signs, physical findings, history, and ECG to determine the likeli-

hood of myocardial infarction; c. application of principle involved making the interpretation (MI), selecting the appropriate course of care (O$_2$, intravenous therapy, nitroglycerin, aspirin), and then delivering that care; d. reassessment of pain, vital signs, and breath sounds constitutes the evaluation phase of the process; e. the run critique provided the opportunity for reflection on action.
(Objective 3)

4. a. Stop and think; b. scan the situation; c. decide and act; d. maintain clear and concise control; e. regularly and clearly reevaluate the patient
(Objective 4)

5. a. Read the patient; b. read the scene; c. react; d. reevaluate; e. revise patient management plan; f. review performance at run critique.
(Objective 6)

6. a. The paramedic must know techniques appropriate within his/her scope of practice that have been approved by medical direction. Paramedics are not expected to make diagnoses. Although in some cases (such as hypoglycemia) paramedics provide definitive care, in most cases definitive care is delivered at the hospital. The paramedic must recognize that personal values may be different from the patient's.
(Objective 1)

7. c. Each of the other choices represents a possible disadvantage of protocols, standing orders, and patient care protocols.
(Objective 2)

8. a. Concept formation involves the process of gathering elements to determine the "what" of the patient story. Data interpretation occurs when data are gathered and interpreted to form a field impression.
(Objective 3)

9. d. The patient has two concurrent serious problems whose treatments are in conflict with one another. The paramedic must use critical thinking to resolve the problem.
(Objective 5)

10. c. In some situations medical direction is either not available or not available in a timely manner to provide assistance in situations that require rapid clinical decision making.
(Objective 6)

● CHAPTER 16
COMMUNICATIONS

1. c.
(Objective 3)

2. i.
(Objective 3)

3. a.
(Objective 3)

4. j.
(Objective 3)

5. b.
(Objective 3)

6. e.
(Objective 3)

7. k.
(Objective 3)

8. h.
(Objective 3)

9. a. Occurrence of the event; b. detection of the need for emergency services; c. notification and emergency response; d. EMS arrival, treatment (including consultation with medical direction), and preparation for transport; e. preparation of EMS for the next emergency response
(Objective 1)

10. EMS response is initiated by bystanders by telephone to a communications center or public safety answering point. The communications specialist obtains the necessary information (often accompanied by digital information) about the origin of the call. The call taker then passes the information by digital technology (if available) to the telecommunicator, who dispatches appropriate emergency personnel and equipment. The EMS crew notifies the communications center while en route and obtains additional information. The EMS crew notifies the communications center on arrival to scene. The EMS crew contacts medical direction for orders and reports. Care is rendered and the patient is prepared for transport; the EMS crew notifies the communication center when they depart from the scene and arrive at the receiving facility. The ambulance is made ready for the next emergency call and communications is notified when it is available for another call.
(Objective 2)

11. Mountains, dense foliage, and tall buildings
(Objective 4)

12. a. To receive calls for EMS assistance; b. dispatch and coordinate EMS resources; c. relay medical information; and d. coordinate with public safety agencies
(Objective 5)

13. a. Name and call-back number of individual who placed the call; b. address of emergency and directions including specific landmarks because of the possible rural location; c. the nature of the emergency (is the victim trapped, how seriously is he or she injured, and is he or she accessible to the EMS crew?)
(Objective 5)

14. Licensing and frequency allocation, establishing technical standards for radio equipment, and establishing and enforcing rules and regulations
(Objective 6)

15. Speak 2 to 3 inches away from and across the microphone, speak slowly and clearly, speak without emotion, be brief, avoid codes (unless approved by system), and advise the receiving party when the transmission has been completed
(Objective 7)

16. City Unit 7, paramedic Smith calling City Hospital. We are on the scene at an industrial site with a patient who fell approximately 20 feet onto a grassy area. The patient is a 30-year-old male weighing approximately 100 kg. Patient's chief complaint is back pain. Also complaining of bilateral heel pain. Patient states he became dizzy and fell. Past medical history of back pain for which he takes ibuprofen. Patient is awake, alert, and oriented ×3. Lungs are clear bilaterally; skin is warm and dry. Tenderness to palpation in lumbar region of back and bilaterally on heels. Soft tissue swelling present bilaterally at calcaneus. Distal pulse, sensation, and movement present in all extremities. V/S are BP 120/80, P 116, R 20. Patient placed on 100% oxygen by complete nonrebreather mask and immobilized on a backboard with cervical collar. Private physician is Dr. Jones. ETA will be 15 minutes. Standing by for any additional orders, over.
(Objective 7)

17. b. Decoding is interpretation of a message. Feedback is the response to the initial idea. Receiving indicates the receiver got the message.
(Objective 2)

18. c. The word *people* was mistakenly interpreted as *patients.*
(Objective 2)

19. c. All other equipment listed is part of a complex system.
(Objective 4)

20. c. A decibel is a unit of measurement for signal power levels. Frequency modulation is a deviation in carrier frequency resulting in less noise. A tone is a unique carrier wave used to signal a receiver selectively.
(Objective 3)

21. b. Amplitude modulation is a radio frequency that fluctuates according to the applied audio. Range refers to the general perimeter of signal coverage. A watt measures power output.
(Objective 3)

22. d. Coverage refers to the area where radio communication exists. A hotline is a dedicated line activated by merely lifting the receiver. Patching permits communication between different communication modes.
(Objective 3)

23. b. These tones can be set to all call for efficient disaster communication. Cellular telephones are used for ambulance-to-hospital contact in some areas.

Satellite dishes and microwave transmitters extend transmission distance.
(Objective 4)

24. d. Mobile transceivers are usually mounted on the vehicle and operate at lower outputs than base stations. Portable radios are hand-held devices used when working away from the emergency vehicle. Remote center consoles are located away from base stations and connected by dedicated telephone line, microwave, or other radio means.
(Objective 4)

25. d. Voting systems automatically select the strongest or best audio signal among numerous satellite receivers.
(Objective 4)

26. d. Remote consoles control all base station functions and are connected by dedicated telephone lines.
(Objective 4)

27. c. No dedicated cell channels exist for EMS so lines may be busy when an emergency call is being made. In some areas the cell coverage is not good and communication may be abruptly terminated. This does not allow simultaneous communication.
(Objective 4).

28. d. This is the physician medical director's job.
(Objective 5)

29. c. Prearrival instructions complement EMS care but do not include call screening.
(Objective 5)

30. c. They also are responsible for licensure and allocation of frequencies. They establish technical standards for radio equipment and establish and enforce rules and regulations for equipment operation.
(Objective 6)

31. b. You should speak 2 to 3 inches from the microphone, converse without emotion, and be brief.
(Objective 7)

32. c. Plan of patient management is the forth component.
(Objective 7)

● CHAPTER 17 DOCUMENTATION

1. At 14:00 4017 arrived to the scene of a residence. Found a 20-year-old female supine on the lawn saying inappropriate words. Her husband states she is a diabetic. He found her in the yard confused. Patient's skin is pale, cool, and diaphoretic. Vital signs are: BP 110/70, P 120/min., R 20/min. with clear breath sounds. Blood glucose determined to be 50 mg/dl. 14:06 IV 250 ml NS initiated in the right antecubital space by paramedic Ward. 14:08 25 g (50 ml) D50W given IVP by paramedic McKenna. 14:10 Patient states: "why are you here?" 14:12 Patient is alert and oriented to person, place, and time. Patient states she took 10 units of regular and 20 units of lente insulin at 07:00 today. 14:13 Ambulance en route to General hospital. Report called to Dr. Smith. No further orders requested. 14:16 BP 118/74, P 96/min., R 20/min. Skin is pink, warm and dry. 14:20 Arrival to General hospital. 100 ml NS infused. On some patient report forms, check boxes or tables will permit documentation of many of the items included in this narrative report. In that instance, it is often unnecessary to repeat the information on the narrative.
(Objectives 3, 4, 5)

2. Medical continuity of care, quality improvement, legal record, supply tracking, performance evaluation, state reporting, education, and skill tracking.
(Objective 2)

3. a. Document the patient's level of consciousness, your advice to the patient, medical direction advice to the patient, signatures of the patient and/or witnesses as required in your system, a narrative description of your exam and the events that occurred. b. Note the name of the person/agency that canceled your response, and the time the response was terminated. Ensure that this falls within the scope of your departmental policies. c. Document care on the appropriate MCI forms (often on triage tags). Record patient condition and disposition on appropriate tracking form (may be done by sector leader). d. Note the purpose of the revision or correction, and why the information did not appear on the original document as soon as possible using the appropriate departmental form. Ensure the correction is made by the original author. Send a copy of the revision to the appropriate parties.
(Objective 6)

4. a. If tetanus vaccine is administered to the patient in the hospital, he will likely have an allergic reaction and be harmed. You could face legal repercussions. b. If additional lidocaine is administered at the hospital, the patient may have a toxic reaction. When the chart is audited for quality purposes, it will appear that you did not perform a procedure that was indicated. If drug inventory is tracked from the patient report, it will not be replaced and you may run short. If the patient's bill is itemized, he or she will not be charged for this intervention and your department may lose revenue needed for operations. c. The patient's condition could deteriorate quickly and the medical staff would not recognize the increased risk of bleeding. You could face legal repercussions. d. If the patient alleges that the numbness developed

as a result of your care, you would have no documentation to substantiate your claim that the patient was symptomatic before your care; you could be sued.
(Objective 8)

5. d. All these elements should be recorded in an accurate, legible, understandable manner.
(Objective 1)

6. c. The records should be maintained confidentially and only released to parties other than the hospital after patient consent is given.
(Objective 2)

7. b. This is documented on the appropriate department incident report.
(Objective 3)

8. c. In a court of law the assumption is that if it is not documented, it was not done.
(Objective 4)

9. a. Advice to the patient, including risks of refusal and benefits of treatment, should be noted. Additionally, you should document that the patient was instructed to call back if the condition worsened, or if he or she reconsidered. A detailed examination is not generally performed on a patient who refuses (document it if it is done).
(Objective 6)

10. a. A special form may be required to document these situations. You should always keep a record in case subsequent liability results.
(Objective 6)

11. b. Some agencies and states require separate reports. Patient care information should only be completed by the paramedic on the call. Corrections and revisions should be made as soon as possible.
(Objective 7)

● CHAPTER 18
TRAUMA SYSTEMS/MECHANISM OF INJURY

1. b
(Objective 3)

2. e
(Objective 3)

3. a
(Objective 3)

4. c
(Objective 3)

5. a. Lacerations of the brain, brainstem, upper spinal cord, heart, aorta, and other large vessels; injury-prevention programs. b. Subdural or epidural hematoma, hemopneumothorax, ruptured spleen, lacerated liver, pelvic fracture, and numerous injuries associated with significant blood loss; decreasing time from injury to definitive care, which must be brief. c. Sepsis, infection, and multiple organ failure; early recognition and treatment of life-threatening injury in the field, with adequate fluid resuscitation and aseptic technique
(Objective 1)

6. a. The vehicle strikes the abutment, the passenger strikes the inside of the vehicle, and the internal organs pull forward rapidly and strike the bony structures inside the body. b. Dislocated knees, patellar fractures, fractured femurs, posterior fracture or dislocation of the acetabulum, vascular injury, and hemorrhage.
(Objective 1)

7. Whether the car struck remains stationary (injuries likely on the side of the impact) or moves away from the point of impact (injuries likely on the side opposite the impact).
(Objective 4)

8. b. The velocity that produces damage is determined by calculating the difference between the speed of the two vehicles. In example a it is 70 − 50 = 20, and in example b it is 40 − 5 = 35.
(Objective 3)

9. a. Intracerebral hemorrhage and cervical fracture; b. ruptured aorta; c. kidney, liver, and spleen lacerations
(Objective 4)

10. a. Pneumothorax could be caused by displaced rib fractures that puncture a lung or by a paper-bag injury, in which impact occurs after the patient has inhaled against a closed glottis. b. Lacerated spleen, liver, or kidney; rupture of the bladder, diaphragm, gallbladder, duodenum, colon, stomach, and small bowel
(Objective 4)

11. a. Laying the bike down; b. head-on (up and over the handle bars); c. angular
(Objective 7)

12. a. Fractures of the lower legs, femur, pelvis, thorax, and spine; injuries to the intraabdominal or intrathoracic contents; and head and spinal injuries
b. Fractures of the femur and pelvis; abdominopelvic and thoracic trauma; and head and neck injuries
(Objective 8)

13. Energy forces involved, body part to which energy is transferred, speed of acceleration and deceleration, forces involved (compression, twisting, hyperextension, hyperflexion), protective gear
(Objective 9)

14. a. Hearing loss, pulmonary hemorrhage, cerebral air embolism, thermal injuries, abdominal hemorrhage, and bowel perforation; b. lacerations, contusions, fractures, and impaled objects; c. fractures and abdominopelvic, thoracic, head and spine injuries
(Objective 9)

15. a. The paramedic should evaluate: the distance fallen; the body position of the patient on impact; and the type of landing surface. b. Children and elderly are more likely to fall. c. An adult is more likely to land on her feet.
(Objective 9)

16. a. Length and width of knives determine the depth and extent of the injury. With bullets, missile damage increases if the bullet is designed to rotate, flatten, or fragment during or after impact. b. Kinetic injury increases with increased speed, and tissue damage increases with increased energy applied. c. As the range increases, the damage decreases because of decreased velocity. Close-range injuries produce more damage because of the direct injury of gases from combustion and the explosion of powder.
(Objective 10)

17. b. Trauma is the fifth leading cause of death overall.
(Objective 1)

18. d. Community education and legislation are pre-incident interventions, and decreasing scene time is a post-injury intervention.
(Objective 1)

19. d. The other components are injury prevention, prehospital care, emergency department care, interfacility transportation, definitive care, trauma critical care, data collection, and trauma registry.
(Objective 2)

20. a. Other factors include patient condition, injury severity indices, and available patient care resources.
(Objective 2)

21. c. Kinematics is based on mechanism of injury and force of energy applied. Index of suspicion for certain types of injuries is related to kinematics, the age of the patient, and preexisting illness.
(Objective 3)

22. a. Direct compression or pressure on a structure is the most common type of force applied in blunt trauma.
(Objective 4)

23. b. Because she was struck on the right side, injury to the liver is more likely than injury to the spleen.
(Objective 4)

24. a. All the other injuries can occur in high-speed crashes in which the lap belt is properly applied.
(Objective 5)

25. c. A small number of restrained persons are ejected. Risk of death is six times greater than the risk for those who are not ejected. Ejection typically happens after impact.
(Objective 5)

26. a. The air bag inflates and then rapidly deflates after the first frontal collision.
(Objective 5)

27. d. Head and neck injuries also are common.
(Objective 7)

28. b. This may compound other injuries and cause traumatic amputation.
(Objective 8)

29. b. Falls from more than three times the height of the individual are likely to produce serious injury. Adults who fall from a height greater than 15 feet usually land on their feet.
(Objective 9)

30. a. Children tend to fall head first because their heads are proportionately larger.
(Objective 9)

31. a.
(Objective 10)

32. b. Nonelastic organs do not stretch.
(Objective 10)

● CHAPTER 19
HEMORRHAGE AND SHOCK

1. b.
(Objective 5)

2. g.
(Objective 5)

3. e.
(Objective 5)

4. a.
(Objective 5)

5. d.
(Objective 5)

6. f.
(Objective 5)

7. a. An adequate amount of oxygen is available to red blood cells. There is a sufficient FiO_2, his airway is patent, and his lungs are clear. b. Red blood cells must be circulated to all tissue cells. Based on the history of significant blood loss and the physical findings that indicate decreased cerebral perfusion (anxiety and confusion) and peripheral perfusion (pale, cyanotic lips and nailbeds), it is evident that red blood cell transport is inadequate. c. Red blood cells must be able to off-load oxygen adequately. This seems to be occurring in this situation, although acid-base abnormalities can impair this ability and insufficient information is available to determine this accurately.
(Objective 3)

8. All blood vessels larger than capillaries are surrounded by layers of connective tissue that counter the pressure of blood in the vascular system, have elastic properties to dampen pressure pulsations and minimize flow variations through-

out the cardiac cycle, and contain muscle fibers to control vessel diameter.
(Objective 4)

9. a. systemic; b. systolic; c. diastolic; d. pulse; e. heart (or aorta); f. vena cava
(Objective 4)

10. a. Spinal cord injury results in a loss of sympathetic tone and therefore impairs the ability of the blood vessels to constrict below the level of the injury. This increases the container size, decreasing the effective circulating volume and preload.
b. When blood loss occurs, a situation potentially exists in which the container is the same size but the volume has decreased, reducing the preload. Body compensatory mechanisms attempt to decrease the size of the container by vasoconstriction in an effort to match the container to the volume.
(Objective 4)

11.

Intravenous Fluid	Isotonic, Hypotonic, or Hypertonic	Fluid Movement
D50W	Hypertonic	Into intravascular space
Lactated Ringer's	Isotonic	No net movement
Normal saline	Isotonic	No net movement
0.45% normal saline	Hypotonic	Out of intravascular space
D5W	Isotonic initially but rapidly hypotonic because of glucose metabolism	Out of intravascular space

(Objective 10)

12. a. Oxygen to cells in vasoconstricted areas decreases. Anaerobic metabolism occurs. Leaky capillary syndrome evolves. Pale, sweaty skin; rapid, thready pulse; elevation in blood glucose; and dilation of coronary, cerebral, and skeletal muscle arterioles occur.
b. Precapillary sphincters open. Blood pools and vascular space is greatly expanded, resulting in increased container size. Decreased preload and congestion of the viscera occur. Increased anaerobic metabolism results in increased respiratory rate. Rouleaux formation inhibits perfusion in visceral capillaries and impedes flow. Hypercoagulability develops.
c. Blood coagulates in microcirculation, clogging capillaries and causing congestion; fibrinolytic mechanisms are then overstimulated, causing pulmonary edema and hemorrhage. Cell membrane function is lost, and anaerobic metabolism increases. Water and sodium leak into cells and

potassium leaks out. Cells swell and die. Oxygen absorption and carbon dioxide elimination is impaired in the lungs, and acute respiratory distress syndrome may result.
d. After 1 to 2 hours a dramatic decrease in blood pressure occurs. Cellular metabolism stops. Organ failure occurs and may include liver, kidney, and heart failure; gastrointestinal bleeding; pancreatitis; and pulmonary thrombosis.
(Objective 6)

13. a. Cardiogenic shock: Administer high-flow oxygen, continue assessment, initiate intravenous normal saline to keep the vein open, consider a fluid challenge of 100 to 200 ml of lactated Ringer's solution or normal saline, monitor lung sounds and patient response very carefully, and consider vasopressor drug therapy.
b. Neurogenic shock: Apply cervical spine immobilization, assess the need to assist ventilations, administer high-flow oxygen, initiate intravenous lactated Ringer's solution or normal saline (avoiding excessive amounts), monitor lung sounds frequently, apply and inflate pneumatic antishock garments if local protocol advises, continue assessment, and consider vasopressor drug therapy.
c. Hypovolemic shock: Administer high-flow oxygen, place patient in modified Trendelenberg position, transport rapidly, initiate two large-bore (14- or 16-gauge) intravenous lines with lactated Ringer's solution or normal saline and infuse rapidly, apply pneumatic antishock garment if local protocol advises and prepare to inflate if patient's condition deteriorates.
d. Anaphylactic shock: Ensure a patent airway, administer high-flow oxygen (administer subcutaneous epinephrine), initiate intravenous lactated Ringer's solution or normal saline with a 14- or 16-gauge catheter, consider administration of diphenhydramine HCl (Benadryl).
e. Septic shock: Administer high-flow oxygen, determine whether the patient has preexisting obstructive pulmonary disease, initiate intravenous therapy with a 14- or 16-gauge catheter, and obtain an accurate patient history.
f. Cardiogenic shock: Assess for a patent airway, administer high-flow oxygen, initiate a 16- or 18-gauge intravenous line with normal saline to keep the vein open, institute electrocardiographic monitoring, initiate maneuvers to decrease heart rate based on the electrocardiographic tracing and patient symptoms (drugs, cardioversion), and apply dressing to head wound.
(Objectives 7 and 10)

14. a. Uncompensated shock: The compensatory mechanisms can no longer sustain a normal systolic blood pressure. The pulse pressure is nar-

rowed. Blood oxygenation is decreased as evidenced by cyanosis.

b. Compensated shock: Systolic blood pressure is adequate, but other signs of shock are evident (cool, pale skin and increased pulse and respiratory rate).
(Objective 8)

15. Irreversible shock may occur suddenly or 1 to 3 weeks after the event. Clinical signs include bradycardia; pale, cold, clammy skin; and cardiac arrest.
(Objective 8)

16. Preexisting disease, medication, older or young age
(Objective 8)

17. a. Drug therapy: Neither pneumatic antishock garments nor rapid fluid infusion is considered because this patient is already in heart failure. Therapy should be directed at improving the function of the heart with drugs.

b. Pediatric pneumatic antishock garments (if indicated by local medical direction), rapid fluid replacement, blood transfusions, and intraosseous infusion: The patient has a mechanism of injury for significant blood loss and is exhibiting signs of uncompensated shock. Pneumatic antishock garments may decrease the container size and maximize flow to the vital organs. Rapid fluid infusion may restore circulating volume. Blood transfusion may be necessary on arrival to emergency department to enhance oxygen-carrying capability and restore the vascular volume. Rapid peripheral intravenous therapy may be impossible in this situation, making intraosseous infusion the vascular access method of choice. Rapid transport is essential.

c. Drug therapy: The heart rate is very slow and is likely the reason that this person is exhibiting signs of shock. None of the other interventions increases heart rate.

d. Drug therapy and rapid fluid replacement: The primary cause of the shock state in this patient is probably histamine release. Drug therapy is the only intervention that can arrest and reverse these symptoms. Rapid fluid replacement also may help restore circulating volume until drug therapy is effective .

e. Pneumatic antishock garments, rapid fluid replacement, and blood transfusions: The primary cause of the shock symptoms according to the patient history is loss of blood. Rapid fluid replacement can restore circulating volume. At the emergency department the blood transfusion helps restore oxygen-carrying capacity and circulating volume.

f. Rapid fluid replacement if indicated by local medical direction: At this time the patient is maintaining a normal blood pressure. The pulse and respiratory rate are somewhat elevated, so as as-

sessment continues, the effects of a rapid fluid bolus can be monitored to determine whether the patient has lost a significant amount of blood. Other interventions may be necessary if the patient's condition deteriorates.
(Objective 10)

18. c. Coffee-ground *emesis* indicates gastrointestinal bleeding. *Epistaxis* is bleeding from the nose. *Melena* is dark, black, tarry stools.
(Objective 1)

19. c. A systolic blood pressure less than 90 mm Hg may be normal in certain individuals. Loss of blood volume may lead to shock but does not define it. Shock leads to decreased myocardial blood flow.
(Objective 2)

20. c. The Fick principle states that adequate oxygen must be available to red blood cells through the alveolar cells of the lungs. So that hemoglobin can be oxygenated, red blood cells must be circulated to the tissue cells, and red blood cells must be able to load oxygen at the lungs and unload oxygen at the peripheral cells.
(Objective 3)

21. a. Vessel length and viscosity are relatively constant. Blood volume may influence pressure but not resistance.
(Objective 4)

22. d. As peripheral vascular resistance decreases, vessel capacitance increases and the container size increases. This makes the existing blood volume insufficient to maintain an adequate preload.
(Objective 4)

23. d.
(Objective 4)

24. a.
(Objective 5)

25. d. Leaky capillary syndrome develops after lactate and hydrogen ions build up in the capillaries and their linings lose their ability to retain large molecular structures within their walls.
(Objective 6)

26. b. This fluid loss is caused by the increased hydrostatic pressure created in this situation.
(Objective 6)

27. b. The precapillary sphincter opens, whereas the postcapillary sphincter remains closed, increasing the pressure inside the capillary and forcing fluid out through the already compromised capillary walls.
(Objective 6)

28. b. Anaphylactic shock is caused by the release of chemicals after an antigen-antibody reaction. Hypovolemic shock results from a loss of body fluid (water, plasma, blood). Neurogenic shock is a loss of vasomotor tone.
(Objective 7)

29. b. Loss of vasomotor tone is a contributing factor to shock in each of the other types of shock.
(Objective 9)

30. d. The compensatory mechanisms of vasoconstriction, increased heart rate, and increased contractility are no longer sufficient to maintain adequate blood pressure.
(Objective 8)

31. a. As peripheral vascular resistance increases, diastolic blood pressure also increases.
(Objective 8)

32. b. Use of pneumatic antishock garments is generally not recommended for any of the other situations.
(Objective 10)

33. a. All the others are crystalloid solutions.
(Objective 10)

34. b. Whole blood and packed red blood cells have red cells and therefore the greatest ability to carry oxygen. Packed cells don't contain plasma, therefore have a greater concentration of red blood cells per unit volume. Only a small amount of oxygen is carried dissolved in plasma.
(Objective 10)

35. c. This is the only fluid that contains red blood cells.
(Objective 10)

36. d. Priorities of care always follow the ABCs; therefore oxygen should be first and intravenous therapy should be initiated en route unless a transportation delay exists; in this case definitive care may be expedited.
(Objective 10)

37. b. This position permits better perfusion without compromising respiratory status.
(Objective 10)

38. d. Vasoactive drugs are not indicated for use in the patient with hypovolemic shock until adequate fluid volume has been replaced at the hospital. Pneumatic antishock garments may occasionally be used to treat hypovolemic shock associated with pelvic fractures.
(Objective 10)

39. a. Increased lung congestion indicates that the failing heart cannot deal with the existing fluid volume. Jugular venous distention should increase with fluid overload. Peripheral edema has a slow onset and is not an acute sign evident in the prehospital phase of care. A moderate decrease in heart rate indicates patient improvement.
(Objective 10)

40. b. Epinephrine is the only treatment that rapidly improves all the life-threatening effects of anaphylaxis. Other adjunct therapy may be used after epinephrine has been given.
(Objective 10)

41. a. The shortest catheter with the widest diameter should be selected.
(Objective 10)

42. c. Drops/min = $\dfrac{200 \times 10}{20} = 100$
(Objective 10)

43. a. Control of internal hemorrhage often requires surgical intervention or other definitive care measures available only in the hospital.
(Objective 11)

● **CHAPTER 20**
SOFT TISSUE TRAUMA

1. e.
(Objective 6)

2. f.
(Objective 6)

3. d.
(Objective 6)

4. a.
(Objective 6)

5. c.
(Objective 6)

6. b.
(Objective 6)

7. Connective tissue, elastic fibers, blood vessels, lymphatic vessels, motor and sensory fibers, hair, nails, and glands
(Objective 1)

8. Protection and cushioning against injury, barrier against infection, temperature regulation, and preservation of body fluids
(Objective 1)

9. a. Release of platelet factors at injury site; b. formation of thrombin; c. trapping of red blood cells in fibrin to form a clot
(Objective 2)

10. The warmth and redness is caused by vasodilation and enhanced blood supply to the affected area. Swelling is caused by increased capillary permeability, which allows plasma, plasma proteins, and electrolytes to leak into extracellular space. Pain is secondary to chemicals and increased pressure resulting from fluid buildup.
(Objective 2)

11. a. Corticosteroids; b. NSAIDs; c. penicillin; d. colchicine; e. anticoagulants; f. antineoplastic agents
(Objective 2)

12. a. Wounds to cosmetic regions; b. gaping wounds; c. wounds over tension areas; d. degloving injuries; e. ring finger injuries; f. skin tearing
(Objective 2)

13. a. Contusion or hematoma: Apply ice or cold packs and compression with manual pressure or compression bandage. Assess for underlying injury.

b. Crush syndrome: Provide airway and ventilation support, administer high-flow oxygen, maintain body temperature, rehydrate with expanding intravenous fluids (1 to 1.5 L initial bolus), and administer pharmacological agents such as sodium bicarbonate (to help control hyperkalemia and acidosis), glucose and insulin (to decrease serum potassium), and mannitol (to promote diuresis).

c. Laceration: Control hemorrhage and monitor for signs of hypovolemic shock.

d. Abrasions: Clean gross contaminants from injured surface and lightly cover with sterile dressing.

e. Dog bite: Ensure that animal is contained, control bleeding, rinse off gross contaminants, splint extremity, and obtain a medical history from the pet owner.

f. Penetrating or impaled object: Leave object in place, do not manipulate object unless it is necessary for patient extrication or transport, control bleeding with direct pressure around the impaling object, stabilize the object with bulky dressings, and immobilize the patient. Treat shock if present.

g. Puncture wound: Evaluate wound, elevate affected extremity, immobilize, and transport.

h. Avulsion: Control bleeding, retrieve the avulsed tissue, wrap tissue in gauze that is dry or moistened with lactated Ringer's or saline solution (per local protocol), seal in plastic bag, and place sealed bag on crushed ice.

i. Degloving: Control bleeding, evaluate for hypovolemia, elevate head of stretcher after you rule out mechanism for cervical spine injury.

j. Amputation: Control bleeding, retrieve amputated tissue, and treat as for avulsion.
(Objectives 3 and 9)

14. Assess for pain, paresis, paresthesia, pallor, and pulselessness in the affected extremity. Determine whether there is swelling or tightness of the compartment, tenderness to palpation, weakness in the leg, or pain on passive stretch (early sign).
(Objective 3)

15. A delay in treatment of compartment syndrome can cause nerve death, muscle necrosis, and crush syndrome.
(Objective 3)

16. When did you cut yourself? Was it a dirty place where you got the cut? How did the injury happen? Does anything else hurt? How much blood did you lose? Rate your pain on a scale of 1 to 10 with 1 being no pain and 10 the worst pain you have ever had. Do you take any medicines? Do you have any major illnesses? When was your last tetanus shot?
(Objective 4)

17. Inspect the wound for bleeding, size, depth, presence of foreign bodies, amount of tissue lost, edema, and deformity. Inspect the surrounding area for damage to arteries, nerves, tendons, and muscle. Assess the sensory and motor function of his hand. Evaluate the perfusion of the wound and of the tissues of the hand distal to the wound. Assess capillary refill, distal pulse, tenderness, temperature, edema, and crepitus (if underlying bone injury is suspected).
(Objective 4)

18. a. Apply direct pressure to the wound with a gloved hand or hand-held dressing (4 to 6 minutes) and then secure a pressure dressing firmly if bleeding is controlled.

b. Elevate the affected area above the level of the heart.

c. Apply pressure-point control if other measures have failed. Select the appropriate pressure point proximal to the wound and compress the artery against the underlying bone for at least 10 minutes.

d. Immobilize by splinting. (Immobilization is used as an adjunct to other control devices.) Select the appropriate splint for the body area and apply it to minimize blood flow.

e. Use pneumatic pressure devices. (Devices such as air splints or pneumatic antishock garments serve as adjuncts for pressure control after the bleeding is controlled by other methods.)

f. Use a tourniquet only when other methods are unsuccessful in controlling bleeding and when preservation of life is selected over preservation of the limb. Notify medical control and select a site 2 inches proximal to the wound over the brachial or femoral artery. Place a tourniquet over the artery and a pad over the artery to be compressed. Wind tourniquet twice around the extremity and tie it in a half knot over the pad. Place a windlass on the half knot and secure it with a square knot. Tighten the windlass until the hemorrhage stops and secure it. Note the time of application and mark "TK" on the patient's forehead and notify the receiving hospital.
(Objective 5)

19. a. This wound is likely much more contaminated than one that occurred in a clean indoor setting.
(Objective 8)

20. b. The risk of infection increases in older patients and in those who have preexisting medical conditions.
(Objective 8)

21. b. Injuries of the hand, foot, lower extremity, scalp, and face have a higher than normal risk of infection.
(Objective 8)

22. a. The risk of infection is greater in wounds that are not cleaned and repaired for longer than 8 to 12 hours after the injury.
(Objective 8)

23. a. Injuries associated with a crushing mechanism are more susceptible to infection than those caused by fine cutting forces.
(Objective 8)

24. b. The dermis provides the vascular supply to the epidermis. The sebaceous glands are in the dermis. The subcutaneous tissue lies under the dermis.
(Objective 1)

25. b. Aldosterone aids in body fluid regulation.
(Objective 2)

26. b. Aspirin decreases platelet activity.
(Objective 2)

27. a. Other conditions associated with impaired healing are advanced age, uremia, diabetes, hypoxia, peripheral vascular disease, malnutrition, advanced cancer, hepatic failure, and cardiovascular disease.
(Objective 2)

28. d. A knife wound would be considered high risk if it were contaminated with organic material or if the patient were immunocompromised or had poor circulation.
(Objective 2)

29. c. All the others are open wounds.
(Objective 3)

30. d. There may be only minimal bleeding, numbness, and blanching at the wound site. Surgical intervention is often necessary.
(Objective 3)

31. b. All other interventions could cause further damage.
(Objective 9)

32. c. Bites may be a combination of puncture, laceration, avulsion, and crush injuries heavily laden with infectious organisms.
(Objective 3)

33. c. All others are late findings.
(Objective 3)

34. b. The most common sites are below the knee and above the elbow.
(Objective 3)

35. d. Blood pools in the injured extremity causing hypovolemia. Elevated blood potassium, phosphate and uric acid levels, and low blood calcium levels occur. Myoglobin is filtered in the kidneys, resulting in acute renal failure.
(Objective 3)

36. c. Other air-filled structures that may be affected are the eardrum, sinuses, stomach, and intestines.
(Objective 3)

37. d. All the other injuries have a high potential for impaired wound healing or infection if not treated by a physician.
(Objective 7)

38. b. Tetanus toxoid should not be given to pregnant patients or children younger than 6 weeks.
(Objective 7)

● CHAPTER 21
BURNS

1. c.
(Objective 8)

2. b.
(Objective 8)

3. d.
(Objective 8)

4. a.
(Objective 8)

5. e.
(Objective 8)

6. a. Thermal
b. Electrical
c. Chemical
d. Radiation
(Objective 1)

7. A. Zone of coagulation: nonviable tissue
B. Zone of stasis: seriously injured but potentially viable (Cells will die if no supportive measures are taken within 24 hours.)
C. Zone of hyperemia: increased blood flow caused by inflammatory response (Cells will recover in 7 to 10 days if no shock or infection develops.)
(Objective 2)

8. a. Chemical mediators cause increased capillary permeability and a fluid shift from the intravascular space to burned tissues.
b. The sodium pump in cell walls is damaged, and sodium moves into injured cells and increases swelling.
(Objective 2)

9. a. Decreased venous return, decreased cardiac output, increased vascular resistance (except in zone of hyperemia), hemolysis, and rhabdomyolysis that may lead to renal failure
b. Increased respiratory rate to meet increased metabolic demands
c. Adynamic ileus, vomiting, and stress ulcer
d. Decreased range of motion resulting from edema and immobilization; osteoporosis and demineralization later
e. Increased circulating levels of epinephrine, norepinephrine, and aldosterone
f. Increased basal metabolic rate
g. Increased susceptibility to infection and depressed inflammatory response
h. Pain, isolation, and fear of disfigurement
(Objectives 2 and 4)

10.

Depth	Extent	Severity	Referral
a. Second degree (partial thickness)	36%	Major	Yes
b. Second degree (partial thickness)	22.5%	Moderate	Yes
c. Third degree (full thickness)	9%	Major	Yes (involves feet)

(Objective 3)

11. a. Simultaneously put out the fire and cool the burn while performing initial assessment; monitor vital signs; assess burn depth (third degree), extent (82%), and severity (major); perform a head-to-toe survey; assess lung sounds and distal pulse, movement, sensation, and capillary refill in all extremities.

    b. Cool the burn with clean water; open the airway; intubate as necessary; ventilate with 100% oxygen; prepare to intubate; remove remaining clothing and jewelry; cover the patient to maintain warmth; initiate lactated Ringer's solution intravenously at 820 ml/hour (2 ml/kg/%BSA burned 24 hours [half of daily fluid to be given in first 8 hours]) up to 1640 ml/hour (4 ml/kg/%BSA burned 24 hours) in an unburned extremity; and rapidly transport patient.
    (Objectives 5 and 6)

12. a. Realize that the burns may swell and be associated with airway problems. Raise the head of the stretcher 30 degrees if spinal injury is not suspected. If the ears are burned, do not use a pillow.

    b. Remove jewelry, assess neurovascular status frequently, and elevate extremities.

    c. Monitor distal pulse, movement, sensation, and respirations and rapidly transport the patient to the nearest appropriate facility.
    (Objective 6)

13. His jacket created an enclosed space and he experienced a loss of consciousness.
    (Objective 7)

14. Facial burns, singed nasal hair, and carbonaceous sputum suggests inhalation injury.
    (Objective 7)

15. Increased dyspnea, decreased level of consciousness, hoarseness, and stridor indicate the need for intubation.
    (Objective 7)

16. Above the glottis is the most likely area of injury. The mechanism of injury does not suggest injury below the glottis.
    (Objective 7)

17. a. What type, concentration, and volume of chemical was involved? How did the injury occur? When did the injury occur? Was any first aid given? Does the patient feel any pain?

    b. With appropriate protective clothing, brush most of the powder off and then irrigate profusely (using a shower if available).
    (Objective 7)

18. a. Rust removers, bathroom cleaners, and swimming pool acidifiers

    b. Drain cleaners, fertilizers, heavy industrial cleaners, and cement and concrete

    c. Phenols, creosote, and gasoline
    (Objective 8)

19. a. Amperage, voltage, resistance, type of current, current pathway, duration of current flow

    b. flow (intensity)

    c. force (tension)

    d. 1000 volts

    e. resistivity, size of object pathway, length of object pathway, and temperature

    f. bone

    g. alternating, direct

    h. one

    i. industry

    j. direction

    k. freeze

    l. least resistance

    m. shortest

    n. increases
    (Objective 10)

20. a. direct contact

    b. arc

    c. flash
    (Objective 10)

21. a. Direct contact can create large areas of coagulation necrosis. The entry wound is often a characteristic "bull's-eye" (dry and leathery), and the exit is ulcerated and explosive.

    b. Dysrhythmias and damage to the myocardium may occur. Cardiac arrest is the most common cause of death after electrical injury. Hypertension secondary to increased catecholamine levels is common.

    c. Central nervous system injury may result in coma, seizures, and peripheral nerve injury and may lead to sensory or motor deficits. Brainstem injury may cause respiratory depression or arrest or cerebral edema or hemorrhage, which can lead to death.

    d. Blood vessel necrosis may cause immediate or delayed hemorrhage or thrombosis.

    e. Muscle injury may result in release of myoglobin, which can cause renal failure.

    f. Acute renal failure occurs in 10% of significant electrical injuries.

    g. The patient may have decreased ventilation or respiratory arrest secondary to central nervous system injury or chest wall dysfunction.

    h. Fractures and dislocations can result from direct electrical injury or injury secondary to fall or electrocution.

i. Burns to conjunctiva or cornea and ruptured tympanic membrane are common.
(Objective 10)

22. a. The electrical source must be removed safely from the patient, preferably by interruption of power by the electric company.

b. Perform cervical spine immobilization and ABCDEs. Determine the patient's chief complaint, source of electricity, duration of exposure, level of consciousness before and after injury, and past medical history. Perform a head-to-toe survey, looking for entry and exit burn wounds or trauma associated with fall. Assess distal pulse, movement, sensation, and capillary refill in all extremities and document them. Monitor electrocardiographic rhythm.

c. Immobilize the cervical spine, open the airway, apply 100% oxygen, assess the need to assist ventilations, remove all jewelry, initiate lactated Ringer's solution intravenously at 20 to 40 ml/kg, monitor the vital signs and electrocardiogram, and maintain body warmth.
(Objective 11)

23. Linear, feathery, pinpoint appearance
(Objective 10)

24. a. The patient is usually conscious and may be confused and amnesic, with stable vital signs.

b. Patient may be combative or comatose, with associated injuries from lightning strike, first- and second-degree burns, tympanic membrane rupture (common), and possible internal injuries.

c. The patient may have immediate brain damage, seizures, respiratory paralysis, and cardiac arrest.
(Objective 10)

25. a. Alpha particles are positively charged atoms with minimal penetrability; however, they are very dangerous when internal exposure occurs.

b. Beta particles are positively or negatively charged electrons that have more penetrating power than alpha particles and can permeate subcutaneous tissue.

c. Gamma particles have a much higher penetrating power than alpha or beta rays and require lead shielding to stop penetration. (Protective clothing does not stop these rays.) Exposure may produce local skin burns and extensive internal damage.
(Objective 12)

26. a. Less than 100 rem usually causes no significant acute problems.

b. A total of 100 to 200 rem can cause symptoms such as nausea and vomiting but is not life threatening.

c. Exposure of greater than 450 rem has a 50% mortality rate within 30 days.
(Objective 12)

27. The rescuers and emergency vehicle initially should be positioned 200 to 300 feet upwind of the site. No eating, smoking, or drinking should be permitted at the site. The appropriate local authorities and medical control should be notified of the situation.
(Objective 12)

28. Protective clothing should be worn, if available. The victim should be approached quickly by trained rescue teams. Rescue personnel should trade off frequently until the victim is stabilized sufficiently to remove him or her a safe distance from the contaminated area. If possible, the crew members should position themselves behind any protective barrier available.
(Objective 12)

29. If ventilation is required for the radiation-contaminated victim, an airway adjunct should be used. The patient should be moved away from the radiation source as soon as possible, but lifesaving care should not be delayed if the patient cannot be moved immediately. Intravenous lines should be initiated only if absolutely necessary, and good aseptic technique should be used to minimize the risk of introducing contaminants into the patient's body.
(Objective 12)

30. d. Alkali agents cause chemical burns; ionizing agents cause radiation burns, and arcing is caused by electrical energy.
(Objective 1)

31. b. Men die more frequently than women secondary to burns. Three fourths of burn fatalities occur in the home. Deaths are also common in low-income homes.
(Objective 1)

32. d. This source includes flames, scalds, or contact with hot substances.
(Objective 1)

33. d. The patient hyperventilates to adapt to the increased metabolic rate. The gastrointestinal tract slows and, with large burns, adynamic ileus is a frequent complication.
(Objective 2)

34. b. First-degree burns are usually red, dry, and painful without blisters. Third-degree burns are white, yellow, tan, brown, or black; leathery; and often painless.
(Objective 3)

35. c. Each leg is between 13.5% to 14% BSA.
(Objective 3)

36. c. Evaporation of fluid from the injured area also accounts for significant fluid loss.
(Objective 4)

37. c. The presence of first-degree burns should be noted in the narrative; however, these burns

should not be included in the estimate of percent body surface area burned.
(Objective 3)

38. c. The burn should be cooled rapidly, and then body temperature should be maintained with sheets and blankets.
(Objective 6)

39. c. 2 ml × 60 × 100 = 24,000 ml in the first 24 hours
½ in the first 8 hours = 12,000 ml
12,000 ml ÷ 8 = 750 ml
The formula states that 2 to 4 ml/kg/% BSA burned is given in 24 hours, so the range would be 750 to 1500 ml.
(Objective 6)

40. a. Petroleum products are not associated with inhalation burns unless they occur in an enclosed space or meet one of the other criteria.
(Objective 6)

41. d. Oxygen saturation levels may be normal because the hemoglobin still is saturated (with carbon monoxide, not oxygen), and the oximeter may not differentiate between the two. Intravenous fluid therapy is not helpful in these patients.
(Objective 7)

42. c. Drying the chemical or delaying treatment only prolongs contact with the skin and increases the burn injury. Application of a chemical antidote is recommended only for a few chemicals.
(Objective 8)

43. c. Each other factor has a direct affect on the severity of the injury.
(Objective 7)

44. b. Subcutaneous injection of the calcium gluconate gel under the burn eschar is the most effective method.
(Objective 9)

45. d. An arc occurs when electrical energy "jumps" from its source through the air to another conductive medium. Direct burns result when the current passes through a person. *Alternating* is a description of a type of electrical current.
(Objective 10)

46. d. The most resistance to electrical energy is provided by bone.
(Objective 10)

47. a. All the other pathological conditions can occur secondary to lightning injury but cause death less frequently than cardiac or respiratory arrest.
(Objective 10)

48. c. Gamma rays have 10,000 times the penetrating power of alpha particles and 100 times the penetrating power of beta particles.
(Objective 12)

● CHAPTER 22
HEAD AND FACIAL TRAUMA

1. a.
(Objective 4)

2. c.
(Objective 4)

3. d.
(Objective 4)

4. b.
(Objective 4)

5. e. This nerve is associated with basilar skull fracture.
(Objective 4)

6. b. Injury to the brain affecting the optic nerve may cause blindness in one or both eyes or visual field defects.
(Objective 4)

7. d. Damage involving the facial nerve may cause immediate or delayed facial paralysis and is associated with basilar skull fracture.
(Objective 4)

8. c. Injury affecting the oculomotor nerve can result in double vision because of the inability of the eye to move medially and down and out. Ptosis and pupil dilation or unresponsiveness to light also may occur.
(Objective 4)

9. a. Loss or alteration of sense of smell associated with injury affecting the olfactory nerve is a common finding associated with basilar skull fracture.
(Objective 4)

10. a. Inspect and palpate the head for lacerations, contusions, and deformities. Inspect the face for asymmetry and soft tissue injury. Evaluate the child's vision by holding up fingers and assessing pupil response. Assess for EOMs by asking the child to look up and down and side to side. Look for deformity of the nose and any drainage of blood or CSF. Inspect the oral cavity for bleeding, soft tissue injury, and missing teeth. Palpate the face for crepitus and question the child about tenderness or numbness. Ask the child to open and close the mouth and move the lower jaw from side to side. Gently palpate for loose teeth.
b. Immobilize the C spine and secure the child to the backboard while frequently suctioning the oral cavity. Tilt the backboard to the side and secure it firmly with straps. Suction the oral cavity frequently and instruct the child to signal when he needs additional suctioning or if he has difficulty breathing. Continually reevaluate for life threats.
(Objective 1)

11. Obtain a history to include the exact mode of injury; previous ocular, medical, and drug history, including cataracts, glaucoma, and presence of hepatitis or HIV; use of eye medications; use of corrective glasses or contact lenses; presence of ocular prostheses; and symptoms and treatment in-

terventions that may have been attempted before EMS arrival. Observe the patient for signs of external trauma, discoloration, injury to the lid, fluid or jelly extruding from the eye, bleeding, blood in the anterior chamber, and the presence of contact lenses. Measure visual acuity with a handheld acuity chart or any printed material with small, medium, and large point sizes. Record the distance at which the visual material was held. Measure each eye separately and assess vision with and without corrective lenses. Evaluate pupil reaction to ensure that they constrict in concert when light is applied and dilate in response to darkness. Assess extraocular muscles by asking the patient to track an object with the eyes (without head movement) up, down, right, and left. (Objective 2)

12. a. Injury: foreign body (or corneal abrasion); management: irrigate with normal saline.

b. Injury: lid avulsion; management: assess for underlying injury to the eye; control bleeding with gentle pressure; for transport, cover with a dressing moistened with normal saline and an eye shield.

c. Injury: embedded foreign body; management: patch uninjured eye; stabilize hook and cover with cardboard cup secured with tape.

d. Injury: traumatic hyphema; management: elevate head of ambulance cot or spine board 40 to 45 degrees; instruct patient to avoid straining.

e. Injury: ruptured globe; management: cover affected eye with damp, sterile dressings and an eye shield.

(Objective 2)

13. Bleeding, shock, hematoma, pulse deficit, neurological deficit, dyspnea, hoarseness, stridor, subcutaneous emphysema, hemoptysis, dysphagia, and hematemesis
(Objective 3)

14. Secure airway and breathing. Maintain spine immobilization. Apply firm, direct pressure to the affected vessels and tamponade the vessel by direct pressure with a gloved finger only to the affected vessel(s). If venous injury is suspected, keep the patient supine or in the Trendelenberg position to prevent an air embolism. If air embolism is suspected, turn the immobilized patient on the left side, head lower than feet, to attempt to trap the air embolus in the right ventricle.
(Objective 3)

15. a. Diffuse axonal injury; loss of consciousness (usually less than 5 minutes), retrograde or antegrade amnesia, vomiting, combativeness, transient visual disturbances, and problems with coordination; should all improve, not deteriorate

b. Focal injury; seizures, hemiparesis, aphasia, personality changes, and loss of consciousness (lasting hours, days, or longer)

c. Focal injury; headache, nausea, vomiting, decreasing level of consciousness, coma, abnormal posturing, paralysis, and bulging fontanelles in infants

d. Focal injury; transient loss of consciousness followed by a lucid interval (6 to 18 hours) and a subsequent decreasing level of consciousness, headache, and contralateral hemiparesis (opposite the side of the bleeding); 50% unconscious without improvement

e. Diffuse axonal injury; patients being usually unconscious for prolonged periods; may have posturing and signs of increased ICP
(Objective 5)

16. Headache, nausea, vomiting, altered level of consciousness, increased systolic blood pressure, widened pulse pressure, decreased pulse rate, abnormally slow respiratory pattern, unilateral dilated pupil, and abnormal posturing
(Objective 5)

17. Intubate tracheally (possibly nasally if signs of basilar skull fracture are not present) using spinal precautions. Hyperventilate the lungs with 100% oxygen at a rate of 24 per minute. Consider gastric tube insertion if available. Maintain fluids to keep the vein open unless signs of shock develop. Consider pharmacological agents, such as mannitol and furosemide, in consultation with medical direction. Notify medical direction and transport the patient to the closest appropriate trauma center.
(Objective 6)

18. a. GCS is 12, and RTS is 11.

b. GCS is 8, and RTS is 7.

c. PTS is 7.

(Objective 7)

19. b. "Donkey face" is associated with this injury. Edema, unstable maxilla, epistaxis, numb upper teeth, nasal flattening, and CSF rhinorrhea are also signs of midface fracture.
(Objective 1)

20. c. Neither an endotracheal tube nor a gastric tube should be placed nasally in the patient with midface fracture because they may pass into the cranial vault. Elevation of the head of the cot would be appropriate only after the cervical spine is cleared by radiographs in the ED. CSF drainage often accompanies these injuries and should be allowed to drain freely.
(Objective 1)

21. d. The zygoma commonly is called the *cheekbone*.
(Objective 1)

22. c. Orbital fractures often are associated with other fractures, such as Lefort II and III and zygomatic fractures.
(Objective 1)

23. d. In children minimal displacement may result in growth changes and ultimate deformity.
(Objective 1)

421

24. d. A chance to reimplant does exist, so if possible, the ear should be transported as described. However, ear injuries that involve cartilage often heal poorly and are infected easily.
(Objective 2)

25. b. Nitrous oxide is contraindicated and may increase the pain. Other measures that may help include requests that the patient yawn, swallow, and move the lower jaw.
(Objective 2)

26. d. Milk may be used if a commercial tooth solution, such as Hank's solution, is not available.
(Objective 2)

27. d. Zone II injuries (b) occur more often but are associated with lower mortality.
(Objective 3)

28. c. Stridor indicates that the upper airway is compromised significantly.
(Objective 3)

29. d. Attempting intubation actually may increase the damage associated with the injury and, if unsuccessful, cause partial airway obstruction to become complete.
(Objective 3)

30. b. Contusion is bruising of a specific area of the brain. All other answers reflect injuries that represent diffuse axonal injury.
(Objective 5)

31. a. This is the earliest sign and is consistent with all patients who have increased intracranial pressure.
(Objective 5)

32. d. The patient in diabetic ketoacidosis demonstrates Kussmaul respirations in an attempt to correct acidosis.
(Objective 5)

33. d. Other common signs and symptoms include dizziness, neck stiffness, unequal pupils, vomiting, seizures, and loss of consciousness.
(Objective 5)

34. c. All other interventions are indicated (depending on medical control) to decrease intracranial pressure; however, ventilation at a rate not to exceed 24 per minute is the fastest method with the least risk to the patient. (Objective 6)

35. d. $\dfrac{40 \text{ g} \times 100 \text{ ml}}{20 \text{ g}} = 200 \text{ ml}$

or/ 20 g:100 ml = 40 g: x ml
$$4000 = 20x$$
$$200 \text{ ml} = x$$

36. b. Atropine may be given to children before intubation to counteract the vagal stimulation. Mannitol is an osmotic diuretic given to decrease ICP but usually is not given for this purpose. Midazolam (Versed) is often given during RSI procedures to sedate the patient.
(Objective 6)

● CHAPTER 23
SPINAL TRAUMA

1. e.
(Objective 9)

2. j.
(Objective 9)

3. a.
(Objective 5)

4. k.
(Objective 5)

5. c.
(Objective 5)

6. f.
(Objective 5)

7. b.
(Objective 8)

8. g.
(Objective 8)

9. h.
(Objective 9)

10. d.
(Objective 5)

11. a. Negative
b. Positive
c. Positive
d. Uncertain
e. Uncertain
f. Positive
g. Uncertain
(Objective 2)

12. Damage from spinal injury can either occur more easily or be complicated by one or more of the following: a. Increased age
b. Osteoporosis
c. Spondylosis
d. Rheumatoid arthritis
e. Paget's disease
f. Congenital cord anomalies (fusion, narrow spinal canal)
(Objective 4)

13. a. hyperflexion
b. hyperextension
c. ligamentous complex and joint capsule
d. dislocation (subluxation)
e. whiplash
f. C5 to C7
g. C1 to C2
h. T12 to L2
i. compression
j. teardrop fractures
k. dislocations
(Objective 5)

14. Absence of motor and sensory function below the nipple, relative bradycardia, hypotension, priapism, unstable body temperature, loss of bowel and bladder control, and decreased depth of respiration (loss of inervation of most intercostal muscles)

(Objective 6)

15. To be reliable, she must be calm, cooperative, sober, alert, and oriented. If she exhibits any of the following, she should be considered unreliable: acute stress reaction, brain injury, intoxication, abnormal mental status, distracting injuries, or problems in communication.

(Objective 4)

16. Motor evaluation: Ask the patient to move her arms and legs. Ask her to flex her elbow, grab and squeeze your fingers, and extend her elbows. Have the patient spread the fingers of both hands and keep them apart while you squeeze the second and fourth fingers. A normal exam produces springlike resistance. Support the patient's lower arm and ask her to hold her wrists or fingers out straight while you press down on her fingers. Moderate resistance should be felt. Place your hands at the sole of each foot and ask the patient to push against your hands. Both sides should feel equal and strong. Then, hold the patient's feet (with fingers on her toes) and instruct her to pull them back to her nose. Both sides should feel equal and strong.

(Objectives 4 and 6)

17. Sensory evaluation: Question the patient about pain in the neck or back and any feelings of numbness or tingling in the body. Assess light touch on each hand and each foot (with the patient's eyes closed) and then, if necessary, prick the hands and feet with a sharp object (without breaking the skin).

(Objectives 4 and 6)

18. a. Increasing pain or neurological deficits during movement

b. Resistance to movement

c. Muscle spasm

d. Airway compromise due to repositioning

e. Severe misalignment of head from midline

(Objective 7)

19. A. Rescuer 1 is positioned at the patient's head, providing inline manual stabilization. Rescuers 2 and 3 are positioned at the patient's midthorax and knees.

B. While maintaining immobilization, the rescuers, in one organized move, slowly logroll the patient onto his or her side, perpendicular to the ground.

C. Rescuer 4 positions the long spine board by placing the device flat on the ground or at a 30- to 40-degree angle against the patient's back.

D. In one organized move, the rescuers slowly logroll and center the patient onto the long spine board.

(Objective 7)

20. a. Methylprednisolone 30 mg/kg bolus, followed by 5.4 mg/kg/hour for 23 hours

Other experimental treatments include naloxone and calcium channel blockers (consult medical direction).

b. Dopamine

21. b. In order of frequency of occurrence, they are motor vehicle crashes, falls, penetrating injuries, and sports injuries.

(Objective 1)

22. c. Most single-story homes are more than three times a person's height, which is classified as positive mechanism of injury.

23. d. The patient in (a) may be experiencing a stress reaction. The patient in (b) has a distracting injury. You cannot examine the patient in (c) well enough to rule out spinal injury by clinical criteria because of the language barrier.

(Objective 2)

24. a. The cervical spine allows the head to rotate with an almost 180-degree range of motion, 60 degrees of flexion, and 70 degrees of extension.

(Objective 3)

25. d. Axial loading occurs when the spine is compressed vertically. Distraction results from excessive "pulling" on the spinal cord. Flexion is a bending motion that decreases the angle between two joints, which more often results from anterior/posterior-type motion.

(Objective 2)

26. d. Pain or tenderness of the neck with or without palpation always should indicate immobilization of the spine.

(Objective 4)

27. c. Axial loading is a vertical loading mechanism of injury. A herniated disk occurs when the cartilage surrounding an intervertebral disk ruptures and releases the pulpy elastic substance that cushions the vertebrae above and below, causing pain and damage to nerve roots.[1]

(Objective 5)

28. a. The spinal cord terminates at L2.

(Objective 5)

29. c. C3, 4 would involve sensory loss at the top of the shoulder; T4 at the nipple; and S1 on the lateral foot.

(Objectives 4 and 6)

30. a. Hypotension, priapism, loss of sweating and shivering, poikilothermy, and loss of bowel and bladder control are also signs.

(Objective 6)

31. b. This weakness usually results from hyperextension or hyperflexion injuries.

(Objective 5)

[1]Anderson KN, Anderson LE: *Mosby's medical, nursing & allied health dictionary*, ed 3, St Louis, 1990, Mosby.

32. d. Transection of the cord above C3 usually results in respiratory arrest. Lesions that occur at C4 may result in diaphragmatic paralysis. Lesions at C5-C6 spare the diaphragm but result in loss of significant intercostal muscle function.
(Objective 6)

33. d. Traction should not be applied on the spine in the field. Primary injury occurs at the time the initial forces are applied.
(Objective 7)

34. d. Immobilize the torso first to prevent angulation of the cervical spine
(Objective 7)

35. c. Spinal shock results from a temporary loss of all spinal cord function distal to the injury.
(Objective 8)

36. d. Rotational stress fractures are common at the affected site of spondylosis.
(Objective 9)

● CHAPTER 24
THORACIC TRAUMA

1. Flail chest.
(Objective 2)

2. The pulmonary contusion and injured segment of the chest will not expand; therefore insufficient negative pressure is generated in the chest to draw in a normal amount of air.
(Objective 2)

3. Intubate if the Glasgow coma score is less than 8 or if the patient has severe hypoxia. Assist ventilations with positive pressure (demand valve, bag-valve) with 100% oxygen. Monitor vital signs, electrocardiogram, and oxygen saturation.
(Objective 2)

4. Dyspnea, tachypnea, diminished breath sounds on the affected side, and chest pain on inspiration.
(Objective 3)

5. a. During inspiration, some air will enter the wound instead of the trachea, which decreases air entering the lung for ventilation; b. Seal wound on three sides with occlusive dressing. Administer high-flow oxygen by nonrebreather mask.
(Objective 3)

6. a. Cyanosis, tracheal deviation, tachycardia, hypotension, and distended neck veins. b. Insert a 14-gauge catheter in the midclavicular line of the second or third intercostal space on the side of the pneumothorax. Listen for a rush of air, consider a flutter valve, reevaluate the patient, and repeat these steps en route if the needle clots.
(Objective 3)

7. Hypoxia and hypovolemic shock.
(Objective 3)

8. a. Traumatic asphyxia; b. Oxygenate and maintain airway and ventilation and evaluate for associated injuries.
(Objective 3)

9. a. Myocardial contusion; b. Oxygen administration, electrocardiographic monitoring, and treatment of dysrhythmias per protocol.
(Objective 4)

10. a. Pericardial tamponade; b. Oxygen administration, fluid replacement, rapid transport, consideration of pericardiocentesis (only with authorization and specialized training).
(Objective 4)

11. Upper extremity or generalized hypertension, systolic murmur, paraplegia (rare), and severe shock.
(Objective 4)

12. d. At least 25% of trauma deaths are associated with chest trauma. Falls, crush injuries, blast injuries, and blows to the chest can also cause significant thoracic trauma.
(Objective 1)

13. d. The clavicle is one of the most commonly fractured bones. Rarely, clavicle fracture can be complicated by injury to the subclavian vein or artery from bony fragment penetration. The mechanism typically involves a fall on outstretched arms or the shoulder.
(Objective 2)

14. d. Children have more elastic chests and are less likely to have rib fractures. The first rib is rarely fractured. The pancreas lies protected behind other abdominal organs and is unlikely to be affected by rib fractures.
(Objective 2)

15. d. The damaged tissue often results in significant hypoxia.
(Objective 2)

16. c. The heart lies under the sternum and may be compressed if it is injured.
(Objective 2)

17. c. Excessive pressure on the chest wall can cause pneumothorax (paper-bag effect). Spontaneous pneumothorax occurs when a rupture or tear develops in the lung parenchyma for no apparent reason.
(Objective 3)

18. a. Pneumothorax in a patient with preexisting lung or heart disease can also be lethal.
(Objective 3)

19. b. Hypotension will develop as a result of hypovolemic shock. Tachypnea, deviation to the affected side (rare), and narrowed pulse pressure may also occur.
(Objective 3)

20. c. Inertial effect is a stretching and shearing of alveoli and intravascular structures. When the kinetic wave of energy is partially reflected at the alveolar membrane surface and the remainder

causes a localized release of energy, it is referred to as the *Spalding effect.*
(Objective 3)

21. b. Profound hypoxia can result from abnormal lung function.
(Objective 3)

22. d. Tracheal deviation may be found in some patients with tension pneumothorax.
(Objective 4)

23. e. Laceration of the liver may also occur.
(Objective 4)

24. c. Pulses may be decreased in the lower extremities.
(Objective 5)

25. c. When the bowel moves into the chest, severe respiratory compromise occurs.
(Objective 6)

● CHAPTER 25
ABDOMINAL TRAUMA

1. a. Spleen; b. Referred pain caused by irritation of the diaphragm by a splenic hematoma or blood in the peritoneum (Kehr's sign); c. This child should have a rapid assessment. Oxygen should be applied, and rapid transport to the closest appropriate trauma center should begin immediately. Intravenous therapy using an isotonic solution should be administered at 20 ml/kg during transport. Repeat IV bolus may be indicated based on the reevaluation.
(Objective 2)

2. Sepsis, infection, abscess formation, and peritonitis (resulting from leakage of the contents of hollow organs).
(Objective 2)

3. a. Unexplained shock; b. Bruising and discoloration to the abdomen; c. Abrasions; d. Obvious bleeding; e. Pain, abdominal tenderness, or guarding; f. Abdominal rigidity, distention; g. Evisceration; h. Rib fractures; i. Pelvic fractures.
(Objective 4)

4. d. This injury is caused by stretching organs and blood vessels.
(Objective 1)

5. c. The other organ injured most frequently is the spleen.
(Objective 2)

6. c. Shock also occurs often.
(Objective 2)

7. b. Bleeding can be severe and difficult to detect. Injury can result from anterior or posterior trauma. Urine output may contain blood.
(Objective 2)

8. a. Steering wheel trauma and penetrating trauma are also associated with pancreatic injury.
(Objective 2)

9. a. This may indicate urethral injury that could be complicated by insertion of a catheter.
(Objective 2)

10. b. The patient will often present with signs and symptoms of shock.
(Objective 3)

11. c. In the presence of unexplained shock in the patient with trauma, abdominal injury should always be at the top of your "rule out" list.
(Objective 4)

12. d. Initial exam can be done on the scene. Further examination and IV therapy may be performed en route to the hospital.
(Objective 5)

13. a. The liver is located in the right upper quadrant. The diaphragm extends low so the chest cavity is easily penetrated with these types of injuries.
(Objective 1)

14. d. High concentration oxygen administration and fluid resuscitation are indicated.
(Objective 5)

15. c. Scene safety should always be the priority on every call, especially when a crime has been committed.
(Objective 5)

● CHAPTER 26
MUSCULOSKELETAL TRAUMA

1. g.
(Objective 1)

2. d.
(Objective 1)

3. f.
(Objective 1)

4. i.
(Objective 1)

5. h.
(Objective 1)

6. a.
(Objective 1)

7. c.
(Objective 1)

8. b.
(Objective 1)

9. e.
(Objective 1)

10. f. and g.
(Objective 5)

11. b., d., f., and g.
(Objective 5)

12. b., d., f., and g.
(Objective 5)

13. b., d., and f.
(Objective 5)

14. b., d., and f.
(Objective 5)

15. b. and d.
(Objective 5)
16. a., b., and d.
(Objective 5)
17. c. and e.
(Objective 6)
18. c.
(Objective 6)
19. c. and h.
(Objective 6)
20. b. and d.
(Objective 6)
21. b. and d.
(Objective 6)
22. b.
(Objective 6)
23. a.
(Objective 6)
24. On every patient, you must assess for the presence of life threats in the initial assessment.
(Objective 3)
25. The six "P's" are pain, pallor, paresthesia, pulses, paralysis, and pressure.
(Objective 3)
26. The initials *DCAP-BTLS* refer to deformity, contusions, abrasions, penetrations or punctures, burns, tenderness, lacerations, and swelling.
(Objective 3)
27. The general principles of splinting are: splint joints above and below, as well as bone ends; immobilize open and closed fractures in the same manner; cover open fractures to minimize contamination; check pulses, sensation, and motor function before and after splinting; stabilize the extremity with gentle, inline traction to position of normal alignment; immobilize a long bone extremity in a straight position that can easily be splinted; immobilize dislocations in a position of comfort; ensure good vascular supply; immobilize joints as found; joint injuries are only aligned if there is no distal pulse; apply cold to reduce swelling and pain; apply compression to reduce swelling; and elevate the extremity if possible.
(Objective 4)
28. There is no pulse distal to the injury, which is an indication to attempt realignment in the prehospital setting.
(Objective 8)
29. Administer an analgesic and/or benzodiazepine (with appropriate monitoring) if not contraindicated by other injuries. Apply inline traction along the shaft of the femur with the hip and knee flexed at 90 degrees. Apply slow and steady traction to relax the muscle spasm. Listen for a "pop" with accompanying sudden relief of pain and easy manipulation of the leg to full extension. Immobilize the leg in full extension with patient supine on a

long spine board; reevaluate pulses and neurovascular status. If unsuccessful, immobilize the leg at a flexion not to exceed 90 degrees and immobilize the leg with pillows or blankets; place the patient supine.
(Objective 8)
30. d. Sprains represent injuries to ligaments.
(Objective 1)
31. b. A complete dislocation is a luxation.
(Objective 1)
32. d. Bursitis involves inflammation of the bursa; tendonitis is inflammation of a tendon caused by injury; and arthritis is inflammation of the joint.
(Objective 2)
33. d. The traditional drugs in this group cause gastrointestinal complications and are being replaced by newer agents with fewer side effects.
(Objective 2)
34. a. Treatment is needed for all of the other signs; however, emergent interventions are needed to preserve the limb when distal pulses are absent.
(Objective 3)
35. c. Because of the life threats present in this patient, time would not be taken to treat this isolated injury except to provide full body immobilization on a spine board.
(Objective 3)
36. b. The fifth metacarpal is broken in a Boxer's fracture.
(Objective 5)
37. d. After a hip fracture, the extremity is usually shortened and externally rotated.
(Objective 6)
38. a. It is not indicated for other types of fractures.
(Objective 6)
39. c. Popliteal artery injury is associated with knee trauma.
(Objective 6)
40. a. Ensure that this is reported to the receiving medical personnel and documented in the patient care report. Assess distal pulse and sensation.
(Objective 7)
41. d. The movement necessary to realign the arm could cause further injury to the back.
(Objective 8)
42. b. Instructions about care of the injury should be given to the patient (preferably in writing) before your departure.
(Objective 9)

● **CHAPTER 27**
PULMONARY

1. c.
(Objective 3)
2. a.
(Objective 3)

3. i.
(Objective 3)

4. h.
(Objective 3)

5. b.
(Objective 3)

6. g.
(Objective 3)

7. e.
(Objective 3)

8. d.
(Objective 3)

9. a. This is a problem with diffusion because there is inadequate oxygen to diffuse across the alveolar membrane into the capillaries.
(Objective 1)
b. This represents a problem with ventilation. It is possible that the drugs have depressed the central nervous system and made ventilations inadequate.
c. This is likely to be related to a problem with diffusion from the fluid that has leaked into the interstitial spaces and perfusion because the left side of the heart is not functioning well.
d. These symptoms are likely related to anemia, which causes a problem with perfusion so oxygen cannot be carried to the tissues.
e. Airway obstruction creates a problem with ventilation.
f. These signs and symptoms suggest pulmonary embolism, which creates a problem with perfusion.
g. Flail chest is often accompanied by pulmonary contusion. This would create a problem with ventilation because of the mechanical disruption and diffusion related to the fluid in the pulmonary spaces.

10. Asthma, chronic obstructive pulmonary disease, heart failure, pulmonary edema, pulmonary embolism, bronchiolitis (infants), foreign body aspiration, toxic inhalation, pneumonia, spontaneous pneumothorax, hyperventilation syndrome or lung cancer are some of the conditions that may present with this chief complaint.
(Objective 3)

11. Signs and symptoms that indicate a life threat include: alterations in mental status, severe cyanosis, absent breath sounds, audible stridor, 1- or 2- word dyspnea, tachycardia, pallor and diaphoresis, cardiac dysrhythmias, pulse rate greater than 130 beats per minute, poor, floppy muscle tone, and the presence of retractions and/or the use of accessory muscles.

12. You should ask about the patient's chief complaint and determine if she/he has any chest pain, productive or nonproductive cough, hemoptysis, wheezing, and signs of respiratory infection (e.g., fever or increased sputum production). Inquire about the patient's past history, especially as related to similar problems and his or her perceived severity of this episode. Obtain a medication history and ask if the patient has ever needed intubation to manage this type of illness. The physical examination should begin by noting your general impression of the patient. Note the patient's position, mentation, ability to speak, respiratory effort, and skin color. Observe the heart rate for tachycardia or bradycardia. Note any abnormal respiratory patterns. Assess the face and neck for pursed-lip breathing and use of accessory muscles. Evaluate the neck for jugular venous distention. Inspect the chest for injury, indicators of chronic disease, accessory muscle use, and chest symmetry. Auscultate the lungs for abnormal breath sounds. Assess the extremities for peripheral cyanosis, clubbing of the fingers, and carpopedal spasm. (Objective 2)

13. a. "Blue bloater," chronic cough with production of large amount of sputum, hypercapnia, hypoxemia, cyanosis, pulmonary hypertension, and cor pulmonale; b. "Pink puffer," hyperexpansion of lungs, barrel chest, resistance to air flow (especially on expiration), pursed lip breathing, and thinness.
(Objective 3)

14. Oxygen should be administered initially at 2 L/min if the patient is not in respiratory failure. If rapid improvement does not occur, the flow of oxygen should be increased while the paramedic carefully monitors the patient. If the patient's condition is critical, intubation and assisted ventilation may be necessary.
(Objective 3)

15. Albuterol; metoproterenol.
(Objective 3)

16. Transport patient in a position of comfort, instruct patient to use pursed-lip breathing and minimize physical activity to conserve energy for breathing, calmly reassure and care for the patient, and provide a cool environment for transport.
(Objective 3)

17. During an acute asthma attack, there is reversible airflow obstruction caused by bronchial smooth muscle contraction, hypersecretion of mucus causing bronchial plugging, and inflammatory changes in the bronchial walls.
(Objective 3)

18. Peak expiratory flow rate measurement can help determine the severity of an asthma attack and evaluate the effectiveness of treatment in reversing airway obstruction.
(Objective 3)

19. Albuterol 0.5 ml (2.5 mg) in 2.5 ml normal saline by nebulizer at 6 to 7 L/min O_2.
(Objective 3)

20. Ask the patient if his breathing is easier. Observe the patient for decreased anxiety, changes in level of consciousness, and ability to converse more easily. Note the degree of respiratory distress by observing patient position, use of accessory muscles, and respiratory rate. Monitor vital signs. (Pulse and respiratory rate should decrease, and pulsus paradoxus should decline to below 20 mm Hg. As the patient improves, the inspiratory and then expiratory wheezes should disappear.)
(Objective 3)

21. Status asthmaticus.
(Objective 3)

22. Ensure that oxygen is at 100% and is humidified, increase fluid rate to hydrate patient, administer other medications (such as methylprednisolone, hydrocortisone) as ordered by medical direction, expedite transport, monitor patient closely for signs of respiratory failure, and prepare to intubate if necessary. If intubation is indicated, follow local medical protocols, which may include sedation (ketamine, benzodiazepine, or barbiturates); paralyze patient; intubate; administer 2.5 to 5.0 mg albuterol directly into ET tube; confirm ET tube placement; ventilate at 8 to 10 breaths/min.
(Objective 3)

23. a. Upper airway obstruction: foreign body, epiglottitis; b. lower airway obstruction: asthma, airway edema; c. trauma: inhalation injury, ARDS secondary to pulmonary contusion; d. alveolar pathology: COPD, lung cancer, inhalation injury; e. interstitial space pathology: pulmonary edema, near-drowning.
(Objective 2)

24. Viral, bacterial, mycoplasma, and aspiration.
(Objective 3)

25. Signs and symptoms of bacterial pneumonia include shaking chills, tachypnea, tachycardia, cough with sputum (rust colored, hemoptysis, yellow, green, gray), malaise, anorexia, flank or back pain, vomiting, fever, wheezing, fine crackles, dyspnea, and sore throat.
(Objective 3)

26. Care includes airway support, oxygen administration, ventilatory assistance, IV fluids, cardiac and oxygen saturation monitoring, and transportation. If wheezing is present, bronchodilator therapy may be used.
(Objective 3)

27. a. Adult respiratory distress syndrome; b. Monitor the chest rising and falling to determine the effectiveness of ventilation; note any difficulty or increasing pressure necessary to ventilate patient; fre-

quently assess vital signs, observing for increased heart rate; monitor electrocardiogram, end-tidal CO_2 and oxygen saturation by pulse oximetry; and observe for cyanosis. Ventilate with high-flow oxygen, ventilate with positive end-expiratory pressure using Boehringer valve if trained and authorized by medical direction, and administer steroids and diuretics if ordered by medical direction.
(Objective 3)

28. Extended travel; prolonged bedrest; obesity; older adulthood; burns; varicose veins; surgery of the thorax, abdomen, pelvis, and legs; pelvic or leg fractures; malignancy; use of birth control pills; congenital or acquired coagulopathies; pregnancy; chronic obstructive pulmonary disease; congestive heart failure; sickle cell anemia; cancer; atrial fibrillation; myocardial infarction; previous pulmonary embolism; deep vein thrombosis; infection; diabetes mellitus; and multiple trauma.
(Objective 3)

29. Dyspnea, cough, hemoptysis, pain, anxiety, syncope, hypotension, diaphoresis, increased respiratory rate, increased heart rate, fever, distended neck veins, chest splinting, pleuritic chest pain, pleural friction rub, crackles, and wheezes (localized).
(Objective 3)

30. This typically occurs in tall, thin males between the ages of 20 and 40. It may also be found in patients with COPD, patients with AIDS who have pneumonia, and drug abusers who deeply inhale free-base cocaine, marijuana, or inhalants such as glue or solvents.
(Objective 3)

31. b. Cardiac, genetic, and stress factors are all intrinsic factors.
(Objective 1)

32. b. Adequate blood volume and patent pulmonary capillaries are related to perfusion. Normal interstitial space affects diffusion.
(Objective 1)

33. c. All of the answers represent findings that indicate respiratory distress; however, in the patient with chronic respiratory illness, their reported level of distress is often the best indication of the severity of their condition.
(Objective 2)

34. c. This signs takes a long time to develop. Acutely hypoxic patients may use accessory muscles or pursed lip breathing in an attempt to improve ventilation. Carpopedal spasm is seen secondary to hypocapnia.
(Objective 2)

35. b. All will have wheezing and cough when acutely ill. There is resistance to airflow in all three conditions, although less in emphysema.
(Objective 3)

36. c. The patient is more likely to be tachycardic than bradycardic. Capillary refill is an indicator of perfusion (flow), not oxygenation.
(Objective 3)

37. d. Right heart failure can develop secondary to pulmonary hypertension (cor pulmonale). The right side of the heart is increasingly forced to pump harder to overcome the excess pressure in the pulmonary arteries. Eventually, it cannot force the blood through, and fluid backs up to the venous side of the system.
(Objective 3)

38. d.
(Objective 3)

39. c. Expiratory wheezing indicates narrowing of the smaller airways. As the larger airways become obstructed, inspiratory wheezing will be audible. When the obstruction is so severe that there is almost no air flow, the chest will be silent with diminished breath sounds and no wheezes.
(Objective 3)

40. a. Albuterol is a beta-2 agonist that causes relatively few side effects. Although each of the other drugs do cause bronchodilation, they are rarely used because of their high incidence of side effects.
(Objective 3)

41. a. The PEFR is most helpful when the patient's normal baseline peak flow is known.
(Objective 3)

42. d. The vaccine is 80% to 90% effective in the prevention of *Pneumococcus* bacillus pneumonia.
(Objective 3)

43. c. Altered level of consciousness may impair the gag reflex or the patient's ability to handle secretions.
(Objective 3)

44. d. The death rate is greater than 65% but does not always occur. Disseminated coagulation may occur in some, but not all, patients.
(Objective 3)

45. a. This adjunct combines partial ventilatory support and CPAP.
(Objective 3)

46. d. The size and location of the embolus determine whether mild signs and symptoms or sudden death will occur.
(Objective 3)

47. c. Most upper respiratory infections have no identifiable cause. Good handwashing is an important action to prevent their spread.
(Objective 3)

48. b. Other risk factors for spontaneous pneumothorax include patients with emphysema, persons with AIDS who develop pneumonia, and healthy tall, thin, men between the ages of 20 and 40.
(Objective 3)

49. b. Narcotic overdose is associated with respiratory depression. (Objective 3)

50. a. Heavy smokers have a 25× greater chance of developing lung cancer than nonsmokers.
(Objective 3)

● CHAPTER 28 CARDIOLOGY

1. c
(Objective 2)
2. f
(Objective 2)
3. a
(Objective 2)
4. e
(Objective 2)
5. b
(Objective 2)
6. g
(Objective 2)
7. h
(Objective 2)
8.

Risk Factor	Prevention Strategy	Resource
a. Smoking	Quit smoking with use of medications, hypnosis, behavior modification, health clinic	Private physician, heart association, cancer association, alternative nicotine products
b. Hypercholesterolemia	Diet modification, drugs	Private physician, health clinic, heart association
c. Obesity	Diet, exercise	Private physician, exercise, community health clinic, dietitian, American Heart Association
d. Sedentary lifestyle	Exercise program, leisure activities	Private physician, local health clubs, heart association, local hospital

(Objective 1)

9.

	Sympathetic	Parasympathetic
a. Heart rate	Increase	Decrease
b. Myocardial contractility	Increase	No effect
c. Lungs	Beta-bronchiolar dilation	Constriction
d. Blood vessels (peripheral)	Constriction	No effect

(Objective 2)

10. a. Epinephrine: increased heart rate, contractility, bronchiolar dilation, and blood vessel constriction in skin, kidneys, gastrointestinal tract, and viscera. b. Norepinephrine: peripheral vasoconstriction. (Objective 2)

11. a. magnetic; b. potential; c. permeable; d. potential; e. millivolts; f. negative; g. negatively; h. potential; i. negative; j. −70 to −90; k. potassium; l. potassium; m. proteins; n. permeable; o. excitability; p. depolarization; q. threshold potential; r. action potential; s. depolarization; t. repolarization; u. positive; v. negative; w. depolarization; x. membrane potential. (Objective 3)

12. a. Sodium rushes into the cell through the fast sodium channels; b. The membrane potential drops to approximately 0; c. The slow calcium channels allow calcium to enter the cell while potassium continues to leave, maintaining the membrane potential of 0; d. The membrane potential returns to −90 mV; e. The sodium pump allows the exchange of sodium and potassium to their proper compartments; f. During phase 4, cardiac pacemaker cells slowly depolarize from their most negative membrane potential to a level at which threshold is reached and phase 0 begins. Non–pacemaker cells maintain a stable resting membrane potential and do not depolarize unless stimulated by a sufficiently strong stimulus. (Objective 3)

13. a. action potentials; b. upward; c. automaticity; d. resting membrane potential. (Objective 3)

14. a. Sinoatrial node; b. intranodal pathways; c. atrioventricular node; d. common bundle of His; e. left posterior bundle branch; f. Purkinje fibers; g. left anterior bundle branch; h. right bundle branch. (Objective 4)

15. The next pacemaker (atrioventricular node) should take over and fire. (Objective 4)

16. a. Acceleration of phase 4 depolarization so cells reach their threshold prematurely (may result from digoxin toxicity, increased catecholamine levels, hypoxia, hypercapnia, myocardial ischemia, infarction, increased venous return, hypokalemia, hypocalcemia, heating or cooling of the heart, or atropine administration); b. Reactivation of tissue by a returning impulse. (Objective 4)

17. O—Onset. What were you doing when the pain began? P—Is there anything that makes the pain better or worse? Q—What does the pain feel like? (Is it sharp, dull, crushing, squeezing?) R—Where is the pain? Does it go anywhere else? S—On a scale of 1 to 10, with 1 being no pain and 10 being the worst pain you have ever had, describe your pain. T—When did you first feel the pain? (Objective 5)

18. Chest pain, dyspnea, syncope, and palpitations. (Objective 5)

19. How did you feel before you passed out? What were you doing when you passed out? What position were you in before you passed out (i.e., laying down, sitting, standing)? How long were you unconscious? Do you have a history of heart disease or other significant medical history? What medicines do you take? Do you feel unusual in any other way? How has your health been over the past several days? (Objective 5)

20. Pulse rate and regularity, ECG, vital signs, circumstances of occurrence, duration, associated symptoms, previous history of palpitations, past medical history, and daily medicines. (Objective 5)

21. Major medical illnesses, home medicines, and similar previous episodes. (Objective 5)

22. Atrial fibrillation with a slow ventricular response. (Objective 10)

23. Yes. Digoxin (Lanoxin) or calcium channel blocker (Cardizem) toxicity can cause this presentation. Digitalis toxicity is more likely in the patient who is also taking a diuretic (furosemide). (Objective 5)

24. Neck: jugular venous distention. Chest: implanted pacemaker generator, median sternotomy scar, lung sounds (crackles), heart sounds (S3 gallop), and pulse deficit. Abdomen: generator for automatic implantable cardioverter defibrillator visible. Extremities: edema and ulceration. Back: sacral edema. Medical alert tags or medical information in wallet. (Objective 5)

25.

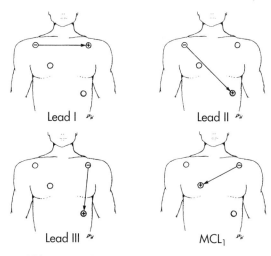

Lead I   Lead II   Lead III   MCL₁

(Objective 6)

26. a. Right arm (right anterior forearm); b. left arm (left anterior forearm); c. right leg (right lower leg); d. left lower leg (left leg); e. V1, fourth intercostal space to the right of the sternum; f. V2, fourth intercostal space to the left of the sternum;

430

g. V4, fifth intercostal space, midclavicular line; h. V3, between V2 and V4; i. V5, anterior axillary line in a straight line with V4; j. V6, midaxillary line, level with V4 and V5 (in women V4–V6 should be placed under the left breast). (Objective 6)

27. a. Excessive body hair: shave; b. diaphoresis: dry area and apply tincture of benzoin; c. poor electrode placement: reapply correctly; d. 60-cycle interference: run monitor on batteries; e. poor cable connections: recheck all connections; f. close proximity to electrical motors. (Objective 6)

28. a. 5; b. 0.04; c. 0.20; d. 3; e. 6. (Objective 6)

29. a. P wave; b. QRS complex; c. T wave; d. PR interval; e. ST segment. (Objective 7)

30. Muscle tremor, AC (60-cycle interference), loose electrodes, patient movement, loss of electrode contact, and external chest compression. (Objective 7)

31. Analyze the QRS complex; analyze the P waves; analyze the rate; analyze the rhythm; analyze the PR interval. (Objective 8)

32. a. Triplicate method (120/min.): Find the R wave on the dark line, count 300-150-100-75 for each next dark line until the next R wave. The R wave falls between 100 and 150. Estimate rate to be 120/min; b. R-R method: 300 ÷ Number of large boxes between R waves = 300 ÷ (almost) 3 = 100/min; c. R-R method: 1500 ÷ Number of small boxes between R waves = 1500 ÷ 13 = 115/min; d. 6-second method: Number of R waves in a 6-second strip × 10 = 12 × 10 = 120/min. (Objective 8)

33. No, this reveals only the rate, not the perfusion status (and the rate is faster than normal for an adult). (Objective 7)

34. a. R-R method (1500 ÷ Number of small boxes between the R waves) or triplicate method (but only if R waves both fall on dark lines). b. The 6-second method is the most accurate and quick estimate for irregular rhythm. (Objective 8)

35. The R-R distance should be equal when measured left to right across an ECG strip (it can vary no greater than 0.16 sec). (Objective 8)

36. a. Conduction through the ventricles is normal; b. Conduction through the ventricles is delayed and may follow an abnormal pathway. (Objective 7)

37. Are they regular? Is there a P wave in front of each QRS? Are they upright or inverted? Do they all look the same? (Objective 8)

38. a. Electrical impulse progressed from the atria to the ventricles through pathways other than the atrioventricular node of the bundle of His; b. Normal conduction from the sinoatrial node through the atrioventricular node; c. Delay in conduction of impulse through the atrioventricular node or bundle of His. (Objective 7)

39. a. QRS: 0.08 sec (normal is less than 0.12 sec); b. P waves: regular, one for each QRS complex, upright, all the same; c. Rate: 75/min (triplicate method); d. Rhythm: regular (R-R intervals =); e. PR interval 0.14 sec. Interpretation: normal sinus rhythm. (Objectives 8 and 9)

40. Patient history, chief complaint, and physical findings. (Objective 10)

41. a. parasympathetic stimulation; b. QRS less than 0.12 sec (unless a conduction delay is present); c. P waves (regular, preceding each QRS, upright, similar); d. PR interval 0.12 to 0.20 sec. (Objective 10)

42. a. Sinus node disease, increased parasympathetic vagal tone, hypothermia, hypoxia, and drug effects (digitalis, propranolol, verapamil); b. Exercise, fever, anxiety, ingestion of stimulants, smoking, hypovolemia, anemia, congestive heart failure, and excessive administration of atropine or vagolytic or sympathomimetic drugs (cocaine, phencyclidine, epinephrine, isoproterenol). (Objective 10)

43. QRS: 0.08 sec. P waves: present, upright, similar. Rate: 50/min. Rhythm: regular. PR interval: 0.16 sec. Interpretation: sinus bradycardia. Distinguishing features: all features of normal sinus rhythm except that rate is less than 60/min. Treatment: stable—observe; unstable—atropine 0.5 to 1.0 mg every 3-5 min to a maximum dose of <2.5 mg (0.03-0.04 mg/kg), transcutaneous pacing, dopamine 5 to 20 mcg/kg/min, epinephrine 2 to 10 mcg/min, isoproterenol 2 to 10 mcg/min. (Objective 10)

44. QRS: 0.06 sec. P waves: present, upright, similar. Rate: 110/min. Rhythm: regular. PR interval: 0.16 sec. Interpretation: sinus tachycardia. Distinguishing features: all features of normal sinus rhythm except that rate is greater than 100/min. Treatment: stable—none; unstable—seek and treat underlying cause. (Objective 10)

45. QRS: 0.08 sec; P waves: present, upright, similar. Rate: 70/min. Rhythm: irregular. PR interval: 0.12 sec. Interpretation: sinus dysrhythmia. Distinguishing features: all features of normal sinus rhythm but irregular rhythm that varies in cycles. Treatment: none. (Objective 10)

46. QRS: 0.08 sec. P waves: normal, upright. Rate: 50/min. Rhythm: irregular. PR interval: 0.16 sec. Interpretation: sinus arrest. Distinguishing features: Normal sinus rhythm until the sinoatrial node fails to fire. Treatment: stable—observe; unstable—atropine and transcutaneous pacing. (Objective 10)

47. a. tissues; b. atria; c. internodal. (Objective 10)

48. a. QRS: normal; b. P waves (if present): different from normal sinus P waves; c. PR interval: abnormal, shortened, or prolonged. (Objective 10)

49. Stress, overexertion, tobacco, caffeine, Wolff-Parkinson-White syndrome, digoxin toxicity, hypoxia, COPD, congestive heart failure, damage to sinoatrial node, rheumatic heart disease, and atherosclerotic heart disease. (Objective 10)

50. QRS: 0.06 sec. P waves: changes from beat to beat. Rate: 75/min. Rhythm: regular. PR interval: variable. Interpretation: wandering atrial pacemaker. Distinguishing features: typically slightly irregular P wave shapes and variable PR interval. Treatment: stable—monitor; unstable secondary to bradycardia—treat as bradycardia. (Objective 10)

51. QRS: 0.06 sec. P waves: present, upright. Rate: 100/min. Rhythm: regular interrupted by premature beats. PR interval: 0.10 sec (premature atrial contraction 0.16 sec). Interpretation: normal sinus rhythm with one premature atrial contraction. Distinguishing features: extra beat occurring earlier than next expected sinus beat; premature atrial contraction has features of sinus beat except that PR interval may be different. Treatment: none. (Objective 10)

52. QRS: 0.06 sec. P waves: unable to determine, may be hidden in T wave. Rate: 180/min. Rhythm: regular. PR interval: unable to determine. Interpretation: supraventricular tachycardia. Distinguishing features: rate greater than 150/min, with complexes originating in atria (QRS complex is <0.12 sec. unless a conduction defect is present.) Treatment: stable—oxygen, intravenous line, 12-lead ECG, consideration of vagal maneuvers, adenosine (6 mg, 12 mg, 12 mg rapid IVP at 1- to 2-minute intervals), diltiazem or verapamil or beta blockers, consider digoxin (Class IIb); unstable—synchronized cardioversion at 50, 100, 200, 300, and 360 joules. (Objective 10)

53. QRS: 0.06 sec. P waves: f-R waves. Rate: 100/min. Rhythm: regular. PR interval: none. FR interval: may vary. Interpretation: atrial flutter with 3:1 conduction. Distinguishing features: flutter waves.

Treatment: stable—(usually no treatment prehospital); with tachycardic rate—diltiazem or verapamil or beta blockers or digoxin to control rate; if impaired cardiac function is present—diltiazem or amiodarone or digoxin; unstable—synchronized cardioversion at 50, 100, 200, 300, and 360 joules. (Objective 10)

54. QRS: 0.06 sec. P waves: none. Rate: 160/min. Rhythm: irregularly irregular. PR interval: none. Interpretation: atrial fibrillation. Distinguishing features: irregularly irregular, no P waves, fibrillation waves. Treatment: calcium channel or beta blocker; impaired cardiac function—diltiazem or amiodarone; acute and associated with serious signs or symptoms—synchronized cardioversion at 100, 200, 300, and 360 joules. (Objective 10)

55. a. junctional (nodal); b. normal; c. may occur before, during, or after QRS or may be absent; inverted in lead II; d. often less than 0.12 sec. (Objective 10)

56. Increased vagal tone on sinoatrial node, pathological slowing of sinoatrial discharge, complete atrioventricular block, digitalis toxicity, damage to the atrioventricular junction, inferior-wall myocardial infarction, and rheumatic fever. (Objective 10)

57. QRS: 0.08 sec. P waves: present, upright, similar in underlying rhythm, absent in premature beats. Rate: 60/min. Rhythm: irregular. PR interval: 0.16 sec (underlying rhythm), none in premature beats. Interpretation: sinus rhythm (borderline bradycardia) with two premature junctional contractions. Distinguishing features: premature beats occurring earlier than next expected sinus beat, lack of P waves, QRS complex within normal limits. Treatment: monitor patient and treat bradycardia if present and symptomatic. (Objective 10)

58. QRS: 0.08 sec. P waves: absent. Rate: 40/min. Rhythm: regular. PR interval: none. Interpretation: junctional escape rhythm. Distinguishing features: rate 40 to 60/min, inverted P waves if present (may occur before, during [absent], or after QRS complex). Treatment: stable—monitor; unstable—atropine 0.5 to 1.0 mg every 5 min to total dose of ≤ 2.5 mg (0.03-0.04 mg/kg), transcutaneous pacing, dopamine 5 to 20 mcg/kg/min, epinephrine 2 to 10 mcg/min, and isoproterenol 2 to 10 mcg/min. (Objective 10)

59. QRS: 0.08 sec. P waves: absent. Rate: 80/min. Rhythm: regular. PR interval: none. Interpretation: accelerated junctional rhythm. Distinguishing features: rate 60 to 100/min, inverted P waves in lead II if present (may be absent or occur before, during, or after QRS complex). Treatment: monitor. (Objective 10)

60. a. 20, 40; b. 100/min; c. 100/min.
(Objective 10)

61. Failure of higher pacemakers, heart block, myocardial ischemia, hypoxia, acid-base or electrolyte imbalance, congestive heart failure, increased catecholamine levels, use of stimulants, medicine toxicity (digitalis, tricyclic antidepressant overdose), sympathomimetic drugs, cardiac trauma, and electrical injury.
(Objective 10)

62. If unstable, all rhythms need cardioversion. If stable:
a. Assess leads I, II, III, MCL1 (V1), and MCL6 (V6) to determine axis deviation. If the QRS complex is negative in leads I, II, and III (extreme right axis or "no-man's land"), and positive in MCL1 (V1), the rhythm is VT; if not, b. Assess the QRS deflection in MCL1 (V1) and MCL6 (V6). Positive QRS deflections with either a single peak, a taller left rabbit ear or an RS complex with a fat r wave or slurred s wave in MCL1 (V1) indicates VT. A negative QS complex, a negative rS complex, or any wide Q wave in MCL6 (V6) also indicates VT; c. If right axis deviation is present (negative QRS complex in lead I; positive QRS complex in leads II and III) and the QRS complex is negative in MCL1 (V1), it indicates VT; d. If all precordial (V) leads are either positive or negative (precordial concordance), it indicates VT; e. If the RS interval is greater than 0.10 sec in any V lead, it indicates VT.
(Objective 10)

63. QRS: 0.16 sec. P waves: absent. Rate: 40/min. Rhythm: regular. PR interval: none. Interpretation: ventricular escape rhythm. Distinguishing features: rate 20 to 40/min, absent P waves, QRS complex greater than 0.12 sec. Treatment: oxygen, transcutaneous pacing, dopamine 5 to 20 mcg/kg/min, epinephrine 2 to 10 mcg/min, isoproterenol 2 to 10 mcg/min.
(Objective 10)

64. QRS: underlying rhythm 0.10 sec. Premature beat: 0.16 sec. P wave: present, upright (except premature beat). Rate: 75. Rhythm: regular interrupted by premature beats. PR interval: 0.16 (underlying rhythm). None: premature beat. Interpretation: normal sinus rhythm with one premature ventricular contraction. Distinguishing features: ectopic beat occurs earlier than next expected sinus beat, wide bizarre QRS complex with T wave deflection opposite QRS complex, no P waves, compensatory pause. Treatment: in presence of hemodynamically compromising PVCs—oxygen, lidocaine 1.0 to 1.5 mg/kg repeated at 0.5- to 0.75-mg/kg doses to a maximum of 3 mg/kg.
(Objective 10)

65. QRS: 0.20 sec. P waves: absent. Rate: 230/min. Rhythm: regular. PR interval: none. Interpretation: monomorphic ventricular tachycardia. Distinguishing features: rate greater than 100/min (usually greater than 150/min), regular, no p waves, QRS equal to or greater than 0.12 sec. Treatment: stable—oxygen, procainamide or sotalol or amiodarone or lidocaine; impaired cardiac function—amiodarone or lidocaine; unstable—synchronized cardioversion at 100, 200, 300, and 360 joules; or unconsciousness, hypotension, or pulmonary edema—defibrillate at 100, 200, 300, and 360 joules or equivalent biphasic energy; pulseless—treat as ventricular fibrillation.
(Objective 10)

66. QRS: none. P waves: none. Rate: none. Rhythm: none, chaotic. PR interval: none. Interpretation: ventricular fibrillation. Distinguishing features: no organized rhythm, chaotic fibrillatory waves. Treatment: rapid defibrillation at 200, 300, and 360 joules or equivalent biphasic energy, cardiopulmonary resuscitation, intubation, epinephrine or vasopressin, amiodarone or lidocaine, magnesium sulfate, and procainamide; consider sodium bicarbonate.
(Objective 10)

67. QRS: none. P waves: none. Rate: none. Rhythm: none. PR interval: none. Interpretation: asystole. Distinguishing features: isoelectric rhythm. Treatment: cardiopulmonary resuscitation, transcutaneous pacing, epinephrine, atropine, and consideration of underlying cause.
(Objective 10)

68. QRS: 0.16 sec. P waves: absent. Rate: 80/min. Rhythm: regular. PR interval: none. Interpretation: ventricular paced rhythm. Distinguishing features: pacemaker spike followed by wide-complex ventricular beat. Treatment: none.
(Objective 10)

69. a. heart blocks; b. conduction system.
(Objective 10)

70. Myocardial ischemia, acute myocardial infarction, increased parasympathetic tone, drug toxicity (digitalis, propranolol, verapamil), and electrolyte imbalance.
(Objective 10)

71. QRS: 0.06 sec. P waves: present, upright. Rate: 60/min. Rhythm: regular. PR interval: 0.32 sec. Interpretation: sinus rhythm with first-degree atrioventricular block. Distinguishing features: PR interval greater than 0.20 sec. Treatment: observe.
(Objective 10)

72. QRS: 0.08 sec. P waves: present, upright, more P waves than QRS complexes. Rate: 60/min. Rhythm: irregular. PR interval: progressively longer until one is not conducted. Distinguishing features: more P waves than QRS complexes, progressively lengthens PR interval until a QRS complex is dropped. Interpretation: second-degree atrioventricular block (Mobitz type I or Wenckebach). Treatment: asymptomatic—observe; if bradycardic with hemodynamic compromise—oxygen, atropine, transcutaneous pacing, dopamine, epinephrine, and isoproterenol. (Objective 10)

73. QRS: 0.06 sec. P waves: present, upright, more P waves than QRS complexes. Rate: 50/min. Rhythm: irregular. PR interval: 0.16 for conducted P waves. Interpretation: second-degree atrioventricular block (Mobitz type II). Treatment: stable—transport for transvenous pacemaker insertion; unstable—oxygen, transcutaneous pacing, dopamine, epinephrine, and isoproterenol. (Objective 10)

74. QRS: 0.08 sec. P waves: present, upright. Rate: 50/min. Rhythm: regular. PR interval: no relationship between P waves and QRS complexes. Interpretation: third-degree (complete) atrioventricular block. Distinguishing features: R-R interval usually regular, more P waves than QRS complexes, no relationship between P waves and QRS complex. Treatment: stable—monitor and transport for transvenous pacemaker insertion; unstable—oxygen, transcutaneous pacing, atropine 0.5 to 1.0 mg (maximum dose 0.04 mg/kg), dopamine 5 to 20 mcg/kg/min, epinephrine 2 to 10 mcg/min, and isoproterenol 2 to 10 mcg/min. (Objective 10)

75. a. QRS equal to or greater than 0.12 sec. QRS complexes produced by supraventricular activity. RSR prime pattern. In V_1, line drawn backward from the J point into the QRS makes a triangle pointing up; b. QRS less than 0.12 sec. QRS complexes produced by supraventricular activity. QS pattern. In V_1, line drawn backward from J point into the QRS makes a triangle pointing down; c. QRS less than 0.12 sec. QRS complexes produced by supraventricular activity and pathologic left axis deviation. A small Q wave followed by a tall R wave in lead I, and a small R wave followed by a deep S wave in lead III; d. Right axis deviation with a normal QRS complex. (Objective 10)

76. a. Any patient with type II AV block; b. Any patient with evidence of disease of both bundle branches; c. Any patient with two or more blocks of any kind. (Objective 10)

77. a. Pulseless electrical activity (the patient has a rhythm but no perfusing pulse); b. Cardiopulmonary resuscitation, intubation, intravenous therapy, epinephrine 1.0 mg every 3 to 5 min; consideration of causes (hypovolemia, pul-

monary embolus, acidosis, tension pneumothorax, cardiac tamponade, hypoxia, hypothermia, hyperthermia, hyperkalemia, massive myocardial infarction, drug overdose) and treatment if causes are found; if rate is slow, administer atropine 1 mg every 3-5 min to a maximum dose of 0.04 mg/kg. (Objective 10)

78. a. QRS normal or wide. Delta wave, onset of QRS complex is slurred or notched; b. PR interval is usually less than 0.12 second. (Objective 10)

79. Patients with WPW are susceptible to PSVTs. Verapamil is contraindicated because it may cause very rapid atrial to ventricular conduction and lead to VF and sudden death. (Objective 10)

80. Atherosclerosis is a process that progressively narrows the lumen of medium and large arteries. Thick hard atherosclerotic plaques called *atheromas* form especially in areas of turbulent blood flow. It is thought to be an endothelial cell response to chronic mechanical or chemical injury. The response includes platelet adhesion and aggregation and proliferation and migration of smooth muscle cells from the media into the intima. Eventually the atheromas become fibrotic and calcified and partially or totally obstruct the involved arteries. Its two major effects are: (1) disruption of the intimal surface causing a loss of vessel elasticity and an increase in thrombogenesis; and (2) a reduction in the diameter of the vessel lumen with resulting decreased blood supply to tissues. (Objective 11)

81. a. Physical exertion; b. emotional stress. (Objective 11)

82. a. Angina typically lasts 1 to 5 min but may last as long as 15 min; b. Relieved by rest, nitroglycerin, or oxygen. (Objective 11)

83. Unless 12-lead ECG interpretation is available, it is impossible to distinguish between these two conditions in the field. Even a negative 12-lead ECG does not exclude AMI. Serial cardiac enzymes and ECGs and other tests such as echocardiograms and stress tests may be needed. Both patients should be managed as though they are having a myocardial infarction (excluding thrombolytic therapy). (Objective 11)

84. Atherosclerotic plaque forms in coronary artery; plaque ruptures; platelets adhere to it and then thrombus forms on the plaque; as thrombus enlarges, it occludes the coronary artery. (Other causes are coronary vasospasm, coronary embolism, severe hypoxia, hemorrhage into diseased arterial wall, and shock.) (Objective 11)

85. (Objective 11)

Area of Heart Injured or Infarcted	Coronary Vessel Involved Most Often	Leads with Visible ST Segment Changes
Anterior	Left coronary	V3, V4
Lateral	Left coronary	V5, V6, I, aVL
Septal	Left coronary	V1, V2
Inferior	Right coronary	II, III, aVF

86. a. 0.1 mV in at least two contiguous leads.
(Objective 11)

87. Left bundle branch block, some ventricular rhythms, left ventricular hypertrophy, pericarditis, ventricular aneurysm, and early repolarization.
(Objective 11)

88. a. Identify rate and rhythm; b. Identify the area of infarct; c. Consider miscellaneous conditions; d. Assess the patient's clinical presentation; e. Recognize the infarction and initiate treatment.
(Objective 11)

89. Lethal dysrhythmias, congestive heart failure, pulmonary edema, cardiogenic shock, and myocardial tissue rupture.
(Objective 11)

90. Nausea; vomiting; diaphoresis; radiation of pain to the neck, jaw, arm, or back; palpitations; dyspnea; and a sense of impending doom.
(Objective 11)

91. ST segment elevation in leads V2, V3, and V4. Possible acute anterior MI.
(Objective 11)

92. Administer oxygen via nasal cannula, minimize physical activity, monitor ECG and oxygen saturation (if pulse oximetry is available), assess vital signs frequently (including lung sounds for crackles), and establish an intravenous line to keep the vein open with normal saline or lactated Ringer's solution.
(Objective 11)

93. Aspirin 162-325 mg; nitroglycerin 0.4 mg sublingually, repeated 2 times; morphine sulfate 2 to 4 mg intravenously titrated to relieve pain.
(Objective 11)

94. a. Patient is alert and able to give informed consent; chest pain or symptoms of acute myocardial infarction for at least 30 min and less than 6 hours; less than 75 years of age; ECG changes consistent with an acute anterior or inferior myocardial infarction; chest pain and ECG changes that persist after the administration of sublingual nitroglycerin. b. History of intracranial bleeding, stroke, ulcer or GI bleeding, pregnancy or postpartum state, uncontrolled hypertension, recent surgery, IV catheters at noncompressible sites, intracranial tumor, thoracic aortic aneurysm, CPR in progress more than 10 minutes, and trauma or any condition that would result in a significant bleeding hazard.
(Objective 11)

95. a. Normal axis; no ST segment elevation, depression. Normal 12-lead ECG; b. QRS 0.14 sec. Pathologic left axis deviation. Left bundle branch block. Cannot detect ST segment elevation in the presence of left bundle branch block; c. Normal axis; ST segment elevation leads II, III, aVF. ST segment depression in leads aVL, V2, V3, V4, V5. Possible inferior MI; d. Normal axis; ST segment elevation leads I, aVL, V2, V3, V4, V5, V6. Extensive anterior MI

96. There is a pathologic left axis deviation. QRS is upright in lead I, and down in leads II and III.
(Objective 10)

97. The triangle should point upward.
(Objective 8)

98. The patient has a left anterior hemiblock (pathologic left axis deviation) and a right bundle branch block (QRS > 0.12 sec and upward triangle).
(Objective 10)

99. The presence of more than one block is known as *bifascicular block* and is associated with a high risk of advancement to complete heart block and increased mortality in the presence of myocardial infarction. This patient's symptoms suggest the potential for myocardial infarction.
(Objective 10)

100. The potential for serious rhythm deterioration should be anticipated. Prophylactic application of defibrillation or pacing pads in this setting may be indicated based on local protocol.
(Objective 10)

101. Left ventricular failure leading to pulmonary edema and possible myocardial infarction.
(Objective 11)

102. Pulmonary edema: orthopnea and frothy blood—tinged sputum. Myocardial infarction: chest pain, radiation of pain, nausea, and vomiting.
(Objective 11)

103. Sinus tachycardia.
(Objective 10)

104.

Drug	Dose	Desired Effect
a. Furosemide	0.5 to 1.0 mg/kg intravenously	Venodilation and diuresis
b. Morphine	2 to 4 mg intravenously	Venodilation, decreased myocardial work, and decreased anxiety
c. Nitroglycerin	0.4 mg sublingually	Peripheral vasodilation and decreased preload and afterload

(Objectives 11 and 13)

105. 3.5
(Objective 13)

106. a. Left heart failure, pulmonary embolism, right ventricle infarct, chronic hypertension, chronic obstructive pulmonary disease and valvular disease; b. Jugular venous distention, tachycardia, enlarged liver or spleen, peripheral and sacral edema, and ascites. (Objective 11)

107. Sinus bradycardia.
(Objective 10)

108. Administer oxygen by nonrebreather mask and give atropine 0.5 mg intravenously.
(Objectives 10 and 13)

109. Cardiogenic shock.
(Objective 11)

110. High-flow oxygen by nonrebreather mask, supine position (if tolerated), intravenous therapy with normal saline—consider fluid challenge (250-500 ml)—dopamine infusion via intravenous piggyback 5 to 15 mcg/kg/min, remove nitroglycerin paste and wipe chest with gauze and monitor ECG for dysrhythmias.
(Objective 11)

111. Expanding or ruptured abdominal aortic aneurysm.
(Objective 11)

112. Palpation in this situation could cause a bulging aneurysm to rupture. If medical direction advises palpation, it should be done very gently.
(Objective 11)

113. No. Increased intraabdominal pressure could cause rupture of the aneurysm.
(Objective 11)

114. Administer oxygen, transport rapidly, apply pneumatic antishock garments (if indicated by protocol) but do not inflate unless the patient's condition deteriorates, initiate two large-bore intravenous lines en route and infuse normal saline or lactated Ringer's solution to keep the vein open unless the patient's condition deteriorates.
(Objective 11)

115. Dissecting thoracic aortic aneurysm.
(Objective 11)

116. Unequal peripheral pulses, neurological deficit, or signs of pericardial tamponade.
(Objective 11)

117. Minimize movement and anxiety, administer high concentration oxygen, initiate a 14- or 16-gauge intravenous line in arm with good pulses (higher blood pressure) to keep the vein open, and monitor vital signs and the ECG frequently.
(Objective 11)

118.

	Embolic	Thrombotic
Causes	Clot breaks loose and travels to narrow area in blood vessel	Clot develops at narrow spot in blood vessel
Onset	Rapid	Gradual
Signs and symptoms	Pulseless extremity pain; decreased motor and sensory function; pallor; cool skin temperature distal to the occlusion; decreased capillary refill; possible shock	Pain in hips, lower limbs, buttocks, leg, and abdomen (depends on affected artery); pain; delayed motor and sensory function; pallor; decreased skin temperature distal to the occlusion; decreased CR; possible shock

(Objective 11)

119. Control bleeding with direct pressure and elevation. The bleeding may be persistent and require hospital management.
(Objective 11)

120. Pain, edema, warmth, erythema, tenderness, and a palpable cord.
(Objective 11)

121. Hypertensive encephalopathy.
(Objective 11)

122. Aphasia, hemiparesis, transient blindness, seizures, stupor, coma, and death.
(Objective 11)

123. Calm patient, apply oxygen and intravenous line to keep the vein open, monitor ECG, and transport rapidly.

124. Nitroglycerin 0.4 mg SL or nitroglycerin paste. Labetalol 10-20 mg IV over 1-2 min.
(Objective 13)

125. Determine unresponsiveness; call for help if no one else is available; open the airway; look, listen, and feel for breathing; if there is none, deliver 2 slow rescue breaths; assess carotid pulse; if there is none, begin cardiopulmonary resuscitation until help arrives.
(Objective 12)

126. a. After intubation, intravenous therapy, and the first dose of epinephrine; b. Yes. Electric shock resulting in injury or death can occur.
(Objective 12)

127. Ventricular tachycardia.
(Objective 10)

128. Defibrillate with 200 joules (then 300 and 360 joules if the rhythm is the same) and then reassess the rhythm and pulse.
(Objective 12)

129. Amount of time patient has been in pulseless ventricular tachycardia (success decreases over time with bystander cardiopulmonary resuscitation), conductive gel applied to paddles, and proper paddle placement.
(Objective 12)

130. Apply conductive gel on the patient's chest (or hands-off defibrillation patches); turn on power

(there is a separate power source for the defibrillator and monitor with some monitors); select correct energy level; place paddles (or patches) in an appropriate position on the patients chest; charge the defibrillator; call "clear" and visually check to ensure that no one is in contact with the patient or cot; lean firmly on paddles (if used) with 20 to 25 lb of pressure; discharge both paddle buttons simultaneously (or depress discharge button on monitor for hands-off defibrillator); and reassess pulse and rhythm.
(Objective 12)

131. Defibrillate at 100, 200, 300, 360 joules.
(Objective 12)

132. It is synchronized with the patient's heartbeat so there is less risk of firing on the relative refractory period and causing ventricular fibrillation.
(Objective 12)

133. Depress the synchronize button before each synchronized shock and hold the paddles firmly on the chest after activation until they discharge.
(Objective 12)

134. a. Third-degree atrioventricular block; b. Inform the patient that he may feel some discomfort; apply the pacing and monitoring pads; ensure adequate upright R wave on monitor; select pacing mode; select pacing rate (70-80/min); set current (mA) at 50 milliamps and slowly increase until capture is observed; reassess patient's vital signs (use right arm for blood pressure); and document and obtain rhythm strips.
(Objective 12)

135. a. Asystole; b. epinephrine 1.0 mg every 3 to 5 min and atropine 1 mg every 5 min until a maximum dose of 0.04 mg/kg is reached; c. transcutaneous pacing.
(Objectives 10 and 12)

136. a. Ventricular fibrillation; b. defibrillation; c. epinephrine 1.0 mg every 3 to 5 min or vasopressin 40 U IV bolus, amiodarone 300 mg IV bolus diluted in 20-30 ml of NS or DSW, or lidocaine 1-1.5 mg/kg intravenously. (Objectives 10 and 13)

137. a. Do not stop resuscitation. Patient is older than 18 years, successfully intubated, last seen 30 minutes (cannot consider for termination). Resuscitation should be considered after 4 rounds of resuscitation drugs; b. Do not stop resuscitation. Patient is older than 18 years, 5 drugs have been given, but intubation was unsuccessful; c. Do not stop resuscitation. Patient is younger than 18 years and has sustained trauma, and you were able to get back a perfusing pulse during the resuscitation; d. Do not stop resuscitation. The patient has met criteria for resuscitation; however, the family objects strongly so efforts should continue.
(Objective 14)

138. d. His identified risk factors are: male sex, age, hypercholesterolemia, diabetes, and hypertension (Acupril is an ACE inhibitor and indapamide is a diuretic).
(Objective 1)

139. c. BP = cardiac output × peripheral vascular resistance.
(Objective 1)

140. c. The circumflex supplies the lateral and posterior portions of the left ventricle and part of the right ventricle. The right coronary artery and the left anterior descending supply most of the right atrium and ventricle and the inferior aspect of the left ventricle.
(Objective 2)

141. b. Aortic valve separates the aorta and left ventricle, the pulmonic valve separates the pulmonary arteries and right ventricle, and the tricuspid valve separates the right atrium and right ventricle.
(Objective 2)

142. d. The electrical charge is the potential difference and is measured in millivolts. Depolarization (electrical conduction) occurs when sodium rushes into the cell, altering the electrical balance.
(Objective 3)

143. c. Potassium is also essential.
(Objective 3)

144. d. Calcium channel blockers selectively block the slow channel and alter the threshold level.
(Objective 3)

145. a. Phase 0 is the rapid depolarization phase; phase 1 is the early rapid depolarization phase; phase 2 is the plateau phase; phase 3 is the terminal phase of rapid repolarization; and phase 4 is the period between action potentials.
(Objective 3)

146. c. This allows complete relaxation of the cardiac muscle before another contraction can be initiated.
(Objective 3)

147. d. The His bundle divides into the right and left bundle branches. The left bundle divides into the anterior and posterior fascicles. A third fascicle of the left bundle branch that innervates the interventricular septum and the base of the heart also has been identified. The bundle branches subdivide and become Purkinje fibers.
(Objective 4)

148. d. The RMP gradually decreases with time until it reaches a critical threshold, at which time depolarization results.
(Objective 4)

149. c. This pause allows the atria to finish contraction and empty before ventricular contraction occurs.
(Objective 4)

150. a. Acetylcholine causes the cell membrane of the SA node to become hyperpolarized, causing a de-

lay in reaching threshold, and therefore it decreases the heart rate. All other answers increase heart rate.
(Objective 4)

151. d. The other answers represent causes of dysrhythmias that result from enhanced automaticity.
(Objective 4)

152. a. Mental status change, abdominal or GI complaints, or vague complaints of ill-being may be presenting symptoms in an older adult patient with a coronary event.
(Objective 5)

153. d. If the heart is unable to pump effectively, blood will back up into the lungs, causing decreased diffusion of gases in the lungs and dyspnea.
(Objective 5)

154. b. Younger patients may experience syncope secondary to increased vagal tone. Nausea or syncope when standing do not predict the incidence of dysrhythmias.
(Objective 5)

155. b.
(Objective 5)

156. c. Peripheral pulses and perfusion would be used to assess strength of myocardial contractions. Placement of patches is usually performed using ribs and gross anatomy.
(Objective 5)

157. b. The ECG does not measure mechanical events.
(Objective 7)

158. c. The others are unipolar leads (a single positive electrode and a reference point).
(Objective 6)

159. d. If the depolarization moves toward a positive electrode, the tracing should show an upward deflection.
(Objective 6)

160. b. These leads all look up onto the inferior portion of the heart.
(Objective 6)

161. d. These leads may help distinguish between supraventricular tachycardia with aberration and ventricular tachycardia and can help diagnose bundle branch blocks.
(Objective 6)

162. c. The negative lead is placed at the lateral end of the left clavicle. The positive lead for MCL6 is placed on the left axillary line at the level of the fifth intercostal space. (Objective 6)

163. a. Many dysrhythmias involve abnormalities of the P wave.
(Objective 6)

164. b. V3 and V4 are anterior leads, and V5 and V6 are lateral precordial leads.
(Objective 6)

165. a. This is used as the baseline.
(Objective 7)

166. b.
(Objective 4)

167. c. The relative refractory period is from the peak of the T wave onward.
(Objective 7)

168. b. In some leads, part of the QRS complex is blended with the baseline and difficult to measure.
(Objective 8)

169. d. $1500 \div 10 = 150/min$.
(Objective 8)

170. b.
(Objective 10)

171. c.
(Objective 10)

172. c.
(Objective 10)

173. a.
(Objective 10)

174. b.
(Objective 10)

175. d.
(Objective 10)

176. a.
(Objective 10)

177. d. Adenosine is not indicated for atrial fibrillation, and verapamil is not indicated when a patient is hypotensive. The patient needs electrical cardioversion because her condition is unstable. Procainamide is indicated for ventricular dysrhythmias.
(Objective 10)

178. a. It originates from tissue other than an intrinsic pacemaker.
(Objective 10)

179. c. Isoproterenol is a beta stimulant, so it will increase the heart rate.
(Objective 10)

180. d. The atria cannot contract to empty. This decreases the blood flow to the ventricles and the cardiac output.
(Objective 10)

181. a.
(Objective 10)

182. d. It is also associated with excessive catecholamine administration, damage to the AV junction, inferior-wall myocardial infarction, and rheumatic fever.
(Objective 10)

183. c. Other causes include failure of higher pacemakers to initiate impulses.
(Objective 10)

184. a. Couplets are 2 PVCs in a row. An idioventricular rhythm originates in the ventricles and supersedes the underlying rhythm. Multifocal PVCs have varied appearance depending on their site of origination.
(Objective 10)

185. a. Precordial concordance with either all positive or all negative deflection in the V leads indicates VT.
(Objective 10)

186. b. Asynchronous (fixed rate) pacemakers stimulate the heart at a set rate regardless of the heart's own action. A dual chamber pacemaker stimulates both the atria and the ventricles.
(Objective 10)

187. d. Bundle branch block occurs when one of the bundles of HIS is blocked. Second-degree AV block type II is an intermittent block.
(Objective 10)

188. d. It yields an initial Q wave in MCL1 (V_1) instead of the normal small R wave. There will be a deep QS pattern that is at least 0.12 sec.
(Objective 10)

189. b. The blockage of 2 of the 3 pathways for ventricular conduction (right BBB with anterior or posterior hemiblock, and left BBB) pose the greatest risk.
(Objective 10)

190. d. Verapamil may cause very rapid atrial to ventricular conduction down the accessory pathway and may lead to VF and sudden death.
(Objective 10)

191. c. Both have the same cause.
(Objective 11)

192. a. Hypotension secondary to pump failure and cardiac rupture can occur but is much less common than lethal dysrhythmias.
(Objective 11)

193. b. A small fluid challenge (250 ml) may be given to a cardiac patient who is hypotensive; however, in the normotensive patient, intravenous fluids should be infused to keep the vein open.
(Objective 11)

194. b. Deep inverted T waves may be present in AMI.
(Objective 11)

195. a. Epinephrine will increase the work and oxygen demands on the heart precipitate lethal dysrhythmias in this patient.
(Objectives 11 and 13)

196. d. Signs include JVD and peripheral edema.
(Objective 11)

197. b. Cardiogenic shock is fatal in up to 70% to 80% of patients.
(Objective 11)

198. b. Decreased systolic pressure is a later sign. Muffled heart sounds are associated with this. Tracheal deviation is seen in tension pneumothorax.
(Objective 11)

199. b. The pain is often described as ripping or tearing and is high intensity.
(Objective 11)

200. a.
(Objective 11)

201. c.
(Objective 11)

202. b. The patient with diabetes is at higher risk for heart disease; however, hypertension does not precipitate diabetes.
(Objective 11)

203. a. The goal is for CPR within 4 min and ACLS treatment within 8 min.
(Objective 12)

204. a. Lower energy levels may be used. There is bidirectional energy flow. Two patches are used.
(Objective 12)

205. b. Anterior-posterior placement is not practical for paddle use. Avoid placing the patch or paddle over the sternum because bone is a poor conductor of electricity. Pediatric paddles are indicated for children under 1 year of age.
(Objective 12)

206. b. The ICDs sequence includes up to 5 shocks in 2 minutes. There is no danger in touching the patients. Strong magnets may inactivate the device.
(Objective 12)

207. d.
(Objective 14)

208. b.
(Objective 14)

209. a.
(Objective 13)

210. c.
(Objective 13)

211. a. Morphine will decrease the preload. It is contraindicated in the patient with head injury. It does not cause bronchodilation.
(Objective 13)

212. a.
(Objective 13)

213. c.
(Objective 13)

214. c. The correct dose is 2 to 10 mcg/g/min.
(Objective 13)

215. a. None of the other criteria should be used to evaluate whether resuscitation should be stopped.
(Objective 14)

● CHAPTER 29
NEUROLOGY

1. a.
2. e.
3. d.
4. b.
5. d.
6. c.
7. e.
8. d.
9. i.
10. j.

11. h.

12. f.

13. c.

14. a.

15. b.

16. k.

(Questions 1-16, Objective 4)

17. a. neuroglia; b. cell body; c. dendrites; d. axon; e. white matter; f. sensory; g. motor; h. interneurons; i. negative; j. positive; k. sodium; l. depolarization; m. nodes of Ranvier; n. quickly; o. synapse; p. norepinephrine, epinephrine, and dopamine.
(Objective 1)

18. Sensory receptor, sensory neuron, interneurons, motor neuron, and effector organ.
(Objective 1)

19. Vertebral arteries and internal carotid arteries.
(Objective 1)

20. a. Decrease; b. decrease; c. decrease; d. decrease
(Objective 2)

21. a. Intracranial bleeding, head trauma, brain tumor, or another space-occupying lesion; b. Anoxia, hypoglycemia, diabetic ketoacidosis, thiamine deficiency, kidney and liver failure, and postictal phase of a seizure; c. Barbiturates, narcotics, hallucinogenics, depressants, and alcohol; d. Hypertensive encephalopathy, shock, dysrhythmias, and stroke; e. Chronic obstructive pulmonary disease and toxic inhalation; f. Meningitis and sepsis.
(Objective 4)

22. a. Why did you call EMS? What happened during the course of this situation? Does the patient have any medical problems such as heart or lung disease, neurological illness, diabetes, or high blood pressure? Does the patient have a history of drug or alcohol abuse or stroke? Has this ever happened to him before? Do you know if he has had any injuries recently?

b. Increased blood pressure, decreased pulse, widened pulse pressure, slow or irregular respiratory rate.

c. He is responsive to verbal stimuli.

d. GCS =13

e. Assess the pupils for shape, size, equality, and response to light. Assess patient's extraocular movements by asking him to follow your finger movements with his eyes (to the extreme left, up and down, to the extreme right, up and down).
(Objective 3)

23. a. Structural; b. toxic-metabolic; c. structural
(Objective 4)

24. Secure the airway and ventilate with 100% oxygen (with inline immobilization of the spine). Assess carotid and radial pulses. Assess vital signs, oxygen saturation, breath sounds, ECG, and pupil response. Scan body for obvious trauma. Draw a blood sample while initiating an IV with 0.9% normal saline. As blood glucose level is less than 80 mg/dl, administer thiamine 100 mg intravenously, reassess, administer 25 g of D50W IV, and reassess. If the blood glucose level had been normal, administer naloxone (Narcan) 2 mg IV and reassess. If no improvement occurs and patient has no gag reflex, she should be intubated (and tube placement verified). Perform ongoing assessment and transport.
(Objectives 3 and 4)

25.

Risk Factor	Modifiable (Yes or No)
a. Age (elderly)	No
b. Race (African-American)	No
c. Gender (male)	No
d. Hypertension	Yes
e. Heart disease (nitroglycerin)	Yes
f. Diabetes (insulin)	Yes
g. Transient ischemic attacks	Yes
h. Cigarette smoking	Yes

(Objective 4)

26. Confusion* or coma, dysarthria*, aphasia, facial droop* or facial numbness, hemiparesis* or hemiplegia, convulsions, incontinence, diplopia, headache, dizziness, ataxia, monocular blindness, or vertigo.
(Objective 4)

27. a. Facial droop, arm drift, and slurred speech; b. patient is older than 45 years; no history of seizures, symptom duration longer than 24 hours, he is not wheelchair bound, blood glucose is normal, and he has obvious asymmetry of smile and arm strength.
(Objective 4)

28. Detection, dispatch, delivery (to a stroke center), door (appropriate hospital for rapid treatment of stroke), data (include CT scan), decision (to identify appropriateness of fibrinolytic therapy), drug.
(Objective 4)

29. Ensure that his airway remains patent, administer supplemental oxygen if his SaO_2 drops below 90% or his condition worsens, monitor vital signs and ECG, elevate head of stretcher 15 degrees, initiate IV LR or NS at 50 ml/hr; protect affected extremities, maintain normal temperature, rapid transport to closest stroke center, control seizures with benzodiazepines if present; comfort and reassure the patient and family.
(Objective 4)

30. Hemorrhagic stroke commonly occurs during stress or exertion. It starts abruptly and often begins with a headache, nausea, vomiting, and progressive deterioration of neurological status. The patient may rapidly lose consciousness or have a seizure. (Objective 4)

31. Stroke, head trauma, toxins, hypoxia, hypoglycemia, infection, metabolic abnormalities, brain tumor, vascular disorders, eclampsia, and drug overdose.
(Objective 4)

32. a. Simple sensory seizure (partial seizure); b. petit mal (generalized seizure); c. Jacksonian seizure (partial seizure); d. grand mal seizure (generalized seizure); e. complex partial seizures (partial seizure).
(Objective 4)

33. History of seizures, including frequency and medication compliance; description of seizure (length, features, incontinence, tongue-biting); history of head trauma; fever, headache, or nuchal rigidity before seizure; medical history, including diabetes, cardiovascular disease, and stroke.
(Objective 4)

34. In the hysterical seizure the following does not occur: trauma to the tongue, incontinence, and response to conventional therapy. Hysterical seizure may, however, stop with a sharp command or sternal rub.
(Objective 4)

35. a. Syncope; b. syncope; c. seizure; d. seizure
(Objective 4)

36. Lorazepam 1 to 2 mg intravenously; or diazepam 5 to 10 mg intravenously every 15 minutes as necessary.
(Objective 4)

37. a. Cluster headache; b. sinus headache; c. tension headache; d. migraine headache.
(Objective 4)

38. a. The internal carotid arteries give rise to the anterior cerebral arteries. The vertebral arteries supply the cerebellum and unite to form the basilar artery.
(Objective 1)

39. d. The Circle of Willis would not protect against a large cerebral bleed, systemic hypoxia, or increased ICP. It can help to maintain blood flow if a clot exists in the vertebral or carotid arteries.
(Objective 1)

40. a. This will decrease cerebral perfusion pressure. CPP will not usually decrease until the ICP exceeds 22 mm Hg (the body will compensate to that level). Fluid in the eye has no influence on CPP. Metabolic rate will increase, but CPP will not be affected with a temperature of 102° F.
(Objective 2)

41. d. Kussmaul respirations occur secondary to metabolic acidosis that occur in diabetic ketoacidosis. Each of the other breathing patterns may be encountered in a patient who has a neurological problem.
(Objective 3)

42. a. Flexion posturing occurs during impairment of cortical regions of the brain. Flaccidity is usually caused by brainstem or cord dysfunction. Dyscon-

jugate gaze is not a posture but an abnormal eye movement.
(Objective 3)

43. c. Barbiturate overdose and medullary injury will more likely present with dilated pupils. Temporal herniation will cause a unilateral dilated pupil.
(Objective 3)

44. d. Airway maintenance is critical. Drug administration would only be indicated if the seizure recurs.
(Objective 4)

45. b. All other choices are risk factors for stroke.
(Objective 4)

46. b. The three components of the stroke scale are facial droop, arm drift, and speech disturbances. All other choices are possible signs or symptoms of stroke but are not included in the stroke scale.
(Objective 4)

47. c. Dystonia refers to an alteration in muscle tone that can cause painful spasms, fixed postures, or strange movement patterns. Inanition refers to starvation or failure to thrive. Palsy is weakness.
(Objective 4)

● CHAPTER 30 ENDOCRINOLOGY

1. a, b, d, e, f, i, j, k
2. b, f, h, i, j
3. b, c, g, i, j
(Questions 1-3, Objective 3)
4. a. Glucagon; b. insulin; c. somatostatin
(Objective 2)
5.

Food	Breakdown Products	Storage
a. Carbohydrates	Glucose	Liver and muscles (excess converted to fat)
b. Proteins	Amino acids	Small amounts in cytoplasm of all cells
c. Fats	Fatty acids, glycerol	Liver and fat cells

(Objective 2)

6. a. Glucose is stored in the liver as glycogen; b. as the blood sugar begins to drop, glucagon is released from the pancreas and stimulates the breakdown of glycogen to glucose.
(Objective 2)

7. Glucagon breaks down glycogen and stimulates gluconeogenesis (formation of glucose from amino acids).
(Objective 2)

8. Glucose cannot be stored in the brain, so when blood sugar drops, no reserves exist. The brain cannot use fats or proteins for energy. (Objective 3)

9. New onset of diabetes is associated with increased fluid intake (polydipsia), increased urine output (polyuria), dizziness, blurred vision, and rapid weight loss. (Objective 3)

10. Long-term complications of diabetes include blindness, kidney disease, peripheral neuropathy, autonomic neuropathy, peripheral vascular disease, heart disease, and stroke. (Objective 3)

11. Assess and protect the airway; place a nasal or oral airway and suction if necessary; evaluate breathing, assist if necessary, and apply oxygen; assess pulse; evaluate vital signs; determine blood glucose level; initiate an IV in the antecubital space; if the blood glucose is less than 80 mg/dl, administer D50W 25 g intravenously; and reassess the patient. (Objective 3)

12. Diabetic ketoacidosis or a pulmonary problem. (Objective 3)

13. Have you had any vomiting or diarrhea? If yes, how much? When did you last eat? What medications do you take and when did you last take them (especially insulin)? How much have you been urinating? Do you feel dizzy when you stand up? Have you lost any weight? Are you thirsty and have you been drinking a lot of fluids? Do you have any abdominal pain? (Objective 3)

14. As you perform your total patient assessment you should assess to see if the patient has warm, dry skin; dry mucous membranes; tachycardia; postural hypotension; fruity breath odor; or decreased level of consciousness. (Objective 3)

15. Oxygen should be applied and the patient monitored for dysrhythmias. An IV of 0.9% normal saline should be initiated. Medical direction will likely advise infusion at a rapid rate, often 250 ml/hr or greater. (Objective 3)

16. Transport rapidly because definitive treatment includes insulin, which is not usually available on EMS units. (Objective 3)

17. Type II diabetes; advanced age; preexisting cardiac or renal disease; inadequate insulin secretion or action; increased insulin requirements (stress, infection, trauma, burns, myocardial infarction); medications such as thiazide diuretics, glucocorticoids, phenytoin, sympathomimetics, propranolol, and immunosuppressives; and parenteral or enteral feedings. (Objective 17)

18.

Disorder	Endocrine gland and hormone affected	Excess or shortage of hormone?	Signs and symptoms	Potentially life threatening?
Graves' disease	Thyroid	Excess	Enlarged thyroid; swollen neck; protruding eyes	Yes, if it progresses to thyroid storm
Thyroid storm	Thyroid	Excess	Tachycardia; heart failure; dysrhythmias; shock; hyperthermia; restlessness; agitation; abdominal pain; coma	Yes
Myxedema	Thyroid (thyroid hormone)	Shortage	Hoarse voice; fatigue; weight gain; cold intolerance; depression; dry skin; hair loss; infertility; constipation; heavy menses	Not unless it progresses to myxedema coma
Cushing's syndrome	Adrenal cortex (corticosteroid hormones)	Excess	Red, round face; obese trunk; wasted limbs; acne; purple stretch marks; inceased facial and body hair; hump on neck; weight gain; hypertension; psychiatric disturbances; insomnia; diabetes	No
Addison's disease	Adrenal cortex (cortisol, aldosterone)	Shortage	Weakness; weight loss; anorexia; hyperpigmented skin; hypotension; hyponatremia; hyperkalemia; GI disturbances	Usually not unless a rapid, acute onset occurs

(Objectives 4 and 5)

19. c. Hormones travel through the blood and may only trigger a receptor site in one organ or throughout the body depending on the hormone. (Objective 1)

20. c. Insulin increases glucose transport into cells, increases glucose metabolism by cells, increases liver glycogen levels, and decreases blood glucose concentration. (Objective 2)

21. c. Insulin is administered by parenteral injection. (Objection 3)

22. b. Most type II diabetics can control the disease with diet and oral hypoglycemic agents. This disease has a slow onset and does not often cause life-threatening emergencies. (Objective 3)

23. d. Glucagon is a pancreatic hormone. Glucosuria is urine that contains glucose. Gluconeogenesis is the formation of glucose by breakdown of fats and fatty acids. (Objective 2)

24. b. If IV access can be established, intravenous D50W should be administered. (Objective 3)

25. d. Thiamine promotes the uptake of glucose in the brain. (Objective 3)

26. c. When an IV cannot be established in a patient with hypoglycemia, glucagon may be given IM.

Glucagon is slower, more expensive, and less effective than D50W. (Objective 3)

27. a. 0.5-1.0 mg IM
(Objective 3)

28. c. There is no ketogenesis in HHNK so there is no acetone (fruity) breath odor as in hyperglycemia. (Objective 3)

29. d. These are caused by adrenergic hyperactivity. (Ojective 4)

● CHAPTER 31
ALLERGIES AND ANAPHYLAXIS

1. a. injection; b. ingestion; c. inhalation; d. absorption; e. antibody; f. hypersensitivity; g. mast cells; h. basophils. (Objective 1)

2. a. Antibiotics (especially penicillin), local anesthetics, cephalosporins, chemotherapeutics, aspirin, nonsteroidal antiinflammatory agents, opiates, muscle relaxants, vaccines, and insulin; b. wasps, bees, and fire ants; c. peanuts, soybeans, cod, halibut, shellfish, egg white, strawberries, food additives, wheat and buckwheat, sesame and sunflower seeds, cotton seed, milk, and mango; d. latex. (Objective 3)

3. a. Histamine release may result in decreased blood pressure, increased gastrointestinal secretions, rhinorrhea, tearing, flushing, urticaria, and angioedema; b. leukotrienes cause wheezing that may precipitate chest pain (resulting from coronary vasoconstriction) and enhance the hypotensive effects of histamine; c. eosinophil chemotactic factor can produce fever, chills, bronchospasm, and pulmonary vasoconstriction. (Objective 3)

4. a. These same signs and symptoms could be caused by asthma, upper airway obstruction, pulmonary edema, or toxic inhalation; b. if the patient takes a beta blocker (such as atenolol, propranolol), it could interfere with the action of epinephrine. If the patient has already self-administered epinephrine (Epi-pen, Ana-pen), determine the time it was administered and whether symptoms have improved or worsened since administration. (Objective 4)

5. Foods such as crab, shrimp, nuts, and egg or food additives are known to cause anaphylaxis. (Objective 3)

6. a. Epinephrine 0.3 to 0.5 mg (1:1000) IM or subcutaneously; b. diphenhydramine (Benadryl) 25 to 50 mg IM or IV and then albuterol (Proventil, Ventolin) updraft. (Objective 4)

7. He may also have stridor, hoarseness, tachypnea, tachycardia, agitation, headache, seizures, decreasing level of consciousness, angioedema, tearing, swelling of the tongue, urticaria, pruritus, sneezing, coughing, tracheal tugging, intercostal retractions, decreased breath sounds, dysrhythmias, chest

tightness, nausea, vomiting, and diarrhea. (Objective 4)

8. Secure the airway, ventilate with 100% oxygen, and intubate. Initiate intravenous therapy with large bore catheter in antecubital space, infuse fluid rapidly, and administer epinephrine 0.1 to 0.5 mg (1:10,000) intravenous over 5 minutes (try to do simultaneously with airway management if resources permit). If necessary, administer diphenhydramine 25 to 50 mg intramuscular or intravenous as a second line drug. Reevaluate the need to administer a second dose of epinephrine if patient has not responded. Consider giving methylprednisolone. (Objective 4)

9. b. An anaphylactic response is a type of life-threatening allergic response. Basophils and mast cells are white blood cells that are involved in the immune response. (Objective 1)

10. b. IgA immunoglobulins are antibodies found in blood, secretions such as tears, and the respiratory system. IgG antibodies are the most common antibodies involved in the immune response. Production of IgM antibodies precedes IgG production in acute infections. (Objective 1)

11. a. Angioedema may be found in local or systemic allergic reactions. All of the other signs or symptoms, if present during an allergic reaction, would be most often associated with a systemic (anaphylactic) reaction. (Objective 2)

12. b. Because no systemic signs or symptoms exist, intramuscular diphenhydramine is indicated. Epinephrine 1:1000 should never be given IVP to treat anaphylaxis. (Objective 2)

13. d. Chemotactic substances cause the attraction of phagocytic cells toward or away from the antigen, leukotactic substances attract leukocytes to the pathogenic agent, and opsonins bind phagocytes to the invading microorganism. (Objective 1)

14. a. All of the other agents are known to cause anaphylaxis. (Objective 3)

15. a. Each of the other problems could cause death, but upper airway obstruction is associated with the most deaths because of anaphylaxis. (Objective 4)

16. b. The skin is usually flushed and warm because of the profound vasodilation. Objective 4)

17. b.
(Objective 2)

18. e.
(Objective 4)

● CHAPTER 32
GASTROENTEROLOGY

1. k
2. l
3. j
4. a

5. e

6. m

7. i

(Questions 1-7, Objective 2)

8. d

(Objective 2 or 3)

9. b

(Objective 3)

10. f

(Objective 3)

11. c

(Objective 2)

12. h

(Objective 2)

13. a. spleen; b. stomach; c. descending colon; d. rectum; e. appendix; f. transverse colon; g. liver; h. diaphragm; i. esophagus.

14. a. No. The pain of pancreatitis is located in the epigastric region or right or left *upper quadrant*; b. no. Pain of cholecystitis is located in the epigastric region or right upper quadrant. It is more common in women under age 50; c. yes. Diverticulitis is one possibility. It is common in older adults, and the pain is often in the left lower quadrant; d. no. Pain from a peptic ulcer would typically be in the epigastric area. (Objective 2)

15. a. Does anything make the pain better or worse? What does the pain feel like (sharp, stabbing, cramping, dull)? Can you show me where the pain is? Does the pain go anywhere else? On a scale of 1 to 10, with 1 being no pain and 10 being the worst pain you have ever had, rate the pain. When did the pain begin? Associated signs and symptoms: Do you have or have you had any nausea, vomiting, diarrhea, constipation, unusual-colored stools, chills, fever, or shortness of breath? Medical history and medications. b. myocardial infarction; abdominal aneurysm could present in a similar manner. (Objective 4)

16. a. Somatic; b. visceral; c. referred. (Objective 4)

17. a. Fever, chills, tachycardia, tachypnea, position (lying on side with knees flexed and pulled in toward the chest), reluctance to move, skin pallor, absent bowel sounds, generalized involuntary guarding, and rigidity of the abdomen. (Objective 4)
b. Oxygen by nonrebreather mask, intravenous 16-gauge catheter with normal saline or lactated Ringer's solution (rate at least 100 ml/hr, determined by patient's vital signs).

18. b. All of the other organs are in the abdominal cavity. (Objective 1)

19. b. Appendicitis would be unusual in this age and would typically not exhibit the symptoms listed. Diverticulosis and peptic ulcer would typically not exhibit the symptoms listed. (Objective 2)

20. b. Her age, time of day, and description of the pain are characteristics of cholecystitis. (Objective 2)

21. c. All disorders listed cause bleeding, but esophagogastric varices rupture usually produces rapid life-threatening bleeding. Bleeding from AV malformations may be minor or severe. Bleeding from diverticulitis may be serious but is not typically an acute life-threatening emergency at onset. Hemorrhoidal bleeding is usually not severe. (Objective 3)

22. b. The patient's age, gender, and description of medical history often discloses more about the cause of the abdominal illness than physical examination. The severity of the patient's present condition is determined by physical examination. (Objective 4)

23. c. Melena (black or maroon stool) indicates the presence of bleeding. Tachycardia can be caused by bleeding, fever, pain, or other fluid loss. (Objective 4)

24. d. Administration of the pain medicines listed is contraindicated in the prehospital setting for undiagnosed abdominal pain. (Objective 5)

● CHAPTER 33
UROLOGY/RENAL

1. e

(Objective 2)

2. c

(Objective 2)

3. b

(Objective 5)

4. h

5. g

6. f

7. d

(Questions 4-7, Objective 2)

8. a. kidney
b. ureter
c. bladder
d. urethra

9. a. Urinary calculus. Initiate intravenous line. Consult with medical direction regarding administration of analgesics such as ketorolac or meperidine; b. testicular torsion. Initiate intravenous line. Apply icepack to scrotum and transport rapidly; c. pyelonephritis. Initiate intravenous line. Transport; d. urinary tract infection. Transport. (Objective 2)

10. Protect the patient's privacy with drapes. Have a paramedic who is the same sex as the patient perform the examination if possible. Have a chaperone present during physical exam of genitalia (if indicated). Explain all actions to the patient and proceed in a calm, caring manner. (Objective 3)

11. a. Trauma, shock, infection, urinary obstruction, and multisystem diseases; b. hypertension, diabetes, congenital condition, and pyelonephritis. (Objective 5)

12. a. Too much fluid taken off in dialysis and bleeding at fistula resulting from pseudoaneurysm (any cause of bleeding is serious because the patient has decreased platelets and is heparinized during dialysis); b. initiate large-bore intravenous line in the arm without the arteriovenous fistula, infuse a small volume initially (200 to 300 ml), and reevaluate the patient for signs of fluid overload (crackles, engorged neck veins, pulmonary edema). (Objective 7)

13.

Disorder	Cause	Affect on Patient	Interventions
Hemorrhage	Decrease in platelet function; anticoagulant use; anemia; bleeding from fistula or graft	Signs and symptoms of shock; dyspnea, angina	Control external bleeding; treat for shock; rapid transport
Hypotension	Hemodialysis because of decreased volume; changes in electrolyte concentration, vascular instability	Decreased blood pressure; signs and symptoms of shock	Small 200 to 300 ml fluid challenge (monitor for S&S of congestive heart failure)
Chest pain	Hypotension and hypoxemia during dialysis	Chest pain, headache, dizziness	Oxygen, fluid replacement, antianginal drugs
Hyperkalemia	Poor diet regulation; missed dialysis	Weakness; may have no symptoms; tall tented T wave; prolonged PRI (K greater than 6 to 6.5 mmol/L); depressed ST segments and loss of P waves (K greater than 7 mmol/L); wide QRS	Suspect if renal patient in arrest; medical direction may order CaCl and NaHCO₃ during arrest
Disequilibrium syndrome	Increase in osmolality of the ECF compared with ICF in brain or CSF	HA, nausea, fatigue; confusion, seizures, coma	Transport; treat seizures with diazepam or lorazepam
Air embolism	Negative pressure in dialysis tubing; malfunction in dialysis machine	Dyspnea, cyanosis, hypotension, respiratory distress	Oxygen, rapid transport; position patient on left side with head down

(Objective 7)

14. a. Epinephrine 1.0 mg IV; NaHCO₃ 1 mEq/kg IV; and atropine 1.0 mg IV. (Objective 7)
b. Epinephrine can increase peripheral vascular resistance and is a sympathomimetic. Sodium bicarbonate should be given because the patient likely has hyperkalemia and severe acidosis related to her chronic renal failure because she missed her dialysis. Atropine is a parasympatholytic and theoretically may help to initiate sinus activity. (Objective 7)
c. Bicarb may inactivate epinephrine, so tubing should be flushed between drugs. (Objective 7)

15. c. Because the twisted testicle blocks the blood supply to the teste, intervention within 4 to 6 hours is essential. (Objective 2)

16. c. Kidney infection is a renal cause, and prostatic enlargement and ureteral strictures are postrenal causes. (Objective 6)

17. a. Do not assess blood pressure or start an IV on the side where the fistula or shunt is placed. Vascular access should not routinely be obtained through the shunt. Rarely, because of an arrest situation, medical direction will authorize vascular access through the shunt. (Objective 5)

18. c. Infection at the site of the catheter insertion is common and may lead to peritonitis. (Objective 7)

19. a. Peaked, tented T waves are associated with hyperkalemia, which is a common electrolyte imbalance. (Objective 7)

20. b. Sodium bicarbonate may temporarily cause movement of potassium out of the vascular space and relieve the cardiac effects until definitive care (dialysis) can be given. (Objective 7)

21. a. Anemia secondary to lack of a substance needed for red blood cell production will decrease the oxygen-carrying capacity of the blood. (Objective 6)

● **CHAPTER 34**
TOXICOLOGY

1. c, g
2. a, b, f, h
3. b, e, g
4. b, d, g
(Questions 1-4, Objective 2)
5. i
(Objective 4)
6. f
(Objective 4)
7. e
(Objectives 4 and 6)
8. c
(Objective 8)
9. g
(Objective 4)
10. b
(Objective 4)
11. j
(Objective 9)
12. a. You should be prepared to tell the poison control center the specific agent ingested, amount of agent ingested, time ingested, age, patient weight, medical condition, and treatment rendered before arrival of EMS personnel.(Objective 3)
b. Ensure adequate airway, ventilation, and circulation. Obtain a history (especially specific to substance ingested) and perform a physical exam. Assess for hypoglycemia. Consult with medical

direction for further treatment guidelines. Monitor vital signs and ECG. Transport rapidly for definitive treatment. (Objective 3)

13. a. Position the patient in the left lateral Trendelenberg (swimmer's) position; b. Rapid sequence endotracheal intubation before orogastric tube intubation if patient has a decreased level of consciousness with an absent gag reflex; c. after assessment for proper tube placement, normal saline (preferably warmed) should be infused into the orogastric tube in 200- to 300-ml boluses, and the tube should be allowed to drain after each bolus. This process is continued until the gastric drainage returns clear. (Objective 3)

14.

	Ingested Poison	Charcoal (Yes/No)	Other Interventions
a.	Bleach	No	Dilution with milk or water (200 to 300 ml for an adult or 15 ml/kg for a child)
b.	Ammonia	No	Dilution with milk or water
c.	Gasoline	No	Initiation of intravenous line, monitoring of airway and electrocardiogram
d.	Methanol	Controversial	Lavage, sodium bicarbonate intravenously (30 to 60 ml), and 80-proof ethanol by mouth
e.	Ethylene glycol	Yes	Lavage, sodium bicarbonate intravenously (30 to 60 ml), 80-proof ethanol by mouth, and (rarely) furosemide, thiamine, and calcium gluconate
f.	Isopropanol	Yes	Lavage
g.	Cyanide	No	Amyl nitrite pearls, 3% sodium nitrite, and 25% sodium thiosulfate

(Objective 4)

15. a. Time varies. Chemical 1 to 2 hours; bacterial toxins 1 to 12 hours; viral or bacterial 12 to 48 hours; b. take universal precautions, maintain airway and breathing, and initiate intravenous therapy with crystalloid solution to treat dehydration and fluid and electrolyte imbalance. (Objective 4)

16. Cholinergic syndrome. (Objective 2)

17. Ask the patient if he still has a sample of the mushroom and what time he took it. If he does not have a sample, have him describe the mushroom. Contact poison control and medical direction (per protocol) for help with identification and treatment information. Prehospital treatment will likely be guided by signs and symptoms rather than specific identification information. (Objective 2)

18. Maintain airway and prepare to suction if needed; administer high-concentration oxygen; monitor ECG and vital signs frequently; initiate an IV line and infuse fluids as ordered by medical direction; and prepare to administer atropine sulfate as ordered by medical direction. (Objective 4)

19. Appropriate personal protective equipment should be worn by rescuers.

Toxic Chemical	Class of Toxin	Signs and Symptoms	Treatment
Copper welding umes	Metal fumes	Chills, fever, myalgias; HA, cough, leukocytosis	Remove patient from source, treat symptoms
Hydrogen sulfide	Chemical asphyxiant	Sudden collapse, rotten egg smell, rapid fatigue	Remove patient from source, oxygenate, sodium nitrate; do not use thiosulfate
Methane gas	Simple asphyxiant	Symptoms of hypoxia without airway irritation	Remove patient from source, oxygenate
Chlorine gas	Irritant	Lacrimation, sore throat, stridor, tracheobronchitis, pulmonary edema	Remove patient from source, humidified oxygen, bronchodilators, airway management

(Objective 6)

20. Ensure personal protection; open airway; administer high-flow oxygen; initiate an intravenous line to keep the vein open; and if pulmonary edema develops, consider administration of diuretics and bronchodilators. (Objective 8)

21. Carbamate or organophosphate. (Objective 9)

22. Pupil constriction, muscle fasciculation, headache, weakness, dizziness, hypotension, bronchoconstriction, anxiety, seizures, and convulsions. (Objective 9)

23. Sinus bradycardia. (Objective 9)

24. Wear protective gear; decontaminate as appropriate; suction oral secretions as necessary; prepare to intubate if patient's condition deteriorates; initi-

ate intravenous therapy with crystalloid to keep the vein open; administer atropine 2 to 4 mg intravenously every 5 to 15 minutes as necessary to induce relative tachycardia, flushing, and decreased secretions; monitor for dysrhythmias; administer pralidoxime; administer diazepam as necessary for seizures.
(Objective 9)

25. a. He took fentanyl or heroin intravenously; b. she was smoking PCP and crack (cocaine); c. they were smoking purified crack cocaine; d. he injected morphine subcutaneously; e. she ingested PCP nasally.
(Objective 10)

26. e
27. g
28. f
29. a
30. b
(Questions 26-30, Objective 11)

31. What was taken? Where is the container? How much was in it and how much is left (may need to estimate based on date prescription issued, amount prescribed daily, and amount left in bottle)? When was the drug taken? Has the patient vomited or taken anything to induce vomiting since the drug was taken? Has any antidote been given to the patient? Ask the patient the following: Why did you do this? Were you trying to hurt or kill yourself?
(Objective 10)

32. 30 to 100 g activated charcoal. (Objective 10)

33.

	Ingested Poison	Charcoal (Yes/No)	Other Interventions
a.	Aspirin	Yes	D50W if patient is hypoglycemic
b.	Acetaminophen	Usually not (varies by medical direction)	Mucomyst (varies by medical direction)
c.	Iron	No	Monitor airway, initiate intravenous line

34. a. Heroin, morphine, and methadone; b. barbiturates (secobarbital, phenobarbital) and benzodiazepines (diazepam, chlordiazepoxide); c. amphetamines and cocaine; d. LSD and phencyclidine (PCP).
(Objective 10)

35. Respiratory depression (partial airway obstruction and decreased minute volume). (Objective 11)

36. Naloxone (Narcan) 2.0 mg intravenously. (Administer enough to ensure adequate airway reflexes and ventilation.)
(Objective 11)

37. Gooseflesh (piloerection), tachycardia, diaphoresis, irritability, insomnia, abdominal cramps, tremors, nausea, vomiting, cold sweats and chills, fever, and diarrhea.
(Objective 11)

38. Bilaterally dilated and slow to react to light.
(Objective 11)

39. Flumazenil (Romazicon).
(Objective 11)

40. Tricyclic antidepressants.
(Objective 11)

41. Cardiac dysrhythmias, seizures, or cerebrovascular accident (secondary to intracranial hemorrhage).
(Objective 11)

42. Personal safety.
(Objective 11)

43. Quiet, calm approach. Interview the patient while minimizing external sensory stimuli (for example, bright lights, noise).
(Objective 11)

44. Euphoria, disorientation, seizures, hypertensive crisis, dysrhythmias, catatonia, unresponsiveness, and bizarre and violent behavior. These patients are extremely difficult to manage and dangerous if found in or provoked into violent behavior.
(Objective 11)

45. No. She is drowsy and her level of consciousness could deteriorate further. Also, more than 20 minutes has passed since ingestion of the drug.
(Objective 11)

46. Sinus tachycardia with delayed ventricular conduction (wide QRS complex).
(Objective 11)

47. Sodium bicarbonate 1 to 2 mEq/kg intravenously.
(Objective 11)

48. Delirium, depressed respirations, hypertension or hypotension, hyperthermia or hypothermia, seizures, coma, and dysrhythmias.
(Objective 11)

49. No. Alcoholics frequently underestimate the number of drinks they have had.
(Objective 13)

50. a. Short-term memory deficit, problems with coordination, and difficulty with concentration can mimic signs and symptoms of head injury; b. nutritional deficiencies can cause muscle cramps, paresthesias, seizures, tremor or ataxia, and poor wound healing; c. chronic dehydration may be difficult to distinguish from a new onset of fluid loss. Patient will decompensate faster if acute fluid loss occurs resulting from trauma; d. clotting factors are suppressed by chronic alcohol abuse, resulting in increased risk of bleeding, especially subdural hematoma, with minor trauma.
(Objective 12)

51. Protect airway (high risk of aspiration); ventilate as necessary; initiate intravenous therapy; draw blood samples per protocol; determine blood glucose levels and if low, administer thiamine 100 mg intravenously and D50W 25 g intravenously; if opiate overdose is suspected or unknown, administer naloxone 2 mg intravenously; monitor airway, breathing, vital signs, and electrocardiogram.
(Objective 13)

52. Manage as in Answer 51 and protect from injury; administer diazepam 2.5 to 5.0 mg or lorazepam 1-2 mg intravenously if additional seizures occur; examine for signs or symptoms of traumatic injury.
(Objective 13)

53. Hyperactive motor, speech, and autonomic activity; confusion; disorientation; delusion; hallucinations; tremor; agitation; insomnia; tachycardia; fever; hypertension; dilated pupils; profuse diaphoresis; and in severe cases, cardiovascular collapse.
(Objective 13)

54. a. Assess for anaphylaxis, apply ice packs, and immobilize and elevate affected extremity; b. scrape or brush off. Do not squeeze because doing so will inject additional venom.
(Objective 14)

55. a. Lyme disease. Early signs are fever, lethargy, muscle pain, and general malaise; late signs are cardiac abnormalities, cranial nerve palsies, and arthritis; b. tick paralysis. Signs include restlessness and paresthesia in hands and feet progressing to ascending symmetric flaccid paralysis, which may include respiratory muscles.
(Objective 14)

56. Apply gloves and grasp tick as close to skin surface as possible (may use tweezers or forceps if available), pull out with steady pressure (avoid squeezing tick), and cleanse wound and observe for any remnants of tick.
(Objective 14)

57. a. Fang marks, pain and edema, weakness, diaphoresis, nausea, vomiting, and paresthesias; b. ensure personal safety from another bite; monitor airway, breathing, and circulation; initiate intravenous therapy in unaffected extremity; immobilize affected extremity in dependent position; and keep patient at rest.
(Objective 14)

58. a. Jellyfish, fire corals, and sea anemones. Rinse wound with seawater; apply vinegar, baking soda, isopropanol, ammonia, meat tenderizer (for 5 to 10 minutes only); remove visible tentacles with forceps; apply shaving cream, gently shave affected area or use knife or spatula to gently scrape remaining tentacles; and rinse again; b. sea urchins, starfish, and sea cucumbers. Remove embedded spines with forceps and immerse affected extremity (and unaffected extremity to prevent thermal injury) in hot water during transport; c. stingrays. Irrigate wound with salt or fresh water; remove venom apparatus if it is visible; and immerse the affected part in hot water.
(Objective 14)

59. b.
(Objective 1)

60. d.
(Objective 2)

61. d. Life threats that will need immediate management will usually be identified by assessing these areas.
(Objective 3)

62. b. Charcoal binds the drug by adsorption. It is often given with a cathartic that speeds the bound drug through the gastrointestinal tract.
(Objective 3)

63. c. Gastric lavage and charcoal are generally considered superior. Ipecac is contraindicated in petroleum distillate ingestions. It is associated with aspiration, Mallory-Weiss tear of the esophagus, pneumomediastinum, and fatal diaphragmatic or gastric rupture. If indicated, it should be given within 20 minutes after ingestion.
(Objective 2)

64. a. Inducing emesis is usually contraindicated for these patients, unless the toxicity of the specific hydrocarbon is so great that the risks of absorption in the gastrointestinal tract outweigh the risks of aspiration.
(Objective 4)

65. c. Methanol and ethylene glycol produce metabolic acidosis, so $NaHCO_3$ is indicated. In a tricyclic antidepressant overdose, it will decrease the toxic cardiac side effects. No metabolic acidosis is usually associated with isopropanol ingestion.
(Objective 4)

66. b. The second most common reported category of poisonings is from plants. Dialysis is not effective for most plant poisonings. Most signs and symptoms occur within several hours after ingestion. Treatment should be based on symptoms and not be delayed until the identity of the plant can be determined.
(Objective 4)

67. a. Salivation and hypotension are likely to accompany the bradycardia. Symptoms vary according to the specific variety of mushroom ingested.
(Objective 4)

68. d. The lower the viscosity, the higher the risk of aspiration.
(Objective 5)

69. d. Huffing or sniffing substances such as carbon tetrachloride, methylene chloride, or aromatic hy-

drocarbons such as benzene and toluene is the most common method. (Objective 8)

70. a. All of the other chemicals are more likely to cause tachycardia. (Objective 9)

71. c. All other interventions are critical; however, rescuer safety should precede treatment because these poisons are readily absorbed through the skin, by ingestion, or by inhalation. (Objective 9)

72. d. $\dfrac{D}{H} \times Q = \text{Volume} \ \dfrac{2 \text{ mg}}{1 \text{ mg}} \times 10 \text{ ml} = 20 \text{ ml}$
(Objective 9)

73. a. All of the others are narcotics. (Objective 11)

74. c. Methamphetamine labs may produce hazards because of booby traps, explosive chemicals, a violent patient, or hazardous material contamination. Scene safety should be the highest priority. (Objective 11)

75. c. Oil of wintergreen contains a large amount of salicylate and has produced many fatal ingestions. (Objective 11)

76. c. Unless patients volunteer information regarding an overdose of acetaminophen, they may be asymptomatic or complain of only mild influenza-like symptoms for the first 24 hours after ingestion. (Objective 11)

77. c. Ingestion of an overdose of iron is often lethal. (Objective 11)

78. c. All of the other drugs are more likely to produce bradycardia, although digoxin can produce bradycardia or tachycardia. (Objective 11)

79. a. The immediate goal is to adsorb the drug and prevent its passage into the small intestine where it can be absorbed into the blood. Later, if signs and symptoms develop, they will be treated. (Objective 11)

80. d. Wernicke-Korsakoff syndrome can lead to irreversible neurological problems and may be avoided by giving thiamine before administration of D50W. (Objective 12)

81. b. The mortality rate has been reported as high as 15% for delirium tremens. It affects about 5% of hospitalized alcoholics undergoing withdrawal and usually occurs 72 to 96 hours after withdrawal of alcohol. Symptoms are associated with autonomic hyperactivity. (Objective 13)

82. b. Diazepam in doses of 5 mg every 5 minutes up to a total of 30 mg may be needed. Lorazepam 1-2 mg IV is an alternative. (Objective 13)

83. d. Anaphylaxis would likely include respiratory distress and urticaria. His reaction was immediate and generalized and involved a large exposure to venom. (Objective 14)

84. a. The brown recluse produces a local reaction leading to delayed skin necrosis. Envenomation from most other spiders typically causes local versus systemic reactions. (Objective 14)

85. c. This description matches a coral snake, which is the only neurotoxic snake listed. (Objective 14)

86. a. Ice or cold packs may increase tissue damage and are not indicated. (Objective 14)

87. c. Isoproterenol may induce or aggravate hypotension and ventricular dysrhythmias and should not be given unless massive beta-blocker poisoning has occurred. (Objective 11)

● CHAPTER 35 HEMATOLOGY

1. h
2. d
3. e
4. b
5. a
6. f
7. c
(Questions 1-7, Objective 1)
8.

Condition	Cause	Signs and Symptoms
Anemia	Iron deficiency; decreased production and survival of RBCs	Fatigue, headaches, sore mouth or tongue, brittle nails, breathlessness, or chest pain
Leukemia	Abnormal chromosomes; disorganized proliferation of WBCs in bone marrow	Bleeding, bone pain, frequent bruising, sternal tenderness, fatigue, headache, weight loss, night sweats; enlarged lymph nodes, liver, spleen, testes; anemia, infections
Lymphomas	Proliferation of cells in lymph tissues (may be genetic link)	Swollen lymph nodes in neck, armpits, groin; fatigue, chills, and night sweats Severe itching, cough, weight loss, dyspnea, chest discomfort
Polycythemia	Unusually large number of red blood cells	Headache, dizziness, blurred vision, generalized itching, hypertension, splenomegaly, platelet disorders, red hands and feet, purple complexion, stroke and development of leukemias
Disseminated intravascular coagulation	Complication of severe injury, trauma, disease; imbalance of clotting mechanisms	Dyspnea, bleeding, hypotension, hypoperfusion

Hemophilia	Inherited bleeding disorder; deficiency of factor VIII or less often factor IX	Spontaneous bleeding (joints, deep muscles, urinary tract, and intracranial sites most common) after injury or during medical procedures
Sickle cell disease	Genetic illness; red blood cells are distorted into sickle shape that is easily destroyed and can clog blood vessels	Episodes of severe pain, fatigue, pallor, jaundice, stroke; delayed growth, development, and sexual maturation; hematuria, priapism, splenomegaly
Multiple myeloma	Malignant neoplasm of bone marrow	Pain, fractures, hypercalcemia, skeletal deformities, kidney failure, anemia, weight loss, rib fractures, recurrent infections

(Objective 2)

9. a. Possibly a vasoocclusive sickle cell crisis; b. dehydration or stress from her illness the day before may have triggered her crisis; c. the spleen may enlarge during a sickle cell crisis, so it should be evaluated; d. you should administer oxygen by nonrebreather mask at 12-15 L per minute. An IV should be initiated and a fluid bolus administered under medical direction. Although analgesia will be a high priority for this patient, medical direction may not order it until the abdomen can be examined to ensure that an urgent surgical condition does not exist. (Objective 2)

10. d. All types of blood cells are formed here. Yellow marrow is composed of connective tissue and fat. (Objective 1)

11. b. Normal hemoglobin ranges from 13.5 to 18 g/100 ml. Normal hematocrit ranges from 38% to 54%. (Objective 1)

12. b. Treatment for aplastic anemia may include blood transfusion, folic acid, and bone marrow transplantation. Iron deficiency anemia is treated with supplemental iron and folic acid. (Objective 2)

13. d. Acute myeloblastic anemia affects middle-age adults. Reed-Sternberg cells are characteristic for Hodgkin's lymphoma. Itching is not a classic symptom. (Objective 2)

14. b. DIC is diagnosed based on clinical history and laboratory values that include clotting studies, platelet count, and fibrin degradation products. Sickle cell anemia is confirmed by laboratory testing. (Objective 2)

15. c. Hodgkin's lymphoma primarily affects lymphoid tissues. (Objective 2)

16. c. The body produces more red cells in an attempt to improve oxygenation in conditions such as high altitude and chronic lung disease. (Objective 2)

17. b. Coagulation inhibition levels are decreased. Platelets and coagulation factors are consumed, and thrombin is formed. (Objective 2)

18. a. Factor VIII is needed to reestablish a normal clotting cascade and stop bleeding. (Objective 2)

19. c. Splenic sequestration occurs in childhood and is caused by blood trapped in the spleen. Aplastic crisis occurs when the bone marrow temporarily stops making red blood cells. In hemolytic crisis, red blood cell breakdown exceeds production. Vasoocclusive sickle cell crisis occurs when the sickle-shaped cells block blood flow to organs and tissues. (Objective 2)

20. d. Hodgkin's disease is a type of lymphoma and affects the lymph tissue. Leukemia is similar to multiple myeloma, but in multiple myeloma, the primary target is bone. (Objective 2)

21. d. Acute or chronic hematological disorders produce tremendous emotional stress on patients and families. You should be empathetic and provide calm support during care and transport. Analgesics and antidysrhythmics may occasionally be indicated. Prehospital blood transfusion is usually only done during interfacility transfers. (Objective 2)

● CHAPTER 36
ENVIRONMENTAL CONDITIONS

1. g
(Objective 1)
2. k
(Objective 1)
3. a
(Objective 3)
4. i
(Objective 1)
5. b
(Objective 5)
6. e
(Objective 6)
7. h
(Objective 3)
8. d
(Objective 5)
9. j
(Objective 1)
10. f
(Objective 5)
11. a. Oxidation of energy sources; b. shivering can increase heat production by 400%; c. increased basal metabolic rate and vasoconstriction. (Objective 1)
12. a. Conduction, convection, and radiation; b. conduction and radiation; c. conduction, radiation,

convection, and evaporation; d. conduction, radiation, convection, and evaporation. (Objective 1)

13. Skin vasodilation (becomes warm and flushed), sweating, decreased hormone secretion, and decreased muscle tone. (Objective 1)

14. Peripheral vasoconstriction (cool, pale skin), goose bumps, shivering, increased voluntary activity, increased hormone secretion, and increased appetite. (Objective 1)

15. a. Heat cramps. Remove patient from hot environment, replace sodium and water, and intravenously infuse saline solution if condition is severe; b. heat exhaustion. Remove patient from hot environment and intravenously infuse saline solution; c. heat stroke. Secure airway, assess breathing, ventilate if indicated, administer high-flow oxygen, move patient to a cool environment, remove all clothing, wet the skin with cool fluid, fan the patient, initiate intravenous fluid therapy with normal saline, consult with medical direction regarding a fluid challenge, and monitor for signs of fluid overload. If seizures recur, administer diazepam, assess for hypoglycemia, and administer D50W if indicated. (Objective 2)

16. Increasing the metabolic rate increases the heart rate and contractility and increases the body's use of oxygen and other nutrients. The patient with preexisting trauma or illness will not tolerate these extra demands, which may compromise organ response to illness or injury. (Objective 3)

17. Assess and secure the airway, assess breathing, and assist with 100% oxygen (warmed and humidified if available); if indicated, assess circulation and begin cardiopulmonary resuscitation only after carefully verifying that no pulse is present. Move the patient to a warm environment and remove all clothing. (Objective 3)

18. a. Cardiopulmonary resuscitation; defibrillation at 200, 300, and 360 joules; intubation; ventilation with warm humid oxygen; intravenous infusion of warm normal saline; and transport to the hospital; b. cardiopulmonary resuscitation, defibrillation at 200, 300, and 360 joules; intubation; ventilation with warm, humid oxygen; intravenous infusion of warm normal saline; intravenous medications as indicated for ventricular fibrillation with a delay between doses; and another defibrillation as core temperature rises. (Objective 3)

19. Resuscitation may be withheld if there are obvious lethal injuries or if the body is frozen, preventing chest compression or airway management. Resuscitation could stop when the patient's core temperature has reached 94°-95° F (34°-35° C) and all resuscitation efforts are still unsuccessful. (Objective 3)

20. Move patient to warm area, remove any wet clothing, and wrap patient in warm blanket. If he is awake and alert, administer warm sugar-sweetened drinks (no alcohol, coffee, or tea). If necessary, apply hot packs wrapped in towels to the neck, armpits, and groin. (Objective 3)

21. a. Atrial fibrillation; b. put the patient at rest and move to a warm environment after ensuring adequate airway, breathing, and circulation. Carefully remove all wet clothing and wrap patient in a blanket. Administer 100% oxygen (heated and humidified if possible) by nonrebreather mask. Initiate intravenous therapy of normal saline (initial fluid challenge of 250 to 500 ml may be ordered by medical direction, and use warmed fluids if available). Transport gently and monitor the patient carefully en route. (Objective 3)

22. In deep frostbite the underlying tissue is hard and not compressible, whereas in superficial frostbite the underlying tissue springs back when palpated. (Objective 3)

23. Lack of protective clothing; preexisting illness or injury (diabetes or vascular insufficiency); fatigue; tobacco; tight, constrictive clothing; alcohol; and medications that cause vasodilation (some antihypertensives). (Objective 3)

24. Elevate and protect the affected extremity, provide rapid transport to a medical facility, and assess for hypothermia. (Objective 3)

25. Temperature of water, length of submersion, cleanliness of water, and age of patient. (Objective 4)

26. Acute respiratory failure, dysrhythmias, decreased cardiac output, cerebral edema leading to central nervous system dysfunction, and renal dysfunction (rare). (Objective 4)

27. Ensure scene safety, initiate cardiopulmonary resuscitation, secure the airway with an endotracheal tube and ventilate with 100% oxygen, assess cardiac rhythm and follow advanced life-support protocols to manage appropriately, assess for hypothermia, and transport to appropriate medical facility. (Objective 4)

28. Ears, sinuses, lungs and airways, gastrointestinal tract, thorax, and teeth. (Objective 6)

29. a. Focal paralysis or sensory changes, aphasia, confusion, blindness or another visual disturbance, convulsion, loss of consciousness, dizziness, vertigo, abdominal pain, and cardiac arrest; b. if the patient's trachea is intubated, fill the balloon with normal saline instead of air; evaluate for

POPS; and transport in the left lateral recumbent position with a 15-degree elevation of the thorax. (Objective 6)

30. a. Decompression sickness; b. administer high-flow oxygen, initiate intravenous therapy, and rapidly transport for recompression (follow local protocol so that patient can reach hyperbaric chamber as quickly as possible). (Objective 6)

31. a. Acute mountain sickness, high-altitude pulmonary edema, and high altitude cerebral edema; b. descent to a lower altitude. (Objective 6)

32. d. Vasoconstriction and vasodilation of the blood vessels in the skin are the major ways the body releases or conserves heat. (Objective 1)

33. d. Based on his symptoms, you suspect heat exhaustion. Because he is nauseated and has orthostatic hypotension, he needs intravenous rather than oral rehydration. He should be moved to a cool environment and not returned to the fire. (Objective 2)

34. d (Objective 2)

35. c. Damage to the body continues as long as the temperature remains elevated. (Objective 2)

36. b. Shivering should continue until the core temperature reaches 86° F (30° C). A tremendous amount of energy is needed for shivering, so glucose and glycogen must be available to fuel this increased muscle activity. (Objective 3)

37. b. Rapid rewarming in warm water is indicated only when sanctioned by medical direction if no chance of refreezing exists. Refreezing is damaging to the tissues. (Objective 3)

38. c. The lack of ventilation causes a buildup of carbon dioxide, which coupled with the lack of oxygen intake (hypoxia) leads to acidosis. (Objective 4)

39. a. Deaths that occur after 24 hours are referred to as *drowning-related deaths.* Submersion is swimming-related distress that is sufficient to require support in the prehospital setting and transportation to a medical facility for further assessment and care. (Objective 4)

40. c. Although each factor listed influences patient outcome after submersion, duration of submersion and degree of hypoxia are the critical elements that determine odds of survival. (Objective 4)

41. a. Dalton's law states that the total pressure of a mixture of gases is equal to the sum of the partial pressures of the component gases. Henry's law states that the amount of gas dissolved in a given volume of fluid is proportional to the pressure of the gas with which it is in equilibrium. Newton's law states that a body at rest will remain at rest until acted on

by an outside force, and a body in motion will remain in motion until acted on by an outside force. (Objective 5)

42. d. As trapped air in the lungs expands on rapid ascent, it ruptures alveoli and allows gas to leak into the subcutaneous tissues. (Objective 6)

43. b. The neurodepressant effects of nitrogen narcosis may lead to diving accidents resulting from impaired judgment. (Objective 6)

44. a. Ataxia signals progression of the illness, and coma may result within 24 hours of its onset. (Objective 6)

● CHAPTER 37
INFECTIOUS AND COMMUNICABLE DISEASES

1. c (Objective 5)

2. g (Objective 7)

3. i (Objective 5)

4. e (Objective 5)

5. h (Objective 9)

6. f (Objective 5)

7. b (Objective 9)

8. j (Objective 9)

9. A pathological agent, a reservoir, a portal of exit from the reservoir, an environment conducive to transmission of the pathogenic agent, portal of entry, and susceptibility of the new host to the infectious disease. (Objective 2)

10. Burns, lacerations, abrasions, intravenous therapy, and urinary catheter. (Objective 3)

11. Human immunodeficiency virus, chemotherapy, and prolonged steroid therapy. (Objective 3)

12. a. Gloves, gown, mask, and eyewear; b. gloves; c. nothing is necessary according to the CDC; however, if bleeding is likely and because prehospital setting is high risk, gloves are indicated; d. gloves, mask, and eyewear; e. gloves, gown, mask, and eyewear; f. gloves. (Objective 1)

13. Hepatitis A, B, or C. (Objective 5)

14. Take HBV vaccination and use strict universal (BSI) precautions as warranted by each situation. (Objectives 1 and 5).

15. Direct introduction of infected blood by needle or transfusion, introduction of serum or plasma through skin cuts, absorption of infected serum or plasma through mucosal surfaces, absorption of saliva or semen through mucosal surfaces, and transfer of infective serum or plasma via inanimate surfaces.
(Objective 5)

16. Yes. If the patient is found to have hepatitis A, you may be given an immune globulin injection. If he has hepatitis B and if you are not immune to the hepatitis B virus, an HBV vaccine will be given to protect against future exposures and hepatitis B immune globulin will be given to provide temporary passive immunity to the hepatitis B virus. No immunization or immune globulin exists that is effective to prevent hepatitis C.
(Objective 5)

17. a. Fever, swollen lymph nodes, and sore throat; b. enlarged lymph nodes; c. bacterial pneumonia, oral lesions, shingles, and pulmonary tuberculosis; d. diarrhea, tumors, dementia, neurological symptoms, and opportunistic infections.
(Objective 5)

18. a. You should take the same precautions you would take with any patient with this type of injury. If no open wounds are present, no BSI is indicated; b. clean the ambulance as you would after any patient.
(Objectives 1 and 5)

19. Periodic skin test with purified protein derivative (of tuberculin) and chest x-ray study if purified protein derivative (of tuberculin) test is positive or other history exists indicating the need.
(Objective 5)

20. a. Gloves and mask (respiratory spread); wear eye shield if risk of splash or spray exists (for example, if the patient vomits or needs to be intubated); b. an exposure should be reported if you did not have appropriate personal protective equipment on or if you had contact with blood or body fluids; c. the need for prophylaxis will be determined by your occupational health provider but is not likely indicated if all BSI precautions were used for the entire call.
(Objective 5)

21. Paresis, wide gait, ataxia, psychosis, and signs of myocardial insufficiency.
(Objective 9)

22. Gloves (mask and protective eyewear if any risk of splash or spray of body fluids exists).
(Objective 1)

23. a. Pubic lice look like crabs or gray-blue spots, and nits appear on abdomen, thighs, eyelashes, eyebrows, and axillary hair; b. head lice have an elongated body with narrow head and three pair of legs, and nits look like dandruff that cannot be brushed off; c. scabies produce bites concentrated around webs of hands and feet, a child's face and scalp, a female's nipples, and a male's penis, as well as vesicles and papules that become easily infected because of scratching.
(Objective 9)

24. Yes. Chickenpox is contagious for 1 to 2 days before the onset of the rash until all of the lesions are crusted and dry.
(Objective 7)

25. 13 to 17 days.
(Objective 7)

26. Varicella can be transmitted 1 to 2 days before eruption of the rash until the lesions have all scabbed over.
(Objective 7)

27. Yes. Blood that came in contact with your mucous membranes is a significant exposure.
(Objective 10)

28. Immediately report the exposure as soon as you arrive at the hospital with the patient. If you did not transport the patient to the hospital, you should go there immediately (or follow your local protocol).
(Objective 10)

29. You should irrigate your eyes immediately after the eye splash exposure.
(Objective 10)

30. No. The ED cannot ignore the patient's request. The patient has the legal right to refuse an HIV test.
(Objectives 5 and 10)

31. Ask if the patient has HIV and assess for risk factors that would indicate the potential for HIV infection (IV drug use, unsafe sex practices).
(Objectives 5 and 10)

32. The ED or occupational medicine staff may still offer you prophylactic drug treatment based on the nature of the exposure and the patient's risk factors (antiviral and possibly protease inhibitor drugs). (Objectives 5 and 10)

33. The benefits to you (risk of HIV infection) versus complications of the prophylaxis therapy based on your personal health status will need to be weighed before you decide whether to take the medicine.
(Objectives 5 and 10)

34. For a year, you will undergo periodic evaluation to determine if you have converted to HIV-positive status. Until that time, you should alter your sexual practices and discontinue breast feeding if you are lactating. This can be a difficult time for paramedics and their significant others, wondering if the next test will be positive. Counseling may provide an opportunity to verbalize those feelings in a healthy manner.
(Objectives 5 and 10)

35. Use of eyeshield and facemask would likely have prevented this exposure.
(Objectives 1 and 15)

36. a. The CDC establishes guidelines that are often adopted by OSHA and incorporated by agencies such as DOH and DOT into other documents (for example, national standard paramedic curriculum). (Objective 1)

37. d. All of the answers reflect something that could break a link in the chain of transmission. Antibiotics can kill the pathogenic agent; cleaning agents with appropriate disinfectants destroy the environment conducive to transmission, immunizations decrease host susceptibility. (Objective 2)

38. b. All other answers are external barriers to infection. (Objective 3)

39. c. Antibodies can fix complement. Killer cells are part of cell-mediated immunity. (Objective 3)

40. c. The communicability period begins when the latent period ends and continues as long as the agent is present and can spread to others. The latent period begins with invasion of the body and ends when the agent can be shed or communicated. The disease period follows the incubation period and has variable lengths. (Objective 4)

41. b. Short- and long-term mortality is higher from hepatitis B. (Objective 2)

42. d. (Objective 2)

43. c. The patient with pneumonia may also have all of the other signs and symptoms. (Objective 5)

44. c. Trismus (lockjaw) often occurs and makes opening the mouth difficult. The patient often has muscle tetany and spasms but not urticaria or seizures. (Objective 6)

45. b. Hydropenia is a lack of water in tissues; polydipsia is increased thirst; and polyuria is increased urination. (Objective 6)

46. d. (Objective 7)

47. b. (Objective 7)

48. c. Antibiotic therapy would only be indicated if a secondary bacterial infection develops. Aspirin is contraindicated for children and patients with chickenpox. Intravenous therapy would only be needed if an acute complication of these viral illnesses develops. (Objectives 7, 8, and 9)

49. c. Influenza and pneumonia can produce cough; however, they do not persist as long as pertussis. (Objective 7)

50. d. Pneumonia is especially true for patients who are elderly or have preexisting lung or heart disease. (Objective 8)

51. d. The enlarged spleen increases the chance of injury if the patient sustains a blow to the abdomen. (Objective 8)

52. d. Syphilis is associated with systemic and chronic signs and symptoms. (Objective 9)

53. d. The virus migrates along the sensory nerve pathways and remains in a latent stage on the ganglion. (Objective 9)

● CHAPTER 38
BEHAVIORAL AND PSYCHIATRIC DISORDERS

1. b
2. g
3. h
4. a
5. c
6. f
(Questions 1-6, Objective 5)

7. Chlorpropamide (Diabinese) indicates that he is diabetic; assess for hypoglycemia or hyperglycemia. Thyroxin is prescribed for thyroid disorders, which can cause behavioral alterations. Treatment with hydralazine suggests he has a history of hypertension or heart disease, so he may have had a transient ischemic attack, stroke, or cardiac dysrhythmia. The ecchymotic area on his head could indicate cerebral injury from trauma, causing his behavior. His warm, moist skin could indicate many problems. If he has a fever, an infectious process will have to be ruled out as a cause for his mental status change. (Objective 2)

8. a. Childhood trauma, parental deprivation, or a dysfunctional family structure; b. war, riots, rape, assault, death of a loved one, economic and employment problems, or prejudice and discrimination. (Objective 2)

9. a. Ensure scene safety; b. contain the crisis; c. render appropriate emergency care; d. transport to the appropriate medical facility. (Objective 3)

10. Look for evidence of violence, substance abuse, a suicide attempt, and any weapons that may be accessible to the patient. (Objective 4)

11. The patient's mental status, name, age, significant medical history, medications, allergies, and the precipitating event for this crisis should be ascertained from the patient, family, or other bystanders. (Objective 4)

12. The need to perform a physical assessment should be guided by your initial patient interview. If no possibility to exacerbate a violent situation arises and no life threat exists, the survey can be deferred until you arrive at the hospital. Bulky clothing and bags should be examined for the presence of weapons by law enforcement before transport. (Objective 4)

13.

Illness	Classification	Clinical Presentation	Treatment (Medical or EMS)
Dementia	Cognitive disorder	General decline in mental funcintioning; ability to provide self-care	Medical interventions
Schizo-phrenia	Schizophrenia	Recurrent psychotic behavior; abnormal thought process, delusions, hallucinations, judgment	Drug therapy; EMS should be friendly but neutral; do not respond to anger or speak to family in hushed tones; be firm, maintain personal safety
Posttraumatic syndrome	Anxiety disorder	Reaction to severe psychosocial event producing depression, sleep disturbances, nightmares, survivor guilt	Psychotherapy; medication
Bipolar disorder	Mood disorder	Alternating depressive and manic behaviors	Medications; EMS should be calm and provide firm emotional support; minimize stimulation (no lights or sirens)
Somatization disorder	Somatoform disorder	Chronic physical complaints without any physical problems identified; associated with anxiety, depression	Psychotherapy
Bulimia nervosa	Eating disorder	Binge-eating followed by purging (vomiting or laxatives), depression, self-deprivation	Medication, psychotherapy, hospitalization

(Objective 5)

14. Talk through the steps (rehearse) of the rescue slowly and calmly with the patient. (Objective 5)

15. Provide calm, firm, emotional support and minimize sensory stimuli. (Objective 6)

16. a. Schizophrenia or paranoia is suggested by this presentation; b. be friendly but neutral; modulate your voice so that it does not get louder if the patient does. Do not talk to the family in whispers.

Use firmness and tact to guide the patient to the ambulance. Consider asking for police assistance if the risk of violence is suspected. (Objective 5)

17. a. Ask, "Why did you do that? Were you trying to kill yourself?" Determine whether she had a plan (did she leave a note or call significant others to say good-bye?); b. ensure safety (protect the patient from escape or injury), listen in a nonjudgmental way, observe the dressing to ensure bleeding is controlled. (Objectives 7, 8, and 9)

18. a. Does the patient have a history of violent, aggressive, or hostile behavior? b. What is the patient's posture? Is he sitting or standing? Does he appear tense or rigid? c. What does his voice sound like? Is his speech loud, obscene, or erratic? d. Is he pacing or agitated or displaying aggressive behaviors?

19. Ask for police assistance. (Objective 14)

20. Look for any objects that the patient could use as a weapon. (Objective 14)

21. A minimum of two rescuers should move swiftly toward the patient and position themselves close to and slightly behind the patient. Each rescuer should then position an inside leg in front of the patient's leg to force the patient into a prone position if needed. The least restrictive restraints needed for a given situation should be used. (Objective 13)

22. Monitor the patient's level of consciousness, airway, breathing, circulation, vital signs, oxygen saturation (if available), and peripheral pulses while the patient remains in restraints. (Objective 13)

23. a. Delusional behavior, neurosis, or psychosis may be present during a behavioral emergency. (Objective 1)

24. c. Many people break laws without demonstrating abnormal behavior. One person (the paramedic) does not establish norms for society. A person may deviate from usual, normal behavior and not meet the standard for abnormal behavior. (Objective 1)

25. c. All of the other questions elicit a yes or no answer and yield limited information. (Objective 5)

26. d. You may acknowledge and label a patient's feelings but do not patronize or give false reassurances. Correct cognitive misconceptions or distortions in a nonconfrontational manner. (Objective 4)

27. a. Common signs and symptoms include inattention, memory impairment, disorientation, clouding of consciousness, and vivid visual hallucinations. (Objective 5)

28. a. In conversion hysteria, painful emotions are unconsciously converted into physical symptoms. (Objective 5)

29. a. The depressed patient has low self-worth, a loss of appetite, and decreased libido and is tense and irritable. (Objective 5)

30. a. Neurosis is a faulty or inefficient way of coping. Paranoia is an abnormal way of thinking, characterized by delusions of persecution or grandeur usually centered on a theme. A phobia occurs when a person transfers feelings of anxiety onto a situation or object in the form of an irrational, intense fear. (Objective 5)

31. c. (Objective 5)

32. a. A small percentage of suicidal patients will also be homicidal. All of the other options are important, but crew safety is your primary responsibility. (Objective 9)

33. b. Women attempt suicide more often but men succeed at a higher rate. All talk or threats of suicide should be taken seriously. When depression lifts, the person may finally have the energy to follow through on a suicide plan. (Objective 7)

34. d. Releasing a patient from restraints en route can place the crew in great danger. (Objective 13)

35. b. Diphenhydramine is an antihistamine and would not be effective in this situation. (Objective 13)

36. d. Be sure you can exit quickly if the situation deteriorates. Do not threaten the patient. Do not allow the patient to be alone or to be alone with an EMS crew member on the scene. Remain a safe distance from the patient until your assessment reveals no danger. (Objective 14)

37. c. Usually the parents can be helpful in the interview and help to relieve anxiety in children (if the situation worsens when they are present immediately remove them). Children can become violent and injure themselves or others. Do not lie to children. (Objective 15)

● CHAPTER 39
GYNECOLOGY

1. e
2. d
3. b
4. f
5. a
6. g
   (Questions 1-6, Objective 2)
7. a. 28; b. 25, 60; c. 4, 6; d. secondary follicles; e. vesicular, graafian follicles; f. ovulation; g. corpus luteum; h. progesterone; i. estrogen; j. zygote; k. chorionic gonadotropin. (Objective 1)

8. Headache, faintness, dizziness, nausea, diarrhea, backache, leg pain, chills, nausea, and vomiting. (Objective 2)

9. a. Have you ever been pregnant? If yes, how many pregnancies and how many have you carried to term? b. Have you ever had a cesarean delivery? c. When was your last menstrual period? How long did it last? Was it normal? Do you have a regular menstrual cycle? Have you had any bleeding between your periods? d. Could you be pregnant now? Is your period late or did you miss one? Do you have any breast tenderness, increased need to urinate, or morning sickness? Have you had any unprotected sexual activity? e. Do you have a history of any gynecologic (female) problems such as bleeding, infections, pain during intercourse, miscarriage, abortion, or ectopic pregnancy? f. Are you having any bleeding now? If you are, what color is it, how many pads have you soaked, and how long have you been bleeding? g. Do you have any vaginal discharge? What color and how much is there? Does it smell bad? h. What kind of birth control do you use? Have you ever forgotten to use it? i. Have you had any injury to your genital area? j. How are you feeling now? (Objective 4)

10. Evaluate vital signs and check for signs of blood loss (skin signs, orthostatic vital signs). Palpate the abdomen to assess for masses, tenderness, guarding, distention, and rebound tenderness. (Objective 4)

11. Pelvic inflammatory disease, ruptured ovarian cyst, dysmenorrhea, endometritis, endometriosis, or appendicitis are all potential causes. Ectopic pregnancy and miscarriage should not be completely discounted because sometimes patients do not give a completely accurate sexual history. (Objective 4)

12. Consider oxygen administration; however, because no signs of shock exist, this may not be necessary. Consider initiating IV therapy. Transport in a position of comfort. (Objective 4)

13. Move to a private, safe location; allow paramedic who is the same sex as the patient to provide care if possible; minimize questions and physical examination as appropriate; and listen and provide comfort. (Objective 5)

14. Handle clothes as little as possible, do not clean wounds, use paper bags for clothing and bag each item separately, ask the victim not to change clothing, and try not to disturb the crime scene. (Objective 6)

15. c. Menstrual flow varies according to each individual. (Objective 1)

16. c. Follicle-stimulating hormone stimulates development of the follicle. Estrogen causes a surge in the production of LH, which initiates the ovarian cycle.
(Objective 1)

17. a. *Chlamydia* organisms and *Chlamydia trachomatis* are also often associated with PID.
(Objective 2)

18. d. All of the other factors often decrease the severity of this condition.
(Objective 2)

19. b. The pain of cholecystitis is usually in the right upper quadrant of the abdomen. All other conditions cause lower abdominal pain.
(Objective 2)

20. a. Urination is usually painful and frequent in cystitis. Flank pain may indicate that the infection has moved to the kidneys.
(Objective 2)

21. d. Endometriosis is an ectopic placement of uterine lining and causes inflammation of the endometrium. It is common in women in their late 30s and is associated with infertility.
(Objective 2)

22. d.
(Objective 2)

23. a. All other answers are nontraumatic causes of vaginal bleeding.
(Objective 3)

24. b. Having a paramedic of the same sex as the patient perform care is desirable but may not always be possible. You should attempt to preserve evidence, but this is not always possible if a life-threatening condition exists that requires rapid intervention. Perform only the necessary history and physical examination.
(Objective 5)

25. c. Bag items separately if possible. The patient should not shower, wash, or have wounds cleansed until evidence can be gathered.
(Objective 6)

● **CHAPTER 40**
OBSTETRICS

1. e
(Objective 9)

2. f
(Objective 9)

3. a
(Objective 9)

4. g
(Objective 9)

5. d
(Objective 9)

6. c
(Objective 9)

7. e
(Objective 9)

8. f
(Objective 8)

9. g
(Objective 9)

10. b
(Objective 9)

11. c
(Objective 8)

12. d
(Objective 9)

13. a. Fifth
b. Fourth
c. Third
d. Sixth
e. Eighth
(Objective 2)

14. The rapid increase in systemic vascular resistance, aortic pressure, and left ventricular and left atrial pressures after placental flow stops, as well as the decrease in pulmonary vascular resistance resulting from expansion of the lungs cause atrioventricular shunts to close within a few hours after birth.
(Objective 2)

15. a. She has had six pregnancies and delivered five children.
b. She has had two or more deliveries.
c. The patient had bleeding after delivery of her baby.
d. You are called to care for a woman who has never delivered and whose pregnancy has reached 40 weeks of gestation.
(Objective 4)

16. a. Decreased tone and motility of the gastrointestinal tract, which leads to slow gastric emptying and relaxation of the pyloric sphincter
b. Decreased P_{CO_2} caused by increased respiratory rate and tidal volume late in pregnancy
c. Pressure that the gravid uterus places directly on the bladder when the fetal head moves down in the pelvis near term
d. Blood pressure decreases 10 to 15 mm Hg during the second semester and gradually increases to prepregnant levels near term (The patient should be questioned about her normal blood pressure.)
e. Impaired venous return resulting from the pressure the uterus exerts
(Objective 3)

17. a. Problems such as maternal nutrition, growth of fetus, maternal diabetes, and preeclampsia would not have been managed; an increased risk of fetal and maternal problems at birth exists.
b. Increased birth weight of the baby may make field

delivery difficult or impossible if cephalopelvic disproportion is present.

c. Vaginal bleeding may indicate abruptio placentae, placenta previa, or uterine rupture. All of these conditions cause an increase in fetal mortality rate and pose a risk of maternal shock and death.

d. Recent maternal narcotic intoxication causes neonatal respiratory depression and increases the risk of complications in the field.
(Objective 4)

18. When did she last feel fetal movement? What other medical problems does she have? What other medications does she take? Is she having any contractions?
(Objective 7)

19. Assess fetal heart tones. (A persistent fetal heart rate of greater than 160 or less than 120 is an early sign of fetal distress and fetal or maternal hypoxia.) Ask the mother to report fetal movement to you.
(Objective 7)

20. Administer 100% oxygen by nonrebreather mask (monitoring oxygen saturation with pulse oximeter, if available). Immobilize the patient on a backboard and roll it to the left side. Consider applying pneumatic antishock garments in case the patient's condition deteriorates (controversial). Initiate intravenous lactated Ringer's solution or normal saline (two large-bore lines) en route to the nearest appropriate trauma center and frequently reassess vital signs, fetal heart tones, and the amount of vaginal bleeding en route.
(Objective 7)

21. Spontaneous abortion
(Objective 9)

22. Retrieve the tissue from the toilet and give it to the emergency department staff so that a pathologist can examine it for completeness.
(Objective 9)

23. 6 sanitary napkins × 20 to 30 ml/pad = 120 to 180 ml of blood lost.
(Objective 9)

24. Pregnant women are often very attached to the fetus and grieve when they know that their baby has died. This fact is especially true if a similar event has happened to the patient in the past.
(Objective 9)

25. a. Vaginal bleeding, shoulder pain, nausea, vomiting, and syncope

b. Administer 100% oxygen by nonrebreather mask. Consider use of pneumatic antishock garments (controversial). While en route, initiate two large-bore intravenous lines and infuse boluses of normal saline or lactated Ringer's solution. Place the patient in modified Trendelenburg position if signs and symptoms of shock do not improve and report her

condition and diagnosis to the receiving hospital so that operative preparations can be made.
(Objective 9)

26. Administer 100% oxygen by a nonrebreather mask. Place the patient in left lateral recumbent position. Initiate precautionary intravenous lactated Ringer's solution or normal saline en route to the hospital. Rapidly transport the patient to the closest appropriate medical center and monitor maternal vital signs and fetal heart tones.
(Objective 6)

27. Preeclampsia
(Objective 8)

28. Left lateral recumbent
(Objective 8)

29. Magnesium sulfate 10% (1 to 4 g slow intravenous infusion) and diazepam (5 mg slow intravenous) over 2 minutes
(Objective 8)

30. Minimized stimulation and gentle patient handling
(Objective 8)

31. Abruptio placentae is a complication, and maternal apnea during a seizure may cause fetal hypoxia.
(Objective 8)

32. How many previous deliveries has she had, and how quickly did they progress? How long has she been in labor, and how close are the contractions?
(Objective 11)

33. Contractions lasting 45 to 60 seconds at 1- to 2-minute intervals; measurement from beginning of one contraction to the beginning of the next; patient who wants to bear down or have a bowel movement; large amount of bloody show; crowning; and mother's feeling that delivery is imminent
(Objective 11)

34. Examine for the presence of a nuchal cord. If this cord is present, gently slip it over the infant's head or, if this is not possible, clamp it in two places and cut between the clamps to release the cord. If the cord is cut, ensure that the rest of the delivery proceeds rapidly because the baby has no source of oxygen. Suction the baby's mouth and nose with a bulb syringe. Deliver the shoulders.
(Objective 11)

35. Clamp 6 to 9 inches from infant in two places. Cut between the clamps with sterile scissors or a scalpel. Examine the cord to ensure that no bleeding exists.
(Objective 11)

36. At 1 minute and 5 minutes of age
(Objective 12)

37. After delivery of the baby, 10 units in 1000 ml of lactated Ringer's solution infused at 20 to 30 gtts/minute on microdrip tubing
(Objectives 11 and 13)

38. If the head does not deliver immediately, place a gloved hand in the vagina with the palm toward the baby's face. Form a V, with the index and middle fingers on either side of the baby's nose, and push the vaginal wall from the face until delivery. If the head does not deliver within 3 minutes, maintain the airway as described and transport the patient to the receiving hospital.
(Objective 14)

39. Position mother on her left side in the knee-chest position. Guide the baby's head downward to allow the anterior shoulder to slip under the symphysis pubis; avoid excess force. Rotate the fetal shoulder girdle into the wider oblique pelvic diameter and deliver the posterior and then the anterior shoulders.
(Objective 14)

40. a. Elevate the mother's hips, administer oxygen, and ask the mother to pant with contractions to avoid bearing down. With gloved hand, gently push the baby's presenting part back into the vagina and elevate it to relieve pressure on the cord. Maintain this position while rapidly transporting the patient to the receiving hospital.
b. No, this baby will have to be delivered by cesarean section. (Objective 14)

41. c.
(Objective 1)

42. d. Although amniotic fluid originates from fetal urine and secretions from the respiratory tract, skin, and amniotic membranes, its primary function is protection.
(Objective 1)

43. b. The ductus arteriosus connects the aorta and pulmonary artery, and the foramen ovale provides a passageway for blood directly from the right to the left atrium. The umbilical cord connects the placenta to the embryo and is its lifeline.
(Objective 2)

44. b.
(Objective 1)

45. a. At week 12, it is just above the symphysis pubis; at week 16, between the symphysis pubis and the umbilicus; and, at week 28, halfway between the umbilicus and the xiphoid. (Objective 5)

46. b. A persistent rate greater than 160 or below 120 is a sign of fetal distress and fetal or maternal hypoxia.
(Objective 5)

47. b. This position prevents pressure from being exerted on the inferior vena cava. (Objective 6)

48. b. Maternal mortality from pregnancy-related causes is very rare. If the patient had abruptio placentae, a healthy delivery would be unlikely. Aortic dissection and congestive cardiomyopathy may cause maternal death, but amniotic fluid embolism is more likely at the time of delivery.
(Objective 6)

49. d. Drug doses and ventilations do not need to be modified. Chest compressions should be performed higher on the sternum.
(Objective 6)

50. d. Edema and hypertension are found in both.
(Objective 8)

51. c. Magnesium can also cause clinically significant hypotension. (Objective 8)

52. c. Uterine inversion also may happen, although less frequently, after a contraction, cough, or sneeze.
(Objective 14)

53. b. During the prodromal period the fetus descends into the birth canal. In the first stage the cervix dilates completely, and in the third stage the placenta is delivered.
(Objective 10)

54. c. Usually the cord can be freed in this manner. If this action fails and the decision is made to cut the cord after your medical direction protocols, delivery must be expedited or the baby will suffer severe hypoxia and risk of death.
(Objectives 11 and 14)

55. c. Weak cry (1); 1 pink body and blue extremities (1); 1 pulse at 128 (2), 1 active movement (2); 1 sneeze (2) = 8
(Objective 12)

56. a. Having the baby suckle stimulates the production of oxytocin.
(Objective 13)

57. b. The premature infant has a large surface-mass ratio and is susceptible to hypothermia. In addition, a potential for cardiorespiratory dysfunction exists because of immaturity.
(Objective 14)

58. c. Other complications include abruptio placentae, postpartum hemorrhage, and abnormal presentation. (Objective 14)

59. b. In this condition the pelvic ring is too small to allow passage of the baby's head.
(Objective 14)

60. d. Pulmonary embolism or, more rarely, amniotic fluid embolism can cause these signs and symptoms. (Objective 14)

61. b. Tearing of the umbilical cord is also a risk.
(Objective 14)

62. c. This condition often occurs after prolonged premature rupture of the membranes.
(Objective 14)

● CHAPTER 41
NEONATOLOGY

1. b
(Objective 1)

2. e
(Objective 1)

3. a
(Objective 1)

4. c

(Objective 1)

5. a. Multiple gestation, inadequate prenatal care, mother's age, history of perinatal morbidity or mortality, post-term gestation, drugs/medication, toxemia, hypertension and diabetes.

b. Premature labor, meconium-stained amniotic fluid, rupture of membranes more than 24 hours before delivery, use of narcotics within 4 hours of delivery, abnormal presentation, prolonged labor or precipitous delivery, prolapsed cord, bleeding

(Objective 1)

6. a. Emptying fluid from the lungs and beginning ventilation

b. Changing the circulatory pattern

c. Maintaining body temperature

(Objective 2)

7. a. Dry the infant's head and body thoroughly; remove any wet coverings; cover the head and body of the baby with warm blankets; turn the heat up high in the ambulance; use chemical warm packs (with blankets between the pack and the infant).

(Objective 3)

8.

Incorrect order	Correct order
Administer epinephrine	Warm, dry, suction, stimulate
Obtain vascular access	Oxygen at 5 L/min
Oxygen at 5 L/min	Ventilate with bag-mask device
Ventilate with bag-mask device	Perform chest compressions
Perform chest compressions	Obtain vascular access
Warm, dry, suction, stimulate	Administer epinephrine

(Objective 4)

9. Initiate positive-pressure breathing with 100% oxygen by bag-mask at 40/min to 60/min

(Objectives 3 and 4)

10. At the brachial artery, at the umbilical cord, or by auscultation

(Objective 3)

11. Continue positive-pressure ventilations for 30 sec; if heart rate does not begin to improve, start chest compressions ½ to ¾ inch at 120/min.

(Objective 4)

12. 2.5 or 3.0

(Objective 4)

13. Initiate a peripheral IV line, an intraosseous line, or an umbilical vein cannulation.

(Objective 4)

14. Epinephrine 0.01 mg/kg (1:10,000)

(Objective 4)

15. a. If breath sounds are audible only on the right, pull back slightly and reevaluate; if tube is in cor-

rect location, secure. If breath sounds are absent, remove the tube and reintubate.

(Objective 5)

b. Suction the tube with a suction catheter and reevaluate.

(Objective 5)

c. Assess for presence of tension pneumothorax, and treat if present. If at hospital, prepare to assist with chest tube placement.

(Objective 5)

16. d. A premature infant refers to a baby born before 37 weeks gestation (weight usually 0.6 to 2.2 kg [1.5 to 5 lb]). The incidence of complications increases as gestational age (and weight) decreases. 7.5 lb is a normal birth weight; 6 hours is not a lengthy labor. Rupture of membranes for more than 24 hours would be a concern.

(Objective 1)

17. a. As the chest recoils during delivery, chemical and temperature changes initiate the first breath. Cutting the umbilical cord initiates changes in fetal circulation.

(Objective 2)

18. c. The torso should be elevated ¾ to 1 inch so the neck is slighted extended.

(Objective 3)

19. b. The mouth should be suctioned before the nose, and then the cord can be cut.

(Objective 3)

20. c. Intravenous fluids are rarely necessary in the normal infant if appropriate resuscitation is done. (Objective 3)

21. a.

(Objective 3)

22. a. Continue the oxygen administration until the color improves (keep the baby warm).

(Objective 3)

23. c. The goal is to stimulate the neonate, without risk of injury.

(Objective 3)

24. b. Often the infant will initiate adequate spontaneous respirations after a brief period of bagging and will not require intubation. Increasing heart rate is a positive indicator.

(Objective 4)

25. c. A heart rate greater than 100/minute is desirable. Chest compressions should be initiated for a persistent heart rate < 80 that does not respond to ventilation.

(Objective 3)

26. b. Decreased chest wall movement, return of bradycardia, unilateral decrease in chest expansion, altered intensity to pitch or breath sounds, and increased resistance to hand ventilation are all signs that may point to tube migration, occlusion, or pneumothorax.

(Objective 5)

27. a. Other causes include narcotic/CNS depressant use, airway or respiratory muscle weakness, oxyhemoglobin dissociation curve shift, septicemia, and metabolic disorders.
(Objective 6)

28. b. Infants are obligate nose breathers; suctioning of mucus from the nasal passages will correct this problem.

29. d. Inadequate ventilations and oxygenation are the most common causes of bradycardia and should be continually reassessed.
(Objective 6)

30. c. Other causes are drugs taken by the mother, congenital diseases or malformations, and intrapartum hypoxemia.
(Objective 6)

31. d. Some vomiting is normal; however, if it is persistent or bile-stained or contains dark blood, a serious underlying illness may exist. Vascular access would not be indicated unless needed to treat dehydration or bradycardia secondary to the vagal stimulation this can produce.
(Objective 6)

32. b. Other causes of diarrhea in the neonate are gastroenteritis, lactose intolerance, neonatal abstinence syndrome, thyrotoxicosis, cystic fibrosis.
(Objective 6)

33. a. The baby should be assessed for clinical signs of dehydration or other signs of illness (fever, lethargy, feeding habits, etc.), but typically this stool pattern is normal in this situation.
(Objective 5)

34. c. All types of seizures in this age group are considered pathologic.

35. a. Hypoglycemia may produce seizure activity. Determining the presence of this condition and correcting it are urgent matters.
(Objective 6)

36. b. Even small temperature elevations in this age group can signal impending sepsis. Febrile seizures are unusual in this age group and would not be expected (especially at this temperature). Ice packs should never be applied to a neonate.
(Objective 6)

37. a.
(Objective 6)

38. d. Brain and hypoxic injuries may occur as well.
(Objective 7)

39. b. Honest, frequent updates about the baby's condition should be given during the resuscitation so that family members can prepare themselves for the outcome.
(Objective 7)

● CHAPTER 42
PEDIATRICS

1. f.
(Objective 7)

2. e.
(Objective 7)

3. h.
(Objective 7)

4. a.
(Objective 7)

5. g.
(Objective 7)

6. c.
(Objective 7)

7. b.
(Objective 7)

8. a. Neonate
   b. Infant, toddler, and preschooler
   c. Neonate
   d. Infant and toddler
   e. Infant, toddler, and school-age child
   f. Young infant, infant, toddler, school-age child, and adolescent (sexual abuse)
   g. Preschooler and school-age child
   h. Adolescent
   (Objective 3)

9. Humidified oxygen by nonrebreather mask, position of comfort (to maximize respiratory efficiency), albuterol 0.01 to 0.03 ml (0.05 to 0.15 mg)/kg/dose to maximum of 0.5 ml/dose diluted in 2 ml of 0.9% NS, or epinephrine 0.01 ml/kg subcutaneous (1:1000), maximum 0.3 ml
(Objective 5)

10. Tachycardia and anxiousness
(Objective 5)

11. Repeat drugs, initiate IV, and continue to reassess.
(Objective 5)

12. Patient will state improvement, respiratory rate will decrease, oxygen saturation will improve, use of accessory muscles will decrease, wheezing will diminish (inspiratory wheeze and then expiratory wheeze should dissipate), and heart rate may decrease (although possibly not because of the effects of beta agonists).
(Objective 5)

13. Drooling, stridor, sudden onset of high fever, and dysphagia
(Objective 5)

14. a. Take the patient into the cool night air or a steam-filled bathroom. b. Allow child to assume position of comfort and administer high-flow oxygen (humidified) by whatever means is least threatening to the child.
(Objective 5)

15. Moderate-to-severe dehydration
(Objective 6)

16. Sinus tachycardia
(Objective 6)

17. Open airway, ventilate with 100% oxygen; initiate lactated Ringer's solution or normal saline intravenously (intraosseously if intravenous line cannot be established), and infuse initial fluid bolus of 20 ml/kg; reassess and repeat until perfusion improves.
(Objective 6)

18. Pulse, 80 to 140; respirations, 30 to 40; and blood pressure, 82/44 mm Hg
(Objective 4)

19. Improved level of consciousness, skin color, and temperature
(Objective 6)

20. Sinus bradycardia, rate 30/min
(Objective 7)

21. Assess ABCs, secure airway, administer 100% oxygen using bag-mask device, perform chest compressions, start an intravenous or intraosseous line, assess vital signs, and if bradycardia continues, administer epinephrine 0.1 ml/kg (1:10,000) intravenously or intraosseously.
(Objective 7)

22. Infuse the medication intraosseously or administer epinephrine 0.1 ml/kg (1:1000) endotracheally diluted to 3 to 5 ml. NOTE: Endotracheal dose is 10 times greater than the intravenous dose.
(Objective 7)

23. Atropine 0.02 mg/kg intravenously to a maximum single dose of 0.5 mg (child) and 1.0 mg (adolescent); minimum dose: 0.1 mg (Objective 7)

24. a. Defibrillate at 2 joules/kg and then at 2 to 4 joules/kg and 4 joules/kg, continue cardiopulmonary resuscitation, administer epinephrine 0.1 ml/kg (1:10,000), defibrillate at 4 joules/kg, and administer amiodarone 5 mg/kg intravenously or intraosseously or lidocaine 1 mg/kg intravenously or intraosseously or magnesium 25 to 50 mg/kg intravenously or intraosseously for torsades de pointes or hypomagnesemia (maximum: 2 g)
b. Epinephrine 0.1 ml/kg (1:1000) intravenously or intraosseously, repeated every 3 to 5 min
(Objective 7)

25. Description of seizure activity, vomiting during seizure, history of epilepsy or another major medical illness, other current medicines, potential for toxic ingestion, recent head injury, and complaints of headache or stiff neck
(Objective 8)

26. Maintain airway and breathing; monitor vital signs, cool child with tepid water and fanning, monitor electrocardiogram and oxygen saturation (if available); depending on patient's vital signs and level of consciousness, initiate lactated Ringer's solution intravenously to keep the vein

open and obtain blood sample; assess blood sugar and treat if it is less than 60 mg/dl
(Objective 8)

27. a. Diazepam 1 mg every 2 to 5 min slow IV; if intravenous or intraosseous infusion is not possible, administer medication rectally at higher dose (0.5 mg/kg).
b. Lorazepam 0.05 to 0.15 mg/kg/dose intramuscularly, intravenously, or intraosseously to maximum dose 4 mg (rectal dose 0.1 to 0.2 mg/kg)
(Objective 8)

28. a. 50% dextrose, 1 to 2 ml/kg/dose or 25% dextrose 2 to 4 ml/kg/dose intravenously (Objective 9)
b. Presenting symptoms of mild hypoglycemia may be hunger, weakness, tachypnea, and tachycardia. Presenting symptoms of moderate hypoglycemia may be sweating, tremors, irritability, vomiting, mood swings, blurred vision, stomachache, headache, and dizziness.
(Objective 9)

29. a. Because a relatively small loss of blood can be devastating, fluid resuscitation should be anticipated for blood volume losses that would seem small in an adult.
b. This makes children susceptible to hypothermia. Measures should be used on the scene to maintain body warmth.
c. This leaves them little reserve for a stressed situation such as shock. Energy and oxygen requirements should be reduced to a minimum by assisting ventilations and using measures to decrease anxiety and promote body warmth.
d. Volume replacement with lactated Ringer's solution or normal saline should be initiated at 20 ml/kg given rapidly and repeated if there is no response. If good response is obtained, the fluids should be continued at a weight-related maintenance rate obtained from medical direction.
e. Intravenous access should first be attempted in a peripheral vein in the arms, hands, or feet. If access cannot be easily established and the patient's condition deteriorates, intraosseous infusion should be used.
(Objectives 6 and 12)

30. Aspiration of marrow may rarely be obtained. The intravenous fluid will run freely with no evidence of infiltration. (Objectives 4 and 6)

31. Occurrence between midnight and 6 AM, male child under 6 months, occurrence between October and March, frothy sputum, wet diaper with stool, second child, and recent mild viral illness.
(Objective 13)

32. Document death as required by protocol, and observe carefully for any obvious external signs of trauma. (Objective 13)

33. Encourage your partner to verbalize, perhaps stating, "It's frightening to go on a call like this when

you have a baby at home." Listen if he wants to talk; if he does not, check on him again in the morning. Initiate the CISD team, following local protocol (if available).
(Objective 13)

34. Protect cervical spine while opening the airway, hyperventilate and consider intubation and hyperventilate with 100% oxygen, verify perfusion with slow pulse; if it is inadequate, initiate cardiopulmonary resuscitation; en route to the hospital, initiate an intravenous or intraosseous lifeline, and administer medicines if indicated.
(Objective 12)

35. The story does not match the physical findings or the child's developmental stage. An 8-month-old child is too young to ride a tricycle. A fall from a tricycle is unlikely to produce an intracerebral bleed. The child had no external signs of head trauma but had bruises at the shoulders that may suggest shaking. The child was dirty (this could be normal).
(Objective 14)

36. Report the suspected abuse to the receiving facility and to other authorities as indicated by local protocol. Carefully document all physical findings and statements made by the mother, using exact quotes if possible. This document is likely to be questioned in court if abuse is suspected.
(Objective 14)

37. Only enough data to address the immediate threats to the health of the sexually abused child should be elicited. The child should be made to feel safe and secure, and the detailed history and physical examination should be performed by child sexual abuse specialists if they are available in your area.
(Objective 14)

38. a. The other 11 components are system approach, education, data collection, quality improvement, injury prevention, prehospital care, emergency care, definitive care, rehabilitation, finance, and ongoing health care from birth to young adulthood.
(Objective 1)

39. b. Have them repeat things back to you in their words to be sure they understand. Give them choices when possible. Anticipate questions about the long-term effect of care, injuries, etc.
(Objective 2)

40. b. Toddlers fear separation and loss of direction, and school-age children fear bodily injury and mutilation but are less likely to interpret words literally.
(Objective 2)

41. b. Asthma is usually not diagnosed until a child is 3 to 5 years of age. Epiglottitis is more common in 3 to 5–year–old children. Foreign body airway obstruction would be unlikely in this age group because children usually do not eat solid food at this age. (Objective 3)

42. c. Each component is important, but information about level of consciousness, color, respiratory effort, and muscle tone can often be assessed by observing children before touching them.
(Objective 4)

43. d. Other signs are use of accessory muscles, nasal flaring, tachypnea, bradypnea, irregular breathing pattern, grunting, and absent or abnormal breath sounds.
(Objective 4)

44. d. It may produce stridor and complete airway obstruction.
(Objective 5)

45. a. The correct dose of epinephrine is 0.01 ml/kg subcutaneously (1:1000), and the correct dose of terbutaline is 0.01 mg/kg of a 1 mg/ml solution subcutaneously.
(Objective 5)

46. d. The child should be permitted to assume a position of comfort, which is typically sitting up with the chin jutted forward to maximize air flow. Examination of the airway can produce obstruction and is contraindicated. Initiation of an intravenous infusion will not improve the child's condition but may cause the child to become agitated and cry, increasing the respiratory distress.
(Objective 5)

47. a. Albuterol can provide temporary symptomatic relief with limited side effects.
(Objective 5)

48. d. Fluid resuscitation should not be delayed until the blood pressure drops, or resuscitating the child may be difficult. The fontanelle would likely be flat, and the skin cool.
(Objective 6)

49. d. The recommended fluid bolus is 20 ml/kg. 20 ml/kg × 20 kg = 400 ml
(Objective 6)

50. c. Crackles and edema are characteristics of congestive heart failure associated with cardiomyopathy.
(Objective 6)

51. b. 44 lb = 20 kg; initial defibrillation is 2 joules/kg; 2 joules × 20 kg = 40 joules
(Objective 7)

52. d. Atropine 0.02 mg/kg to a maximum dose of 0.5 mg in a child
(Objective 7)

53. b. Epinephrine is the first drug of choice in patients with bradycardia with hemodynamic compromise, followed by atropine if no improvement results.
(Objective 7)

54. a. If his condition deteriorates, synchronized cardioversion may be considered.
(Objective 7)

55. c. Unless the dehydration produces severe electrolyte imbalance, it is much more likely to produce shock and death than seizures. (Objective 8)

56. c. Ventilatory equipment should be available, and careful observation of respiratory rate and depth should be performed. If pulse oximetry is available, it should be used. (Objective 8)

57. c. Undiagnosed type I diabetes can manifest in this manner with severe hyperglycemia and ketoacidosis. This child is critical and will need urgent transport with airway management, oxygenation, and fluid resuscitation. (Objective 9)

58. a. Hypoglycemia can lead to death if uncorrected. (Objective 11)

59. d. Tachypnea, GI irritation, hypoglycemia, cardiac dysrhythmias (ventricular), seizure, coma, coagulation defects, and death can occur from salicylate poisoning. (Objective 11)

60. d. Changes in color perception, hallucinations, and blindness can occur, as well as other CNS and GI effects. (Objective 11)

61. b. Epinephrine would only be indicated if cardiac arrest ensues. Aspirin may be given to counteract the platelet aggregation property of cocaine; lorazepam is administered to treat anxiety and/or seizures; and nitroglycerin is used as a vasodilator to treat his chest pain. (Objective 11)

62. d. Sodium bicarbonate may be given to improve myocardial contractility and cardiac output. Lidocaine would be given to treat ventricular dysrhythmias (if present). Normal saline 10 ml/kg bolus may be given to improve cardiac output. Oxygen should be given at high flow based on the patient's physical findings. (Objective 11)

63. a. Other prehospital interventions may include oxygen administration, ventilatory support (if indicated), ECG monitoring, treatment for shock, epinephrine infusion, sodium bicarbonate, and calcium chloride (controversial). (Objective 11)

64. d. Motor vehicle crashes are the leading cause of death and serious injury in children. (Objective 12)

65. a. Other findings include hypertension, bradycardia, and Cheyne-Stokes respirations. (Objective 12)

66. c. (Objective 12)

67. c. Low maternal/paternal age, low socioeconomic group, and rank of second or third in the birth order is associated with increased incidence. (Objective 13)

68. c. Fractures in a child less than 2 years of age should be cause for suspicion. (Objective 14)

69. d. Retinal hemorrhage is a sign of a shaken baby. (Objective 14)

70. d. If suctioning does not improve the situation, removing and replacing the tracheostomy may be necessary. If this is not possible or proves unsuccessful, oral intubation or intubation through the stoma may be necessary. (Objective 15)

71. a. Correcting the hypoxia is the priority. The machine can be checked and fixed after the hypoxia is corrected. (Objective 15)

72. a. If the child develops signs of air embolism, position him on the left side with his head lowered and administer high flow oxygen. (Objective 15)

73. b. If the tube becomes dislodged, the feeding could be delivered to the lung, causing aspiration. (Objective 15)

● CHAPTER 43
GERIATRICS

1. a. Because baseline PaO_2 is lower, there is less ability to compensate if chest trauma is sustained or if the patient is hypoxic because of trauma (for example, inhalation injury). The chest wall is less elastic and more susceptible to injury.

   b. Myocardial contusion can cause pump failure caused by poor cardiac reserve. Decreased ability to increase heart rate can cause decreased ability to compensate for shock, and dysrhythmias can cause syncope and precipitate a fall.

   c. Renal blood flow is decreased, so a sudden traumatic event that causes shock and hypoperfusion to the kidneys can precipitate the onset of renal failure; decreased renal function can make an older adult more susceptible to toxic drug effects, leading to central nervous system depression, disturbances in balance, hypotension, and dysrhythmias, all of which can increase the risk of falls.

   d. Kyphosis may alter balance and predispose a person to falls, and osteoporosis increases the incidence of fractures after falls.

   e. Advancing age can result in decreased peripheral vasoconstriction, lowered metabolic rate, and poor peripheral circulation and can impair the body's ability to regulate temperature effectively, especially during stressful events, such as traumatic injury. Hypothermia may occur rapidly. (Objective 1)

2. a. His multiple illnesses and drugs will make it difficult to assess for new onset of signs or symptoms. **Diabetes:** Impairs pain perception and retards healing. **Heart attack and heart failure:** Cardiac output may be impaired from chronic conditions, and dysrhythmias may be chronic. **Lung disease:** Patient's baseline must be determined. Cyanosis, increased respiratory rate, and abnormal lung sounds may be chronic. **Lanoxin:** Therapeutic effects slow heart rate; patient may

not become tachycardic in response to trauma, and toxic effects may cause dysrhythmias. **Insulin:** Excessive amounts may cause hypoglycemia and produce central nervous system impairment. **Dyazide:** Diuretics may cause an electrolyte imbalance that can affect muscle strength and may precipitate dysrhythmias that can cause syncope and falls. (Objective 2)

b. Dysrhythmias, visual impairment, neurologic disabilities, arthritis, changes in gait, postural hypotension, syncope, cerebrovascular accident or transient ischemic attack, medications, slippery surfaces, loose rugs, objects on floors, poor lighting, pets, low beds or toilet seats, defective walking equipment, and lack of handrails on stairs. (Objective 8)

3. In the older adult, dyspnea and weakness may be the only presenting history for myocardial infarction. Carefully obtain a patient history, perform a physical examination, including 12-lead ECG, and treat with a high index of suspicion for myocardial infarction (these signs and symptoms also accompany pulmonary embolus). (Objective 3)

4. Atrial fibrillation (Objective 3)

5. Cerebrovascular accident and pulmonary embolism (Objective 3)

6. Cholecystitis, colonic diverticular disease, appendicitis, aortic abdominal aneurysm, mesenteric artery occlusion, and mesenteric vein thrombosis (Objective 2)

7. a. Rapid
   b. Variable: It is usually self-limited and can be corrected quickly when the cause is identified.
   c. Electrolyte imbalance, hypoglycemia, hyperglycemia, acid-base imbalance, hypoxia, vital organ failure, and Wernicke's encephalopathy (Objective 3)

8. Hypothyroidism, Cushing's syndrome, vitamin deficiencies, and hydrocephalus (Objective 3)

9. Sinus bradycardia, rate 30/min (Objective 3)

10. a. Atropine 0.5 -1.0 mg intravenously (Objective 3)
    b. Transcutaneous pacing (Objective 3)

11. Acute myocardial infarction, drug toxicity, or vagal response (Objective 3)

12. Sinus tachycardia . (Objective 3)

13. Bacterial pneumonia or pulmonary embolus (Objective 3)

14. No to both: you must treat the patient and her underlying problem. (Objective 3)

15. Administer high-flow oxygen via nonrebreather mask, initiate intravenous therapy, and monitor patient response and vital signs closely en route. (Objective 3)

16. a. Normal sinus rhythm with a premature atrial contraction and a premature ventricular contraction
    b. Continue to monitor the patient and electrocardiogram rhythm.
    c. Assess for limited airflow, increased work of breathing, dyspnea, hypoxemia, or hemodynamic compromise. Measure $EtCO_2$ if available. (Objective 3)

17. a. Junctional rhythm
    b. Observe the patient for any signs of hemodynamic compromise related to the slow rhythm (monitor vital signs and electrocardiogram). Consider drug administration or pacing if unstable.
    c. Functional cells are lost in the SA and AV nodes during aging and contribute to dysrhythmias. (Objectives 2 and 3)

18. Delirium (sudden onset) (Objective 3)

19. Normal sinus rhythm with a premature atrial contraction (Objective 3)

20. There is no reason for this ECG to cause these symptoms. (Objective 3)

21. Intoxication or poisoning, withdrawal from drugs, metabolic disturbances, infectious process, central nervous system trauma, and stroke (Objective 3)

22. Second-degree heart block Mobitz type II (Objective 3)

23. a. Myocardial infarction is the most likely cause. (Objective 3)
    b. Administer high-concentration oxygen. Continue assessment to include breath sounds, and observe for signs of congestive heart failure and head-to-toe survey. Initiate IV therapy at a TKO rate. Prepare to apply transcutaneous pacing. Consult with medical direction regarding administration of sedation (with caution because of dyspnea and hypotension). Provide rapid transport for definitive cardiac care. Perform a 12-lead ECG if available. (Objective 3)

24. Decreased ability to sense changes in ambient temperature, less total body water to store heat, reduced likelihood to become tachycardic to compensate for cold stress, decreased ability to shiver, inability to pay utilities for heat, insufficient insulation, malnutrition, arthritis, drug overdose, hepatic failure, hypoglycemia, infection, Parkinson's disease, stroke, thyroid disease, and uremia. (Objective 6)

25. a. Bleeding problems, increased hemorrhage from trauma, multiple contusions, and allergic reactions
    b. Electrolyte abnormalities (sodium and potassium) and dehydration
    c. Influenza-like symptoms, multiple dysrhythmias, and bradycardia
    d. Dry mouth, tachycardia, ventricular dysrhythmias, seizures, and impaired level of consciousness

e. Impaired perception (increased risk of falls) and decreased level of consciousness with respiratory depression.

f. Decreased heart rate (excessive) and broncho-constriction, mood alteration

g. Tachycardia, dysrhythmias, and central nervous system stimulation

h. Dysrhythmias and clotting abnormalities
(Objective 5)

26. His heart rate is slow relative to the rest of his clinical picture (everything else indicates impending shock or hypoxia).
(Objective 8)

27. He may have a pacemaker or be on medications (for example, digitalis or beta blockers) that prevent his heart rate from becoming tachycardic in response to a decrease in cardiac output.
(Objective 8)

28. Yes, abdominal injuries are frequently lethal in older adults. His perception of pain may be impaired, and this situation could deteriorate quickly especially with signs of shock.
(Objective 8)

29. Ensure a patent airway; deliver high-flow oxygen by nonrebreather mask; apply pneumatic anti-shock garments (if indicated by local protocol); en route to a trauma center, initiate two large-bore intravenous lines, and administer small fluid challenges in consultation with medical direction; frequently monitor vital signs and lung sounds (for increased rales [crackles]) to ensure that the patient is not developing a volume overload.
(Objective 8)

30. a. Follow local protocols and report to appropriate authority (for example, local law enforcement, abuse hotline, medical direction) as indicated, report findings to receiving hospital, and document findings thoroughly on prehospital run report.
b. Yes, daughter lives with parent.
(Objective 9)

31. d. Total lung capacity remains unchanged because the loss of chest wall compliance balances the weakened respiratory muscles. The residual volume increases as a result of variable increases in alveolar diameter and the tendency for distal airways to collapse on expiration.
(Objective 1)

32. a. Lordosis is the normal S curve of the spine. Osteolysis is degeneration of bone. Scoliosis is lateral curvature of the spine usually found in childhood.
(Objective 3)

33. d. The patient has no history of COPD. His history and clinical presentation point to leftsided heart failure. Furosemide would be the drug of choice.
(Objective 3)

34. a. Risk of myocardial infarction increases in postmenopausal women. Myocardial infarction may manifest without pain in elderly patients. Pneumonia is a complication of patients who are immune compromised or who have other chronic illness, and it may have an atypical presentation in older adults. Pulmonary embolus is a higher risk in patients with cancer and bedridden patients.
(Objective 3)

35. a. The other conditions may cause delirium.
(Objective 3)

36. d. These signs can be decreased or eliminated with drug therapy.
(Objective 3)

37. c. This condition results from excessive blood glucose and causes serious dehydration. IV fluids are indicated in the prehospital setting to treat the severe dehydration that accompanies this condition. Sodium bicarbonate may be indicated after arterial blood gas analysis is done or if the patient experiences cardiac arrest.
(Objective 3)

38. a. Thyroid dysfunction may also cause tachydysrhythmias, constipation, weight loss, anemia, or musculoskeletal complaints.
(Objective 3)

39. d. Prostate enlargement is a cause of dysuria commonly found in this age group.
(Objective 3)

40. b. The ulcers often become infected because of the poor blood supply to the area.
(Objective 3)

41. d. Cataracts are a loss in transparency of the lens of the eye. Conjunctivitis is an inflammation of the conjunctiva of the eye. Corneal abrasion is a scraping-off of the outer layer of the cornea.
(Objective 4)

42. d. Some of the older drugs that are prescribed to patients with Parkinson's disease may produce this reaction.
(Objective 5)

43. a. Cyclic antidepressants, antidysrhythmics, and beta blockers may increase the risk of hyperthermia.
(Objective 6)

44. c. This may result from diuretic or other drug therapy and have a very slow onset.
(Objective 7)

45. b. It may be caused by physiological or psychological factors.
(Objective 7)

46. b. The venous blood of a subdural hematoma takes longer to fill the larger space between the skull and brain.
(Objective 8)

47. c.
(Objective 8)

48. a. Sedative hypnotics place the older patient at greater risk for falls.
(Objective 8)

● CHAPTER 44
ABUSE AND NEGLECT

1. Request and await police to help assess and maintain scene safety. Domestic violence calls are very dangerous.
(Objective 4)

2. Move the patient to the ambulance as soon as possible. Do not ask about the violence until you have the patient alone. Have police remain with the alleged abuser while you perform your examination.
(Objective 4)

3. The patient may fear for the safety of herself or her children if she leaves. Victims often believe that the offender's behavior will change. She may not have money or emotional support to help her leave. She may believe that she is the cause of the behavior or that abuse is a normal part of marriage.
(Objective 2)

4. Often the perpetrator is released from jail within several hours. A woman who leaves is 75% more likely to be killed by her partner. A woman who leaves should be directed to community support agencies that can maximize her safety. Sometimes it is more prudent for her to stay and carefully plan a safe departure than to leave suddenly.
(Objective 4)

5. Accept her decision, and support her by confirming she is not at fault and doesn't deserve to be abused. Give her written information (preferably on something small enough to hide) about community resource agencies that can provide financial, emotional, safety-related, and legal resources to assist her. Help her prepare a quick way out. Identify safety precautions for her.
(Objective 4)

6. The victim is a widow who is over 75 years of age. She has multiple chronic health problems and lives with a child.
(Objective 7)

7. The patient seems hesitant to confirm the source of the injury and has aging bruises.
(Objective 5)

8. If you suspect abuse, you should report your suspicions to medical direction and call the agency mandated by law to report suspected elder abuse.
(Objective 6)

9. This child is with a parent, and alcohol abuse is evident, which greatly increases the risk of physical abuse. You also have received many calls to this home.
(Objective 7)

10. The burns involve both extremities and the buttocks and are circumferential, indicating that the child was probably forcibly held in the hot water.
(Objective 8)

11. The child does not mind separation from the parents, appears fearful, and does not like to be touched.
(Objective 7)

12. This case should be reported to the appropriate state agency for child abuse on arrival to the hospital (refer to local reporting protocols).
(Objective 7)

13. a. Take steps to preserve evidence.
b. Do not allow the patient to urinate, defecate, douche, or bathe.
c. Do not remove evidence from areas of sexual contact.
d. Notify law enforcement immediately.
e. Maintain a chain of evidence with clothing and other items.
(Objective 10)

14. a. Abrasions or bruises on the upper limb, head, and neck
b. Forcible signs of restraint
c. Petechiae of the face and conjunctiva
d. Broken teeth, swollen jaw or cheekbone, or eye injuries
e. Muscle soreness or stiffness of the shoulder, neck, knee, hip, or back
(Objective 9)

15. b. Battering may include physical abuse (assault) or psychological abuse such as intimidation, isolation, or threats to control another person.
(Objective 1)

16. d. This is known as the *honeymoon phase.*
(Objective 2)

17. a. All these fears usually exist, but children are usually the most compelling reason for the victim to stay.
(Objective 2)

18. a. Abusers may feel that abuse is a form of discipline. Abusers or victims often have an intense need for love and affection and are unable to set personal boundaries.
(Objective 2)

19. a. Abusive injuries are more commonly found on the face, head, neck, breasts, and abdomen.
(Objective 3)

20. a. The partner may be reluctant to leave the victim alone and may need to be distracted for you to be able to conduct an effective history. If the victim does not volunteer information, you could say something nonthreatening, such as, "I'm concerned for you because I've seen these types of injuries in people who have been hit by others." Do not intimidate or accuse the victim. You cannot insist on transport if the adult patient is competent.
(Objective 4)

21. c. Sexual molestation is physical abuse, theft is financial or material abuse, and withholding food is neglect.
(Objective 5)

22. b. Report it to the authorities so that they will have complete information if a pattern of abuse exists.
(Objective 6)

23. a. Most perpetrators are a parent, female, and under 40.
(Objective 7)

24. c. If the child volunteers the same story as the parents without prompting, and the story is consistent with the injuries you are seeing, abuse is not likely. You will likely not have time in the field to assess the family or check police records.
(Objective 8)

25. d. About 49,000 men report sexual assault each year. Rape is a crime of violence, not a sexual act. Threats of harm or use of weapons for intimidation is common.
(Objective 9)

26. c. Abused children should understand that the assault was not their fault, and they won't be punished. False reassurances serve no purpose.
(Objective 10)

● CHAPTER 45
PATIENTS WITH SPECIAL CHALLENGES

1. b
2. e
3. h
4. f
5. a
6. c
7. d
(Objective 3)
8. a, b, c, d
(Objective 1)
9. c, e
(Objective 1)
10. b, c, d, e
(Objective 1)
11. c, d
(Objective 2)
12. b, c, d
(Objective 2)
13. b, d (Objective 2)
14. b, c, e
(possibly) (Objective 3)
15. c, d, e
(Objective 3)
16. c, d
(Objective 3)
17. c, d
(Objective 3)
18. c, d
(Objective 3)
19. c, d
(Objective 3)

20. c
(Objective 6)

21. d. Speak in low tones into the patient's ear if residual hearing exists. Otherwise, if the patient reads lips, speak at a regular speed in view of the patient.
(Objective 1)

22. b.
(Objective 1)

23. b. The safety of the patient, crew, and bystanders should always be prioritized.
(Objective 2)

24. a. Anxiety can produce a host of symptoms that mimic serious medical illness.
(Objective 2)

25. d. The arthritic pain and deformity can make spinal immobilization challenging.
(Objective 3)

26. b. Ataxia is a loss of coordination and balance. Diplegic cerebral palsy affects all four limbs, the legs more severely than the arms. Mucoviscidosis is cystic fibrosis.
(Objective 3)

27. d. These patients often have excessive secretions, and the paramedic should anticipate the need for suctioning.
(Objective 3)

28. b. Individual beliefs exist even within specific cultures. People may choose to have their own beliefs about the cause of their illness despite your explanations. You need not agree with all aspects of a patient's cultural beliefs, but do not let your opinion interfere with patient care or interaction.
(Objective 4)

29. c. Some families will not be fully prepared for the death regardless of the length of illness. The paramedic should support the patient and family with honest and empathetic care. Talking to the patient and family should be encouraged if the patient's condition permits.
(Objective 5)

30. c. There is no reason not to mention the disease to the patient, but the condition should remain confidential with regard to others. Use BSI as you would for any other patient care situation. The dignity of each patient is an important part of prehospital patient care delivery.
(Objective 6)

31. c. The patient may worry about receiving poor credit ratings, adding to a mounting debt, and being a deadbeat. Offer constructive suggestions related to their financial concerns rather than empty statements.
(Objective 7)

● CHAPTER 46
ACUTE INTERVENTIONS FOR THE HOME HEALTH CARE PATIENT

1. The hypoxic patient may be restless, confused, tachycardic, hypertensive, dyspneic, cyanotic or have a headache. When you monitor the patient, you may find a low SaO$_2$ or cardiac dysrhythmias. (Objective 3)

2. If he appears to be in distress, immediately begin ventilation with a bag-valve device and 100% O$_2$. Then you can evaluate the problem with the equipment. Determine the need for suctioning. (Objective 3)

3. Check the ventilator for disconnected tubing, power cords, and settings, and check to ensure that the tracheostomy tube is in the proper place and the balloon is adequately inflated. (Objective 3)

4. Reassure the patient that the problem is fixed, perhaps showing him how you fixed it. Tell him you will remain with him for several minutes after you place him back on the ventilator to ensure that everything continues to work properly. (Objective 3)

5. Assess the patient's level of consciousness and level of distress; respiratory rate and lung sounds; neck for signs of JVD; skin color, temperature, and moisture; and vital signs. (Objective 4)

6. Slow the infusion to a keep-open rate. Provide high-concentration oxygen. Elevate the patient's head. Maintain body warmth. Monitor vital signs. Reassess. If her condition does not improve, consider the need for a diuretic. (Objective 4)

7. The need to transport depends on the patient's response to your interventions, other anticipated complications based on the contents of the infusion, and the patient's wishes with regard to transport. The decision should be made in consultation with medical direction. (Objective 4)

8. The wound has many signs of infection and necrosis. (Objective 6)

9. A properly healing wound should have a pink or red wound bed, clear or serosanguinous drainage, and no odor. (Objective 6)

10. The surrounding skin should be assessed for color, warmth, and swelling. (Objective 6)

11. The red, warm surrounding skin suggests infection. (Objective 6)

12. A full assessment is necessary. Specifically, vital signs, including temperature and lung sounds, should be evaluated. (Objective 6)

13. His physical examination suggests systemic infection. You should administer high-concentration oxygen, initiate IV fluids, and transport. (Objective 6)

14. A full assessment is indicated, including initial assessment, vital signs, blood glucose, and ECG and oxygen saturation monitoring. (Objective 7)

15. Infantile apnea may be caused by hypoglycemia, hypocalcemia, hypothermia, sepsis, pneumonia, meningitis, CNS hemorrhage, hypoxic injury, seizures, respiratory distress, hyaline membrane disease, and obstruction. (Objective 7)

16. Keep the baby warm. Administer dextrose if the glucose level is low. Administer high-concentration oxygen by mask or blow-by. Initiate an intravenous line (in consultation with medical direction). Continually monitor breathing, color, oxygen saturation, and ECG monitor and transport. (Objective 7)

17. Ensure that resuscitation equipment is within easy reach. Open the appropriate size bag-mask for the child and connect it so it is easily accessible should another apneic episode occur. (Objective 7)

18. d. The immigrant migration to large cities stimulated the growth of nurse-provided home care for the poor. (Objective 1)

19. c. The home health field may continue to expand, perhaps offering these services in the future. (Objective 1)

20. a. These factors occur in three phases: preinjury, injury, and postinjury. (Objective 1)

21. d. The same precautions should be used as in the hospital setting. (Objective 1)

22. d. Environmental assessments include infectious waste, pets, and hazards. (Objective 2)

23. c. Life-threats should be identified before further assessment. (Objective 2)

24. c. The patient should keep an oxygen cylinder on hand in case this happens. (Objective 3)

25. d. Cuff leak and disconnected tubing produce a low pressure alarm. The oxygen alarm will sound if oxygen supply is inadequate. (Objective 3)

26. c. The rest are central venous access devices. (Objective 4)

27. d. Although a site infection is not an immediate life threat, it can cause sepsis and possibly death if it spreads and becomes systemic. (Objective 4)

28. c. Fever is a sign of infection. Distended neck veins and pulmonary congestion are signs of fluid overload. Other signs and symptoms of embolus include cyanosis; weak, rapid pulse; and a loss of consciousness. (Objective 4)

29. b. (Objective 4)

30. c. Urosepsis is managed with antibiotic therapy. (Objective 5)

31. c. Excessive diarrhea can cause rapid skin breakdown and dehydration and electrolyte imbalances. A change in the volume or type of tube feeding may remedy the problem. (Objective 5)

32. c. The foreskin should be retracted to visualize the urethra. The balloon should be inflated with 3 to 5 ml of sterile water. Excessive force should not be necessary and may cause injury to the urethra. (Objective 5)

33. c. An adequate blood supply and sufficient oxygen and nutrition are also essential. (Objective 6)

34. c. Fever and abdominal pain are the most common signs and symptoms of postpartum hemorrhage. (Objective 7)

35. d. Some women who suffer from this condition fantasize about harming their babies. All the other symptoms should be assessed after the physical well-being of the mother and baby are ensured. (Objective 7)

36. b. Further evaluation is necessary, but his clinical presentation suggests severe dehydration that will require immediate fluid resuscitation and rapid transport. (Objective 7)

37. c. This condition can also be caused by chromosomal abnormalities and major organ system defects. (Objective 7)

38. c. Palliative care customizes treatment for patients and their families, providing pain and symptom management if needed and mental and spiritual guidance with a goal of improving quality of life. (Objective 8)

● CHAPTER 47
ASSESSMENT-BASED MANAGEMENT

1. a. Hypoglycemia
   b. Stroke
   c. Age (stroke more common in elderly), history (patient in *a* had history of diabetes).
   (Objective 1)

2. a. Ectopic pregnancy
   b. Appendicitis
   c. Sex (male in *b* would not have gynecologic complaints), age (appendicitis common in this age group), clinical signs (shock in ectopic pregnancy versus fever in appendicitis).
   (Objective 1)

3. a. Nephrolithiasis (kidney stone)
   b. Abdominal aortic aneurysm
   c. Age (aneurysm more common in men 60-70), clinical signs/symptoms (hematuria is common in kidney stones; urge to defecate, cool extremity, and signs of shock consistent with aneurysm).
   (Objective 1)

4. a. SIDS or child abuse
   b. Drug or alcohol toxicity or suicide
   c. Age (SIDS and abuse more common in infants; suicide and drug abuse or overdose more common in teens).
   (Objective 1)

5. a. Myocardial infarction
   b. Myocardial contusion
   c. Age (MI more common in older patients; history of *a* consistent with risk factors of MI; mechanism of injury in *b* consistent with myocardial injury).
   (Objective 1)

6. Your attitude, the patient's willingness to cooperate, and labeling or tunnel vision (the expectation that her signs and symptoms were related to alcohol intoxication) may have contributed to your decision. (Objective 2)

7. Chronic alcoholism can impair the clotting mechanisms, putting the patient at risk for bleeding. Poor coordination secondary to intoxication increases the risk of injury (falls) in alcoholic patients. (Objective 2)

8. a. The team leader establishes contact and begins dialogue with the patient, obtains the history, and performs the physical examination.
   b. The patient care person provides scene cover (watches the crowd), gathers scene information (size/type of weapon), obtains vital signs, and performs skills.
   (Objective 3)

9. When moving into a volatile situation such as this one, minimal equipment should be taken; the drug box would not be indicated based on the dispatch information. (Objective 4)

10. The resuscitative approach is necessary because a life threat exists. (Objective 5)

11. a. The presence of distracting injuries (the chest wound)
    b. The environment (dangerous and dark)
    (Objective 2)

12. The patient is conscious, and breath sounds are present and equal bilaterally.
(Objective 6)

13. a. Initial assessment and ongoing assessment are both components of assessment-based management.
(Objective 1)

14. c. The field impression is based on a careful history, physical examination, and then analysis and evaluation based on the paramedic's knowledge and past experiences.
(Objective 2)

15. b. Alcohol or drug intoxication, hypovolemia, and head injury or concussion are other physiological problems that may cause a patient to be uncooperative.
(Objective 3)

16. d. This becomes especially important when multiple units respond to a scene.
(Objective 4)

17. c. Taking notes keeps you from forgetting critical information that will be necessary when you complete your patient care report later.
(Objective 5)

18. b. The contemplative approach is appropriate only when immediate intervention to manage a life threat is not needed.
(Objective 5)

19. a. All the other conditions represent life-threatening problems associated with hyperventilation, your examination should therefore be tailored to rule out those problems first.
(Objective 5)

20. a. An inadequate or inaccurate report can result in delayed patient care related to room or resource (medical staff, equipment) unavailability.
(Objective 6)

21. d. Ideally, the report should be concise, follow a standard format, and include pertinent positive and negatives. The patient's name should not be included if radio communication is used.
(Objective 6)

● CHAPTER 48 OPERATIONS

1. a. KKK A-1822
b. AMD 001-009
(Objective 1)

2. a. Supplies (airway, vascular access, dressings)
b. Medications (number and expiration dates, oxygen supply)
c. Equipment (including routine maintenance, battery loads, supplementary supplies)
(Objective 2)

3. a. The patient may aspirate and die.
b. You will be unable to defibrillate until another unit arrives, and the patient may deteriorate into asystole and die.
c. You will be unable to determine whether the altered consciousness is due to hypoglycemia. If you administer glucose and the patient's altered level of consciousness is related to a stroke, this action may worsen his condition.
d. You will have to search for other appropriate supplies, wasting time to care for the patient and baby. What will you use to cut the cord and then clamp it?
e. The patient's hypoxia may worsen, resulting in death.
(Objective 2)

4. a. National response time standards
b. Geographical area
c. Population and patient demand
d. Traffic conditions
Others include time of day and appropriate placement of vehicles.
(Objective 3)

5. a. Ensure that the police follow at a safe distance. Use a different siren tone than the police.
b. Slow the ambulance to a safe speed, and use the low beam lights.
c. Be aware that not all drivers will hear your sirens or see your lights. Stop and look to ensure that all traffic is stopping (make eye contact if possible). Use the yelp mode of the siren, and remain vigilant as you proceed.
(Objective 4)

6. Your patient is critical and requires specialized resources, and you are far from a hospital.
(Objective 6)

7. Advise the flight crew that you are at an MVC with a critically ill child. Let them know the location of the landing zone and any prominent landmarks or hazards.
(Objective 6)

8. The landing zone should be 75 × 75 feet. It should have few vertical structures and be relatively flat and free of high grass, crops, debris, or rough terrain (check local standards for specific variations).
(Objective 6)

9. As many patient care procedures as possible should be done, depending on the ETA of the helicopter. The airway should be secured, and the patient ventilated appropriately. The patient should be secured to a long spine board with straps and cervical immobilization. Vascular access should be obtained and other patient assessment and care (maintain warmth) continued until arrival of the helicopter.
(Objective 6)

10. Do not approach the aircraft unless directed by the crew. Approach from the front of the aircraft, and stay clear of the tail rotor. Allow a minimal num-

ber of people to help load. Secure loose objects. Walk in a crouched position. Carry objects at waist height. Depart from the front in view of the pilot. Wear eye protection.
(Objective 6)

11. b. The AMD 001-009 performance standards are incorporated in the latest KKK standards.
(Objective 1)

12. c. Lack of or failure of essential patient equipment could mean the difference between life and death.
(Objective 2)

13. a. A number of factors will affect those times, and they can vary by time of day and other variables. This should be monitored on a continual basis.
(Objective 3)

14. c. Paramedics driving an ambulance should remain at or below the speed limit except in extreme circumstances. For maximal safety, the paramedic attendant should also be restrained except when patient care requires movement. Lights and sirens should be used only on emergency responses (as dictated by policy) and when a critical patient is being transported.
(Objective 4)

15. a. Ideally, the ambulance should be on the same side of the road as the crash. Emergency lights should be left on. Ambulances should be parked uphill and upwind from hazardous materials incidents.
(Objective 4)

16. b. Some air medical services require training in specialized airway and vascular access techniques and expanded medication administration knowledge. This varies by agency.
(Objective 5)

17. b. Unless inclement weather or impassable roads prohibit transport, all the other patients could be appropriately transported by ground ALS service.
(Objective 6)

18. d. No one should approach the aircraft until a crew member signals that it is OK. A minimal number of people should approach the aircraft. No objects should be held up.
(Objective 6)

● CHAPTER 49
MEDICAL INCIDENT COMMAND

1. e
(Objective 1)

2. a
(Objective 1)

3. g
(Objective 1)

4. b
(Objective 1)

5. A rapid scene assessment should be performed. Communication should be established with the communications center or emergency operations center (as dictated by local policy). Additional units should be requested as soon as the need has been identified.
(Objective 7)

6. a. Command is determined by the preplanned system of arriving emergency units. The person assuming command must be familiar with ICS structure and the operating procedures of responding units.
(Objective 7)

b. It will likely be a unified command involving EMS, fire/rescue, and police. Some communities have public safety departments that incorporate all three functions. In that instance, a single command will likely be used.
(Objective 4)

7. Assuming an effective command position that has a good vantage point and is away from any danger of the bleachers, transmitting initial radio reports to the communications center; evaluating the scene rapidly (visually and with reports of other first responders); developing a strategy to safely extricate, triage, treat, transport, and provide security on scene; requesting additional equipment and personnel resources and assigning command roles; assigning sectors and identifying objectives in cooperation with section chiefs; evaluating information to determine progress of the event; sending units no longer needed back into service; terminating command at an appropriate time; and evaluating the effectiveness of operations (may be done retrospectively).
(Objective 4)

8. Incident command organizational charge completed.
(Objective 3)

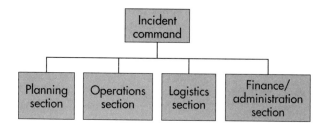

9. a. Procuring and distributing supplies (medicine, food, water, protective gear) and resources (heavy equipment, special tools)

b. Designating and staffing a safe helicopter landing zone and designating and staffing a staging area where all arriving apparatus will report and be assigned to areas where needed

c. Triaging victims and moving them to designated treatment area, securing necessary experts to determine the safest extrication procedures for this structure, coordinating physical rescue operations (including direction of heavy equipment), and ensuring scene safety

d. Selecting a site in close proximity but safely removed from actual collapse site, categorizing patients on arrival and designating them to the appropriate segment of treatment area or immediate or delayed zones, providing patient care and stabilization until transport can be provided, and communicating frequently with transportation sector so that appropriate patient transfers can be facilitated

e. Coordinating patient transport with staging and treatment sectors, communicating with receiving hospitals so that appropriate resources can be selected, and assigning patients to ambulances or helicopters and directing them to the appropriate facilities.
(Objective 8)

10. Effective communications can be enhanced by using a common frequency (command frequency) for interdisciplinary communication when necessary; using the radio frequencies designated in the plan; using different frequencies for fire, EMS, and other support agencies; ensuring that common terminology is being used; ensuring clear, concise radio traffic; preparing messages before transmitting; limiting use of radios; and identifying the speaker only by sector.
(Objective 7)

11. a. Air medical transport because of heavy traffic and heavy equipment to extricate victims from under bleachers.
(Objective 8)
b. The preplan should identify the availability and location of specialized resources that may be needed during an MCI situation.
(Objective 2)

12. a. Delayed, yellow (may be upgraded after retriage in treatment sector)
b. Critical, red
c. Critical, yellow
d. Delayed, green
e. Critical, red
f. Dead/dying, black
(Objective 10)

13. The airway may be opened if necessary, and hemorrhage controlled.
(Objective 10)

14. a. The ICS should be adaptable to small or large situations involving one or multiple jurisdictions as the need arises.
(Objective 1)

15. d. Preidentification of resources ensures rapid deployment by logistics during a disaster.
(Objective 2)

16. c. Command, finance, logistics, operations, and planning (C-FLOP) are the foundations on which the ICS is built.
(Objective 3)

17. c. The priority is always the safety of the emergency responders and the public.
(Objective 4)

18. b. The incident commander has overall responsibility. The section chiefs should be directing staff within their sector, not performing physical tasks or providing patient care.
(Objective 3)

19. b. Rehab sector falls under the command of the logistics section.
(Objective 3)

20. d. In most city EMS systems, this type of patient situation should not overwhelm the system and necessitate a mass casualty plan.
(Objective 6)

21. c. Triage sorts patients, opens airways, and controls hemorrhage.
(Objective 8)

22. b. Physicians are probably not appropriately trained for command. Their services may be more useful in assisting with triage and providing emergency surgery to facilitate extrication (all extrication sector responsibilities). A physician may also be assigned to the treatment sector.
(Objective 3)

23. a. As much verbal communication as possible should take place during the mass casualty incident to permit essential communication on the airwaves.
(Objective 7)

24. b.
(Objective 9)

25. d. Abnormal vital signs, obvious anatomic injury, and other obvious preexisting illnesses and injuries should be considered when triaging patients.
(Objective 10)

26. b. A respiratory rate greater than 30 indicates critical status in the START triage method. This patient obviously has a serious anatomic injury and abnormal physiological signs, indicating that urgent care is necessary.
(Objective 10)

27. a. The patient should also be asked to state his name and the current date, including year.
(Objective 10)

28. d. Patient identification, transporting unit, and hospital destination should also be noted.
(Objective 10)

29. c. The services provided depend on the local CISM team.
(Objective 11)

1. Drowning, foot/extremity entrapment, hypothermia, recirculating current
(Objective 4)

2. Defusing immediately after the incident if the emotional impact is high; critical incident stress debriefing 24 to 72 hours after the incident; follow up to ensure specific crew members are recovering; specialty debriefing to the people with the patient (if your team provides that service)

3. Rescue truck, possibly specialized hazardous materials team, high-angle rescue specialists
(Objective 2)

4. Asphyxiation, toxic inhalation, trauma, drowning, and exposure (depending on time of year)
(Objective 5)

5. Toxic gas may exist or oxygen levels may be low, and these may vary at different levels in the pipe.
(Objective 5)

6. It may be difficult to maneuver in the pipe with a standard air tank, and the time required for the rescue may exceed the tank capacity.
(Objective 5)

7. The line may kink or tangle, or the equipment may fail.
(Objective 5)

8. High angle rescue will likely be necessary to retrieve the patient.
(Objective 7)

9. During arrival and scene size-up, you should look for environmental risks, number of patients, and the need for medical care and/or rescue, and then request additional resources.
(Objectives 2 and 6)

10. Information was limited to location and the fact there was a crash. No additional equipment was dispatched (or has arrived).
(Objective 2)

11. Immediately delegate several crowd members to move the crowd to a safe distance to allow for patient care and arrival of additional equipment. Call for law enforcement officers to take charge of crowd control.
(Objective 2)

12. Advanced life-support ambulance, rescue truck, pumper, and law enforcement officers.
(Objective 2)

13. Hazards identified are a crowd and the gasoline spill.
(Objective 2)

14. Ensure that no one is smoking in close proximity to the crash. Disconnect the vehicle battery cables.
(Objective 2)

15. Begin initial patient assessment and airway management (if indicated).
(Objective 8)

16. Protect the patient with blankets, shields, or flame-retardant coverings.
(Objective 8)

17. Securing an open airway, protecting the cervical spine, and assisting ventilations with high-concentration oxygen if possible.
(Objective 8)

18. Disentanglement entails removal of the wreckage from the patient. Rescuers must protect the patient and maintain the airway, cervical spine immobilization, and breathing to the best of their ability. Packaging entails immobilization and removal of the patient from the scene to the emergency response vehicle. Rescuers must protect the patient's spine, splint or bandage injuries if appropriate (based on the acuteness of the patient's condition), and ensure that the patient is adequately secured before removal begins. The paramedic should oversee safe transport of the patient by the rescue team to the ambulance.
(Objective 2)

19. a. Contact utility workers to move downed wires or shut off power, keep bystanders away, and secure energized wires with a dry fire hose or other appropriate means.
b. Advise occupants to stay in the car.
(Objective 6)

20. Ropes, air bags, pry bars, jacks, wedges, cutters, spreaders, and winches.
(Objective 6)

21. c. Other than safety, the patient is the primary focus of the rescue.
(Objective 1)

22. c. Unless responding as part of a specialized fire/rescue team, the paramedic is not responsible for coordinating the rescue, serving as the safety officer, or operating equipment. Although everyone on the scene should be alert for overall safety considerations, the paramedic's responsibilities are to recognize when a rescue is safe before arrival of specialized teams and to provide patient care and monitoring during a rescue situation.
(Objective 1)

23. b. Initial efforts should ensure that the crew is uninjured so that their EMS functions can be maintained.
(Objective 1)

24. c. The dispatch call can provide the first information needed to size up a rescue situation and respond to it with the appropriate safety measures.
(Objective 2)

25. d. Moving all standardized equipment into the rescue area is not practical. Basic assessment and stabilization should be attempted until the patient

is in the ambulance. In certain situations, in which the surroundings are unsafe or the patient is not accessible, delivering care may not be possible. (Objective 2)

26. a. Ear and eye protection may also be necessary. A face mask with supplemental air or oxygen would be needed only in situations where inadequate oxygen or toxic fumes exist. (Objective 2)

27. a. Although ear plugs are helpful during the response, they may impair communications on a rescue. (Objective 3)

28. b. Walking in swift water could result in a foot becoming trapped, and the paramedic could be dragged under the water's surface. (Objective 4)

29. a. Alcohol and drug use also contribute to drowning. Properly worn PFDs decrease the risk of drowning. (Objective 4)

30. d. Survival after cold water drowning is difficult to predict except when rigor mortis, dependent lividity, or putrefaction is present. (Objective 4)

31. b. If the person is close enough, the rescuer should reach out with a long device. The next measure would be to throw a device to the person. Then, if this is unsuccessful, a boat should be taken to rescue the person. Finally, if no other option exists, a trained rescuer with appropriate PPE should enter the water in an attempt to rescue. (Objective 4)

32. b. High oxygen concentrations create a risk of rapid combustion to fuel fire or explosion. Concentrations less than 19.5% are considered an atmospheric hazard. (Objective 5)

33. b. Personnel on the scene may be helpful and give you that information also. (Objective 5)

34. c. Rescuer safety should be the primary concern. (Objective 5)

35. d. Flares would be dangerous in the presence of a gasoline leak. Apparatus should be staged off the highway if possible. Placing one large apparatus in front of the scene so safe loading can occur may be helpful. Use warning lights cautiously, and ensure that headlights are not pointed at oncoming traffic. (Objective 6)

36. d. In some cases the battery may be left connected. The other measures would be unnecessary in the absence of flames. (Objective 6)

37. d. Class A is used to extinguish ordinary combustibles; class B, flammable liquids; and class C, energized electrical equipment. (Objective 6)

38. b. The other tools are used for disentanglement. (Objective 6)

39. b. The steering column should not be cut. (Objective 6)

40. c. Both the rescuers and patient are at risk for falls during rescue from hazardous terrain. (Objective 7)

41. c. *High-angle* refers to cliffs or the sides of buildings or other structures; rope or aerial apparatus is needed for such rescues. Flat terrain with obstacles may include large rocks, loose soil, and waterbeds or creeks. (Objective 7)

42. a. Ideally, team cooperation is a standard on all scenes. Hostile or unstable patients are not unique to rescue situations. (Objective 8)

43. c. When the muscles are crushed, they release their pigment (myoglobin), which can cause renal failure. Hypotension and metabolic acidosis may also occur. (Objective 8)

● CHAPTER 51
HAZARDOUS MATERIALS INCIDENTS

1. i (Objective 1)
2. e (Objective 1)
3. h (Objective 1)
4. a (Objective 1)
5. f (Objective 1)
6. d (Objective 1)
7. c (Objective 1)
8. k (Objective 1)
9. g (Objective 1)
10. b (Objective 1)
11. j, e (Objective 5)
12. f, d (Objective 5)
13. g (Objective 5)
14. a (Objective 5)

15. j, e
(Objective 5)

16. i
(Objective 5)

17. h, j, e
(Objective 5)

18.

Category	Description
a. First responder awareness	May witness or discover hazardous materials release but does not have emergency-response duties pertaining to hazardous material as part of the job duties
b. First responder operations	Responds to hazardous materials releases to protect nearby persons, property, or the environment without trying to stop the release
c. Hazardous material technician	Responds to hazardous materials situations to stop the release
d. Hazardous material specialist	Has a direct or specific knowledge of various hazardous substances and provides support to hazardous materials technicians
e. On-scene incident commander	Trained to assume control of a hazardous materials event

(Objective 2)

19. a. Placards on trucks, shipping papers, and material safety data sheets
b. Visual indicators (vapor), container characteristics, company name on truck, and smell
(Objective 3)

20. Hazardous materials texts; poison control centers; CHEMTREC; federal agencies; commercial agencies; subject experts; site coordinators; regional, state, and local agencies
(Objective 3)

21. a. Chemical splash protective clothing to protect the skin and eyes from direct chemical contact
b. Structural firefighting clothing, including helmet, positive-pressure self-contained breathing apparatus, turnout coat and pants, gloves and boots, and a protective hood of fire-resistant material.
c. Vapor-protective clothing (suit with a self-contained breathing apparatus worn inside or outside the suit or a supplied air breathing apparatus with emergency escape capabilities).
(Objective 4)

22. a. Irritants damage the upper and lower respiratory tracts and irritate the eyes.
b. Asphyxiants deprive the body tissues of oxygen.
c. Nerve gases, anesthetics, and narcotics act on the nervous system, causing disruption of cardiorespiratory function.

d. Hepatotoxins destroy the liver's ability to function in a normal capacity.
e. Cardiotoxins may induce myocardial ischemia and cardiac dysrhythmias.
f. Neurotoxins may cause cerebral hypoxia or neurological or behavioral disruption.
g. Hemotoxins cause destruction of red blood cells, resulting in hemolytic anemia.
h. Carcinogens are cancer-causing agents.
(Objective 5)

23. Confusion, anxiety, dizziness, visual disturbances, changes in skin color, shortness of breath or burning of the upper airway, tingling or numbness of extremities, loss of coordination, seizures, nausea and vomiting, abdominal cramps, diarrhea, unconsciousness
(Objective 5)

24. Apply protective gear, remove contact lenses, and flush with copious amounts of water, normal saline, or lactated Ringer's solution.
(Objective 6)

25. A. The hot zone is the area that includes the hazardous material and any associated wastes. Only specially trained and clothed personnel may enter this area.
B. The warm zone is the area that can become contaminated if the hot zone is unstable. Decontamination and patient care activities take place here.
C. The cold zone is the area around the warm zone. Minimal protective clothing is required. The command post and other support agencies are located here.
(Objective 7)

26. En route to the emergency scene, the EMS crew should attempt to identify the hazardous material and obtain preliminary information regarding the potential hazards and recommended safety equipment, initial first aid, and a safe distance factor for response to the area. Medical control should be notified so that appropriate measures can be taken at the hospital for potential victims. If a positive identification of the involved substance is made, the dispatching agency should contact the appropriate authorities and other experts, such as CHEMTREC, to get additional information and support. The scene should be approached from uphill and upwind, and the EMS crew should call for additional help as needed. The arriving crew should be alert to any fire hazards and leakage of gas or liquid from the involved cars and remain clear of all vapors and spills.
(Objective 7)

27. Nonambulatory patients should be removed from the hot zone by trained personnel who have adequate protective clothing. All patients in the hot zone should be considered contaminated. Patient care in the hot zone should consist only of airway and breathing management, spinal immobilization, and control of hemorrhage. Intravenous lines should be avoided unless absolutely necessary to prevent internal introduction of contaminants. Decontamination should be attempted only with adequate protection of the rescue workers; often, removal of the victim's clothing removes most of the contaminant, with the remainder being washed with copious amounts of water and mild detergent soap. All contaminated clothing from the patient and rescuers should be left in the decontamination area. Further patient care should be provided in the support area before transport. The patient should be wrapped tightly in blankets. (Objective 9)

28. Presuit examination: Assess baseline vital signs, and instruct rescuers of possible symptoms to anticipate if contamination or exposure occurs. Postentry examination: Assess vital signs and monitor rescuer for signs or symptoms of exposure or heat-related illness. (Objective 8)

29. Outer gloves and boots should be removed and placed in a receptacle. Remove contaminated breathing apparatus. Remove protective clothing, and assess the need to remove outer clothing (based on type of chemical). Shower and wash twice. Put on clean clothing. Obtain medical evaluation. (Objective 8)

30. b. External hazards refer to materials that produce external damage, whereas internal hazards cause internal damage. Not all hazmat substances are IDLH. (Objective 1)

31. d. The Ryan White laws pertain to infectious disease exposure. (Objective 2)

32. d. The categories are first responder awareness, first responder operations, hazardous material technician, hazardous materials specialist, and on-scene incident commander. (Objective 2)

33. d. All other responses are informal means of recognizing and identifying hazardous materials. (Objective 3)

34. d. The U.S. Department of Transportation governs hazardous materials in transit. (Objective 3)

35. c. The others would not usually be associated with this type of exposure. (Objective 5)

36. b. The other signs described are systemic effects, which are not the most common findings in external exposure to corrosive chemicals. (Objective 6)

37. e. A high index of suspicion for rescuer exposure should always be maintained. (Objective 5)

38. d. This ensures that hazardous gases and liquids are moving away from the ambulance. (Objective 7)

39. b. (Objective 8)

40. a. Safety overrides all considerations.

41. d. Shaving may permit internal entry of chemicals. Clothing should be left at the exit point and appropriately cleaned or discarded. (Objective 9)

● **CHAPTER 52**
CRIME SCENE AWARENESS

1. Scene size-up for danger should begin during response and be based on dispatch information, knowledge of the area, and physical assessment of the scene during the approach. (Objective 1)

2. a. Past history of problems or violence
   b. Known drug or gang area
   c. Loud noises indicating violent activity
   d. Presence of alcohol or drug use
   e. Presence of dangerous pets
   f. Unusual silence or darkened residence
   (Objective 2)

3. a. Avoid use of lights and sirens as you get close, use unconventional pathways to approach the house, avoid positioning yourself between the ambulance lights and the residence, listen for signs of danger before entry, and stand on the doorknob side of the entry door. (Objective 2)
   b. One crew member should approach the car while the other remains in the ambulance, ambulance lights should be used to light the vehicle, approach should be made from the passenger side, and the paramedic should not walk between the ambulance and other vehicle. Observe for unusual activity in the rear seat, and do not move forward from post C if a threat is suspected. If there are any warning signs of danger, retreat until law enforcement secures the scene. (Objective 3)

4. a. Avoidance should be used. The EMS crew should stage their ambulance at a safe distance until law enforcement officers indicate that the scene is safe enough to proceed.
   b. Tactical retreat should be used, and cover should be sought. The paramedics should immediately retreat to a safe area of cover for protection against the projectiles and the possibility of further crowd violence.
   c. Cover and concealment should immediately be sought. Seek cover behind a solid object that will not allow penetration of a bullet, and conceal

yourself from the perpetrator until the scene is safe or retreat can be done safely.

d. Distraction and evasive maneuvers may be attempted during retreat. Try to move something between you and the patient to slow his attack as you quickly retreat. (Objective 6)

5. a. Fingerprints
b. Footprints
c. Blood or other body fluids
d. Hair
e. Carpet fibers
f. Clothing fibers
(Objective 8)

6. d. Locations of unsafe scenes may be known, as may the presence of crowds, intoxicated people on the scene, violence on the scene, or weapons. (Objective 1)

7. a. Other indications of a potentially dangerous residence are history of violence, known drug or gang area, loud noises, witnessing acts of violence, alcohol or drug use, or dangerous pets. (Objective 2)

8. a. Lights should be left on, and only one crew member should approach to leave the second crew member to call for help if needed. (Objective 3)

9. c. Police may lose control of the scene, causing danger for you, your partner, and the patient. Leave the scene as quickly as possible. Angry people may target violence at uniformed paramedics. (Objective 4)

10. d. Gang-related activity varies by region. All these agencies may provide you with information that can alert you to danger related to gang activities. (Objective 5)

11. c. This production process can produce hazardous gases, explosive forces, or fires. (Objective 5)

12. d. Injuries that aren't consistent with the history or mechanism of injury should be viewed with suspicion. Inaccurate medical history may reflect poor patient knowledge. Excessive nervous talking may be related to many factors. (Objective 5)

13. a. Avoidance requires alertness to detect and avoid dangerous situations. (Objective 6)

14. c. The other choices provide concealment but can easily be penetrated by a bullet and therefore should not be used for cover. (Objective 6)

15. d. The boxer stance and clenched fists are also signs of increasing aggression. (Objective 6)

16. c. High-velocity rifle bullets or thin- or dual-edged weapons, such as ice picks, may penetrate the body armor. (Objective 7)

17. a. Other areas of training include hostage survival, care under fire, weapons and ballistics, medical threat assessment, forensic medicine, assessment under special situations, safe searches, dental injury management, medical issues related to drug lab raids, and rescue and extraction. (Objective 7)

18. b. Document only objective findings. Try not to disturb any evidence. Save patient items in a paper bag. (Objective 8)

EMERGENCY DRUG INDEX

1. Actions: suppress acute or chronic inflammation and potentiate relaxation of vascular smooth muscle by β-adrenergic agonist. Indications: anaphylaxis, asthma, shock, and spinal cord injury. Adverse reactions: hypertension, sodium and water retention, hypokalemia, hypocalcemia, alkalosis, and HA

2. a. Onset: 1 to 2 hours. Duration: 8 to 24 hours. Dose: 40 to 125 mg intravenously (in spinal cord injury, initial dose of 30 mg/kg, followed by IV infusion of 5.4 mg/kg/hour)
b. Onset: 4 to 8 hours. Duration: 24 to 72 hours. Dose: 4 to 24 mg intravenously

3. Diphenhydramine (Benadryl). **Class:** antihistamine. **Description:** drug that prevents histamine from reaching H_1 and H_2 receptor sites. **Indications:** allergic reactions, anaphylaxis, and acute extrapyramidal reactions. **Contraindications:** asthma attacks, patients taking monoamine oxidase inhibitors, hypersensitivity, narrow-angle glaucoma, newborns, and nursing mothers. **Adverse reactions:** drowsiness, sedation, disturbed coordination, hypotension, palpitations, tachycardia or bradycardia, thickening of bronchial secretions, and dry mouth and throat. **Onset:** maximal effects in 1 to 3 hours. **Duration:** 6 to 12 hours. **Dose:** adult—25 to 50 mg deep intramuscular or intravenous injection; pediatric—5 mg/kg/day in divided doses intravenously or intramuscularly. **Special considerations:** pregnancy category C.

4. Vasopressin (Pitressin). **Class:** naturally occurring antidiuretic hormone. **Description:** direct stimulation of smooth muscles; when given in high doses acts as a nonadrenergic peripheral vasoconstrictor. **Indications:** adult shock—refractory VF; vasodilatory shock. **Contraindications:** responsive patients with coronary artery disease. **Adverse reactions:** ischemic chest pain, abdominal distress, sweating, nausea, vomiting, tremors. **Onset:** immediate. **Duration:** variable. **Dose:** adult cardiac arrest: 40 U IV push one time. Pediatric: not recommended. **Special considerations:** May cause cardiac ischemia and angina. May be given IO.

5. Glucagon. **Class:** pancreatic hormone and insulin antagonist. **Description:** drug used to elevate

blood glucose level if sufficient stores of glycogen are available; also has a positive inotropic effect on the heart. **Indications:** altered level of consciousness resulting from hypoglycemia if glucose administration not possible. Calcium channel blocker or β-blocker toxicity. **Contraindications:** hypersensitivity to proteins. **Adverse reactions:** tachycardia, hypotension, nausea, vomiting, and urticaria. May potentiate the effects of oral anticoagulants. **Onset:** within 1 minute. **Duration:** 60 to 90 minutes. **Dose:** adult—0.5 to 1.0 mg intramuscularly; pediatric—0.025 to 1.0 mg intramuscularly (may repeat in 7 to 10 minutes). Calcium channel blocker or β-blocker toxicity, adult 1 to 5 mg over 2 to 5 min. **Special considerations:** not first-line choice for hypoglycemia.

6. a. Procainamide (Pronestyl). **Class:** antidysrhythmic (class 1-A). **Description:** drug that reduces automaticity of ectopic pacemakers and suppresses reentry dysrhythmias by slowing intraventricular conduction. **Indications:** suppression of premature ventricular contractions refractory to lidocaine, suppression of ventricular tachycardia (with a pulse) refractory to lidocaine, suppression of ventricular fibrillation refractory to lidocaine, and paroxysmal supraventricular tachycardia with wide-complex tachycardia of unknown origin (especially if Wolff-Parkinson-White syndrome is present). **Contraindications:** second- and third-degree atrioventricular block, complete heart block, tricyclic antidepressant toxicity, digitalis toxicity, and torsades de pointes. **Adverse reactions:** hypotension, bradycardia, reflex tachycardia, atrioventricular block, widened QRS complex, prolonged PR or QT interval, premature ventricular contractions, ventricular tachycardia, ventricular fibrillation, asystole, central nervous system depression, confusion, and seizure. **Onset:** 10 to 30 minutes. **Duration:** 3 to 6 hours. **Dose:** adult—20 mg/minute slow IV infusion (100 mg IV push in refractory VF) to maximum dose 17 mg/kg, maintenance infusion after resuscitation or after initial bolus; 1 g mixed in 250 ml of solution infuse at (1 to 4 mg/minute). **Special considerations:** administration should be discontinued if dysrhythmia is suppressed, hypotension develops, the QRS complex widens by 50% of its original width, or a total of 17 mg/kg has been given; use caution with patients with asthma, digitalis-induced dysrhythmias, AMI, or cardiac, renal, or hepatic insufficiency. Do not use in combination with other drugs that prolong the QT interval.

b. Amiodarone (Cordarone). **Class:** class III antidysrhythmic. **Description:** multiple mechanisms of action; prolongs action potential and refractory period; α-alpha adrenoreceptor and calcium channel blocker. **Indications:** treatment and prophylaxis of frequently recurring VF and unstable VT. **Contraindications:** pulmonary congestion, cardiogenic shock, hypotension, sensitivity to amiodarone. **Adverse reactions:** hypotension, bradycardia, headache, dizziness, AV conduction abnormalities, flushing, abnormal salivation. **Onset:** within minutes. **Duration:** variable. **Dose:** adult cardiac arrest—300 mg IV push. Supplemental bolus for cardiac arrest: 150 mg IV push in 3-5 min. Loading infusion after reestablishment of spontaneous circulation: 360 mg (diluted) over 6 hours.

7. Nitroglycerin (Nitrostat). **Class:** vasodilator. **Description:** drug that dilates peripheral venous and arteriolar blood vessels and reduces cardiac workload and oxygen demand. **Indications:** ischemic chest pain, pulmonary hypertension, hypertensive emergencies, and congestive heart failure. **Contraindications:** hypersensitivity, hypotension, head injury, and cerebral hemorrhage. **Adverse reactions:** headache, postural syncope, reflex tachycardia, hypotension, nausea, vomiting, and diaphoresis. **Onset:** 1 to 3 minutes. **Duration:** 30 to 60 minutes. **Dose:** tablet: 0.3 to 0.4 mg sublingually that may be repeated in 5 minutes, 2 times; metered spray: 0.4 mg/spray, 1 sublingual spray that may be repeated in 5 minutes, twice; **Infusion**— 200 to 400 mcg/ml at a rate of 10 to 20 mcg/minute; increase by 5 to 10 mcg/minute every 5 to 10 minutes to desired effect. **Special considerations:** the drug must be kept in an airtight container protected from light; older adults have an increased risk of hypotension.

8. Lidocaine (Xylocaine). **Class:** antidysrhythmic, local anesthetic (class 1-B). **Description:** drug that suppresses premature ventricular contractions and raises ventricular fibrillation threshold. **Indications:** ventricular fibrillation, ventricular tachycardia, significant ventricular ectopy in the presence of myocardial ischemia or infarction; wide complex tachycardia of unknown origin. **Contraindications:** hypersensitivity, Stokes-Adams syndrome, and second- or third-degree heart block in the absence of an artificial pacemaker. **Adverse reactions:** lightheadedness, confusion, blurred vision, hypotension, cardiovascular collapse, bradycardia, and central nervous system depression (including seizures) with high doses. **Onset:** 30 to 90 seconds. **Duration:** 10 to 20 minutes. **Dose:** adult—administration intravenously or via endotracheal bolus (at 2 to 2½ times IV dose) followed by a continuous infusion: for ventricular fibrillation, 1.0 to 1.5 mg/kg IV repeated in 3 to 5 minutes to a total loading dose of 3 mg/kg; for ventricular ectopy or stable ventricular tachycardia, 1 to 1.5 mg/kg intravenously repeated in 5 to 10 minutes at 0.5 to 0.75 mg/kg to a total dose of 3 mg/kg; given via infusion: dilution of 1 g of

lidocaine in 250 ml of D_5W and infusion at 2 to 4 mg/minute; pediatric—1 mg/kg/dose IV or IO; infusion: 20 to 50 mcg/kg/minute. **Special considerations:** the drug has a short half-life; if bradycardia is present with premature ventricular contractions, the bradycardia is treated first with atropine; high doses can result in coma or death; decrease dose in elderly. Avoid lidocaine in reperfusion dysrhythmias after thrombolytic therapy; use extreme caution in patients with hepatic disease, heart failure, marked hypoxia, severe respiratory depression, hypovolemia, or shock.

9. Ketorolac tromethamine (Toradol). **Class:** nonsteroidal antiinflammatory. **Description:** an antiinflammatory that also exhibits peripherally acting nonnarcotic analgesic activity by inhibiting prostaglandin synthesis. **Indications:** Short-term management of moderate to severe pain. **Contraindications:** Hypersensitivity; allergies to aspirin or other nonsteroidal antiinflammatory drugs; bleeding disorders; renal failure; active peptic ulcer disease. **Adverse reactions:** anaphylaxis from hypersensitivity, edema, sedation, bleeding disorders, rash, nausea, and headache. **Onset:** within 10 minutes. **Duration:** 6 to 8 hours. **Dose:** adult—IM: 30 to 60 mg, followed by 15 to 30 mg q6h prn up to 5 days; IV: 30 mg over 1 minute (patients <65 yo); one-half dose (15 mg) for patients >65 yo and those with renal impairment. **Special considerations:** pregnancy category B safety; clear, slightly yellow solution; use with caution and reduce dose in elderly.

10. Naloxone (Narcan). **Class:** synthetic opioid antagonist. **Description:** a competitive narcotic antagonist used to manage and reverse overdoses caused by narcotics and synthetic narcotic agents. **Indications:** complete or partial reversal of narcotic depression and ventilatory depression resulting from opioids, including narcotic agonists (heroin, morphine sulfate, hydromorphone [Dilaudid], methadone, meperidine [Demerol], paregoric, fentanyl [Sublimaze], oxycodone [Percodan], and codeine), narcotic agonist/antagonists (butorphanol tartrate [Stadol], pentazocine [Talwin], propoxyphene [Darvon], and nalbuphine [Nubain]); decreased level of consciousness, coma of unknown origin, and circulatory support in refractory shock (investigational), PCP, and ETOH ingestion (investigational). **Contraindications:** hypersensitivity and caution with narcotic-dependent patients, who may experience withdrawal syndrome. **Adverse reactions:** tachycardia, hypertension, dysrhythmias, nausea, vomiting, blurred vision, withdrawal, and diaphoresis. **Onset:** within 2 minutes. **Duration:** 30 to 60 minutes. **Dose:** adult—0.4 to 0.8 mg intravenously or intramuscularly; 0.8 mg subcuta-

neously may be repeated in 5-minute intervals to a maximum of 10 mg; infusion: mix 8 mg in 1000 ml of D_5W and infuse at ⅔ of the reversal dose titrated to desired effect; pediatrics <5 years old or <20 kg—0.1 mg/kg/dose intravenously, intramuscularly, or subcutaneously or via endotracheal administration (diluted). **Special considerations:** seizures have been reported; drug may not reverse hypotension and may cause withdrawal syndrome; use caution if patient is a suspected narcotic addict. Narcan has shorter duration than some narcotics, monitor patient carefully after administration.

11. Midazolam hydrochloride (Versed). **Class:** short-acting benzodiazepine. **Description:** benzodiazepine that may be administered for conscious sedation to relieve apprehension or impair memory before tracheal intubation or cardioversion. **Indications:** premedication for trachea intubation or cardioversion. **Contraindications:** hypersensitivity to midazolam; glaucoma; shock; coma; alcohol intoxication (relative); depressed vital signs; concomitant use of barbiturates, alcohol, narcotics, or other CNS depressants. **Adverse reactions:** respiratory depression, hiccough, cough, oversedation, pain at injection site, nausea and vomiting, headache, blurred vision, fluctuations in vital signs, hypotension, and respiratory arrest. **Onset:** 1 to 3 minutes. **Duration:** 2-6 hours, dose dependent. **Dose:** adult—1 to 2.5 mg slow IV (over 2 to 3 minutes); repeat prn in small increments (total maximum dose not to exceed 0.1 mg/kg); elderly—0.5 mg slow IV (maximum of 1.5 mg in a 2-minute period); pediatric—loading dose 0.05 to 0.2 mg/kg, followed by continued infusion at 1 to 2 mcg/kg/minute. **Special considerations:** pregnancy category D; continuously monitor respiratory and cardiac function; have resuscitation equipment and medication readily at hand; never administer medication as IV bolus.

12. Atropine sulfate (Atropine and others). **Class:** anticholinergic agent. **Description:** drug that inhibits the action of acetylcholine at postganglionic parasympathetic receptor sites; blocks vagus nerve and causes increased heart rate and enhanced AV conduction. **Indications:** hemodynamically significant bradycardia, asystole, PEA, organophosphate or nerve-gas poisoning, and exercise-induced pulmonary disorders. **Contraindications:** tachycardia, hypersensitivity, unstable cardiovascular status in acute hemorrhage and myocardial ischemia, and narrow-angle glaucoma, obstructive disease of the GI tract, obstructive uropathy, and thyrotoxicosis. **Adverse reactions:** tachycardia; paradoxical bradycardia when pushed slowly or when used at doses less than 0.5 mg; palpitations; dysrhythmias; headache; dizziness; anticholinergic effects (dry

mouth, nose, skin, photophobia, blurred vision, urine retention); nausea; vomiting; flushed, hot, dry skin; and allergic reactions. **Onset:** rapid. **Duration:** 2 to 6 hours. **Dose:** bradydysrhythmias: adult—0.5 to 1.0 mg intravenously every 3 to 5 minutes as needed (maximum total dose 0.03 to 0.04 mg/kg); pediatric—0.02 mg/kg/dose intravenously or intraosseous (minimum total dose dose 0.1 mg; maximum single dose 0.5 mg for a child and 1.0 mg for an adolescent; may repeat in 5 minutes for maximum total dose of 1.0 mg child and 2.0 mg adolescent). Asystole: adult—1.0 mg IV/ET; repeat to total dose 0.03 to 0.04 mg/kg; pediatric—same dose as bradycardia. PEA: if absolute or relative bradycardia, same dose as asystole. Anticholinesterase poisoning: adult—2 mg intravenously every 5 to 15 minutes to dry secretions, repeated as needed; pediatric—0.05 mg/kg/dose (usual dose 1 to 5 mg) intravenously, repeated as needed every 20 minutes until atropine effect is observed. **Special considerations:** potential adverse effects when given with digitalis, cholinergics, and neostigmine; effects of atropine may be enhanced by antihistamines, procainamide, quinidine, antipsychotics, antidepressants, and benzodiazepines.

13. Epinephrine (Adrenalin). **Class:** sympathomimetic. **Description:** drug that stimulates α- and β-receptors; causes bronchodilation and, when administered via rapid intravenous injection, causes rapid increases in systolic pressure, ventricular contractility, and heart rate; causes vasoconstriction of the arterioles of the skin, mucosa, and splanchnic areas; and antagonizes the effects of histamine. **Indications:** bronchial asthma, acute allergic reactions, asystole, PEA, ventricular fibrillation, and pulseless ventricular tachycardia. **Contraindications:** hypersensitivity, hypovolemic shock, coronary insufficiency (should be used with caution). **Adverse reactions:** headache, restlessness, weakness, dysrhythmias, hypertension, and precipitation of angina pectoris and tachycardia. **Onset:** 5 to 10 minutes (subcutaneously), 1 to 2 minutes (intravenously). **Duration:** 5 to 10 minutes. **Dose:** asystole, PEA, pulseless ventricular tachycardia, or ventricular fibrillation: adult—1 mg intravenous push repeated every 3 to 5 minutes; pediatric—first dose: standard (0.1 ml/kg 1:10,000) intravenously or intraosseously, high (0.1 ml/kg 1:1000) via endotracheal administration (diluted to 3 to 5 ml); second and subsequent doses: high (0.1 ml/kg 1:1000) intravenously or intraosseously, high (0.1 ml/kg 1:1000) via endotracheal administration. Bradycardia refractory to other interventions: adult—2 to 10 mcg/minute (1 mg 1:1000 in 500 ml of normal saline or D_5W); pediatric—dilute 0.6 mg/kg to create 100 ml solution; begin infusion at 1 ml/hour

(0.1 mcg/kg/minute) and adjust every 5 minutes for desired effect (0.1 to 1.0 mcg/kg/minute). Anaphylactic reaction or bronchoconstriction: adult—mild to moderate: 0.3 to 0.5 ml (1:1000) subcutaneously; severe: 1 to 2 ml (1:10,000) slow intravenous injection; pediatric—0.01 ml/kg SQ (1:1000), maximum of 0.3 ml. **Special considerations:** syncope has been reported after administration in children; it may increase myocardial oxygen demand.

14. Nitrous oxide: oxygen (50:50) (Nitronox). **Class:** gaseous analgesic and anesthetic. **Description:** drug that depresses the central nervous system and causes anesthesia. **Indications:** moderate to severe pain. **Contraindications:** impaired level of consciousness, head injury, chest trauma, inability to comply with instructions, decompression sickness, undiagnosed abdominal pain, bowel obstruction, hypotension, shock, and COPD. **Adverse reactions:** dizziness, apnea, cyanosis, nausea, vomiting, and malignant hyperthermia. **Onset:** 2 to 5 minutes. **Duration:** 2 to 5 minutes. **Dose:** adult—invert cylinder several times before use and instruct the patient to inhale deeply through the mask or mouthpiece, which the patient must hold; pediatric—same. **Special considerations:** the drug increases the incidence of spontaneous abortion; it diffuses into gas-filled pockets trapped in the patient (for example, pneumothorax, intestinal obstruction) and may cause rupture; nitrous oxide is a nonexplosive gas.

15. Sodium bicarbonate. **Class:** buffer, alkalinizing agent, electrolyte supplement. **Description:** drug that reacts with hydrogen ions to form water and carbon dioxide to buffer metabolic acidosis. **Indications:** known pre-existing metabolic acidosis, tricyclic antidepressant overdose, and alkalinization for treatment of specific intoxications. **Contraindications:** patients with chloride loss from vomiting or gastrointestinal suction, metabolic and respiratory alkalosis, hypernatremia, hypokalemia, hypocalcemia, and abdominal pain of unknown origin. **Adverse reactions:** metabolic alkalosis, hypoxia, rise in intracellular P_{CO_2} and increased tissue acidosis, hypernatremia, seizures, and tissue sloughing at injection site. **Onset:** 2 to 10 minutes. **Duration:** 30 to 60 minutes. **Dose:** Urgent forms of metabolic acidosis: adult—1 mEq/kg intravenously repeated in 5 minutes with 0.5 mEq/kg every 10 minutes; pediatric—same. **Special considerations:** if possible, arterial blood gas analysis should guide administration of this drug; it may increase edematous or sodium-retaining states; it may initially worsen cellular acidosis; it may worsen congestive heart failure.

16. a. Thiamine (Betaxin). **Class:** vitamin (B_1). **Description:** drug necessary for carbohydrate metab-

olism. **Indications:** coma of unknown origin (with administration of dextrose 50% or naloxone), delirium tremens, beriberi, and Wernicke's encephalopathy. **Contraindications:** none significant. **Adverse reactions:** hypotension (from rapid injection or a large dose), anxiety, diaphoresis, nausea, vomiting, and allergic reaction (rare). **Onset:** rapid. **Duration:** depends on degree of deficiency. **Dose:** adult—100 mg slow intravenous or intramuscular injection. **Special considerations:** anaphylactic reactions have been reported.

b. Dextrose 50%. **Class:** carbohydrate and hypertonic solution. **Description:** the principal carbohydrate used in the body. **Indications:** hypoglycemia, altered level of consciousness, coma of unknown etiology, seizure of unknown etiology. **Contraindications:** intracranial hemorrhage, increased ICP, or suspected CVA in the absence of hypoglycemia. **Adverse reactions:** warmth, pain, burning from medication infusion, thrombophlebitis. **Onset:** less than 1 minute. **Duration:** depends on degree of hypoglycemia. **Dose:** adult—12.5 to 25 g slow intravenous injection (may repeat once); pediatric—0.5 to 1 g/kg/dose IV/IO. 1 to 2 ml/kg 50%; 2 to 4 ml/kg 25%; 5 to 10 ml/kg 10%. **Special considerations:** blood glucose analysis should be performed before administration, if possible; extravasation may cause tissue necrosis; it may sometimes precipitate severe neurological symptoms (Wernicke's encephalopathy) in patients with thiamine depletion, such as alcoholics; high-risk groups should receive thiamine before D50.

17. Diazepam (Valium and others). **Class:** benzodiazepine. **Description:** drug that raises the seizure threshold in the cerebral cortex and acts on the limbic, thalamic, and hypothalamic regions of the brain to potentiate the effects of inhibitory neurotransmitters. **Indications:** acute anxiety states, acute alcohol withdrawal, muscle relaxation, seizure activity, and premedication to countershock or transcutaneous pacing. **Contraindications:** hypersensitivity, substance abuse, coma, shock, CNS depression secondary to head injury, respiratory depression. **Adverse reactions:** hypotension, reflex tachycardia, respiratory depression, ataxia, psychomotor impairment, confusion, and nausea. **Onset:** 1 to 5 minutes (intravenously); 15 to 30 minutes (intramuscularly). **Duration:** 15 minutes to 1 hour (intravenously), 15 minutes to 1 hour (intramuscularly). **Dose:** seizure activity: adult—5 mg intravenously over 2 minutes (may give up to 10 mg for most adults); pediatric—infants >30 days to 5 years 0.2 to 0.5 mg slow intravenously or intraosseous every 2 to 5 minutes as necessary (maximum total dose 5 mg); children >5 years: 1 mg every 2 to 5 min to max 10 mg slow IV. Premedication for car-

dioversion: adult—5 to 15 mg intravenously 5 to 10 minutes before procedure. **Special considerations:** it may cause local venous irritation; dose should be reduced by 50% in older adults; resuscitation equipment should be readily available; anticonvulsant effect has a short duration.

18. Albuterol (Proventil, Ventolin). **Class:** sympathomimetic bronchodilator. **Description:** a β₂-specific sympathomimetic stimulant that relaxes bronchiolar smooth muscle and peripheral vasculature. **Indications:** relief of bronchospasm in patients with reversible obstructive airway disease and prevention of exercise-induced bronchospasm. **Contraindications:** hypersensitivity, cardiac dysrhythmias associated with tachycardia. **Adverse reactions:** restlessness, apprehension, dizziness, palpitations, increased blood pressure, and dysrhythmias. **Onset:** 5 to 15 minutes via inhalation. **Duration:** 3 to 4 hours via inhalation. **Dose:** bronchial asthma: adults—via metered dose inhaler, 1 to 2 inhalations (90 to 180 mcg) every 4 to 6 hours (5 minutes between inhalations); via inhalation, 2.5 mg (0.5 ml of 0.5% solution) diluted to 3 ml with 0.9% NaCl administered over 5 to 15 minutes; pediatric—via solution, 0.01 to 0.03 ml (0.05 to 0.15 mg)/kg/dose to a maximum of 0.5 ml/dose diluted in 2 ml of 0.9% normal saline (may be repeated every 20 minutes, 3 times). **Special considerations:** sympathomimetics may exacerbate adverse cardiac effects; drug may potentiate hypokalemia; it may precipitate angina pectoris and dysrhythmias; it should be used with caution with patients with diabetes mellitus, hyperthyroidism, prostatic hypertrophy, cardiovascular disorder or seizure disorder; it should be administered only by inhalation in prehospital care.

19. Aspirin (ASA, Bayer, Ecotrin, St. Joseph, others). **Class:** analgesic, antiinflammatory, antiplatelet, antipyretic. **Description:** drug that blocks pain impulses in the CNS, dilates peripheral vessels, and decreases platelet aggregation. **Indications:** mild to moderate pain or fever; prevention of platelet aggregation in ischemia and thromboembolism; unstable angina; prevention of myocardial infarction or reinfarction. **Contraindications:** hypersensitivity to salicylates; GI bleeding; active ulcer disease; hemorrhagic stroke; bleeding disorders; children. **Adverse reactions:** stomach irritation, heartburn or indigestion, nausea or vomiting, allergic reaction. **Onset:** 15 to 30 minutes. **Duration:** 4 to 6 hours. **Dose:** adult—mild pain or fever: 325 to 650 mg po q4hour; myocardial infarction: 160 to 325 mg PO (chew).

20. Adenosine (Adenocard). **Class:** endogenous nucleotide, miscellaneous antidysrhythmic agent. **Description:** drug that slows tachycardia associ-

ated with the atrioventricular node via modulation of the autonomic nervous system without causing negative inotropic effects and acts directly on sinus pacemaker cells and vagal nerve terminals to decrease chronotropic and dromotropic activity. **Indications:** treatment of SVT. **Contraindications:** second- or third-degree atrioventricular block, sick sinus syndrome, and hypersensitivity to adenosine; atrial flutter, atrial fibrillation, and ventricular tachycardia will not be converted by adenosine. **Adverse reactions:** lightheadedness, paresthesia, headache, diaphoresis, palpitations, chest pain, hypotension, dyspnea, nausea, and metallic taste. Transient sinus bradycardia, sinus pause, brady-asystole ventricular ectopy. **Onset:** immediate. **Duration:** 10 seconds. **Dose:** adult—initial, 6 mg over 1 to 3 seconds, if no response in 1 to 2 minutes, administration of 12 mg over 1 to 3 seconds, 12-mg dose repeated once as necessary; pediatric—0.1 mg/kg rapid intravenous injection; may be doubled once (maximum single dose 12 mg). **Special considerations:** methylxanthines antagonize the action of adenosine; dipyridamole potentiates the effect of adenosine; carbamazepine may potentiate the atrioventricular-nodal blocking effect of adenosine; may produce broncho-constriction in patients with asthma or broncho-pulmonary disease; asystole (up to 15 seconds) followed by normal sinus rhythm is common after administration.

21. a. Morphine sulfate (Astramorph PF and others). **Class:** opioid analgesic. **Description:** drug that increases peripheral venous capacitance and decreases venous return; promotes analgesia, euphoria, and respiratory and physical depression; decreases myocardial oxygen demand; a schedule II drug. **Indications:** chest pain associated with myocardial infarction, moderate to severe acute or chronic pain, and pulmonary edema with or without pain. **Contraindications:** hypersensitivity to narcotics, hypovolemia, hypotension, head injury or undiagnosed abdominal pain, and patients who have taken monoamine oxidase inhibitors within 14 days; increased intracranial pressure; and severe respiratory depression. **Adverse reactions:** hypotension, tachycardia, bradycardia, palpitations, syncope, facial flushing, respiratory depression, euphoria, bronchospasm, dry mouth, and allergic reaction. **Onset:** 1 to 2 minutes. **Duration:** 2 to 7 hours. **Dose:** adult—2 to 4 mg intravenously every 5 to 30 minutes titrated to relief of pain; pediatric—0.1 to 0.2 mg/kg/dose intravenously (maximum 15 mg total dose). **Special considerations:** narcotics rapidly cross the placenta; drug should be used with caution with older adults, patients with asthma, and patients susceptible to CNS depression; naloxone should be readily avail-

able; drug may worsen bradycardia or heart block in inferior MI (vagotonic effect).

b. Meperidine (Demerol). **Class:** opioid analgesic. **Description:** an opioid agonist that produces analgesia, euphoria, and respiratory and CNS depression. **Indications:** moderate to severe pain, preoperative medication, OB analgesia. **Contraindications:** hypersensitivity to narcotics, concurrent use of monoamine oxidase inhibitors or selective serotonin reuptake inhibitors, labor or delivery of a premature infant, and head injury. **Adverse reactions:** respiratory depression, euphoria, delirium, agitation, hallucination, seizures, headache, visual disturbances, coma, facial flushing, hypotension, circulatory collapse, dysrhythmias, allergic reaction, nausea, and vomiting. **Onset:** 10 to 45 minutes (intramuscularly), within 5 minutes (intravenously). **Duration:** 2 to 4 hours. **Dose:** adult—50 to 100 mg q 3 to 4 hours (intramuscularly), 15 to 35 mg (intravenously); pediatric—1 to 2 mg/kg/dose (intramuscularly) every 3 to 4 hours. **Special considerations:** drug should be used with caution in patients with asthma and chronic obstructive pulmonary disease and may aggravate seizures in patients with convulsive disorders; nalaxone should be readily available.

22. Labetalol (Normodyne, Trandate). **Class:** α- and β-adrenergic blocker. **Description:** competitive α_1-receptor blocker as well as a nonselective β-receptor blocker used to lower blood pressure in hypertensive crisis. **Indications:** hypertensive emergencies. **Contraindications:** bronchial asthma (relative), uncompensated CHF, second- and third-degree heart block, bradycardia, cardiogenic shock, pulmonary edema. **Adverse reactions:** dose-related orthostatic hypotension, headache, dizziness, edema, fatigue, vertigo, ventricular dysrhythmias, dyspnea, allergic reaction, facial flushing, diaphoresis. **Onset:** within 5 minutes. **Duration:** 3 to 6 hours. **Dose:** adult—10 mg slow IV bolus over 2 minutes; additional injections at 10-minute intervals prn (maximum 150 mg); infusion: mix 200 mg in 250 ml D$_5$W (0.8 mg/ml) and infuse at a rate of 2 to 8 mg/minute, titrated to supine blood pressure (maximum 300 mg). **Special considerations:** pregnancy safety category C; monitor blood pressure, pulse, ECG continuously; observe for signs of CHF, bradycardia, bronchospasm; administer with patient in supine position.

23. Activated charcoal (Actidose-Aqua, Liqui-char). **Class:** adsorbent, antidote. **Description:** drug that binds and adsorbs ingested toxins. **Indications:** many oral poisonings and medication overdoses. **Contraindications:** corrosives, GI bleeding, caustics, and petroleum distillates. **Adverse reactions:** nausea (indirectly), vomiting, and constipation.

Onset: immediate. **Duration:** continual in gastrointestinal tract. **Dose:** prepared in a slurry and administered by mouth or slowly by gastric tube; adult—30 to 100 g; pediatric—15 to 30 g; infant <1 yr—1 g/kg. **Special considerations:** drug does not adsorb all drugs and toxic substances (for example, phenobarbital, aspirin, cyanide, lithium, iron, lead, and arsenic).

24. Magnesium sulfate. **Class:** electrolyte, anticonvulsant. **Description:** drug that reduces striated muscle contractions and blocks peripheral neuromuscular transmission by reducing acetylcholine release at the myoneural junction. **Indications:** seizures resulting from eclampsia, torsades de pointes, refractory ventricular fibrillation, or suspected hypomagnesemia. **Contraindications:** heart block or myocardial damage. **Adverse reactions:** diaphoresis, facial flushing, hypotension, depressed reflexes, hypothermia, reduced heart rate, circulatory collapse, diarrhea, and respiratory depression. **Onset:** (IV) immediate. **Duration:** 30 minutes. **Dose:** seizures associated with pregnancy: 1 to 4 g (8 to 32 mEq) IV; maximum dose of 1.5 ml/minute. Pulseless arrest (torsades de pointes, or hypomagnesemic state): adult—1 to 2 g in 10 ml of D_5W IV over 1 to 2 minutes; pediatric—25 to 50 mg/kg over 10 to 20 minutes. **Special considerations:** other central nervous system depressants may enhance central nervous system depressant effects; drug should not be administered in the 2 hours before delivery; calcium gluconate or calcium chloride should be available as antagonist; drug may be needed for up to 48 hours after delivery; use with caution in patients with renal failure.

25. Dopamine (Intropin). **Class:** sympathomimetic. **Description:** drug that acts on α_1- and β-adrenergic receptors, increasing systemic vascular resistance and exerting a positive inotropic effect on the heart, and dilates renal and splanchnic vasculature at low doses (dopaminergic effect), maintaining blood flow. **Indications:** hemodynamically significant hypotension in the absence of hypovolemia. **Contraindications:** tachydysrhythmias, ventricular fibrillation, and patients with pheochromocytoma. **Adverse reactions:** dose-related tachycardias, hypertension, and increased myocardial oxygen demand. **Onset:** 2 to 4 minutes. **Duration:** 10 to 15 minutes. **Dose:** adult—begin infusion at 2 to 5 mcg/kg/minute; IV (titrated to patient response); final dosage range of 5 to 20 mcg/kg/minute recommended; low dose: 1 to 5 mcg/kg/minute; cardiac dose: 5 to 20 mcg/kg/minute; vasopressor: 10 to 20 mcg/kg/minute; pediatric—2 to 20 mcg/kg/minute; IV/IO titrated to patient response (not to exceed 20 mcg/kg/minute). **Special considerations:** drug should be infused through a large stable vein to avoid extravasation injury; patient should be monitored for signs of compromised circulation; infusion pump recommended.

26. Verapamil (Isoptin). **Class:** calcium channel blocker (class IV antidysrhythmic). **Description:** antidysrhythmic, antianginal, antihypertensive; inhibits the movement of calcium ions across cell membranes, decreases atrial automaticity, reduces atrioventricular conduction velocity, prolongs the atrioventricular nodal refractory period, decreases myocardial contractility, reduces vascular smooth muscle tone, and dilates coronary arteries and arterioles. **Indications:** paroxysmal supraventricular tachycardia (unresponsive to adenosine), atrial flutter with rapid ventricular response, and atrial fibrillation with a rapid ventricular response; vasospastic and unstable angina; chronic stable angina. **Contraindications:** hypersensitivity, sick sinus syndrome (unless the patient has a pacemaker), second- or third-degree heart block, hypotension, cardiogenic shock, severe congestive heart failure, Wolff-Parkinson-White syndrome with atrial fibrillation or flutter, patients receiving intravenous β-blockers, wide-complex tachycardias. **Adverse reactions:** dizziness, headache, nausea, vomiting, hypotension, bradycardia, complete atrioventricular block, and peripheral edema. **Onset:** 2 to 5 minutes. **Duration:** 30 to 60 minutes. **Dose:** adult—2.5 to 5.0 mg intravenous bolus over 2 minutes; repeat with 5 to 10 mg in 15 to 30 minutes, as necessary (maximum of 30 mg). **Special considerations:** vital signs should be monitored closely; be prepared to resuscitate the patient; atrioventricular block or asystole may occur because of slowed atrioventricular conduction; decrease dose when administering to elderly or borderline hypotensive patients.

27. Furosemide (Lasix). **Class:** loop diuretic. **Description:** drug that inhibits reabsorption of sodium and chloride in the proximal tubule and loop of Henle. IV doses can increase venous capacitance and decrease preload. **Indications:** pulmonary edema associated with congestive heart failure, and hepatic or renal disease. **Contraindications:** anuria, hypersensitivity; states of severe electrolyte depletion; dehydration; known allergy to sulfonamides. **Adverse reactions:** hypotension, electrocardiogram changes, dry mouth, hypercalcemia, hypochloremia, hypokalemia, hyponatremia, and hyperglycemia; may cause hearing loss if too rapid infusion of large doses. **Onset:** vascular effects within 5 minutes intravenously; diuresis, 15 to 20 minutes. **Duration:** 2 hours. **Dose:** adult—0.5 to 1.0 mg/kg slow intravenous injection (not to exceed 20 mg/minute); if no response, double dose to 2 mg/kg slow over 2 minutes; pediatric—1 mg/kg/dose. **Special consider-**

ations: drug has been known to cause fetal abnormalities; it should be protected from light.

28. Oxytocin (Pitocin). **Class:** pituitary hormone. **Description:** drug that indirectly stimulates uterine smooth muscle contractions, which transiently reduce uterine blood flow, and stimulates the mammary gland to increase lactation. **Indications:** postpartum hemorrhage after infant and placental delivery; induces labor at term (not a prehospital indication). **Contraindications:** presence of a second fetus; hypertonic or hyperactive uterus. **Adverse reactions:** tachycardia, hypertension, dysrhythmias, angina pectoris, anxiety, seizure, nausea, vomiting, allergic reaction, and uterine rupture (excessive dose). **Onset:** intravenous—immediate; intramuscular—3 to 5 minutes. **Duration:** intravenous—20 minutes; intramuscular—30 to 60 minutes. **Dose:** intramuscular—3 to 10 units after delivery of the placenta; intravenous—mix 10 units in 1000 ml normal saline or lactated Ringer's solution and infuse at 20 to 30 drops/minute, titrated to the severity of bleeding and uterine response. **Special considerations:** vasopressors may potentiate hypertension; vital signs and uterine tone should be monitored closely.

29. b. Dopamine is used to increase stroke volume.

30. d. Narcotic analgesics and nitrous oxide are contraindicated in undiagnosed abdominal pain because they may mask symptoms.

31. a. Epinephrine 1:10,000 intravenously is indicated for all other conditions listed.

32. b. Adenosine, β-blockers (atenolol), and calcium blockers (diltiazem) are Class III recommendations to control rate in atrial fibrillation/flutter in the presence of WPW.

33. d. Calcium and pacemaker are used to treat calcium channel blocker overdose.

34. a. It causes vasoconstriction at high doses.

35. a. Aspirin and oxygen should be administered. The patient's legs should be elevated and a fluid bolus administered in an attempt to increase the BP. His ECG and clinical presentation suggest the probability of right ventricular infarction, so nitroglycerin would not be given. Morphine would not be given until the blood pressure increases. Verapamil is not indicated in this setting.

36. a. Hydralazine is an antihistamine used to treat nausea. Morphine is a narcotic analgesic. Nifedipine is a calcium channel blocker used to treat hypertension.

37. c. All others are β-agonists.

38. b. Verapamil vasodilates and further decreases blood pressure.

39. d.

40. b. It dilates blood vessels and decreases peripheral vascular resistance and blood pressure.

41. a. The other drugs listed increase the plasmin in the blood, which causes degradation of fibrin threads and fibrinogen.

42. c. Naloxone is administered to reverse potential narcotic intoxication. Thiamine promotes uptake of glucose in the brain and prevents the development of Wernicke's encephalopathy when glucose is administered. D50W corrects underlying hypoglycemia.

43. b. It is an osmotic diuretic and pulls excess fluid from the brain, temporarily decreasing intracranial pressure.

44. a.

45. d. Oxytocin should be administered only after delivery of all the babies.

46. b. Benadryl causes thickening of the bronchial secretions and exacerbates an asthma attack.

47. c. Syrup of ipecac is contraindicated in patients without gag reflexes because aspiration may occur. Compazine is an antiemetic and decreases the effect of the ipecac. Hydrocarbons such as gasoline pose a large risk of aspiration, so ipecac is not indicated.

48. d. It is not effective against barbiturates.

49. c. It also may cause hypotension.

50. a. Magnesium would be given if there were a prolonged QT interval. β-blockers would be an option for polymorphic VT. Procainamide would be indicated in the absence of signs of congestive heart failure.

51. d.

52. b.

53. d. Furosemide decreases intravascular volume and causes vasodilation, which causes decreased preload and therefore less fluid to back up in the lungs.

54. d. Adenosine is not a calcium channel blocker and is not used to treat atrial flutter.

55. a. Atropine would increase the heart rate and the work of the heart and make the patient's condition worse.

56. b. Vistaril or phenergen often is ordered concurrently to prevent this side effect.

57. a. Haloperidol (Haldol) is a major tranquilizer.

58. d.

Illustration Credits and Acknowledgments

Fig. 6-1 Thibodeau GA: *Structure & function of the body,* ed 9, St Louis, 1992, Mosby.

Figs. 6-4, 6-5, 6-13, 6-14 *A:* Thibodeau GA: *Structure & function of the body,* ed 9, St Louis, 1992, Mosby (Illustrator E.W. Beck).

Figs. 6-6, 6-8 Seeley R, Stephens T, Tate P: *Anatomy & physiology,* ed 2, St Louis, 1992, Mosby (Illustrator David J. Mascaro & Associates).

Fig. 6-18 Thibodeau GA: *Structure & function of the body,* ed 9, St Louis, 1992, Mosby (Illustrator Branislav Vidic).

Figs. 6-10, 6-11 Thibodeau GA: *Structure & function of the body,* ed 9, St Louis, 1992, Mosby (Illustrator Christine Oleksyk).

Fig. 6-15 Seeley R: *Anatomy & physiology,* ed 2, St Louis, 1992, Mosby (Sims/ Illustrator Jody L. Fulks).

Fig. 6-16 Thibodeau GA: *Structure & function of the body,* ed 9, St Louis, 1992, Mosby (Illustrator Barbara Cousins).

Fig. 6-17 Thibodeau GA: *Structure & function of the body,* ed. 9, St Louis, 1992, Mosby (Illustrator William Ober).

Figs. 28-1, 28-3 Cotton S: *Mosby's paramedic study guide,* St Louis, 1989, Mosby.

Figs. 28-4, 28-12 Huszar R: *Basic dysrhythmias,* ed 2, St Louis, 1994, Mosby.

NATIONAL REGISTRY OF EMT-PARAMEDIC EXAMINATION SKILL SHEETS

Courtesy the National Registry of Emergency Medical Technicians, Columbus, Ohio

National Registry of Emergency Medical Technicians
Advanced Level Practical Examination

PATIENT ASSESSMENT - TRAUMA

Candidate: _____ Examiner: _____

Date: _____ Signature: _____

Scenario # _____

Time Start: _____ NOTE: Areas denoted by "**" may be integrated within sequence of Initial Assessment	Possible Points	Points Awarded
Takes or verbalizes body substance isolation precautions	1	
SCENE SIZE-UP		
Determines the scene/situation is safe	1	
Determines the mechanism of injury/nature of illness	1	
Determines the number of patients	1	
Requests additional help if necessary	1	
Considers stabilization of spine	1	
INITIAL ASSESSMENT/RESUSCITATION		
Verbalizes general impression of the patient	1	
Determines responsiveness/level of consciousness	1	
Determines chief complaint/apparent life-threats	1	
Airway -Opens and assesses airway (1 point)　　　　-Inserts adjunct as indicated (1 point)	2	
Breathing -Assess breathing (1 point) -Assures adequate ventilation (1 point) -Initiates appropriate oxygen therapy (1 point) -Manages any injury which may compromise breathing/ventilation (1 point)	4	
Circulation -Checks pulse (1point) -Assess skin [either skin color, temperature, or condition] (1 point) -Assesses for and controls major bleeding if present (1 point) -Initiates shock management (1 point)	4	
Identifies priority patients/makes transport decision	1	
FOCUSED HISTORY AND PHYSICAL EXAMINATION/RAPID TRAUMA ASSESSMENT		
Selects appropriate assessment	1	
Obtains, or directs assistant to obtain, baseline vital signs	1	
Obtains SAMPLE history	1	
DETAILED PHYSICAL EXAMINATION		
Head -Inspects mouth**, nose**, and assesses facial area (1 point) -Inspects and palpates scalp and ears (1 point) -Assesses eyes for PERRL** (1 point)	3	
Neck** -Checks position of trachea (1 point) -Checks jugular veins (1 point) -Palpates cervical spine (1 point)	3	
Chest** -Inspects chest (1 point) -Palpates chest (1 point) -Auscultates chest (1 point)	3	
Abdomen/pelvis** -Inspects and palpates abdomen (1 point) -Assesses pelvis (1 point) -Verbalizes assessment of genitalia/perineum as needed (1 point)	3	
Lower extremities** -Inspects, palpates, and assesses motor, sensory, and distal circulatory functions (1 point/leg)	2	
Upper extremities -Inspects, palpates, and assesses motor, sensory, and distal circulatory functions (1 point/arm)	2	
Posterior thorax, lumbar, and buttocks** -Inspects and palpates posterior thorax (1 point) -Inspects and palpates lumbar and buttocks area (1 point)	2	
Manages secondary injuries and wounds appropriately	1	
Performs ongoing assessment	1	

Time End: _____　　　　　　　　　　　　　　　　　　　　　　**TOTAL**　　43

CRITICAL CRITERIA

____ Failure to initiate or call for transport of the patient within 10 minute time limit
____ Failure to take or verbalize body substance isolation precautions
____ Failure to determine scene safety
____ Failure to assess for and provide spinal protection when indicated
____ Failure to voice and ultimately provide high concentration of oxygen
____ Failure to assess/provide adequate ventilation
____ Failure to find or appropriately manage problems associated with airway, breathing, hemorrhage or shock [hypoperfusion]
____ Failure to differentiate patient's need for immediate transportation versus continued assessment/treatment at the scene
____ Does other detailed/focused history or physical exam before assessing/treating threats to airway, breathing, and circulation
____ Orders a dangerous or inappropriate intervention

You must factually document your rationale for checking any of the above critical items on the reverse side of this form.

National Registry of Emergency Medical Technicians
Advanced Level Practical Examination

PATIENT ASSESSMENT - MEDICAL

Candidate: _____ Examiner: _____

Date: _____ Signature: _____

Scenario: _____

	Possible Points	Points Awarded
Time Start: _____		
Takes or verbalizes body substance isolation precautions	1	
SCENE SIZE-UP		
Determines the scene/situation is safe	1	
Determines the mechanism of injury/nature of illness	1	
Determines the number of patients	1	
Requests additional help if necessary	1	
Considers stabilization of spine	1	
INITIAL ASSESSMENT		
Verbalizes general impression of the patient	1	
Determines responsiveness/level of consciousness	1	
Determines chief complaint/apparent life-threats	1	
Assesses airway and breathing -Assessment (1 point) -Assures adequate ventilation (1 point) -Initiates appropriate oxygen therapy (1 point)	3	
Assesses circulation -Assesses/controls major bleeding (1 point) -Assesses skin [either skin color, temperature, or condition] (1 point) -Assesses pulse (1 point)	3	
Identifies priority patients/makes transport decision	1	
FOCUSED HISTORY AND PHYSICAL EXAMINATION/RAPID ASSESSMENT		
History of present illness -Onset (1 point) -Severity (1 point) -Provocation (1 point) -Time (1 point) -Quality (1 point) -Clarifying questions of associated signs and symptoms as related to OPQRST (2 points) -Radiation (1 point)	8	
Past medical history -Allergies (1 point) -Past pertinent history (1 point) -Events leading to present illness (1 point) -Medications (1 point) -Last oral intake (1 point)	5	
Performs focused physical examination [assess affected body part/system or, if indicated, completes rapid assessment] -Cardiovascular -Neurological -Integumentary -Reproductive -Pulmonary -Musculoskeletal -GI/GU -Psychological/Social	5	
Vital signs -Pulse (1 point) -Respiratory rate and quality (1 point each) -Blood pressure (1 point) -AVPU (1 point)	5	
Diagnostics [must include application of ECG monitor for dyspnea and chest pain]	2	
States field impression of patient	1	
Verbalizes treatment plan for patient and calls for appropriate intervention(s)	1	
Transport decision re-evaluated	1	
ON-GOING ASSESSMENT		
Repeats initial assessment	1	
Repeats vital signs	1	
Evaluates response to treatments	1	
Repeats focused assessment regarding patient complaint or injuries	1	
Time End: _____		
TOTAL	48	

CRITICAL CRITERIA

_____ Failure to initiate or call for transport of the patient within 15 minute time limit

_____ Failure to take or verbalize body substance isolation precautions

_____ Failure to determine scene safety before approaching patient

_____ Failure to voice and ultimately provide appropriate oxygen therapy

_____ Failure to assess/provide adequate ventilation

_____ Failure to find or appropriately manage problems associated with airway, breathing, hemorrhage or shock [hypoperfusion]

_____ Failure to differentiate patient's need for immediate transportation versus continued assessment and treatment at the scene

_____ Does other detailed or focused history or physical examination before assessing and treating threats to airway, breathing, and circulation

_____ Failure to determine the patient's primary problem

_____ Orders a dangerous or inappropriate intervention

_____ Failure to provide for spinal protection when indicated

You must factually document your rationale for checking any of the above critical items on the reverse side of this form.

Candidate:_____ Examiner:_____

Date: _____ Signature: _____

NOTE: If candidate elects to ventilate initially with BVM attached to reservoir and oxygen, full credit must be awarded for steps denoted by "**" so long as first ventilation is delivered within 30 seconds.

	Possible Points	Points Awarded
Takes or verbalizes body substance isolation precautions	1	
Opens the airway manually	1	
Elevates tongue, inserts simple adjunct [oropharyngeal or nasopharyngeal airway]	1	
NOTE: Examiner now informs candidate no gag reflex is present and patient accepts adjunct		
**Ventilates patient immediately with bag-valve-mask device unattached to oxygen	1	
**Hyperventilates patient with room air	1	
NOTE: Examiner now informs candidate that ventilation is being performed without difficulty and that pulse oximetry indicates the patient's blood oxygen saturation is 85%		
Attaches oxygen reservoir to bag-valve-mask device and connects to high flow oxygen regulator [12-15 L/minute]	1	
Ventilates patient at a rate of 10-20/minute with appropriate volumes	1	
NOTE: After 30 seconds, examiner auscultates and reports breath sounds are present, equal bilaterally and medical direction has ordered intubation. The examiner must now take over ventilation.		
Directs assistant to pre-oxygenate patient	1	
Identifies/selects proper equipment for intubation	1	
Checks equipment for: -Cuff leaks (1 point) -Laryngoscope operational with bulb tight (1 point)	2	
NOTE: Examiner to remove OPA and move out of the way when candidate is prepared to intubate		
Positions head properly	1	
Inserts blade while displacing tongue	1	
Elevates mandible with laryngoscope	1	
Introduces ET tube and advances to proper depth	1	
Inflates cuff to proper pressure and disconnects syringe	1	
Directs ventilation of patient	1	
Confirms proper placement by auscultation bilaterally over each lung and over epigastrium	1	
NOTE: Examiner to ask, "If you had proper placement, what should you expect to hear?"		
Secures ET tube [may be verbalized]	1	
NOTE: Examiner now asks candidate, "Please demonstrate one additional method of verifying proper tube placement in this patient."		
Identifies/selects proper equipment	1	
Verbalizes findings and interpretations [compares indicator color to the colorimetric scale and states reading to examiner]	1	
NOTE: Examiner now states, "You see secretions in the tube and hear gurgling sounds with the patient's exhalation."		
Identifies/selects a flexible suction catheter	1	
Pre-oxygenates patient	1	
Marks maximum insertion length with thumb and forefinger	1	
Inserts catheter into the ET tube leaving catheter port open	1	
At proper insertion depth, covers catheter port and applies suction while withdrawing catheter	1	
Ventilates/directs ventilation of patient as catheter is flushed with sterile water	1	
TOTAL	27	

CRITICAL CRITERIA

_____ Failure to initiate ventilations within 30 seconds after applying gloves or interrupts ventilations for greater than 30 seconds at any time
_____ Failure to take or verbalize body substance isolation precautions
_____ Failure to voice and ultimately provide high oxygen concentrations [at least 85%]
_____ Failure to ventilate patient at a rate of at least 10/minute
_____ Failure to provide adequate volumes per breath [maximum 2 errors/minute permissible]
_____ Failure to pre-oxygenate patient prior to intubation and suctioning
_____ Failure to successfully intubate within 3 attempts
_____ Failure to disconnect syringe **immediately** after inflating cuff of ET tube
_____ Uses teeth as a fulcrum
_____ Failure to assure proper tube placement by auscultation bilaterally **and** over the epigastrium
_____ If used, stylette extends beyond end of ET tube
_____ Inserts any adjunct in a manner dangerous to the patient
_____ Suctions the patient for more than 15 seconds
_____ Does not suction the patient

You must factually document your rationale for checking any of the above critical items on the reverse side of this form.

p303/8-003k

Candidate: _____ Examiner: _____

Date: _____ Signature: _____

NOTE: If candidate elects to initially ventilate with BVM attached to reservoir and oxygen, full credit must be awarded for
steps denoted by "**" so long as first ventilation is delivered within 30 seconds.

	Possible Points	Points Awarded
Takes or verbalizes body substance isolation precautions	1	
Opens the airway manually	1	
Elevates tongue, inserts simple adjunct [oropharyngeal or nasopharyngeal airway]	1	
NOTE: Examiner now informs candidate no gag reflex is present and patient accepts adjunct		
**Ventilates patient immediately with bag-valve-mask device unattached to oxygen	1	
**Hyperventilates patient with room air	1	
NOTE: Examiner now informs candidate that ventilation is being performed without difficulty		
Attaches oxygen reservoir to bag-valve-mask device and connects to high flow oxygen regulator [12-15 L/minute]	1	
Ventilates patient at a rate of 10-20/minute with appropriate volumes	1	
NOTE: After 30 seconds, examiner auscultates and reports breath sounds are present and equal bilaterally and medical control has ordered insertion of a dual lumen airway. The examiner must now take over ventilation.		
Directs assistant to pre-oxygenate patient	1	
Checks/prepares airway device	1	
Lubricates distal tip of the device [may be verbalized]	1	
NOTE: Examiner to remove OPA and move out of the way when candidate is prepared to insert device		
Positions head properly	1	
Performs a tongue-jaw lift	1	

☐ USES COMBITUBE®	☐ USES PTL®		
Inserts device in mid-line and to depth so printed ring is at level of teeth	Inserts device in mid-line until bite block flange is at level of teeth	1	
Inflates pharyngeal cuff with proper volume and removes syringe	Secures strap	1	
Inflates distal cuff with proper volume and removes syringe	Blows into tube #1 to adequately inflate both cuffs	1	
Attaches/directs attachment of BVM to the first [esophageal placement] lumen and ventilates		1	
Confirms placement and ventilation through correct lumen by observing chest rise, auscultation over the epigastrium, and bilaterally over each lung		1	
NOTE: The examiner states, "You do not see rise and fall of the chest and you only hear sounds over the epigastrium."			
Attaches/directs attachment of BVM to the second [endotracheal placement] lumen and ventilates		1	
Confirms placement and ventilation through correct lumen by observing chest rise, auscultation over the epigastrium, and bilaterally over each lung		1	
NOTE: The examiner confirms adequate chest rise, absent sounds over the epigastrium, and equal bilateral breath sounds.			
Secures device or confirms that the device remains properly secured		1	
TOTAL		20	

CRITICAL CRITERIA

_____ Failure to initiate ventilations within 30 seconds after taking body substance isolation precautions or interrupts ventilations for greater than 30 seconds at any time
_____ Failure to take or verbalize body substance isolation precautions
_____ Failure to voice and ultimately provide high oxygen concentrations [at least 85%]
_____ Failure to ventilate patient at a rate of at least 10/minute
_____ Failure to provide adequate volumes per breath [maximum 2 errors/minute permissible]
_____ Failure to pre-oxygenate patient prior to insertion of the dual lumen airway device
_____ Failure to insert the dual lumen airway device at a proper depth or at either proper place within 3 attempts
_____ Failure to inflate both cuffs properly
_____ **Combitube** - failure to remove the syringe immediately after inflation of each cuff
        PTL - failure to secure the strap prior to cuff inflation
_____ Failure to confirm that the proper lumen of the device is being ventilated by observing chest rise, auscultation over the epigastrium, and bilaterally over each lung
_____ Inserts any adjunct in a manner dangerous to patient

You must factually document your rationale for checking any of the above critical items on the reverse side of this form.

Candidate: _____ Examiner _____

Date: _____Signature:_____

NOTE: If candidate elects to ventilate initially with BVM attached to reservoir and oxygen, full credit must be awarded for steps denoted by "******" so long as first ventilation is delivered within 30 seconds.

	Possible Points	Points Awarded
Takes or verbalizes body substance isolation precautions	1	
Opens the airway manually	1	
Elevates tongue, inserts simple adjunct [oropharyngeal or nasopharyngeal airway]	1	
NOTE: Examiner now informs candidate no gag reflex is present and patient accepts adjunct		
**Ventilates patient immediately with bag-valve-mask device unattached to oxygen	1	
**Hyperventilates patient with room air	1	
NOTE: Examiner now informs candidate that ventilation is being performed without difficulty and that pulse oximetry indicates the patient's blood oxygen saturation is 85%		
Attaches oxygen reservoir to bag-valve-mask device and connects to high flow oxygen regulator [12-15 L/minute]	1	
Ventilates patient at a rate of 20-30/minute and assures adequate chest expansion	1	
NOTE: After 30 seconds, examiner auscultates and reports breath sounds are present, equal bilaterally and medical direction has ordered intubation. The examiner must now take over ventilation.		
Directs assistant to pre-oxygenate patient	1	
Identifies/selects proper equipment for intubation	1	
Checks laryngoscope to assure operational with bulb tight	1	
NOTE: Examiner to remove OPA and move out of the way when candidate is prepared to intubate		
Places patient in neutral or sniffing position	1	
Inserts blade while displacing tongue	1	
Elevates mandible with laryngoscope	1	
Introduces ET tube and advances to proper depth	1	
Directs ventilation of patient	1	
Confirms proper placement by auscultation bilaterally over each lung and over epigastrium	1	
NOTE: Examiner to ask, "If you had proper placement, what should you expect to hear?"		
Secures ET tube [may be verbalized]	1	
TOTAL	17	

CRITICAL CRITERIA

_____ Failure to initiate ventilations within 30 seconds after applying gloves or interrupts ventilations for greater than 30 seconds at any time
_____ Failure to take or verbalize body substance isolation precautions
_____ Failure to pad under the torso to allow neutral head position or sniffing position
_____ Failure to voice and ultimately provide high oxygen concentrations [at least 85%]
_____ Failure to ventilate patient at a rate of at least 20/minute
_____ Failure to provide adequate volumes per breath [maximum 2 errors/minute permissible]
_____ Failure to pre-oxygenate patient prior to intubation
_____ Failure to successfully intubate within 3 attempts
_____ Uses gums as a fulcrum
_____ Failure to assure proper tube placement by auscultation bilaterally **and** over the epigastrium
_____ Inserts any adjunct in a manner dangerous to the patient
_____ Attempts to use any equipment not appropriate for the pediatric patient

You must factually document your rationale for checking any of the above critical items on the reverse side of this form.

p305/8-003k

National Registry of Emergency Medical Technicians
Advanced Level Practical Examination

DYNAMIC CARDIOLOGY

Candidate: _____ Examiner: _____

Date: _____ Signature: _____

SET #_____

Level of Testing: □ NREMT-Intermediate/99 □ NREMT-Paramedic

Time Start:_____	Possible Points	Points Awarded
Takes or verbalizes infection control precautions	1	
Checks level of responsiveness	1	
Checks ABCs	1	
Initiates CPR if appropriate [verbally]	1	
Attaches ECG monitor in a timely fashion or applies paddles for "Quick Look"	1	
Correctly interprets initial rhythm	1	
Appropriately manages initial rhythm	2	
Notes change in rhythm	1	
Checks patient condition to include pulse and, if appropriate, BP	1	
Correctly interprets second rhythm	1	
Appropriately manages second rhythm	2	
Notes change in rhythm	1	
Checks patient condition to include pulse and, if appropriate, BP	1	
Correctly interprets third rhythm	1	
Appropriately manages third rhythm	2	
Notes change in rhythm	1	
Checks patient condition to include pulse and, if appropriate, BP	1	
Correctly interprets fourth rhythm	1	
Appropriately manages fourth rhythm	2	
Orders high percentages of supplemental oxygen at proper times	1	
Time End: _____ **TOTAL**	24	

CRITICAL CRITERIA

_____ Failure to deliver first shock in a timely manner due to operator delay in machine use or providing treatments other than CPR with simple adjuncts

_____ Failure to deliver second or third shocks without delay other than the time required to reassess rhythm and recharge paddles

_____ Failure to verify rhythm before delivering each shock

_____ Failure to ensure the safety of self and others [verbalizes "All clear" and observes]

_____ Inability to deliver DC shock [does not use machine properly]

_____ Failure to demonstrate acceptable shock sequence

_____ Failure to order initiation or resumption of CPR when appropriate

_____ Failure to order correct management of airway [ET when appropriate]

_____ Failure to order administration of appropriate oxygen at proper time

_____ Failure to diagnose or treat 2 or more rhythms correctly

_____ Orders administration of an inappropriate drug or lethal dosage

_____ Failure to correctly diagnose or adequately treat v-fib, v-tach, or asystole

You must factually document your rationale for checking any of the above critical items on the reverse side of this form.

National Registry of Emergency Medical Technicians
Advanced Level Practical Examination

STATIC CARDIOLOGY

Candidate: _____ Examiner: _____

Date: _____ Signature: _____

SET #_____

Level of Testing: ☐ NREMT-Intermediate/99   ☐ NREMT-Paramedic

Note: No points for treatment may be awarded if the diagnosis is incorrect.
Only document incorrect responses in spaces provided.

Time Start:_____

	Possible Points	Points Awarded
STRIP #1		
Diagnosis:	1	
Treatment:	2	
STRIP #2		
Diagnosis:	1	
Treatment:	2	
STRIP #3		
Diagnosis:	1	
Treatment:	2	
STRIP #4		
Diagnosis:	1	
Treatment:	2	

Time End: _____   **TOTAL**   **12**

p307/8-003k

National Registry of Emergency Medical Technicians
Advanced Level Practical Examination

INTRAVENOUS THERAPY

Candidate: _____ Examiner: _____

Date: _____ Signature: _____

Level of Testing: ❏ NREMT-Intermediate/85   ❏ NREMT-Intermediate/99   ❏ NREMT-Paramedic

Time Start: _____

	Possible Points	Points Awarded
Checks selected IV fluid for: -Proper fluid (1 point) -Clarity (1 point)	2	
Selects appropriate catheter	1	
Selects proper administration set	1	
Connects IV tubing to the IV bag	1	
Prepares administration set [fills drip chamber and flushes tubing]	1	
Cuts or tears tape [at any time before venipuncture]	1	
Takes/verbalizes body substance isolation precautions [prior to venipuncture]	1	
Applies tourniquet	1	
Palpates suitable vein	1	
Cleanses site appropriately	1	
Performs venipuncture -Inserts stylette (1 point) -Notes or verbalizes flashback (1 point) -Occludes vein proximal to catheter (1 point) -Removes stylette (1 point) -Connects IV tubing to catheter (1 point)	5	
Disposes/verbalizes disposal of needle in proper container	1	
Releases tourniquet	1	
Runs IV for a brief period to assure patent line	1	
Secures catheter [tapes securely or verbalizes]	1	
Adjusts flow rate as appropriate	1	
TOTAL	**21**	

Time End: _____

CRITICAL CRITERIA
____ Failure to establish a patent and properly adjusted IV within 6 minute time limit
____ Failure to take or verbalize body substance isolation precautions prior to performing venipuncture
____ Contaminates equipment or site without appropriately correcting situation
____ Performs any improper technique resulting in the potential for uncontrolled hemorrhage, catheter shear, or air embolism
____ Failure to successfully establish IV within 3 attempts during 6 minute time limit
____ Failure to dispose/verbalize disposal of needle in proper container

NOTE: Check here (_____) if candidate did not establish a patent IV and do not evaluate IV Bolus Medications.

INTRAVENOUS BOLUS MEDICATIONS

Time Start: _____

Asks patient for known allergies	1	
Selects correct medication	1	
Assures correct concentration of drug	1	
Assembles prefilled syringe correctly and dispels air	1	
Continues body substance isolation precautions	1	
Cleanses injection site [Y-port or hub]	1	
Reaffirms medication	1	
Stops IV flow [pinches tubing or shuts off]	1	
Administers correct dose at proper push rate	1	
Disposes/verbalizes proper disposal of syringe and needle in proper container	1	
Flushes tubing [runs wide open for a brief period]	1	
Adjusts drip rate to TKO/KVO	1	
Verbalizes need to observe patient for desired effect/adverse side effects	1	
TOTAL	**13**	

Time End: _____

CRITICAL CRITERIA
____ Failure to begin administration of medication within 3 minute time limit
____ Contaminates equipment or site without appropriately correcting situation
____ Failure to adequately dispel air resulting in potential for air embolism
____ Injects improper drug or dosage [wrong drug, incorrect amount, or pushes at inappropriate rate]
____ Failure to flush IV tubing after injecting medication
____ Recaps needle or failure to dispose/verbalize disposal of syringe and needle in proper container

You must factually document your rationale for checking any of the above critical items on the reverse side of this form.

National Registry of Emergency Medical Technicians
Advanced Level Practical Examination

PEDIATRIC INTRAOSSEOUS INFUSION

Candidate: _____ Examiner: _____

Date: _____ Signature: _____

Time Start:_____	Possible Points	Points Awarded

Checks selected IV fluid for:
    -Proper fluid (1 point)
    -Clarity (1 point)
	2	

Selects appropriate equipment to include:
    -IO needle (1 point)
    -Syringe (1 point)
    -Saline (1 point)
    -Extension set (1 point)
	4	

Selects proper administration set	1	
Connects administration set to bag	1	
Prepares administration set [fills drip chamber and flushes tubing]	1	
Prepares syringe and extension tubing	1	
Cuts or tears tape [at any time before IO puncture]	1	
Takes or verbalizes body substance isolation precautions [prior to IO puncture]	1	
Identifies proper anatomical site for IO puncture	1	
Cleanses site appropriately	1	

Performs IO puncture:
    -Stabilizes tibia (1 point)
    -Inserts needle at proper angle (1 point)
    -Advances needle with twisting motion until "pop" is felt (1 point)
    -Unscrews cap and removes stylette from needle (1 point)
	4	

Disposes of needle in proper container	1	
Attaches syringe and extension set to IO needle and aspirates	1	
Slowly injects saline to assure proper placement of needle	1	
Connects administration set and adjusts flow rate as appropriate	1	
Secures needle with tape and supports with bulky dressing	1	

Time End: _____   **TOTAL**   23

CRITICAL CRITERIA

_____ Failure to establish a patent and properly adjusted IO line within the 6 minute time limit
_____ Failure to take or verbalize body substance isolation precautions prior to performing IO puncture
_____ Contaminates equipment or site without appropriately correcting situation
_____ Performs any improper technique resulting in the potential for air embolism
_____ Failure to assure correct needle placement before attaching administration set
_____ Failure to successfully establish IO infusion within 2 attempts during 6 minute time limit
_____ Performing IO puncture in an unacceptable manner [improper site, incorrect needle angle, etc.]
_____ Failure to dispose of needle in proper container
_____ Orders or performs any dangerous or potentially harmful procedure

You must factually document your rationale for checking any of the above critical items on the reverse side of this form.

p310/8-003k

National Registry of Emergency Medical Technicians
Advanced Level Practical Examination

SPINAL IMMOBILIZATION (SEATED PATIENT)

Candidate:_____ Examiner:_____

Date: _____ Signature:_____

Time Start: _____	Possible Points	Points Awarded
Takes or verbalizes body substance isolation precautions	1	
Directs assistant to place/maintain head in the neutral, in-line position	1	
Directs assistant to maintain manual immobilization of the head	1	
Reassesses motor, sensory, and circulatory function in each extremity	1	
Applies appropriately sized extrication collar	1	
Positions the immobilization device behind the patient	1	
Secures the device to the patient's torso	1	
Evaluates torso fixation and adjusts as necessary	1	
Evaluates and pads behind the patient's head as necessary	1	
Secures the patient's head to the device	1	
Verbalizes moving the patient to a long backboard	1	
Reassesses motor, sensory, and circulatory function in each extremity	1	
Time End: _____ **TOTAL**	12	

CRITICAL CRITERIA

_____ Did not immediately direct or take manual immobilization of the head
_____ Did not properly apply appropriately sized cervical collar before ordering release of manual immobilization
_____ Released or ordered release of manual immobilization before it was maintained mechanically
_____ Manipulated or moved patient excessively causing potential spinal compromise
_____ Head immobilized to the device **before** device sufficiently secured to torso
_____ Device moves excessively up, down, left, or right on the patient's torso
_____ Head immobilization allows for excessive movement
_____ Torso fixation inhibits chest rise, resulting in respiratory compromise
_____ Upon completion of immobilization, head is not in a neutral, in-line position
_____ Did not reassess motor, sensory, and circulatory functions in each extremity after voicing immobilization to the long backboard

You must factually document your rationale for checking any of the above critical items on the reverse side of this form.

National Registry of Emergency Medical Technicians
Advanced Level Practical Examination

SPINAL IMMOBILIZATION (SUPINE PATIENT)

Candidate:_____Examiner:_____

Date: _____Signature:_____

Time Start: _____	Possible Points	Points Awarded
Takes or verbalizes body substance isolation precautions	1	
Directs assistant to place/maintain head in the neutral, in-line position	1	
Directs assistant to maintain manual immobilization of the head	1	
Reassesses motor, sensory, and circulatory function in each extremity	1	
Applies appropriately sized extrication collar	1	
Positions the immobilization device appropriately	1	
Directs movement of the patient onto the device without compromising the integrity of the spine	1	
Applies padding to voids between the torso and the device as necessary	1	
Immobilizes the patient's torso to the device	1	
Evaluates and pads behind the patient's head as necessary	1	
Immobilizes the patient's head to the device	1	
Secures the patient's legs to the device	1	
Secures the patient's arms to the device	1	
Reassesses motor, sensory, and circulatory function in each extremity	1	
Time End: _____ TOTAL	14	

CRITICAL CRITERIA

_____ Did not immediately direct or take manual immobilization of the head
_____ Did not properly apply appropriately sized cervical collar before ordering release of manual immobilization
_____ Released or ordered release of manual immobilization before it was maintained mechanically
_____ Manipulated or moved patient excessively causing potential spinal compromise
_____ Head immobilized to the device **before** device sufficiently secured to torso
_____ Patient moves excessively up, down, left, or right on the device
_____ Head immobilization allows for excessive movement
_____ Upon completion of immobilization, head is not in a neutral, in-line position
_____ Did not reassess motor, sensory, and circulatory functions in each extremity after voicing immobilization to the device

You must factually document your rationale for checking any of the above critical items on the reverse side of this form.

p312/8-003k

BLEEDING CONTROL/SHOCK MANAGEMENT

Candidate: _____ Examiner: _____

Date: _____ Signature: _____

	Possible Points	Points Awarded
Time Start:_____		
Takes or verbalizes body substance isolation precautions	1	
Applies direct pressure to the wound	1	
Elevates the extremity	1	
NOTE: The examiner must now inform the candidate that the wound continues to bleed.		
Applies an additional dressing to the wound	1	
NOTE: The examiner must now inform the candidate that the wound still continues to bleed. The second dressing does not control the bleeding.		
Locates and applies pressure to appropriate arterial pressure point	1	
NOTE: The examiner must now inform the candidate that the bleeding is controlled.		
Bandages the wound	1	
NOTE: The examiner must now inform the candidate that the patient is exhibiting signs and symptoms of hypoperfusion.		
Properly positions the patient	1	
Administers high concentration oxygen	1	
Initiates steps to prevent heat loss from the patient	1	
Indicates the need for immediate transportation	1	
Time End: _____ **TOTAL**	10	

CRITICAL CRITERIA

_____ Did not take or verbalize body substance isolation precautions
_____ Did not apply high concentration of oxygen
_____ Applied a tourniquet before attempting other methods of bleeding control
_____ Did not control hemorrhage in a timely manner
_____ Did not indicate the need for immediate transportation

You must factually document your rationale for checking any of the above critical items on the reverse side of this form.

p313/8-003k

oxytocin

Generic Name

Generic Name

Generic Name

● FLASHCARD 52

Trade Name: _____

Class: _____

Descriptions: _____

_____

Indications: _____

_____

Contraindications: _____

_____

Adverse Reactions: _____

_____

Onset: _____

Duration _____

Dosage: _____

_____

_____

_____

Special Considerations: _____

_____

_____

● FLASHCARD 51

Question 28

Trade Name: _____

Class: _____

Descriptions: _____

_____

Indications: _____

_____

Contraindications: _____

_____

Adverse Reactions: _____

_____

Onset: _____

Duration _____

Dosage: _____

_____

_____

_____

Special Considerations: _____

_____

_____

● FLASHCARD 54

Trade Name: _____

Class: _____

Descriptions: _____

_____

Indications: _____

_____

Contraindications: _____

_____

Adverse Reactions: _____

_____

Onset: _____

Duration _____

Dosage: _____

_____

_____

_____

Special Considerations: _____

_____

_____

● FLASHCARD 53

Trade Name: _____

Class: _____

Descriptions: _____

_____

Indications: _____

_____

Contraindications: _____

_____

Adverse Reactions: _____

_____

Onset: _____

Duration _____

Dosage: _____

_____

_____

_____

Special Considerations: _____

_____

_____

magnesium sulfate

dopamine

verapamil

furosemide

● FLASHCARD 48

Question 25

Trade Name: _____

Class: _____

Descriptions: _____

_____

Indications: _____

_____

Contraindications: _____

_____

Adverse Reactions: _____

_____

Onset: _____

Duration _____

Dosage: _____

_____

_____

_____

Special Considerations: _____

_____

_____

● FLASHCARD 47

Question 24

Trade Name: _____ N/A _____

Class: _____

Descriptions: _____

_____

Indications: _____

_____

Contraindications: _____

_____

Adverse Reactions: _____

_____

Onset: _____

Duration _____

Dosage: _____

_____

_____

_____

Special Considerations: _____

_____

_____

● FLASHCARD 50

Question 27

Trade Name: _____

Class: _____

Descriptions: _____

_____

Indications: _____

_____

Contraindications: _____

_____

Adverse Reactions: _____

_____

Onset: _____

Duration _____

Dosage: _____

_____

_____

_____

Special Considerations: _____

_____

_____

● FLASHCARD 49

Question 26

Trade Name: _____

Class: _____

Descriptions: _____

_____

Indications: _____

_____

Contraindications: _____

_____

Adverse Reactions: _____

_____

Onset: _____

Duration _____

Dosage: _____

_____

_____

_____

Special Considerations: _____

_____

_____

morphine sulfate

meperidine

labetalol

activated charcoal

● FLASHCARD 44

Question 21b

Trade Name: _____

Class: _____

Descriptions: _____

_____

Indications: _____

_____

Contraindications: _____

_____

Adverse Reactions:_____

_____

Onset: _____

Duration _____

Dosage:_____

_____

_____

_____

Special Considerations: _____

_____

_____

● FLASHCARD 43

Question 21a

Trade Name: _____

Class: _____

Descriptions: _____

_____

Indications: _____

_____

Contraindications: _____

_____

Adverse Reactions:_____

_____

Onset: _____

Duration _____

Dosage:_____

_____

_____

_____

Special Considerations: _____

_____

_____

● FLASHCARD 46

Question 23

Trade Name: _____

Class: _____

Descriptions: _____

_____

Indications: _____

_____

Contraindications: _____

_____

Adverse Reactions:_____

_____

Onset: _____

Duration _____

Dosage:_____

_____

_____

_____

Special Considerations: _____

_____

● FLASHCARD 45

Question 22

Trade Name: _____

Class: _____

Descriptions: _____

_____

Indications: _____

_____

Contraindications: _____

_____

Adverse Reactions:_____

_____

Onset: _____

Duration _____

Dosage:_____

_____

_____

_____

Special Considerations: _____

_____

_____

diazepam

albuterol

aspirin

adenosine

● FLASHCARD 40

Question 18

Trade Name: _____

Class: _____

Descriptions: _____

_____

Indications: _____

_____

Contraindications: _____

_____

Adverse Reactions: _____

_____

Onset: _____

Duration _____

Dosage: _____

_____

_____

Special Considerations: _____

_____

_____

● FLASHCARD 39

Question 17

Trade Name: _____

Class: _____

Descriptions: _____

_____

Indications: _____

_____

Contraindications: _____

_____

Adverse Reactions: _____

_____

Onset: _____

Duration _____

Dosage: _____

_____

_____

_____

Special Considerations: _____

_____

_____

● FLASHCARD 42

Question 20

Trade Name: _____

Class: _____

Descriptions: _____

_____

Indications: _____

_____

Contraindications: _____

_____

Adverse Reactions: _____

_____

Onset: _____

Duration _____

Dosage: _____

_____

_____

_____

Special Considerations: _____

_____

● FLASHCARD 41

Question 19

Trade Name: _____

Class: _____

Descriptions: _____

_____

Indications: _____

_____

Contraindications: _____

_____

Adverse Reactions: _____

_____

Onset: _____

Duration _____

Dosage: _____

_____

_____

_____

Special Considerations: _____

_____

nitrous oxide

sodium bicarbonate

thiamine

dextrose 50%

● FLASHCARD 36

Question 15

Trade Name: _____ N/A _____

Class: _____

Descriptions: _____

_____

Indications: _____

_____

Contraindications: _____

_____

Adverse Reactions:_____

_____

Onset: _____

Duration _____

Dosage:_____

_____

_____

_____

Special Considerations: _____

_____

_____

● FLASHCARD 35

Question 14

Trade Name: _____

Class: _____

Descriptions: _____

_____

Indications: _____

_____

Contraindications: _____

_____

Adverse Reactions:_____

_____

Onset: _____

Duration _____

Dosage:_____

_____

_____

_____

Special Considerations: _____

_____

_____

● FLASHCARD 38

Question 16b

Trade Name: _____ N/A _____

Class: _____

Descriptions: _____

_____

Indications: _____

_____

Contraindications: _____

_____

Adverse Reactions:_____

_____

Onset: _____

Duration _____

Dosage:_____

_____

_____

_____

Special Considerations: _____

_____

● FLASHCARD 37

Question 16a

Trade Name: _____

Class: _____

Descriptions: _____

_____

Indications: _____

_____

Contraindications: _____

_____

Adverse Reactions:_____

_____

Onset: _____

Duration _____

Dosage:_____

_____

_____

_____

Special Considerations: _____

_____

naloxone

midazolam
hydrochloride

atropine sulfate

epinephrine

● FLASHCARD 32

Question 11

Trade Name: _____

Class: _____

Descriptions: _____

_____

Indications: _____

_____

Contraindications: _____

_____

Adverse Reactions: _____

_____

Onset: _____

Duration _____

Dosage: _____

_____

_____

_____

Special Considerations: _____

_____

_____

● FLASHCARD 31

Question 10

Trade Name: _____

Class: _____

Descriptions: _____

_____

Indications: _____

_____

Contraindications: _____

_____

Adverse Reactions: _____

_____

Onset: _____

Duration _____

Dosage: _____

_____

_____

_____

Special Considerations: _____

_____

_____

● FLASHCARD 34

Question 13

Trade Name: _____

Class: _____

Descriptions: _____

_____

Indications: _____

_____

Contraindications: _____

_____

Adverse Reactions: _____

_____

Onset: _____

Duration _____

Dosage: _____

_____

_____

_____

Special Considerations: _____

_____

● FLASHCARD 33

Question 12

Trade Name: _____

Class: _____

Descriptions: _____

_____

Indications: _____

_____

Contraindications: _____

_____

Adverse Reactions: _____

_____

Onset: _____

Duration _____

Dosage: _____

_____

_____

_____

Special Considerations: _____

_____

amiodarone

nitroglycerin

lidocaine

ketorolac
tromethamine

● FLASHCARD 28

Question 7

Trade Name: _____

Class: _____

Descriptions: _____

_____

Indications: _____

_____

Contraindications: _____

_____

Adverse Reactions: _____

_____

Onset: _____

Duration _____

Dosage: _____

_____

_____

_____

Special Considerations: _____

_____

_____

● FLASHCARD 27

Question 6b

Trade Name: _____

Class: _____

Descriptions: _____

_____

Indications: _____

_____

Contraindications: _____

_____

Adverse Reactions: _____

_____

Onset: _____

Duration _____

Dosage: _____

_____

_____

_____

Special Considerations: _____

_____

_____

● FLASHCARD 30

Question 9

Trade Name: _____

Class: _____

Descriptions: _____

_____

Indications: _____

_____

Contraindications: _____

_____

Adverse Reactions: _____

_____

Onset: _____

Duration _____

Dosage: _____

_____

_____

_____

Special Considerations: _____

_____

_____

● FLASHCARD 29

Question 8

Trade Name: _____

Class: _____

Descriptions: _____

_____

Indications: _____

_____

Contraindications: _____

_____

Adverse Reactions: _____

_____

Onset: _____

Duration _____

Dosage: _____

_____

_____

_____

Special Considerations: _____

_____

_____

diphenhydramine

vasopressin

glucagon

procainamide

● FLASHCARD 24
Question 4

Trade Name: _____

Class: _____

Descriptions: _____
_____

Indications: _____
_____

Contraindications: _____
_____

Adverse Reactions: _____
_____

Onset: _____

Duration _____

Dosage: _____
_____
_____
_____

Special Considerations: _____
_____
_____

● FLASHCARD 23
Question 3

Trade Name: _____

Class: _____

Descriptions: _____
_____

Indications: _____
_____

Contraindications: _____
_____

Adverse Reactions: _____
_____

Onset: _____

Duration _____

Dosage: _____
_____
_____

Special Considerations: _____
_____
_____

● FLASHCARD 26
Question 6a

Trade Name: _____ N/A _____

Class: _____

Descriptions: _____
_____

Indications: _____
_____

Contraindications: _____
_____

Adverse Reactions: _____
_____

Onset: _____

Duration _____

Dosage: _____
_____
_____
_____

Special Considerations: _____
_____

● FLASHCARD 25
Question 5

Trade Name: _____

Class: _____

Descriptions: _____
_____

Indications: _____
_____

Contraindications: _____
_____

Adverse Reactions: _____
_____

Onset: _____

Duration _____

Dosage: _____
_____
_____
_____

Special Considerations: _____
_____

72.

QRS:_____ P wave: _____

Rate: _____ Rhythm:_____ PRI: _____

Interpretation:____**Second-degree atrioventricular block (Mobitz type I or Wenckebach)**_____

Distinguishing features: _____

Treatment: _____

_____

73.

QRS:_____ P wave: _____

Rate: _____ Rhythm:_____ PRI: _____

Interpretation:____**Second-degree atrioventricular block (Mobitz type II)**_____

Distinguishing features: _____

Treatment: _____

_____

74.

QRS:_____ P wave: _____

Rate: _____ Rhythm:_____ PRI: _____

Interpretation:____**Third-degree (complete) atrioventricular block**_____

Distinguishing features: _____

Treatment: _____

_____

FLASHCARD 20

Fig. 28-27

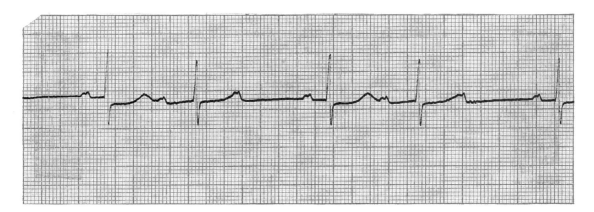

● **FLASHCARD 21**

Fig. 28-28

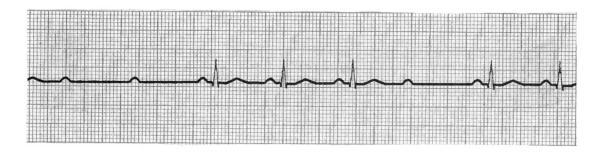

● **FLASHCARD 22**

Fig. 28-29

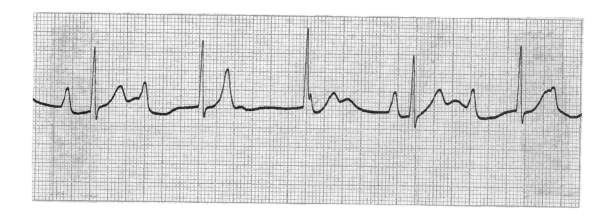

67.

QRS:_____ P wave:_____

Rate:_____ Rhythm:_____ PRI:_____

Interpretation:___**Asystole**_____

Distinguishing features:_____

Treatment:_____

_____

- -

68.

QRS:_____ P wave:_____

Rate:_____ Rhythm:_____ PRI:_____

Interpretation:___**Ventricular paced rhythm**_____

Distinguishing features:_____

Treatment:_____

_____

- -

71.

QRS:_____ P wave:_____

Rate:_____ Rhythm:_____ PRI:_____

Interpretation:___**Sinus rhythm with first-degree atrioventricular block**_____

Distinguishing features:_____

Treatment:_____

_____

● **FLASHCARD 17**

Fig. 28-24

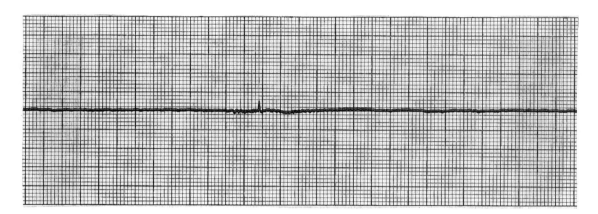

● **FLASHCARD 18**

Fig. 28-25

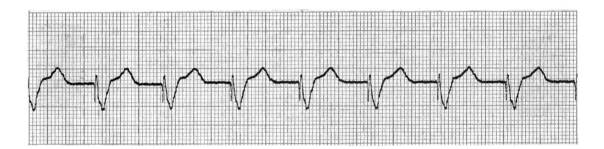

● **FLASHCARD 19**

Fig. 28-26

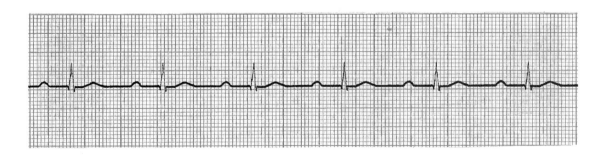

64.

QRS:_____ P wave: _____

Rate: _____ Rhythm:_____ PRI: _____

Interpretation:____**Normal sinus rhythm with one premature ventricular contraction**_____

Distinguishing features: _____

Treatment: _____

_____

- -

65.

QRS:_____ P wave: _____

Rate: _____ Rhythm:_____ PRI: _____

Interpretation:____**Monomorphic ventricular tachycardia**_____

Distinguishing features: _____

Treatment: _____

_____

- -

66.

QRS:_____ P wave: _____

Rate: _____ Rhythm:_____ PRI: _____

Interpretation:____**Ventricular fibrillation**_____

Distinguishing features: _____

Treatment: _____

_____

● FLASHCARD 14

Fig. 28-21

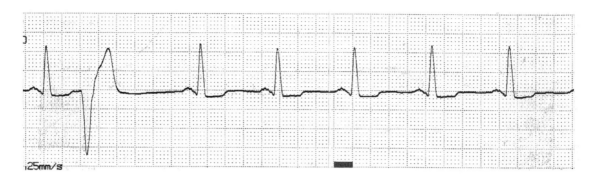

● FLASHCARD 15

Fig. 28-22

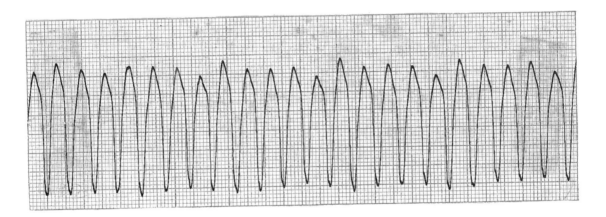

● FLASHCARD 16

Fig. 28-23

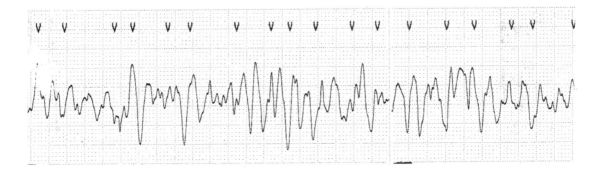

58.

QRS:_____ P wave: _____

Rate: _____ Rhythm:_____ PRI: _____

Interpretation:_____**Junctional escape rhythm**_____

Distinguishing features: _____

Treatment: _____

_____

59.

QRS:_____ P wave: _____

Rate: _____ Rhythm:_____ PRI: _____

Interpretation:_____**Accelerated junctional rhythm**_____

Distinguishing features: _____

Treatment: _____

_____

63.

QRS:_____ P wave: _____

Rate: _____ Rhythm:_____ PRI: _____

Interpretation:_____**Ventricular escape rhythm**_____

Distinguishing features: _____

Treatment: _____

_____

● **FLASHCARD 11**

Fig. 28-18

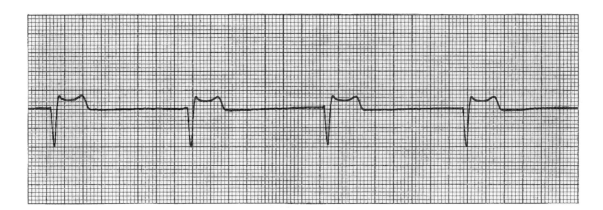

● **FLASHCARD 12**

Fig. 28-19

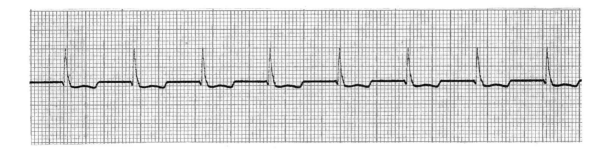

● **FLASHCARD 13**

Fig. 28-20

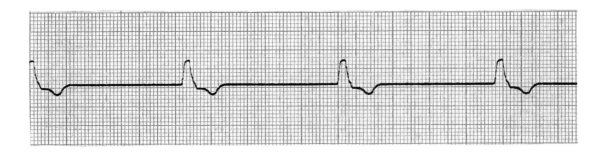

53.

QRS:_____ P wave: _____

Rate: _____ Rhythm:_____ PRI: _____

Interpretation:___**Atrial flutter with 3:1 conduction**_____

Distinguishing features: _____

Treatment: _____

_____

54.

QRS:_____ P wave: _____

Rate: _____ Rhythm:_____ PRI: _____

Interpretation:___**Atrial fibrillation**_____

Distinguishing features: _____

Treatment: _____

_____

57.

QRS:_____ P wave: _____

Rate: _____ Rhythm:_____ PRI: _____

Interpretation:___**Sinus rhythm (borderline bradycardia) with two premature junctional contractions**___

Distinguishing features: _____

Treatment: _____

_____

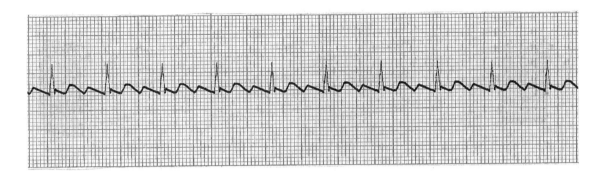
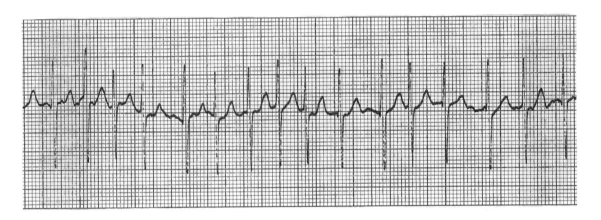

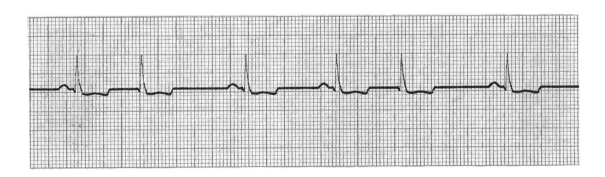

50.

QRS:_____ P wave: _____

Rate: _____ Rhythm:_____ PRI: _____

Interpretation:___**Wandering atrial pacemaker**_____

Distinguishing features: _____

Treatment: _____

_____

51.

QRS:_____ P wave: _____

Rate: _____ Rhythm:_____ PRI: _____

Interpretation:___**Premature atrial contraction**_____

Distinguishing features: _____

Treatment: _____

_____

52.

QRS:_____ P wave: _____

Rate: _____ Rhythm:_____ PRI: _____

Interpretation:___**Supraventricular tachycardia**_____

Distinguishing features: _____

Treatment: _____

_____

Fig. 28-12

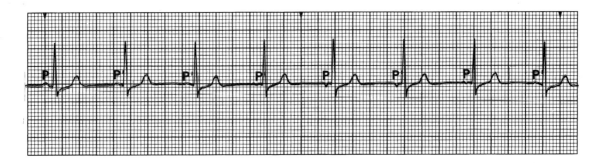

Fig. 28-13

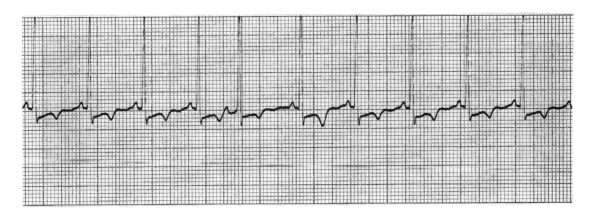

Fig. 28-14

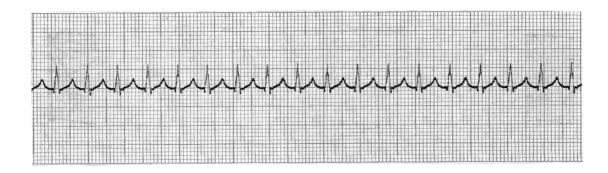

44.

QRS:_____ P wave: _____

Rate: _____ Rhythm:_____ PRI: _____

Interpretation:___**Sinus tachycardia**_____

Distinguishing features: _____

Treatment: _____

_____

- -

45.

QRS:_____ P wave: _____

Rate: _____ Rhythm:_____ PRI: _____

Interpretation:___**Sinus dysrhythmia**_____

Distinguishing features: _____

Treatment: _____

_____

- -

46.

QRS:_____ P wave: _____

Rate: _____ Rhythm:_____ PRI: _____

Interpretation:___**Sinus arrest**_____

Distinguishing features: _____

Treatment: _____

_____

● FLASHCARD 2

Fig. 28-9

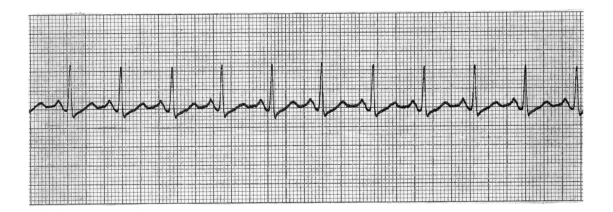

● FLASHCARD 3

Fig. 28-10

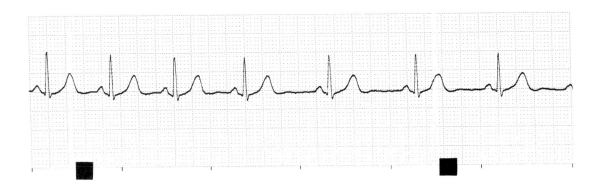

● FLASHCARD 4

Fig. 28-11

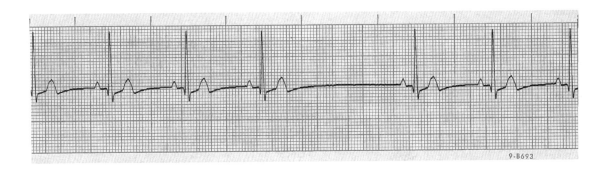

The following ECG strips and drug flashcards are included to make the task of studying easier. The cards should be comp[...]
in accordance with the questions on pages 206-214. However, they are not designed to be used in just those areas.

Challenge yourself and use the drug cards:
- With a fellow student as flashcards to study
- To review drugs in subsequent chapters
- In the cardiovascular section to enhance your instructor's lecture
- While on clinical sites as an easy reference
- Before final examinations as a quick, portable review

The ECG cards may be helpful:
- During ECG study, group them according to their similarities, and later, as you master them, mix them up and identify each one
- To make up scenarios in study groups
- When practicing for cardiac algorithm practicals
- To bring along during hospital and field clinicals as an easy reference

Be creative and invent your own uses for these flashcards. They are here so you can improve your knowledge and enhance success in study.

● **FLASHCARD 1**

Fig. 28-8

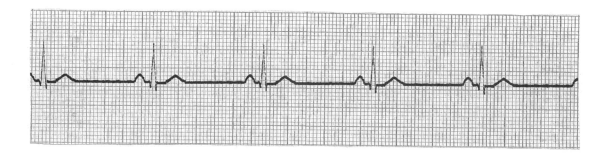

S: _____ P wave: _____

te: _____ Rhythm: _____ PRI: _____

erpretation: **Sinus bradycardia** _____

Distinguishing features: _____

reatment: _____

_____